ADVANCED BIOMATERIALS

ADVANCED BIOMATERIALS

Fundamentals, Processing, and Applications

Edited by

Bikramjit Basu, Dhirendra Katti, and Ashok Kumar

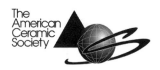

WILEY

A JOHN WILEY & SONS, INC., PUBLICATION

Published by John Wiley & Sons, Inc., Hoboken, New Jersey.
Published simultaneously in Canada.

For general information on our other products and services or for technical support, please contact our Customer Care Department within the United States at (800) 762-2974, outside the United States at (317) 572-3993 or fax (317) 572-4002.

Wiley also publishes its books in a variety of electronic formats. Some content that appears in print may not be available in electronic formats. For more information about Wiley products, visit our web site at www.wiley.com.

Library of Congress Cataloging-in-Publication Data:

International Conference on Design of Biomaterials (2006 : Indian Institute of Technology Kanpur)
    Advanced biomaterials fundamentals, processing, and applications / [edited by] Bikramjti Basu, Dhirendra S. Katti, and Ashok Kumar.
        p. ; cm.
    This volume is an outcome of the International Conference on Design of Biomaterials, organized at Indian Institute of Technology Kanpur, India during 8–11th December, 2006.
    Includes bibliographical references and index.
    ISBN 978-0-470-19340-2 (cloth)
    1. Biomedical materials—Congresses.   I. Basu, Bikramjti. II. Katti, Dhirendra S. III. Kumar, Ashok, Dr. IV. Title.
    [DNLM: 1.   Biocompatible Materials—therapeutic use–Congresses. 2.   Blood Substitues—therapeutic use–Congresses. 3.   Nanostructures–therapeutic use–Congresses. 4.   Tissue Engineering–Congresses.   QT 37 I614a 2009]
    R857.M3I525 2009
    610.28–dc22

                                                                                                2008041827

Printed in the United States of America.

10 9 8 7 6 5 4 3 2 1

CONTENTS

Foreword (by Prof. Larry L. Hench)   ix

Preface   xi

Contributors   xv

About the Editors   xxi

SECTION I

**1 FUNDAMENTALS OF BIOMATERIALS
AND BIOCOMPATIBILITY**   3
Bikramjit Basu and Shekhar Nath

**2 FUNDAMENTALS OF HYDROXYAPATITE AND RELATED
CALCIUM PHOSPHATES**   19
*Racquel Zapanta LeGeros, Atsuo Ito, Kunio Ishikawa,
Toshiro Sakae, and John P. LeGeros*

3 MATERIALS FOR ORTHOPEDIC APPLICATIONS   53
Shekhar Nath and Bikramjit Basu

**4 THE MICRO MACROPOROUS BIPHASIC CALCIUM PHOSPHATE
CONCEPT FOR BONE RECONSTRUCTION AND
TISSUE ENGINEERING**   101
Guy Daculsi, Franck Jegoux, and Pierre Layrolle

**5 SCIENCE AND TECHNOLOGY INTEGRATED TITANIUM DENTAL
IMPLANT SYSTEMS**   143
Yoshiki Oshida and Elif Bahar Tuna

v

6 INJECTABLE HYDROGELS AS BIOMATERIALS   179
Lakshmi S. Nair, Cato T. Laurencin, and Mayank Tandon

7 NANOMATERIALS FOR IMPROVED ORTHOPEDIC AND
BONE TISSUE ENGINEERING APPLICATIONS   205
*Lijie Zhang, Sirinrath Sirivisoot, Ganesh Balasundaram, and
Thomas J. Webster*

SECTION II

8 INTRODUCTION TO PROCESSING OF BIOMATERIALS   245
*Dhirendra S. Katti, Shaunak Pandya, Meghali Bora, and
Rakesh Mahida*

9 LASER PROCESSING OF ORTHOPEDIC BIOMATERIALS   277
Rajarshi Banerjee and Soumya Nag

10 FUNCTIONALLY GRADED ALL CERAMIC HIP JOINT   323
*Omer Van der Biest, Guy Anné, Kim Vanmeensel, and
Jef Vleugels*

11 MEDICAL DEVICES BASED ON BIOINSPIRED CERAMICS   357
*Pío González, Julián Martínez-Fernández,
Antonio R. de Arellano-López, and Mrityunjay Singh*

12 IONOMER GLASSES: DESIGN AND CHARACTERIZATION   411
Artemis Stamboulis and Fei Wang

13 DESIGNING NANOFIBROUS SCAFFOLDS FOR
TISSUE ENGINEERING   435
Neha Arya, Poonam Sharma, and Dhirendra S. Katti

14 DESIGN OF SUPERMACROPOROUS BIOMATERIALS
VIA GELATION AT SUBZERO
TEMPERATURES—*CRYOGELATION*   499
*Fatima M. Plieva, Ashok Kumar, Igor Yu. Galaev, and
Bo Mattiasson*

SECTION III

15 BIOMATERIAL APPLICATIONS 535
Ashok Kumar, Akshay Srivastava, and Era Jain

16 CELL-BASED NANOCOMPOSITES AND BIOMOLECULES FOR BONE TISSUE ENGINEERING 551
Michelle Ngiam, Susan Liao, Casey Chan, and S. Ramakrishna

17 ORTHOPEDIC INTERFACE TISSUE ENGINEERING: BUILDING THE BRIDGE TO INTEGRATED MUSCULOSKELETAL TISSUE SYSTEMS 589
Helen H. Lu, Kristen L. Moffat, and Jeffrey P. Spalazzi

18 CELLS OF THE NERVOUS SYSTEM AND ELECTRICAL STIMULATION 613
Carlos Atico Ariza and Surya K. Mallapragada

19 PLACENTAL UMBILICAL CORD BLOOD: A TRUE BLOOD SUBSTITUTE 643
Niranjan Bhattacharya

20 SUPPORTED CELL MIMETIC MONOLAYERS AND THEIR BLOOD COMPATIBILITY 663
K. Kaladhar and Chandra P. Sharma

21 TITANIUM NITRIDE AND DIAMOND LIKE CARBON COATINGS FOR CARDIOVASCULAR APPLICATIONS 677
C.V. Muraleedharan and G.S. Bhuvaneshwar

INDEX 707

FOREWORD

It is nearly 40 years since the first batch of bioactive glass (45S5 Bioglass) implants were made and implanted in the femurs of rats. Six weeks later, scientists discovered that the glass implants bonded to bone—a strong, living interfacial bond. This finding, along with discoveries of tissue compatibility of new polymers, demonstrated that novel materials could be designed and processed to achieve special types of bioactive behavior with tissues. Millions of patients worldwide have benefited from this revolution in thinking; that is, the design of materials to function *with* the body instead of being isolated *from* the body. However, the rapid increase in the worldwide population of ageing people requires an ever-increasing lifetime of prostheses. Innovations in the design, processing, and applications of all classes of biomaterials are needed to meet this challenge of longer implant survivability.

The goal of this book, "Advanced Biomaterials: Fundamentals, Processing and Applications," is to provide the reader with a good overview of novel biomaterials research and development in 2007–2008. The editors and authors have succeeded in meeting this goal. Much has changed during the 40 years since the first bioactive glass implants used in rat femurs, as shown by many chapters in this book. Two important themes of inquiry emerge in this book: 1) nanotechnology and 2) gradient structures. Both of these innovative directions of research offer great promise for future improvements of survivability. In several chapters, the scale of structure being investigated has been decreased to the nano-scale, in keeping with the scale of natural occurring nano-composites. Biomimetic principles of self-organization of three dimensional structures at the nano-scale are described and the principles involved are reviewed.

Nearly all tissues exhibit gradient interfaces that are critical for transferring stress across cell boundaries. Replicating such gradients in both the structure and the properties of man-made biomaterials is difficult but, as shown herein, progress is being made. Also, a goal throughout the last 40 years has been to achieve improved blood–biomaterials interactions. Advances in this area are also reviewed. A broad cross section of biomaterials studies throughout the world is represented in this book and I thereby recommend it to readers, both those at beginning and those at advanced levels of interest and competence in the field.

Larry L. Hench
March 4, 2008

PREFACE

Biomaterials as well as their applications as artificial organs are widely recognized as an emerging area for material scientists, biotechnologists, chemists, engineers and medical professionals. Recent developments in the areas of material science and biological science have enabled impressive progress in the attempts to develop new biomaterials. The development of new biocompatible materials (bulk or coating) and/or refinement of existing material composition/processing techniques are expected to broaden the diversity of applications of biomaterials in the coming years. The progress in biomaterials research clearly requires an improved understanding in multiple disciplines, as well as the development of new design methodologies in order to obtain better properties in terms of physical and biological performance. In the above context, an International Conference on Design of Biomaterials (BIND-06, url: http://home.iitk.ac.in/~bikram/bind06.htm) was organised at Indian Institute of Technology Kanpur, India during 8–11 December, 2006. The advances in areas such as Tissue Engineering, cell-biomaterial interaction, Bioceramics, Polymeric Biomaterials, orthopedic biomaterials, cardiovascular biomaterials, Nanobiomaterials, ophthalmic biomaterials, dental biomaterials and biomaterial applications were largely discussed in the symposium. BIND-06 was jointly organized by Society for Biomaterials and Artificial Organs-India (SBAOI, url: www.sbaoi.org) and Indian Institute of Technology Kanpur (IIT-K, url: http://www.iitk.ac.in/). SBAOI is a member of the International Union of Societies for Biomaterial Sciences and Engineering (IUSBSE).

This edited volume on "Advanced Biomaterials: Fundamentals, Processing and Applications" is the outcome of the International Conference on Design of Biomaterials. The book primarily consists of three broad sections, namely: Fundamentals; Processing; and Applications of Biomaterials. Each of these sections contains a number of chapters that discuss specific topics pertaining to state-of-the-art aspects within the respective area. The current book has contributions by some of the renowned scientists, engineers and clinicians, which is a hallmark of interdisciplinary areas, such as biomaterials science.

In first section on **fundamentals**, the basic aspect of structure, processing and properties as well as approaches to develop or design new biomaterials is presented. For example, the chapter by Bikramjit Basu and co-workers broadly discusses the various methods to optimize the processing conditions/material composition to design biomaterials based on metals, ceramics and polymers. Considering the fact that inorganic component of the natural cortical bone is calcium phosphate (CaP-) compound, rich with hydroxyapatite (HA) phase, the chapter contributed by Racquel Z. Legeros and co-workers described the fundamental crystal structure and properties of HA, calcium-deficient apatite (CDA) and other biologically relevant apatites. The chapter contributed by Lakshmi S. Nair and co-workers report their recent work on developing various *in situ* gelling stimuli sensitive (light, temperature and pH) polymeric systems as drug and cell delivery vehicles. The feasibility of developing injectable composites by combining the thermogelling solution with hydroxyapatite has also been discussed. In the context of interfacial tissue engineering, the chapter by Helen H. Lu and co-authors discusses the functional integration of soft tissue grafts as well as model scaffold systems, based on biodegradable polymers and calcium phosphate composites for tendon-to-bone integration. The potential mechanism for *ex vivo* development and *in vivo* translation of integrated musculoskeletal tissues with biomimetic complexity and functionality has also been presented in this chapter. In the chapter by C. P. Sharma and co-author, a novel biomimetic approach is presented to develop thin solid films by self-assembling amphiphiles for the purpose of surface modification of biomaterials and related devices. The chapter contributed by Thomas J. Webster and co-workers demonstrates how the cross-fertilisation of ideas from nanotechnology and bone-tissue engineering can be drawn to develop metals, ceramics or polymer based nanophase materials for orthopedic applications. In the chapter by Artemis Stamboulis and co-author, the results of a number of state-of-art characterization tools, including Magic Angle Spinning Nuclear Magnetic Resonance (MAS-NMR), are presented to provide evidences for amorphous phase separation (APS) during crystallisation of Apatite stoichiometric ionomer glasses (SiO_2-Al_2O_3-P_2O_5-CaO-CaF_2).

Under the **processing section**, some emerging manufacturing techniques, like Laser Engineered Net Shaping (LENS™), as well as processes involved in designing of bioactive scaffolds, polymeric drug delivery system have been covered. The chapter written by R. Banerjee and co-workers demonstrates how novel near-net shape processing technologies, such as LENS can be utilized to rapidly manufacture custom-designed functionally-graded implants with site-specific properties. The chapter by Omer Van Der Biest and his co-workers largely focuses on the design principles of Electrophoretic deposition as a novel processing route to develop functionally gradient materials (FGM) based on biocompatible ceramics. The chapter by Yoshiki Oshida presents how one can achieve better osseointegration property in Titanium-based new dental implants by introducing functionality. In the chapter by Fatima Pliena and Ashok Kumar in the area of the soft biomaterials, a novel approach of designing supermacroporous cryogels has been discussed.

Under the section on **applications**, various aspects of tissue engineering, synthetic heart valve, and blood substitutes have been discussed. The contribution by Seeram Ramakrishna and co-workers presented the results of the biomimetic mineralization of nanofibrous composites, especially those made of collagen and nano-hydroxyapatite. It has been concluded that an effective bone regeneration approach using tissue-engineered constructs loaded with growth factors, that create a favorable environment *in vivo*, can revolutionize the clinical management of bone-related diseases and orthopedic applications. The chapter contributed by Surya K. Mallapragada and co-workers demonstrates how micropatterned biodegradable polymer films furnish a combination of physical, chemical and biological cues in order to facilitate peripheral nerve regeneration. In the chapter written by Pio González and co-workers, the development of a new generation of bimorphic silicon carbide ceramics, fabricated from bio-derived cellulose templates, to mimic structure/properties of natural bone is presented. The chapter written by G. S. Bhuvaneshwar and co-worker presents the development of DLC and TiN coating materials with an emphasis on better coating properties with respect to hemocopatibility and inherent mechanical stability for a wide range of cardiovascular applications. Based on clinical trials, it has been concluded that DLC-coated UHMWPE could be an excellent material for use as a bearing in all rotating cardiovascular appliances, such as centrifugal blood pumps, cell separators and implantable cardiovascular pumps. The chapter by Guy Daculsi and co-worker describes various concepts to develop micro- and macro-porous biphasic calcium phosphate (BCP) bioceramics (an optimum balance between the more stable HA phase and more soluble TCP) for better osteogenic and osteoinductive properties for tissue engineering of hybrid bone. The chapter by Niranjan Bhattacharya demonstrates that freshly-collected and properly-screened placental umbilical cord blood, following the birth of a healthy baby, can be an ideal and true blood substitute, in contrast to the current generation of artificial blood (poor RBC substitutes).

The above described layout of the book as well as the succession of the chapters is primarily meant for easy understanding for both students and experts pursuing the area of biomaterials science. In particular, this edited volume has the following major important features:

a) Integration of fundamentals-processing-application, enabling the possibility of using this book as a text book for teaching, academic, and research purposes,

b) Coverage of broader range of topics, while providing contemporary and exciting areas, such as nanobiomaterials, interface tissue engineering, emerging manufacturing techniques and new polymeric materials, and

c) A basic book for a large number of active researchers from various disciplines of biological sciences, metallurgy and materials science, ceramics, polymers, biotechnology as well as engineers, manufacturers, dentists and surgeons.

Although this book is meant for readers who have been introduced to the broad area of biomaterials, the introductory chapters to each section have been designed to facilitate readers who do not have a background in the area of biomaterials science. While conceiving the content of this book, the editors desired to motivate young researchers as well as to provide experts with a healthy balance of topics for teaching and academic purposes. It is expected that this book, if used as a text, would benefit senior undergraduate and postgraduate students.

It is important to reiterate here that this book is an outcome of the International conference on design of biomaterials and therefore the editors (organisers of BIND-06) would like to take this opportunity to acknowledge the financial support received from both government and private agencies, including Air Force Office of Scientific Research (AFOSR), Asian office of Aerospace Research and Development (AOARD), Council of Scientific and Industrial Research (CSIR), Department of Biotechnology (DBT), Defence Research and Development Organization (DRDO), Department of Science & Technology (DST), Indian Council of Medical Research (ICMR), Indo-US Science and Technology Forum (IUSSTF) for organising this conference. We would also like to thank IIT Kanpur administration as well as the local, national and international organising committee members of BIND-06 conference, in particular Dr. M. Singh, NASA Glenn Research Center Cleveland, USA. We express our gratitude to all the contributors of various book chapters and give special thanks to Prof. Larry Hecnh for writing the foreword of this book. In closing, the Editors would like to thank their respective families for their constant support and encouragement.

Bikramjit Basu

Dhirendra S. Katti

Ashok Kumar

Kanpur, India

August 2009

To view supplemental material for this book, including color versions of figures, please visit ftp://ftp.wiley.com/public/sci_tech_med/advanced_biomaterials.

CONTRIBUTORS

Guy Anné

Department of Metallurgy and Materials Engineering, Katholieke Universiteit Leuven, Kasteelpark ARENBERG nr 44, B-3001 HEVERLEE-LEUVEN, Belgium

Carlos Atico Ariza

Chemical and Biological Engineering, Iowa State University, Ames, Iowa, USA

Neha Arya

Department of Biological Sciences and Bioengineering, Indian Institute of Technology Kanpur, Kanpur-208016, UP, India

Ganesh Balasundaram

Divisions of Engineering and Orthopedics, Brown University, Providence, Rhode Island, USA

Rajarshi Banerjee

Department of Materials Science and Engineering, University of North Texas, Denton, Texas, USA

Bikramjit Basu

Department of Materials and Metallurgical Engineering, Indian Institute of Technology Kanpur, Kanpur-208016, UP, India

Niranjan Bhattacharya

Advisor, Biomedical Research and Consultant, Advanced Medical Research Institute (AMRI) Hospitals, Gol Park, B.P. Poddar Hospitals, Alipore, Apollo Gleneagle Hospital, and Vidyasagore Hospital, Calcutta, India

G. S. Bhuvaneshwar

Division of Artificial Organs, Biomedical Technology Wing, Sree Chitra Tirunal Institute for Medical Sciences & Technology, Thiruvananthapuram, India

Meghali Bora
Department of Biological Sciences and Bioengineering, Indian Institute of Technology Kanpur, Kanpur-208016, UP, India

Casey Chan
Division of Bioengineering, Faculty of Engineering, National University of Singapore, Singapore, and Department of Orthopedic Surgery, Yong Loo Lin School of Medicine, National University of Singapore, Singapore

Guy Daculsi
INSERM, Université de Nantes, UMR U791, Faculté de Chirurgie Dentaire, Place Alexis Ricordeau, 44042 Nantes Cedex 01, France, and CHU de Bordeaux/INSERM, CIC-Innovations Technologiques Biomatériaux, Bortdeaux, France

Julián Martínez-Fernández
Departamento de Física de la Materia Condensada-ICMSE, University of Seville, Av. Reina Mercedes, Seville, Spain

Igor Yu. Galaev
Department of Biotechnology, Center for Chemistry and Chemical Engineering, Lund University, SE–22100 Lund, Sweden

Pío González
Departamento de Física Aplicada, ETSII, University of Vigo, Campus Lagoas-Marcosende, 36310 Vigo, Spain

Kunio Ishikawa
Faculty of Dental Sciences, Kyushu University, Fukuoka, Japan

Atsuo Ito
National Institute of Advanced Industrial Science and Technology, Tsukuba, Japan

Era Jain
Department of Biological Sciences and Bioengineering, Indian Institute of Technology Kanpur, Kanpur-208016, UP, India

Franck Jegoux
INSERM, Université de Nantes, UMR U791, Faculté de Chirurgie Dentaire, Place Alexis Ricordeau, 44042 Nantes Cedex 01, France, and CHU Pontchaillou Service ORL et chirurgie maxillofaciale, Rennes, France

K. Kaladhar
Biosurface Technology Division, Biomedical Technology Wing, Sree Chithra Tirunal Institute for Medical Science and Technology, Thiruvananthapuram, Kerala, India

Dhirendra S. Katti
Department of Biological Sciences and Bioengineering, Indian Institute of Technology Kanpur, Kanpur-208016, UP, India

Ashok Kumar
Department of Biological Sciences and Bioengineering, Indian Institute of Technology Kanpur, Kanpur-208016, UP, India

Cato T. Laurencin
Department of Orthopedic Surgery, and Department of Chemical, Materials and Biomolecular Engineering, University of Connecticut, Connecticut, USA

Pierre Layrolle
INSERM, Université de Nantes, UMR U791, Faculté de Chirurgie Dentaire, Place Alexis Ricordeau, 44042 Nantes Cedex 01, France

John P. LeGeros
Calcium Phosphate Research Laboratory, Department of Biomaterials & Biomimetics, New York University College of Dentistry, New York, New York, USA

Racquel Zapanta LeGeros
Calcium Phosphate Research Laboratory, Department of Biomaterials & Biomimetics, New York University College of Dentistry, New York, New York, USA

Susan Liao
Division of Bioengineering, Faculty of Engineering, National University of Singapore, Singapore, and Department of Orthopedic Surgery, Yong Loo Lin School of Medicine, National University of Singapore, Singapore

Antonio R. de Arellano-López
Departamento de Física de la Materia Condensada-ICMSE, University of Seville, Av. Reina Mercedes, Seville, Spain

Helen H. Lu
Department of Biomedical Engineering, Columbia University, New York, New York, USA

Rakesh Mahida
Department of Biological Sciences and Bioengineering, Indian Institute of Technology Kanpur, Kanpur-208016, UP, India

Surya K. Mallapragada

Iowa State University, Chemical and Biological Engineering, Ames, Iowa, USA

Bo Mattiasson

Department of Biotechnology, Center for Chemistry and Chemical Engineering, Lund University, SE–22100 Lund, Sweden

Kristen L. Moffat

Biomaterials and Interface Tissue Engineering Laboratory, Department of Biomedical Engineering, Columbia University, New York, New York, USA

C. V. Muraleedharan

Division of Artificial Organs, Biomedical Technology Wing, Sree Chitra Tirunal Institute for Medical Sciences & Technology, Thiruvananthapuram, India

Soumya Nag

Department of Materials Science and Engineering, Ohio State University, Columbus, Ohio, USA

Lakshmi S. Nair

Department of Orthopedic Surgery, and Department of Chemical, Materials and Biomolecular Engineering, University of Connecticut, Connecticut, USA

Shekhar Nath

Department of Materials and Metallurgical Engineering, Indian Institute of Technology Kanpur, Kanpur-208016, UP, India

Michelle Ngiam

National University of Singapore (NUS), Graduate Program in Bioengineering, NUS Graduate School (NGS) for Integrative Sciences and Engineering, Center for Life Sciences (CeLS), Singapore

Yoshiki Oshida

Indiana University School of Dentistry, Professor Emeritus, Syracuse University College of Engineering, Research Professor, L. C. Smith College of Engineering, Department of Mechanical and Aerospace Engineering, Syracuse University, Syracuse, New York, USA

Shaunak Pandya

Department of Biological Sciences and Bioengineering, Indian Institute of Technology Kanpur, Kanpur-208016, UP, India

Fatima M. Plieva

Protista Biotechnology AB, SE-22370 Lund, Sweden and Department of Biotechnology, Center for Chemistry and Chemical Engineering, Lund University, SE–22100 Lund, Sweden

Stijn Put

Department of Metallurgy and Materials Engineering, Katholieke Universiteit Leuven, Kasteelpark ARENBERG nr 44, B-3001 HEVERLEE-LEUVEN, Belgium

S. Ramakrishna

Division of Bioengineering, Faculty of Engineering, National University of Singapore, Singapore, and Department of Mechanical Engineering, Faculty of Engineering, National University of Singapore, Singapore, and National University of Singapore Nanoscience & Nanotechnology Initiative, Singapore

Toshiro Sakae

Nihon University School of Dentistry, Matsudo, Japan

Chandra P. Sharma

Biosurface Technology Division, Biomedical Technology Wing, Sree Chithra Tirunal Institute for Medical Science and Technology, Thiruvananthapuram, Kerala, India

Poonam Sharma

Department of Biological Sciences and Bioengineering, Indian Institute of Technology Kanpur, Kanpur-208016, UP, India

Mrityunjay Singh

Ohio Aerospace Institute, Ceramics Branch, NASA Glenn Research Center, Cleveland, Ohio, USA

Sirinrath Sirivisoot

Divisions of Engineering and Orthopedics, Brown University, Providence, Rhode Island, USA

Jeffrey P. Spalazzi

Biomaterials and Interface Tissue Engineering Laboratory, Department of Biomedical Engineering, Columbia University, New York, New York, USA

Akshay Srivastava

Department of Biological Sciences and Bioengineering, Indian Institute of Technology Kanpur, Kanpur-208016, UP, India

Artemis Stamboulis

University of Birmingham, Metallurgy and Materials, Edgbaston, Birmingham, UK

Mayank Tandon

Department of Biomedical Engineering, University of Virginia, Virginia, USA

Elif Bahar Tuna

Istanbul University Faculty of Dentistry, Department of Pediatric Dentistry, Capa Istanbul, Turkey

Omer Van der Biest

Department of Metallurgy and Materials Engineering, Katholieke Universiteit Leuven, Kasteelpark ARENBERG nr 44, B-3001 HEVERLEE-LEUVEN, Belgium

Kim Vanmeensel

Department of Metallurgy and Materials Engineering, Katholieke Universiteit Leuven, Kasteelpark ARENBERG nr 44, B-3001 HEVERLEE-LEUVEN, Belgium

Jef Vleugels

Department of Metallurgy and Materials Engineering, Katholieke Universiteit Leuven, Kasteelpark ARENBERG nr 44, B-3001 HEVERLEE-LEUVEN, Belgium

Fei Wang

University of Birmingham, Metallurgy and Materials, Edgbaston, Birmingham, UK

Thomas J. Webster

Divisions of Engineering and Orthopedics, Brown University, Providence, Rhode Island, USA

Lijie Zhang

Divisions of Engineering and Orthopedics, Brown University, Providence, Rhode Island, USA

ABOUT THE EDITORS

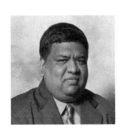

Bikramjit Basu, Ph.D.

Bikramjit Basu received his Ph.D. in Metallurgy and Materials Engineering from Katholieke Universiteit Leuven, Belgium in 2001. After a brief stint of post-doctoral research at UC, Santa Barbara, he joined Indian Institute of Technology Kanpur, India, where he is currently Associate Professor at Department of Materials and Metallurgical Engineering. He held visiting positions at University of Warwick, Seoul National University and UPC, Barcelona. At present, his primary research activities are in designing biomaterials for hard tissue replacement with a primary focus on establishing processing-structure-property relationship. He has authored or co-authored more than 100 research papers in peer-reviewed international journals. In recognition of his outstanding contribution in Ceramic Science, he received several noteworthy National awards, including those from Indian National Academy of Engineering and Indian National Science Academy. Recently, he has been selected to receive the prestigious Coble Award for Young Scholars of the American Ceramic Society. He is currently an editorial board member of *Journal of Korean Ceramic Society, Journal of Materials Engineering Innovation* and *Materials Science and Engineering C*.

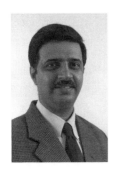

Dhirendra S. Katti, Ph.D.

Dhirendra S. Katti received his Ph.D. in Chemistry from Bombay University in 1999. He was then a post-doctoral fellow and Research Assistant Professor at Drexel University, Philadelphia. He then moved on to be Assistant Professor (Tenure Track) at the Department of Orthopaedic Surgery and the Department of Biomedical Engineering at The University of Virginia. Currently, he is Associate Professor at the Department of Biological Sciences and Bioengineering at Indian Institute of Technology Kanpur, India. His current research interests are in the area of Biomaterials, Controlled Drug Delivery Systems, Tissue Engineering and Nanobiotechnology. He is an editorial board member of *Journal of Biomedical Nanotechnology*.

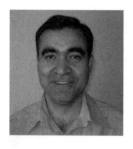

Ashok Kumar, Ph.D.

Ashok Kumar received his Ph.D. in Biotechnology in 1994 jointly from Institute of Genomics and Integrative Biology, Delhi, and Indian Institute of Technology, Roorkee, India. He spent his post-doctoral time at Nagoya University, Japan and Lund University, Sweden. He continued as faculty at Lund University, Sweden and also worked in a biotechnology company in Sweden. He is currently Associate Professor at the department of Biological Sciences and Bioengineering, Indian Institute of Technology, Kanpur. His current research interests are in the area of biomaterials, tissue engineering, bioprocess engineering and environmental biotechnology. He has published about 100 peer-reviewed research papers in international journals, has written six book chapters, and has several patents. He is the editor of a book on cell separations and is presently working on editing two more books in the area of biomaterials. He is the associate editor of *Nanoscale Research Letters* and is on the editorial board of three other biological journals.

Section I

1

FUNDAMENTALS OF BIOMATERIALS AND BIOCOMPATIBILITY

Bikramjit Basu and Shekhar Nath

Department of Materials and Metallurgical Engineering, Indian Institute of Technology Kanpur, Kanpur, India

Contents

1.1 Overview	4
1.2 Introduction	4
1.3 Some Useful Definitions and Their Implications	5
1.3.1 Biomaterial	5
1.3.2 Biocompatibility	7
1.3.3 Host Response	7
1.4 Cell–Material Interactions	8
1.5 Experimental Evaluation of Biocompatibility	12
1.5.1 *In Vitro* Tests	12
1.5.2 *In Vivo* Tests	14
1.6 Steps for Characterizations of Biomaterials	15
1.7 Broad Overview of Fundamentals Section	16
References	17

Advanced Biomaterials: Fundamentals, Processing, and Applications, Edited by Bikramjit Basu, Dhirendra S. Katti, and Ashok Kumar
Copyright © 2009 The American Ceramic Society

1.1 OVERVIEW

In last two decades, impressive progress has been recorded in terms of developing new materials or refining existing material composition and microstructure in order to obtain better performance of designed materials in biomedical applications. The success of such large efforts clearly demands better understanding of various concepts such as biocompatibility, host response, and cell-biomaterial interaction. This chapter reviews the fundamentals for understanding biomaterials development.

1.2 INTRODUCTION

One of the most exciting and rewarding research areas of materials science involves the applications of materials to health care, especially to reconstructive surgery. The importance of biomaterials can be well realized from an economical aspect, that is, in terms of an estimate of total health care expenditure around the world. In the most developed country of the world, the United States, total health care expenditure in the year 2000 was approximately 14 billion US dollars. It was also reported that the US market for biomaterials in 2000 was 9 billion US dollars. It can be further noted that the respective annual expenses in other countries of the world are typically around two-to-three times that of the US expenses[1]. With continuous changes in lifestyle as well as in global scenarios in the health sector, such expenses are definitely on a much higher side today in both developed and, more importantly, developing nations, than at the beginning of this century. To this end, the development of biomaterials and related devices is important.

The field of biomaterials is multidisciplinary, and the design of biomaterials requires the synergistic interaction of materials science, biological science, chemical science, medical science and mechanical science. Such interaction has been schematically illustrated in Figure 1.1. Also shown in Figure 1.1 is the necessity to develop cross-disciplinary approaches in designing new biomaterials. Among different kinds of biomaterials[2], metals and metallic alloys are used in orthopedics, dentistry and other load-bearing applications; ceramics are used[3] with emphasis on either their chemically inert[4] nature or their high bioactivity[5]; polymers are used for soft tissue replacement and research is also being pursued for application in hard tissue replacement. To achieve better biological properties and mechanical strength, composite materials of metals, ceramics and polymers are being developed and clinically assessed to a limited extent. Broadly, all biomaterials are being developed to maintain a balance between the mechanical properties of the replaced tissues and the biochemical effects of the material on the tissue. Both areas are of great importance as far as the clinical success of materials is concerned. However, in most (if not all) biological systems, a range of properties is required, such as biological activity, mechanical strength, chemical durability, and so forth. Therefore, a clinical need often can only be fulfilled by a designed material that exhibits a complex combination of some of the above mentioned properties. Figure 1.2 shows the different organs of a living human body that can

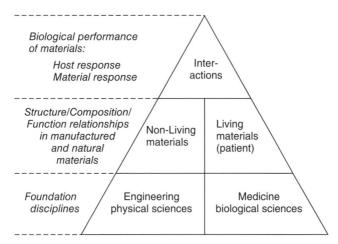

Figure 1.1. Concept triangle illustrating the synergistic interaction of Engineering and Biological science disciplines, involved in designing biomaterials. The schematic also demonstrates the multidisciplinary approach of the science and technology of biomaterials. [Reproduced from, J Black, in chapter: Biocompatibility: Definition and Issues, Biological Performance of Materials: Fundamentals of Biocompatibility, CRC Press, US, 2006.]

be replaced by various biomaterials. In living humans, most orthopedic/prosthetic joints and dental restorations demand the use of hard tissue/cortical bone or analogue materials, such as high-strength metals or high-hardness ceramics. To this end, the use of softer polymeric materials is restricted to the cranial area, blood vessels, heart valves, intraocular lenses, and so on.

In this section, the structure of this introductory chapter has been presented. Section 1.3 discusses necessary biological terms and their importance as well as the materials classification with respect to host response. Specially, in subsections 1.3.1 and 1.3.2, the two important terms *biomaterials* and *biocompatibility* have been defined and their implications are provided. In the subsequent subsection (1.3.3), the host tissue response with biomaterials has been assessed critically. In section 1.4, the cell-material interaction has been discussed with an aim to provide a fundamental idea about the interactions of a specific cell line with implanted materials. The next section (1.5) demonstrates the various *in vitro* and *in vivo* experiments to determine the biocompatibility of the materials. In the subsequent section (1.6), the steps involved in characterizing biomaterials are discussed. At the close, the brief highlights of the various book chapters under 'Fundamentals' section is presented in section 1.7.

1.3 SOME USEFUL DEFINITIONS AND THEIR IMPLICATIONS

1.3.1 Biomaterial

Broadly, biomaterials can be defined as synthetic materials, which have been designed to induce a specific biological activity[6]. The major difference of

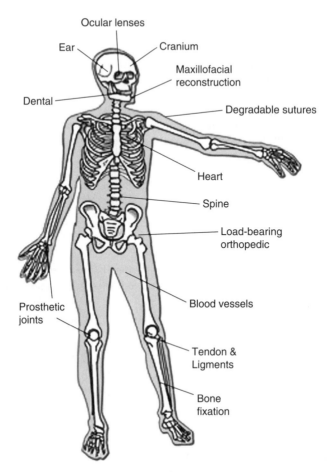

Figure 1.2. A schematic of the various human body parts, which can be potentially replaced by synthetic biomaterials. [Reproduced from, J Black, in chapter: Biocompatibility: Definition and Issues, Biological Performance of Materials: Fundamentals of Biocompatibility, CRC Press, US, 2006.]

biomaterials from other classes of materials is their ability to remain in a biological environment without damaging the surroundings and without getting damaged in that process[7]. Therefore, biomaterials require both biological and materials properties to suit a specific application. It must be emphasized here that biological properties/responses of a material in physiological environments are, by far, the most important consideration, as opposed to superior mechanical properties, for selecting/defining biomaterials. From the health care perspective, it is desirable that a biocompatible material interrupts normal body functions as little as possible. The most important aspect of a biomaterial is, therefore, how a biomaterial interacts when implanted in a human or animal body.

1.3.2 Biocompatibility

The fundamental requirement of any biomaterial concerns the ability of the material to perform effectively with an appropriate host response for the desired application, that is, the material and the tissue environment of the body should coexist without having any undesirable or inappropriate effect on each other. This has also been mentioned in Figure 1.1. Such a requirement is broadly described by the concept known as 'biocompatibility'[8]. Broadly, biocompatibility is defined as 'the ability of a material to perform with an appropriate host response in a specific application.' From a biological point of view, biocompatibility arises from the acceptability of non-living materials (synthetic biomaterial) in a living body (mammal/human). There are three important aspects of biocompatibility that a candidate biomaterial seeks to achieve in diverse environments, such as bone, blood vessel and the eye. In the first place, biomaterials must be biochemically compatible, non-toxic, non-irritable, non-allergenic and non-carcinogenic; second, biomechanically compatible with surrounding tissues; and third, a bioadhesive contact must be established between the materials and living tissues. It needs to be emphasized here that the biocompatibility depends on place of applications. For example, a specific material could be biocompatible in bone replacement, but the same material may not be biocompatible in direct blood contact application. However, as will be discussed later, a range of *in vitro/in vivo* tests are suggested to completely describe the biocompatibility property. It must be emphasized hence that for a given biomedical application, only a selected set of relevant tests, among various tests mentioned in section 1.6, should be carried out on potential implant materials.

1.3.3 Host Response

In order to develop new materials, it is desirable to understand the *in vivo* host response of various biomaterials. Ideally, biomaterials should not induce any change or provoke undesired reaction in the neighboring or distant tissues. An important aspect of host response involves the formation of a structural and biological bond between the material and host tissues. When the biocompatibility is lacking, materials cause tissue reactions, which may be systemic or local. Systemic responses can be toxic or allergic and triggered by the products of metallic corrosion and polymer degradation, release of micro particles from materials, and the presence of contaminants.

Different human systems (such as respiratory, circulation, or digestive) respond in different ways to contact with foreign bodies or materials. Depending on the biocompatibility and host reaction, biomaterials can be broadly classified into three main categories on the basis of various types of host responses of biomaterials after implantation into the living body[2]:

a) **Bioinert / biotolerant:** Bioinert materials are biocompatible materials, but cannot induce any interfacial biological bond between implants and bone.

b) **Bioactive:** Bioactive materials are a group of biocompatible materials that can attach directly with body tissues and form chemical and biological bonds during early stages of the post implantation period.

c) **Bioresorbable:** Bioresorable materials are the type of biocompatible materials that are gradually resorbed before they finally disappear and are totally replaced by new tissues *in vivo*.

When a bioinert material is implanted, a capsule-like layer forms on the surface of the implant to keep it isolated from the living part of the body. For example, bioinert ceramics, such as alumina or zirconia, develop fibrous capsules at their interface when implanted. However, it is important to note that the thickness of an interfacial fibrous layer depends upon motion and the extent of required fit at the interface. Therefore, a bioinert material is not useful for long-term application. The most significant class of biomaterial is bioactive material, which can potentially behave as the part of a living body. A few examples of bioactive materials are 45S5 bioglass and calcium phosphates (HA). For bioactive materials, the interfacial bond prevents motion between the implant–tissue interfaces and imitates the type of interface found when natural tissues repair themselves[9]. The third kind of material is bioresorable or degradable, which degrades with time inside the body's environment. The degradation rate should be such that the regeneration rate of new tissue will be same as the material resorption rate. Tricalcium Phosphate (TCP) and bone cement are the two examples of bioresorable materials.

1.4   CELL–MATERIAL INTERACTIONS

The interaction between biomaterials and natural tissues is an important scientific issue and understanding this issue is essential to designing new biocompatible materials. In understanding the interaction and integration of biomaterials in a human body, it is worthwhile to mention the physicochemical conditions of the human body's environment. For example, nominal pH values vary over a wide range of 1.0 (gastric content) to 7.4 (blood)[10]. Additionally, pH values can change depending on health conditions (disease, etc.). The temperature of the normal core of human body is around 37.4 °C; however, deviations over a range of temperature 20–42.5 °C have been reported for diseased patients[10]. As far as the inorganic composition of the human body is concerned, total body burden of Ca, Na, Cl ions is much higher and also traces of Mg, Fe, Zn, Cu, Al, and so on, are present in cytoplasm.

Biologically, a cell is defined as a self-duplicating unit, given the proper nutrients and environment. A cell can alternatively be described as a collection of self-replicating enzymes and structural proteins. In Figure 1.3a, the anatomy of a typical mammalian eukaryotic cell has been provided. Various important organelles can be identified in Figure 1.3a and important organelles include mitochondrion (energy warehouse), Golgi apparatus, Endoplasmic Reticulum (ER), etc. It can be mentioned here that rough ER is one of the preferred locations for protein

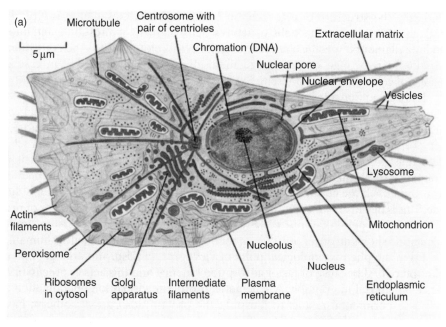

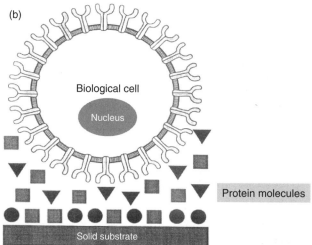

Figure 1.3. Schematic illustration showing the anatomy of an eukaryotic animal cell (a) [Reproduced from Bruce Alberts, Alexander Johnson, Julian Lewis, Martin Raff, Keith Roberts, Peter Walter, Introduction to the Cells in "Molecular Biology of The Cell".] and the fundamental mechanisms involved in biomaterial-cell interaction, established by the adsorbed proteins (circles, boxes and triangles) with the integrin proteins of a biological cell (b) [Reproduced from BD Ratner, AS Hoffman, FJ Schoen, JE Lemons, Biomaterials Science—An Introduction to Materials in Medicine, 2nd edition, Academic Press, New York, 2004.].

synthesis. The structure of cytoskeleton is also visible. Cytoskeleton is typically made up of three proteinaceous structures: actin filament, microtubule and inter-mediate filaments. Specific chatrcaterisitcs of cytoskeleton allows the constituent proteins to rearrange or reorganize themselves when desired, e.g., in case of change of cell shape in response to external stimulation.

It is critical that any implant material must, to a minimum extent, elicit a toxic response, that kills cells in the surrounding tissues or releases chemicals that can migrate within tissue fluids and cause systemic damage to the patient. Therefore, it is important, in the first place, to understand biomaterial–cell interaction. A sche-matic illustration of the fundamental mechanisms involved in biomaterial–cell in-teraction is shown in Figure 1.3b. It can be recalled that once a material is implanted in an animal, a large number of protein molecules are adsorbed on biomaterial sur-face. This is because of the abundance of protein as an order of 10^9 number of pro-tein molecules per eukaryotic cell is estimated in the human body. Also, a simple calculation shows an order of 10^{14} number of eukaryotic cells in a healthy human.

From the phenomenological point of view, protein adsorption on an implant takes place first because of faster adsorption kinetics, and this acts as precursor to the cell–material interaction. A schematic of protein adsorption phenomenon as well as experimental results to illustrate the protein adsorption isotherm have been provided in Figure 1.4. Therefore, a material does not "see" a cell directly

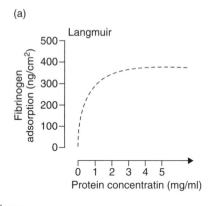

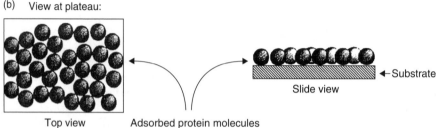

Figure 1.4. Schematic illustration showing the anatomy of a eukaryotic animal cell (a) and the fundamental mechanisms involved in biomaterial-cell interaction, established by the adsorbed proteins (circles, boxes and triangles) with the integrin proteins of a biological cell (b). [Reproduced from BD Ratner, AS Hoffman, FJ Schoen, JE Lemons, Biomaterials Science— An Introduction to Materials in Medicine, 2nd edition, Academic Press, New York, 2004.]

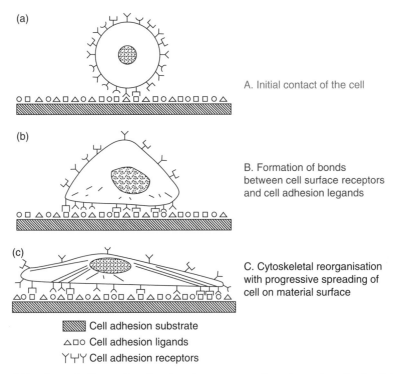

(a)

A. Initial contact of the cell

(b)

B. Formation of bonds
between cell surface receptors
and cell adhesion legands

(c)

C. Cytoskeletal reorganisation
with progressive spreading of
cell on material surface

▨▨▨ Cell adhesion substrate
△▢○ Cell adhesion ligands
Υ⋎Υ Cell adhesion receptors

<u>Figure 1.5.</u> Schematic illustration showing the anatomy of a eukaryotic animal cell (a) and the fundamental mechanisms involved in biomaterial-cell interaction, established by the adsorbed proteins (circles, boxes and triangles) with the integrin proteins of a biological cell (b). [Reproduced from BD Ratner, AS Hoffman, FJ Schoen, JE Lemons, Biomaterials Science—An Introduction to Materials in Medicine, 2nd edition, Academic Press, New York, 2004.]

and the initial interaction is established through the interaction of cell surface receptors with adsorbed protein ligands. Such protein-to-protein binding importantly helps a cell to spread on the material surface.

Subsequent spreading to cover entire implant surface is also facilitated by cytoskeletal reorganization, as shown schematically in Figure 1.5.

After implantation of a biomaterial, a monolayer of protein molecules gets absorbed on the material surface within a minute. Subsequently, the transport of various cell types towards the biomaterial surface occurs and the interaction of the integrin proteins of cell surface with the absorbed protein of biomaterials surface is established. The secretion of cell enzymes of various cell type form an extra cellular matrix (ECM). Depending on cell biomaterial interaction, various cell types can adhere in a self-organized manner to form a tissue. To this end, an important event is the formation of the small blood vessels (angiogenesis) as well as formation of large blood vessels (vasculogenesis) within the newly-formed tissue layer. Such formation is necessary for the supply of nutrients locally to various cell types as well as for the removal of waste from ECM.

1.5 EXPERIMENTAL EVALUATION OF BIOCOMPATIBILITY

Any research program of assessment on biomaterials must include a range of *in vitro* and *in vivo* tests, as stated by various standard agencies (for example, International Organization for Standardization [ISO]). ISO guidelines are also available and such guidelines are followed to select the tests for the biological evaluation of materials and medical as well as dental devices. It may be worthwhile to remember the difference between *in vitro* and *in vivo* tests. *In vitro* tests are lab scale simulated experiments, which are rapid and are a must as initial screening tests. From the results of the *in vitro* tests, one cannot obtain any information of inflammation and immune response of the materials. Also, most of the *in vitro* experiments use single cell lines, which do not reflect the actual tissue interaction (involving multiple cell types) *in vivo*. Although the *in vitro* experiments are inexpensive, such tests do not provide appropriate representation of physiological conditions. These tests, nevertheless, are effective as the first step of biocompatibility evaluations. On the other hand, *in vivo* experiments produce a better approximation to the human environment. Here, the material comes in contact with different cell types and the effect of hormonal factors can be analyzed. Also, *in vivo* tests provide interactions with extracellular matrix, blood-borne cells, protein and molecules. These experiments can be regarded as the second step prior to clinical use.

1.5.1 *In Vitro* Tests

In order to harmonize the existing guidelines, ISO has prepared the guideline document 'Biological testing of Medical Devices—Part 1: Guidance on Selection of Test' (ISO 10933-1), which incorporates all the national and international documents. ISO 10993 requirements for long-lasting tissue/bone implants require various biological tests and the following are the major *in vitro* tests:

- **Cytotoxicity:** This is an *in vitro* test of cell toxicity. The cytotoxicity experiments determine whether the material is toxic in contact with some particular cell lines. The test is generally done in a laboratory using some standard/relevant cell lines and the cells are seeded on the materials. As far as the experimental evaluation of biocompatibility is concerned, the cytotoxicity tests are widely cited as the primary assessment of biocompatibility and therefore are discussed in more detail below.

    As a first step, the sterilization of the samples is carried out in order to remove other micro-organisms, if present on the surface. Depending on type of implant materials (i.e., chemistry and chemical composition), the sterilization is either carried out in steam autoclave (15 psi, 121 °C, 20 minutes) or using γ-ray irradiation. The culture medium used for cell culture testing is DMEM (Dulbecco's modified Eagles' medium), containing 10% serum, 1% antibiotic cocktail. The samples are incubated in the culture solution containing mammalian cells (direct contact) for 24 hours at 37.4 °C (human body temperature).

The choice of cell types depends on desired application of a given biomaterial. For example, if the material under investigation is to be used as bone analogue material, then human osteoblast (HOB) cell lines are to be used. Nevertheless, as per ISO guidelines, fibroblast cells, which are normally contained in living connective tissue, are to be used for primary assessment of cell adhesion. This is because of the fact that these cells can easily proliferate on material surfaces and also they come in contact at wound/injured area (e.g., implant zone) at the initial stage. Another parameter for cell culture testing is the time of culture. Usually, the tests are widely reported to be carried out for 24 hours; however, slowly growing cells, like HOB, need to be cultured for three to seven days. In order to quantify the number of attached cells or to study cell–material or cell–cell interactions using light/electron microscopy, the cells were fixed in glutaraldehyde/formaldehyde. Before fixing, these are washed twice in PBS (Phosphate buffer saline) to completely remove the culture medium. The formaldehyde solution is (4%) diluted in PBS and it is kept for 20 minutes. Finally, the samples are stored in PBS at 4 °C. Afterward, the samples will be dried in a critical point dryer using liquid CO_2.

MTT assay is a standard colorimetric assay (an assay which measures changes in color) to quantify cellular proliferation (cell growth). It is used to determine cytotoxicity of potential medicinal agents and other toxic materials. Yellow MTT (3-(4,5-Dimethylthiazol-2-yl)-2,5 diphenyltetrazolium bromide, a tetrazole) is reduced to purple formazan in the mitochondria of living cells. A solubilization solution (usually either dimethyl sulfoxide or a solution of the detergent sodium dodecyl sulfate in dilute hydrochloric acid) is added to dissolve the insoluble purple formazan product into a colored solution. The absorbance of this colored solution can be quantified by measuring at a certain wavelength (usually between 500 and 600 nm) by a spectrophotometer. This reduction takes place only when mitochondrial reductase enzymes are active, and therefore, conversion is directly related to the number of viable (living) cells.

- **Genotoxicity:** In this *in vitro* experiment, it is primarily observed whether any genetic mutation occurs in the cells in direct contact with the biomaterial surface.
- **Hemocompatibility:** Hemocompatibility evaluates the material's compatibility with red blood cells. In particular, thrombogenic property or changes in RBC content in a blood stream flowing over the biomaterials are assessed and a better thrombus material should ideally show limited thrombus formation. Such evaluation is a must for cardiovascular implant materials. The examples of hemocompatibile materials are PolyTetra Flouro Ethylene (PTFE), Diamond Like Carbon (DLC), and so on.

1.5.2 *In Vivo* Tests

The different *in vivo* tests include:

- **Sensitization:** This is an *in vivo* test, where materials are kept in the subcutaneous region of an animal and the observations are the change in skin color, allergic effect, or some other irritations.
- **Implantation:** Implantation is an *in vivo* experiment, where a sample of a predefined shape is placed in the long bone of a mammal (rabbit, rat and mouse). After a specified time frame, the samples and surrounding tissues are examined histopathologically to determine the *in vivo* response of the materials. In general, short term implantation tests are conducted for up to 12 weeks and long term tests for up to 78 weeks. Since the animals are sacrificed, the number of animals is limited to a minimum number from an animal welfare point of view.
- **Carcinogenicity:** Carcinogenicity is a long term *in vivo* experiment, which determines any cancerous effect on the cells in contact with materials. The examples of carcinogenic materials are Pb, Sn, and so on.

ISO-10993 draft categorizes the devices by the nature of their contact with the body:

a) Surface-containing devices, such as electrodes, compression bandages, contact lenses, urinary catheters, and so on.
b) External communicating devices, such as dental cements, arthroscopes, intravascular catheters, dialysis tubing, and so on.
c) Implant devices, such as hip and knee prosthesis, pacemakers, artificial tendons, heart valves, and so on.

Furthermore, ISO-10993 document groups the implants according to the duration of their interaction with the body [limited exposure (<24h), prolonged exposure (>24h and <30 days) or permanent contact (>30 days)]. The interaction duration and contact type between the device and tissues affect the selection of the test to asses the device compatibility.

Sufficient knowledge about the biodegradation[11] of biomaterials is essential in the evaluation of local or systemic effects, which can be caused in patients. For example, the corrosion of orthopedic alloys causes the release of various metal elements in human tissue and has to be assessed with respect to levels, kinetics, and chemical state of the ions. Currently, there are no standard practices, methods or guideline for the evaluation of corrosion of orthopedic alloys, and of the products formed from corrosion. Other important tests for load-bearing implants include friction and wear tests. Besides evaluation of frictional and wear resistance properties, the wear debris particles need to be analyzed in terms of size/ size distribution and chemistry. This analysis is critical as far as asceptic loosening or osteolysis is concerned. In addition, *in vitro* dissolution tests assess the weight change or deposition of any mineralized phase (such as CaP-rich) on the surface of biomaterial. In the absence of prescribed ISO guidelines, all the above mentioned tests are carried out in simulated body fluid solution, such as Ringer's solution or Hank's balanced salt solution (HBSS). Depending on the intended use of biomaterials, different proteins such as bovine serum albumin (BSA) or other serum proteins are added to SBF. During corrosion/wear/*in vitro* dissolution tests, the pH of 7.4 and temperature of 37 °C are closely maintained during the entire test duration. In case of tests with dental restorative material, such as glass-ceramics, *in vitro* dissolution tests are carried out in artificial saliva.

1.6 STEPS FOR CHARACTERIZATIONS OF BIOMATERIALS

In order to evaluate the cell/tissue interactions for biomaterials, certain specific experiments have to be followed. These include:

a) The first step is the material development and its characterization. Previous experience and literatures help in choosing the appropriate system to evaluate a material for a specific application.

b) After evaluating the physical properties and some other necessary tests, the material goes to microbiology section, where the material is sterilized by ethanol or gamma ray or some other techniques. Depending on the desired biomedical application of the materials under investigation, it goes to thrombosis lab and tissue culture lab, to evaluate the *in vitro* properties of materials. In thrombosis lab, materials are tested in contact with blood. The tests are platelet count, platelet adhesion, hematology, coagulation test, and immunology. In tissue culture lab, the interaction of cells as well as different tissues with materials is observed. The tests are cell proliferation and cell adhesion and *in vitro* toxicity. Depending on end use, a specific property of a material is evaluated. For orthopedic implant applications, cell adhesion is mostly desirable, but cell adhesion assessment is not desirable for heart valve materials. For the latter, the desirable property is thromboresistance.

c) Subsequently, material goes to the *in vivo* toxicity lab. Here, materials extract is injected into animal bodies or material is placed in the animal body. After a long-term observation, the animal is sacrificed and the contacting body parts of the animal are taken to the histopathology lab for further experiments

d) In the histopathology lab, animal tissues are prepared for microscopic analysis. Special techniques are adopted to make the sample for optical, scanning and transmission electron microscopy.

e) There are some important aspects to choose the animal for *in vivo* experiments. The animal welfare committee and ethical committee decide the number of animals and the type of animals for particular *in vivo* experiments. Some guidelines need to be followed.

f) When the material is successfully selected for a particular application, it goes to implant biology section to shape the material into final use. Rapid prototyping using CAD-CAM technology is the new technique for developing these materials.

g) The other important aspects of biocompatibility testing are clean room practice and microbiological evaluation of materials. The laboratory environment should be free from dust and microbes and totally sterilized. Distilled water maintenance plays an important role, because in every step the quality the distilled water, dictates the perfection in experiments.

1.7 BROAD OVERVIEW OF FUNDAMENTALS SECTION

In the **Fundamentals section of this book (section I)**, the topics will cover the structure and properties of calcium phosphates, mechanical properties of bones, interaction of cells with nanobiomaterials, interface tissue engineering, blood compatibility, and polymer-ceramic biocomposites. In particular, the fundamental aspect of structure, processing and properties of the natural bone as well as those related to various approaches to develop or design new biomaterials is presented in the chapters under this section. For example, the chapter by **Bikramjit Basu** and co-workers broadly discusses the various approaches to optimize the processing conditions or material composition to design biomaterials in metals, ceramics and polymeric materials for hard tissue replacement. Limited discussion is also made on biocompatible coatings. It is well known that the inorganic component of the natural cortical bone is calcium phosphate (CaP) compounds, rich with hydroxyapatite (HA) phase. In view of this, concerted research efforts were invested in understanding the structure and properties of HA and subsequently to modify or refining the structure and properties of HA to improve the physical/ biological properties. In this context, the chapter contributed by **Racquel Z. Legeros** describes, among many aspects, the fundamental crystal structure of HA and calcium-deficient apatite (CDA). The results obtained with various characterization tools in precisely describing the structure of such complex inorganic compounds are provided. Following the substitution of anion (OH^-) by F^- or Cl^-, $(CO3)^{-2}$ and similarly, incorporation of Sr, Ba, Pb to substitute (Ca^{+2}) cation are discussed along with their implication on structure and properties in reference of stoichiometic HA.

The aspect of synthesis of various types of biologic apatites, including ACP, DCPDTCP, OCP, TTCP is mentioned briefly along with the existing/potential biomedical applications of CaP-compounds. The chapter by **Guy Daculsi** describes the processing strategies to develop micro- and macro-porous biphasic calcium phosphate (BCP) bioceramics (an optimum balance between the more stable HA phase and more soluble TCP) for better osteogenicity and osteoinductive properties. The clinical applications requiring better control of biomaterial resorption and bone substitution are highlighted along with the existing commercial use of BCP blocks/particulates/designed matrices with bone marrow or mesenchymal stem cells for tissue engineering (hybrid bone). Overall musculoskeletal joint motion depends largely on the synchronized interactions and integration between bone and soft tissues such as ligaments, tendons or cartilage. Therefore an important consideration in the current functional tissue engineering effort is how to achieve tissue–to–tissue integration and as a consequence, the focus in the field of tissue engineering has shifted from tissue formation to tissue function, in particular on regenerating the anatomic interface between various soft tissues and bone.

In the context of interfacial tissue engineering, the chapter by **Helen H. Lu** discusses the following aspects: design considerations in interface tissue engineering and recent research results using the anterior cruciate ligament–to–bone interface model system. It is posited that functional integration of soft tissue grafts can be achieved through the regeneration of the characteristic fibrocartilage interface found between soft tissue and bone. Some model scaffold systems based on biodegradable polymers and calcium phosphate composites for tendon–to–bone integration have been discussed, along with a discussion of the potential mechanism for *ex vivo* development and *in vivo* translation of integrated musculoskeletal tissues with biomimetic complexity and functionality.

The chapter by **Yoshiki Oshida** presents how better osseointegration property in Titanium-based new dental implants can be achieved by introducing functionality. The aspects of biological, mechanical and morphological compatibilities at the ti-implant/hard tissue interface have been utilized and described along with the related processing strategies. Since the last decade, nanotechnology offers exciting alternatives to traditional implants since human tissues are composed of constituent nanostructured entities. The cross-fertilisation of ideas drawn from nanotechnology and bone-tissue engineering offers the opportunity to closely biomimi the cortical bone properties, in terms of the combination of the structure–property–biological performance correlationship.

In this context, the chapter contributed by **T. J. Webster** focuses on the contemporary development of nanomaterials for orthopedic applications. After briefly reviewing the existing problems with the existing orthopedic implants (osteolysis, fractures etc.), the results obtained with synthesized novel nanophase composites (that is, materials with dimensions less than 100 nm in at least one direction) of metals, ceramics, biodegradable polymers, injectable hydrogels are presented. It is demonstrated that the increased regeneration of bone, cartilage, vascular, and bladder tissue *in vivo* is achievable on nanophase compared to conventional materials.

REFERENCES

1. B. D. Ratner, A. S. Hoffman, F. J. Schoen and J. E. Lemons, Biomaterials Science-An Introduction to Materials in Medicine, 2nd edition, pp.526, Academic Press, New York, 2004.

2. Joon B. Park, Joseph D. Bronzino, Biomaterials: Principles and Applications, CRC press, New York, 2003.

3. L. L. Hench, J. Wilson, An Introduction to Bioceramics, Vol. 1, World Scientific, 1993.

4. C. Piconi and G. Maccauro, "Zirconia as a ceramic biomaterial," Biomaterials, **20** [1] 1–25 (1999).

5. L. L. Hench, "Bioceramics," J. Am. Ceram. Soc., **81** [7] 1705–1728 (1998).

6. D. F. Williams, Consensus and definitions in biomaterials: Advances in Biomaterials, Elsevier Publishers, Amsterdam, The Netherlands, 1988.

7. M. S. Valiathan, and V. K. Krishnan, "Biomaterial: An Overview", Nation. Med. J. Ind., **12** [6] 270–74 (1999).

8. D. F. Williams, Definitions in Biomaterials, Progress in Biomedical Engineering, Elsevier Publishers, Amsterdam, The Netherlands, 1987.

9. C. P. Sharma, "Biomaterials and Artificial Organs–Current Status," Biomaterials, Biomedical Technology & Quality System, Published by IIPC, SCTIMST, 2004.

10. F. H. Silver, and D. L. Christiansen, Biomaterials Science and Biocompatibility, Springer publication, London, UK, 1999.

11. M. F. Harman, A. Naji and P. Gonfrier, "*In vitro* Study of Biomaterials Biodegradation using Human Cell Cultures," Clini. Mater., **15** 281–85 (1994).

2

FUNDAMENTALS OF HYDROXYAPATITE AND RELATED CALCIUM PHOSPHATES

[1]Racquel Zapanta LeGeros, [2]Atsuo Ito, [3]Kunio Ishikawa, [4]Toshiro Sakae, and [1]John P. LeGeros

[1]*Calcium Phosphate Research Laboratory, Department of Biomaterials & Biomimetics New York University College of Dentistry, New York, New York, USA*
[2]*National Institute of Advanced Industrial Science and Technology, Tsukuba, Japan*
[3]*Faculty of Dental Sciences, Kyushu University, Fukuoka, Japan*
[4]*Nihon University School of Dentistry, Matsudo, Japan*

Contents

2.1 Overview 20
2.2 Introduction 20
2.3 Fundamentals of Hydroxyapatite 23
    2.3.1 Structure and Properties of Hydroxyapatite, HA and Calcium-Deficient Apatite, CDA 23
    2.3.2 Substitutions in the Apatite Structure 25
        2.3.2.1 Fluoride or Chloride Incorporation 25
        2.3.2.2 Carbonate Incorporation 27
        2.3.2.3 Simultaneous Incorporation of Carbonate and Fluoride 33
        2.3.2.4 Incorporation of Cations Substituting for Calcium Ions 34
        2.3.2.5 Incorporation of Anions Substituting for the Phosphate Ions 34

Advanced Biomaterials: Fundamentals, Processing, and Applications, Edited by Bikramjit Basu, Dhirendra S. Katti, and Ashok Kumar
Copyright © 2009 The American Ceramic Society

2.4 Related Calcium Phosphates   35
    2.4.1 Amorphous Calcium Phosphates (ACP)   35
    2.4.2 Dicalcium Phosphate Dihydrate (DCPD)   36
    2.4.3 Octacalcium Phosphate (OCP)   38
    2.4.4 Tricalciumphosphate (α-TCP, β-TCP)   38
    2.4.5 Tetracalcium Phosphates (TTCP)   39
2.5 Biologic Apatites and Related Calcium Phosphates   39
2.6 Calcium Phosphate-Based Biomaterials   40
    Acknowledgments   45
    References   46

2.1 OVERVIEW

Several types of calcium phosphates occur in nature and in biologic systems. These apatites or tricalcium phosphates incorporate different ions. In biologic systems, besides the carbonate apatite which comprise the mineral phase of the calcified tissues (enamel, dentin, cementum, bone), there are other calcium phosphates (amorphous calcium phosphate, dicalcium phosphate, octacalcium phosphate and magnesium-substituted tricalcium phosphates.) Calcium phosphates of synthetic or biologic origin are used as bone graft materials or as coatings on orthopedic and dental implants.

A brief review of the physico-chemical properties of hydroxyapatite and related calcium phosphates and their medical and dental applications are presented in this chapter.

2.2 INTRODUCTION

Calcium phosphates occur in biologic systems (Table 2.1) and in nature (Table 2.2). Apatites (specially, substituted apatites) are the most commonly occurring calcium phosphate compounds. For example, most of the mineral apatites incorporate fluoride (F-apatite), chloride (Cl-apatite), carbonate (dahllite) or fluoride and carbonate (staffellite), with few occurrences of unsubstituted calcium hydroxyapatite, HA (Table 2.2). The mineral phase of calcified human tissues (for example, enamel, dentin, cementum, bone), previously idealized as calcium hydroxyapatite, HA or fluor-apatite [5,19,50] is associated with minor constituents such as magnesium, sodium, and carbonate, and has been determined as a carbonate-substituted apatite, CHA [57,59,64,107]. The mineral phases of some fish enameloids and special shells are CHA or carbonate and F-substituted apatite (CFA) [72,86].

Mixtures of CHA and other calcium phosphates occur in pathologic calcifications, for example, kidney or urinary stones, dental calculus, vascular calcifications and other soft-tissue calcifications (lung, skin, joints), calcified deposits found in heart valves prostheses, and so on. [64,112]. CHA and other calcium phosphates also occur in diseased states (for example, tooth enamel or dentin caries) [63,97].

TABLE 2.1. Calcium Phosphates in Biologic Systems

Calcium phosphate	Chemical formula	Occurrence
Carbonate apatite, Carbonate-F-apatite	$(Ca,Z)_{10}(PO_4,Y)_6(OH,Z)_2$	enamel, dentin, bone, fish enameloids, special shells, pathologic calcifications (dental calculus, urinary stone, sof-tissue calcifications), fossil teeth & bones, calcification on heart valve prostheses
Octacalcium phosphate, OCP	$Ca_8H_2(PO_4)_6.5H_2O$	pathologic calcifications (dental calculus urinary stones)
Brushite, dicalcium phosphate dihydrate, DCPD	$CaHPO_4.2H_2O$	pathologic calcifications:dental calculus, chondrocalcinosis, crystalalluria; human enamel and dentin caries
Whitlockite, Mg-substituted beta tricalcium phosphate, β-TCMP	$(Ca,Mg)_3(PO_4)_2$	pathologic calcifications: dental calculus urinary stones, arthritic cartilage, soft tissue calcifications; arrested dentin caries.
Amorphous calcium phosphate, ACP	$(Ca,Mg)_x(PO_4,Y')_y$	soft tissue calcification (skin, joint) associated with uremia
Calcium pyrophosphate Dehydrate, CPPD	$Ca_2P_2O_7.2H_2O$	pseudo-gout deposits in synovium fluid

Z = Na, Mg, K, Sr, etc; Y = CO3, HPO4; X = Cl, F; Y′ = P2O7, CO3. [57,63,64,68,72,86,89,90,97,112]

Calcium phosphates occurring in biologic systems (Table 2.1) include: carbonate apatite (CHA), amorphous calcium phosphate (ACP), dicalcium phosphate dihydrate (DCPD), dicalcium phosphate anhydrous (DCPA), octacalcium phosphate (OCP), magnesium-substituted tricalcium phosphate (β-TCMP), and calcium pyrophosphate dihydrate (CPPD) [13,64,112]. Other non-phosphatic compounds that also occur in urinary stones with or without calcium phosphates include calcium oxalates, struvite (magnesium ammonium phosphate) or uric acid.

Synthetic apatites and biologically relevant calcium phosphates (for example, ACP, DCPD, OCP, β-TCP) have been extensively studied in the early 1950s and 1960s to gain insights into:

(a) the formation of the bone mineral;

(b) demineralization-remineralization of tooth mineral (enamel or dentin) associated with dental caries;

(c) ways of preventing formation of different types of calcium phosphates associated with pathologic calcifications (for example, dental calculus, urinary stones, soft tissue calcifications (heart, lung, joint, skin), or calcification of prostheses (for example, heart valve prosthesis).

TABLE 2.2. Lattice Parameters of Mineral, Synthetic and Biologic Apatites

Apatite	Substituent	Lattice parameters (± 0.003Å)	
		a-axis	c-axis
Mineral			
OH-Apatite (Holly Springs)	—	9.422	6.880
F-Apatite (Durango, Mex)	F-for-OH	9.375	6.880
Dahllite (Wyoming)	CO_3-for-PO_4	9.380	6.889
Staffelite (Staffel, Germany)	CO_3-for-PO_4, F-for-OH	9.345	6.880
Marine phosphorites (USA)	CO_3-for-PO_4, F-for-OH	9.322	6.882
Synthetic (non-aqueous)[a]			
OH-apatite	—	9.422	6.882
F-apatite	F-for-OH	9.375	6.880
Cl-apatite	Cl-for-OH	9.646	6.771
CO_3-apatite	CO_3-for-OH (Type A)	9.544	6.859
Synthetic (aqueous[b])			
OH-apatite	—	9.438	6.882
OH-apatite	HPO_4-for-PO_4	9.462	6.879
F-apatite	F-for-OH	9.382	6.880
(Cl,OH)-apatite	Cl-for-OH	9.515	6.858
CO_3-apatite	CO_3-for-PO_4 (Type B)	9.298	6.924
CO_3-F-apatite	CO_3-for-PO_4 (Type B) and F-for-OH	9.268	6.924
Sr-apatite	Sr-for-Ca	9.739	6.913
Pb-apatite	Pb-for-Ca	9.894	7.422
Ba-apatite	Ba-for-Ca	10.162	7.722
Biologic apatite			
Human enamel	(CO_3, HPO_4)-for PO_4	9.441	6.882
Shark enameloid	CO_3-for-PO_4 (Type B) and F-for-OH	9.382	6.880

[57,64]

The first application of calcium phosphate for bone repair was reported in 1920 [1]. It was not until the early 1970s, but especially in the 1980s and 1990s, that extensive studies on apatites (particularly calcium hydroxyapatite, HA) and some calcium phosphates (especially β-TCP) have been investigated for their potential use as bone substitute materials [2,18,46]. Commercial calcium phosphate products used for bone repair, augmentation or as scaffolds for tissue engineering include: apatites (HA and calcium-deficient apatites), β-TCP, biphasic calcium phosphates, BCP (intimate mixtures of HA and β-TCP) [2,12,15,18,20,46,54,62, 64,70,75]. HA is also used to deposit bioactive coatings on orthopedic and dental implants [30,82]. Experimental apatites (CHA, CFA) and other calcium phosphates (e.g., OCP, Mg- or Zn-substituted β-TCP) are investigated as possible bone graft materials, implant coatings, or therapies in bone disease such as osteo-porosis [4,39,47,49,56,71,85,95,105,111,114].

Different types of calcium phosphates (for example, α-TCP, β-TCP, ACP, tetracalcium phosphate, TTCP) are used in the preparation of calcium phosphate cements [11,74,101]; other calcium phosphates (HA, BCP, CHA) are used in polymer/calcium phosphate composites [8,43,93].

This chapter provides a brief review of hydroxyapatite (HA), substituted apatites, and related calcium phosphates, and their properties and applications as biomaterials. Particular emphasis has been made on carbonate apatites since bone and tooth mineral consists of carbonate apatite. This chapter covers a brief description of the fundamentals of hydroxyapatite (structure and properties of unsubstituted and substituted apatites) and related calcium phosphates; calcium phosphates occurring in biologic systems (normal and pathologic calcifications); and calcium phosphate based biomaterials for medical and dental applications.

2.3 FUNDAMENTALS OF HYDROXYAPATITE

2.3.1 Structure and Properties of Hydroxyapatite, HA and Calcium-Deficient Apatite, CDA

The name "Apatite" (from the Greek word, "apatit", meaning to deceive) was given to mineral apatites because they were often mistaken for precious gems like topaz, aquamarine, amethyst [17]. The name 'apatite' describes a family of compounds having similar structure (hexagonal system, with space group, $P6_3/m$) in spite of a wide range of composition. The structures of calcium hydroxyapatite (HA), $Ca_{10}(PO_4)_6(OH)_2$; calcium fluor-apatite (FA), $Ca_{10}(PO_4)_6F_2$; and calcium chlor-apatite (ClA), $Ca_{10}(PO_4)_6Cl_2$; are well established from analyses of mineral FA apatite single crystals [5] and synthetic apatite single crystals [50,124]. The similarity of the x-ray diffraction (XRD) patterns of enamel, dentin and bone to those of mineral apatites together with chemical analyses showing calcium and phosphate as principal constituents led to the conclusion as early as 1926 that the inorganic phases of bones and teeth are basically a calcium hydroxyapatite, HA, idealized as $Ca_{10}(PO_4)_6(OH)_2$ [19]. Association of carbonate in biologic apatite led to speculation of the similarity between bone mineral and mineral carbonate-containing apatites (that is, dahllite) [98], Combined studies on mineral, biologic and synthetic apatites provided experimental evidence that established that bio-logic apatites are carbonate apatites [57,59,107].

Crystallographically, HA and FA belong to the hexagonal system while ClA belongs to the monoclinic system. The apatite hexagonal system, space group $P6_3/m$, is characterized by a six-fold a-axis perpendicular to three equivalent a-axes (a1, a2, a3) at angles 120° to each other. The unit cell, the smallest building unit containing a complete representation of the apatite crystal, contains ten cal-cium (Ca), six phosphate (PO_4) and two hydroxyl (OH) groups closely packed together in an arrangement shown in Figure 2.1 [124]. The ten calcium atoms are

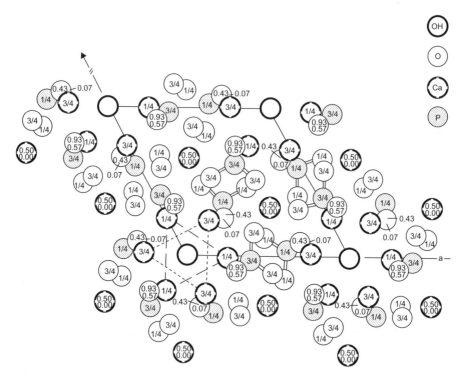

<u>Figure 2.1.</u> The arrangement of the atoms of calcium hydroxyapatite, $Ca_{10}(PO_4)_6(OH)_2$, in a hexagonal unit cell. The OH ions located in the corners of the unit-cell are surrounded by two sets of Ca(II) atoms arranged in a triangle at appositions z = 1/4 and ¾, by two sets of PO_4 tetrahedra also in triangular positions; and by hexagonal array of Ca(I) atoms at the outermost distance [124].

defined as Ca(I) or Ca (II) depending on their environment. Four Ca atoms occupy the Ca (I) positions at levels z = 0 and two at z = ½ (0.5). Six Ca atoms occupy the Ca(II) positions one set of three Ca atoms located at z = ¼ (0.25), the other set of three at z = ¾ (0.75), surrounding the OH groups located at the corners of the unit cell. The six tetrahedral PO_4 groups are arranged in sets of three at levels z = 0.25 and at z = .75. The network of PO_4 groups provides the skeletal framework of the apatite and gives great stability to the apatite structure.

Calcium-deficient apatite (CDA) is obtained by precipitation or hydrolysis methods at temperatures 25 °C to 95 °C [34,57,64,102]. CDA differs from stoichiometric hydroxyapatite (HA) in several properties. Compared to HA, CDA has:

(a) a lower Ca/P molar ratio (ranging from 1.4 to 1.66 for CDA, 1.67 for HA);

(b) lower crystallinity (reflected by lower diffraction intensities and broader diffraction peaks;

(c) greater *a*-axis dimension of CDA (9.438 to 9.461 A versus 9.422 A for HA), probably due to the incorporation of HPO_4 (partial HPO_4-for-PO_4 substitution) [64, Table 2.2];

(d) appearance of IR absorption band at about 864 cm^{-1} (attributed to P-O-H vibration band of the HPO_4 group) and broad band at 3400 to 3600 (attributed to the H-O-H vibration band of adsorbed H_2O).

In addition, heating or sintering CDA above 800 °C results in the transformation of CDA to β-TCP or mixtures of HA and β-TCP (with differing HA/β-TCP ratios), depending on the Ca/P of the CDA before sintering and on the sintering temperature, 900 to 1100 °C [57,64,84].

2.3.2   Substitutions in the Apatite Structure

The apatite structure, $Ca_{10}(PO_4)_6(OH)_2$, is a very hospitable one allowing the substitutions of many other ions for the Ca^{2+}, PO_4^{3-}, or OH^- groups. Such substitutions cause changes in the crystallographic, physical and chemical properties of apatites: for example, lattice parameters (*a*- and/or *c*-axis dimensions), spectral properties, color, morphology (crystal size and shape), solubility and thermal stability. The extent of the change is proportional to the amount and size of the substituting ion (Table 2.2). Substitution in the apatite also affects the *in vitro* cell response [29,36,122,123].

Studies on properties of unsubstituted and substituted apatites have been based on apatites prepared by precipitation, hydrolysis of other calcium phosphates (for example, DCPD, DCPA, OCP, α-TCP), hydrothermal reactions or by solid state reactions at high temperatures [3,7, 9,21,22,27,31,32,41,57,58,60,64,71, 73,76–81,83,87,89.91,92,103,106–109,115–118,121,126].

Stoichiometric HA (Ca/P ratio = 1.67) is obtained by solid state reactions. Biologic apatites and synthetic apatites obtained by precipitation or hydrolysis (for example, DCPD or DCPA in NaOH solution) methods are usually calcium deficient (Ca/P ratio <1.67). Single crystals of HA can be obtained by hydrothermal reactions [3].

2.3.2.1   Fluoride or Chloride Incorporation.   Substitution of F-for-OH or Cl-for-OH does not significantly change the atomic arrangements in the apatite structure. However, while F-substitution does not change the hexagonal symmetry of the apatite, Cl-substitution results in changing the symmetry from hexagonal to monoclinic symmetry because of the much larger Cl atom substituting for the OH group, affecting the relative position of the Cl with respect to the Ca triangle, as shown in Figure 2.2 [124]. F-for-OH (F ionic radius < OH) substitution causes a contraction in the *a*-axis dimension with no significant change in the *c*-axis while Cl-for-OH substitution causes expansion in both *a*- and *c*-axis dimensions compared to F- or Cl-free apatites (Table 2.2 and Table 2.3).

Full or partial F-for-OH substitution in synthetic apatites depends on the F concentration in the solution [57,59,72]. Incorporation of F in synthetic or

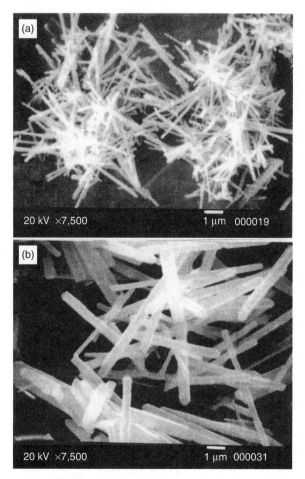

Figure 2.2. Effect of incorporation of fluoride (F⁻) ions on crystal size of apatite: causes larger and thicker apatite crystals [59,64].

biologic apatite causes growth of larger and thicker apatite crystals as shown in Figure 2.2 [59,64,79] and are less soluble than the F-free apatites [45,59,64,100].

Full or partial Cl-for-OH substitution in the apatite structure depends on the method of preparation. Partial Cl-for-OH substitution, $Ca_{10}(PO_4)_6(OH,Cl)_2$, is obtained from aqueous systems at low temperatures (37 °C to 95 °C [58,64,109] while full substitution, $Ca_{10}(PO_4)_6Cl_2$, can only be obtained from non-aqueous systems at temperatures 1000 °C or above [22,64]. The forming apatite from solution highly discriminates against the incorporation of the Cl ions. This explains why biologic apatite contains very low Cl concentration in spite of the high Cl concentration in the biologic fluid.

Thermal stability of apatites decreases in the order: FA > HA > ClA [124] while solubility decreases in the following order: ClA > HA > FA [52].

TABLE 2.3. Comparative data on F-apatite, OH-apatite and Cl-apatite

	F-Ap	OH-Ap	Cl-Ap
Ionic radius (A)	F = 1.36	OH = 1.53	Cl = 1.81
Ca-F, -OH, -Cl distance (A)	2.29	2.89	2.80
Unit cell volume (A^3)	523	530	545
Lattice parameters (±0.003A)			
a-axis	9.375	9.422	9.647
c-axis	6.880	6.882	6.771

[124]

2.3.2.2 Carbonate Incorporation. Early studies on carbonate-containing apatite were prompted by the need to understand the nature of carbonate incorporation in biologic apatite (particularly bone and tooth mineral). Such studies demonstrated that carbonate $(CO_3)^{2-}$ can substitute in the apatite structure either for the $(OH)^-$ or the $(PO_4)^{3-}$ group, referred to as Type A or Type B substitution, respectively [7]. The first synthetic carbonate-substituted apatite with Type A substitution prepared at high temperatures (1000 °C) was first reported by Elliott [21] and Bonel [7]. Apatite with Type B carbonate substitution prepared at low temperatures (25 °C to 95 °C) was first reported by LeGeros [57,87,126] and was demonstrated to be more similar to the carbonate substitution in biologic apatite [57,59,83]. The type of substitution depends on the method of preparation of the carbonate apatite. Type B substitution (CO_3-for-PO_4) is obtained when prepared from solution (either by precipitation or hydrolysis method at 25 °C to 95 °C [57,81,87,126], or by hydrothermal reactions at 200 °C and 200 psi [41,57,117,118,121]. When prepared at high temperature (1000 °C), Type A substitution (CO_3-for-OH) is obtained [7,21]. Simultaneous Type A and Type B carbonate substitutions have also been reported when prepared by hydrothermal conversion of flux growth (Table 2.4) [24–26,115,116,118,121]. In the presence of Na^+ ions in solution, a coupled substitution Na-for-Ca and CO_3-for-PO_4 occurs [26,57,59,64,126]. For this report, apatite with CO_3-for-PO_4 substitution (Type B) will be referred to as CHA; with CO_3-for-OH (Type A) substitution, as CA.

The two types of substitution have opposite effects on the lattice parameters. Type A substitution, in which larger planar CO_3 group substitutes for OH group, causes an expansion in the a-axis and contraction in the c-axis dimensions. Type B substitution in which a smaller planar CO_3 group substitutes for the larger tetrahedral PO_4 group causes a contraction in the a-axis and expansion in the c-axis dimensions (Figure 2.3). CO_3-apatite prepared by hydrothermal reactions appear to allow simultaneous CO_3-for-OH and CO_3-for-PO_4 substitution, as evidenced by the larger a-axis for similar amount of CO_3 incorporation compared to the a-axis dimension of CHA. Changes in infrared (IR) spectral characteristics are specific for the two types of CO_3 substitution (Figure 2.4) [22,83].

In terms of amount of CO_3 substitution, Type A substitution allows for the complete substitution of OH (1 mole CO_3 for 1 mole OH), while Type B

TABLE 2.4. Hydrothermal and Flux Growth of Carbonate Apatite

Starting Material	Method*	Temp. (°C)	Pressure (MPa)	Product	Ref.
DCPA-H_2O-CO_2	h	180–290	—	$Ca_{9.64}H_{0.35}(PO_4)_6[(CO_3)_{0.14}(OH)_{1.36}(H_2O)_{0.35}$	[41]
$CaCO_3$-$(NH_4)_2HPO_4$-H_2O	h, f	250–900	13–137	CO_3 replacing OH and PO_4	[110]
αTCP-$(NH_4)_2CO_3$-H_2O	h	200	137	CO_3 replacing PO_4	[121]
$CaSO_4$-$(NH_4)_2CO_3$	h	200	137	CO_3 replacing PO_4	[118]
TCP-$Ca(OH)_2$-$CaCO_3$-H_2O	h	750–900	69–137	$Ca_{9.9}[(PO_4)_{5.8}(CO_3)_{0.2}](OH)_2$	[110]
$CaCO_3$-$NH_4H_2PO_4$-H_2O	h	250	100	$Ca_{9.50}(NH_4)_{0.10}(PO_4)_{5.05}(CO_3)_{0.95}(OH)_2$	[44]
TCP-$CaCO_3$	f	1400	55	$Ca_{9.8}[(PO_4)_{5.6}(CO_3)_{0.4}]CO_3$	[116]
DCPD-$Ca(OH)_2$-$CaCO_3$-Na_2CO_3	f	1200	1000	$Ca_{9.13}Na_{0.87}[(PO_4)_{5.05}(CO_3)_{0.95}][(CO_3)_{0.86}OH_{0.28}$	[26]
$Ca_2P_2O_7$-CaO-$CaCO_3$	f	1400	2000	$Ca_{10}(PO_4)_6[(CO_3)_{0.75}OH_{0.5}]$	[25]

*h: hydrothermal method, f: flux method.

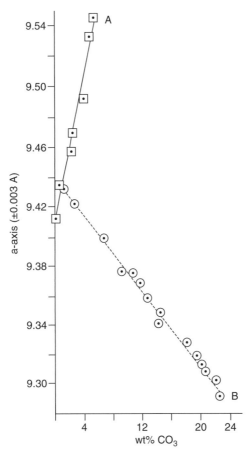

Figure 2.3. Effect of two types of substitution on the *a*-axis dimensions of synthetic carbonate apatites. Type A (CO_3-for-OH) causes an expansion and Type B (CO_3-for-PO_4), a contraction of the *a*-axis dimension compared to carbonate-free apatites [7,21,57,59,64,81,126].

substitution allows only partial substitution (maximum of 3 moles CO_3 for 3 moles PO_4) [57,57,64,126]. In addition to the effects on lattice parameters, substitution of CO_3 (Type B) in the apatite structure causes changes in morphology, in crystallite size (Figure 2.5A) and in dissolution properties [57,64,73,81,92]. In synthetic apatites prepared at 60 °C to 95 °C′ morphological changes were observed: from needle-like or acicular crystals to rod-shaped to equi-axed crystals, depending on the amount of carbonate incorporated in the apatite (Figure 2.5B) [64,81,92]. When prepared at 37 °C, increasing the amount of carbonate incorporation decreases crystallite size (reflected in the broadening of the diffraction peaks) and eventually promotes the formation of ACP (Figure 2.6).

Crystal size of carbonate apatite also depends on the preparation method and temperature of preparation: nano-crystals of CHA, similar to bone apatite [Figures 2.7A and 2.7B], are obtained by precipitation method at 25 °C or 37 °C;

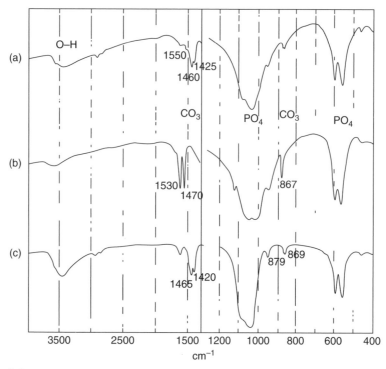

Figure 2.4. IR spectra of synthetic carbonate apatite, Type B (C) and Type A (B) compared to that of biologic apatite, enamel apatite (C). The spectra of Type B carbonate apatite, CO_3-for-PO_4 coupled with Na-for-Ca (A) is more similar to that of biologic apatite (C) [21,57,59,64,83].

larger crystals (similar to tooth enamel apatite) are obtained by precipitation or hydrolysis method at 80 to 95 °C [57,59,64]. Larger size crystals are obtained by hydrothermal reactions (Figure 2.5) [41]. Single crystals of carbonate apatite with one or both type of CO_3 substitution are obtained from high pressure solution growth methods, typically, hydrothermal and flux methods (Table 2.4).

Solubility of the apatite increases as the amount of carbonate in the apatite increases regardless of the type of substitution: Type A [40] or Type B [73]. Incorporation of one CO_3^{2-} per unit cell in hydroxyapatite by the CO_3-for-OH substitution increased the solubility product by $10^{15.9}$ [40].

X-ray structure analysis using flux-grown carbonate apatite single crystals revealed that planar CO_3 in CO_3-for-PO_4 substitution are located close to the sloping oxygen triangle consisting of the O(1), O(2) and O(3) of the PO_4 group in hydroxyapatite [25,26] confirming earlier inferences from polarized IR study [22]. The sloping angle that is defined by the angle between the normal to the CO_3 plane and the c-axis varied depending on the Na-substitution of adjacent Ca site. Planar CO_3 groups in CO_3-for-OH substitution are located at the height nearly the same as that of Ca (I) ($z = 0, 1/2$) or hydroxyapatite with the CO_3 plane being parallel [115] or nearly parallel (canting less than 12 °) to the c-axis [Ito-16,17].

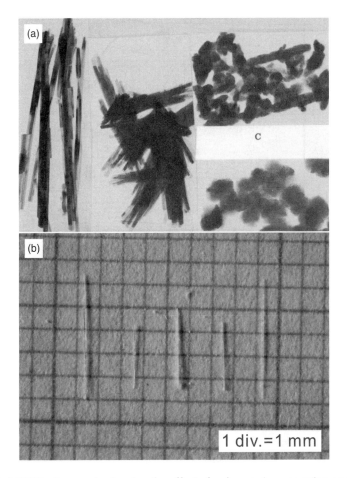

Figure 2.5. (a) TEM micrographs showing the effect of carbonate incorporation on the crystal size and morphology of apatite. Apatites prepared by hydrolysis method containing (in wt % CO_3): 0.5 (A) 2.5 (B) 12.5 (C) and 17.2 (D) [81,82]. (b) Single crystals of carbonate apatite crystals obtained by hydrothermal reaction [41].

However, lateral position and direction of the CO_3 triangle are three-differently reported:

(i)   the C atom and one of the three O atoms are located on the c-axis, thus bisector of CO_3 plane coincides with the c-axis [115];

(ii) the two of the three 0 atoms are located near the c-axis, thus bisector of CO_3 triangle is nearly normal to the c-axis [Ito 15–17];

(iii) bisector of CO_3 triangle is nearly parallel to the c-axis but the CO_3 triangle rotated about the horizontal axis so that the apical oxygen atom is displaced slightly off the c-axis [24].

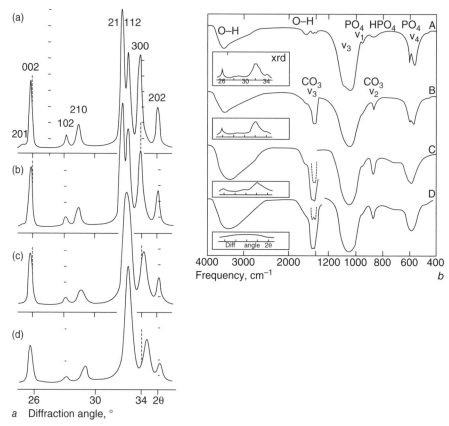

Figure 2.6. X-ray diffraction profiles of apatites prepared at 95 °C (6a) and 37 °C (6b) with increasing ion concentrations in solution and in the apatite. With apatites prepared at 95 °C (a), increasing carbonate, broadening of x-ray diffraction peaks indicate decrease in crystallite size and shift in diffraction peaks indicate changes in lattice parameters caused by CO_3 incorporation in the apatite. At 37 °C, high carbonate concentration promotes the formation of carbonate containing amorphous calcium phosphate, ACP, shown by the absence of diffraction peaks and lack of resolution in the phosphate band (6bD) [55,59,87,126].

The type (i) and (ii) carbonate configuration are associated with the conventional type A infrared carbonate absorption bands at 1451 and 1540 cm^{-1}, while the type (iii) configuration is associated with carbonate absorption bands at 1506 and 1571 cm^{-1} (Figure 2.4) [22,24,57,83]. The type (iii) configuration is a high-pressure feature. On the other hand, Rietvelt X-ray structure analysis using hydrothermally synthetic carbonate apatite powders indicated that CO_3 planes are parallel to the c-axis in CO_3-for-PO_4 substitution [44].

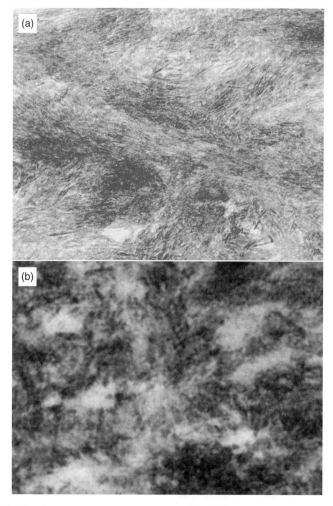

Figure 2.7. TEM micrographs of cow bone apatite (7A) compared to carbonate apatite precipitated at 37 °C (7B).

2.3.2.3 Simultaneous Incorporation of Carbonate and Fluoride. Mineral (staffellite, marine phosphorites), and biologic apatites (from fossil bones and teeth, some fish enameloids and special shells contain both F^- and CO_3^{2-} ions [17,57,59,72,86]. Simultaneous incorporation of carbonate (CO_3-for-PO_4) and fluoride (F-for-OH) in synthetic apatites is obtained by precipitation or hydrolysis methods [64]. The contributions of these ions to the lattice parameters and dissolution property of F-and CO_3-containing apatite (CFA) are additive. Thus, the a-axis of CFA is much shorter than that of CHA since the incorporation of either CO_3^{2-} and F^- ions causes contraction of the a-axis and CFA is less soluble than CHA because of the stabilizing effect of F^- ions but more soluble than FA because of the de-stabilizing effect of CO_3^{2-} in CFA [73]. In addition the crystallite size of CFA (from precipitation or hydrolysis preparation) is larger than that of CHA but smaller than that of FA since CO_3 incorporation causes the growth of smaller apatite crystals while F incorporation causes the growth of larger crystals.

Indirect methods of preparing CFA are by suspension of CHA in F-containing solutions and heating the F-treated CHA at 700 °C [114]; treatment of bovine bone in F-solutions and heating at temperatures 600 °C or above [28], hydrolysis of calcium carbonate, $CaCO_3$. (calcite or aragonite forms) in F-containing solutions, hydrolysis of CaF_2 in CO_3-containing solutions, hydrolysis of non-apatitic calcium phosphates (e.g., DCPD, DCPA, OCP, α-TCP, β-TCP, or calcium monophosphate, $CaH_4(PO_4)_2.H_2O$) in solutions containing both F and CO_3 ions [64,78]. In these cases, the efficacy of conversion of the calcium phosphate, calcium carbonate or calcium fluoride depends on reaction pH and temperature [78].

2.3.2.4 Incorporation of Cations Substituting for Calcium Ions.
Several cations can substitute for the calcium (Ca) ions in the apatite structure, $Ca_{10}(PO_4)_6(OH)_2$. For example, strontium (Sr), barium (Ba) and lead (Pb) can completely substitute for the Ca^{2+} ions to yield $Sr_{10}(PO_4)_6(OH)_2$, $Ba_{10}(PO_4)_6(OH)_2$ or $Pb_{10}(PO_4)_6(OH)_2$, respectively [27,57,64,80,91]. Because Sr^{2+}, Ba^{2+} and Pb^{2+} have larger ionic radii compared to Ca^{2+}, such substitutions result in expanded a- and c-axes compared to unsubstituted calcium hydroxyapatite (Table 2.2). Colors (purple, blue, green, pink, brown, etc.) of mineral or synthetic apatites are caused by incorporation of small amounts of some cations such as manganese (Mn^{2+}), copper (Cu^+, Cu^{2+}), cobalt iron (Fe, Fe) [91,125]. Limited incorporation of sodium (Na^+) ions Na-for Ca can be obtained when precipitation or hydrolysis or hydrothermal reactions are performed in the presence of Na-containing solution [26,91,125]. Because of the similarity in ionic radius between Na^+ and Ca^{2+}, no significant effect on lattice parameters are observed.

Mg, a minor but important constituent in biologic apatites, is incorporated only to a very limited extent in synthetic apatites obtained by precipitation or hydrolysis methods [57,59,60,64,77,89]. Limited amount of zinc (Zn) can be incorporated in the apatite [64,76].

Incorporation of Sr^{2+} or Mg^{2+} in apatite increases its solubility [64,80,89]. Simultaneous incorporation of Mg and CO_3 in apatite has additive effects in decreasing crystal size and increasing the extent of dissolution in acidic buffer [89,103].

2.3.2.5 Incorporation of Anions Substituting for the Phosphate Ions.
Besides the CO_3-for-PO_4 substitution discussed above, other anions can substitute for the PO_4 ions in the apatite structure. These anions include sulfate, manganate, borate, silicate, etc. [31,64,91]. Like any other substitutions in the apatite structure, these substitutions will affect the properties of the apatite.

2.4   RELATED CALCIUM PHOSPHATES

Apatites and other calcium phosphates that occur in biologic systems are listed in Table 2.1. The crystallographic properties of synthetic calcium phosphate are summarized in Table 2.5. In biologic or synthetic systems, non-apatitic calcium phosphates (e.g., ACP, DCPD, DCPA, OCP, β-TCP) can transform to apatites and substituted apatites or to other calcium phosphates by dissolution-precipitation processes as represented in Figure 2.8 [64].

Non-apatitic calcium phosphates are found in pathologic calcifications but not in normal mineralized tissues (mineral phases of teeth and bones). Non-apatitic calcium phosphates, except tricalcium phosphate (TCP) and tetracalcium phosphate (TTCP), can be prepared directly by precipitation or in gel systems (Figure 2.9) or indirectly by hydrolysis methods [64,69]. From solutions of similar Ca/P molar ratios, different types of calcium phosphates are obtained depending on the solution pH, temperature and composition [57,64]. In the presence of F$^-$ ions, apatite can form even from solutions with low pH. (e.g., pH 4 at 95 °C).

The different types of calcium phosphates are characterized by their Ca/P molar ratios (Table 2.5), their characteristic morphology and dissolution properties (Figure 2.10) [22,64,66] However, the morphology and crystal size can be affected by other ions present in solution (Figure 2.9). For example, the usual platy morphology of DCPD appears as smaller thick rods in the presence of $P_2O_7^{4-}$ ions [64,69]; OCP can assume a platy or ribbon-like morphology [61,64].

The different types of calcium phosphates also differ in their solubilities (Figure 2.10) decreasing in the order:

$$ACP > DCPD > OCP > \beta\text{-TCP} > CDA > HA.$$

2.4.1   Amorphous Calcium Phosphates (ACP)

ACP can be represented by the formula, $(Ca, X)_x(PO_4, Y)_y.H_2O$, where $X = Mg^{2+}$, Zn^{2+}, Sn^{2+} or Al^{3+} ions; $Y = CO_3^{2-}$, or $P_2O_7^{4-}$ ions [57,59,64,76,77,90,91]. Depending on the composition, the Ca/P molar ratio can range from 1.3 to 2.5. At room temperature or 37 °C, ACP can form under any of the following solution (containing Ca^{2+} and PO_4^{3-} ions) conditions: high pH (pH .10), high CO_3/P molar ratios, Mg/Ca molar ratio greater than 0.4, Zn/Ca molar ratio greater than 0.4, small concentrations of $P_2O_7^{4-}$, critical concentrations of Sn^{2+}, Al^{2+} [64,76,77,91]. ACP is characterized by absence of diffraction peaks in x-ray diffraction profiles except for a broad peak with a maximum at about 30.40° 2θ (e.g., shown in Figure 2.6). The FT-IR spectra of ACP shows lack of resolution of the PO_4 absorption bands. ACP compounds are represented by hollow spheres in transmission electron micrographs [64,90]. Ions that promote formation of ACP can act synergistically, e.g., $Mg^{2+} + CO_3^{2-}$ or $+P_2O_7^{4-}$ [64,90]. ACP incorporating other ions besides calcium and phosphate ions remain stable even after heating at 400 °C [64,90]. Stability of ACP in solution depends on the ACP composition or solution composition [64,90].

TABLE 2.5. Crystallographic Properties of Synthetic Calcium Phosphates

Calcium Phosphates	Molecular formula	Crystal habit	Space group	Ca/P molar ratio
*Monocalcium phosphate Monohydrate, MCPM	$Ca(H_2PO_4)_2.H_2O$	triclinic $a = 5.626$ A $b = 11.889$ $c = 6.4728$		0.5
Dicalcium phosphate dihydrate DCPD or brushite	$CaHPO_4.2H_2O$	monoclinic $a = 5.182$ A $b = 15.18$ $c = 6.239$ $B = 116.25°$	C2/c	1.0
*Dicalcium phosphate anhydrous Monetite	$CaHPO_4$	triclinic $a = 6.91$ A $b = 6.63$ $c = 6.99$	PI	1.0
Octacalcium phosphate, OCP	$Ca_8H_2(PO_4)_6.5H_2O$	triclinic $a = 19.87$ A $b = 9.63$ $c = 6.87$	PI	1.33
*Tricalcium phosphate, β-TCP Whitlockite	$Ca_3(PO_4)_2$	hexagonal $a = 10.428$ A $c = 37.378$	R3c	1.50
**Tricalcium phosphate, β-TCMP Mg-substituted	$(Ca,Mg)_3(PO_4)_2$	hexagonal $a = 10.32$ A $c = 37.00$	R3c	1.50
*Tetracalcium phosphate, TTCP	$Ca_4(PO_4)_2O$	monoclinic $a = 7.023$ A $b = 11.986$ $c = 9.473$	$P2_1$	2.0
*Hydroxyapatite, HA	$Ca_{10}(PO_4)_6(OH)_2$	hexagonal $a = 9.422$ A $c = 6.880$	$P6_3/m$	1.67
*Fluoroapatite, FA	$Ca_{10}(PO_4)_6(F)_2$	hexagonal $a = 9.377$ A $c = 6.880$	$P6_3/m$	1.67
*Chloroapatite, ClA	$Ca_{10}(PO_4)_6(Cl)_2$	monoclinic $a = 9.632$ A $c = 7.00$	C2/c	1.67

[22,64].*Does not occur in biologic systems. **(Ca+Mg)/P.[22,64].

2.4.2 Dicalcium Phosphate Dihydrate (DCPD)

DCPD also referred to as brushite is represented by the formula $CaHPO_4.2H_2O$. It can be prepared by precipitation at 25–60 °C at pH 4 to 6 or from gel systems (Figure 2.9) [64,69]. DCPD, but not DCPA (dicalcium phosphate anhydrous,

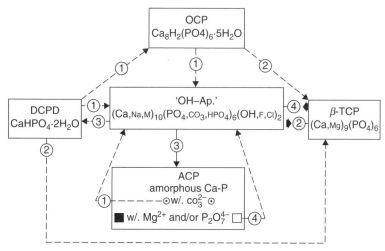

Figure 2.8. Schematic presentation of the transformation of one type of calcium phosphate to another [59,64].

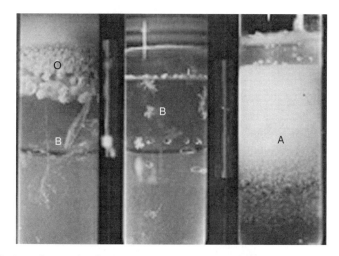

Figure 2.9. Crystal growth of calcium phosphates in gel system. (silica gel incorporating phosphate ions, calcium ions diffusing into the gel), 37 °C, solution Ca/P molar ratio, 1/1. (1) pH 6.5, OCP (O) spheres grew on the top layer and DCPD platy crystals grew on the bottom layer of the gel' (2) same pH but in the presence of $P_2O_7^{4-}$ ions, OCP growth was inhibited, DCPD crystal size reduced and change in shape observed; (3) in the presence of F^- ions, growth of OCP and DCPD were suppressed, growth of (F,OH)-apatite needle-like crystals was promoted [59,64,69].

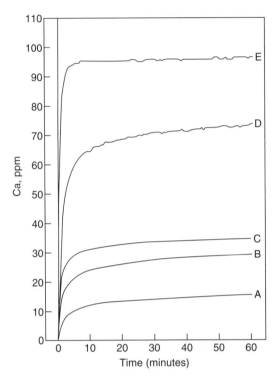

Figure 2.10. Comparative dissolution of different calcium phosphates in acidic buffer. [64]. The calcium phosphates were prepared by precipitation. (A) Mg-substituted tricalcium phosphate, β-TCMP; (B) CHA; (C) Mg-substituted CHA; (D) OCP; (E) DCPD.

CaHPO$_4$), occur in biologic systems (Table 2.1). Both DCPD and DCPA are used in the preparation of apatites (calcium deficient apatites, CDA) or substituted apatites or substituted beta-tricalcium phosphate (e.g., Mg-TCP or Zn-TCP) in the presence of the appropriate ions in solution during the hydrolysis of DCPD or DCPA.

2.4.3   Octacalcium Phosphate (OCP)

OCP is structurally similar to apatite and has been speculated to be precursors to biologic apatite [10]. OCP is formed by hydrolysis of DCPD or directly by precipitation, or in gel systems [61,64]. It can also be formed by electrochemical deposition on metallic substrate [56,94]. OCP can transform to carbonate apatite in the presence of CO_3^{2-} ions, to F-apatite in the presence of F$^-$ ions.

2.4.4   Tricalciumphosphate (α-TCP, β-TCP)

Pure beta tricalcium phosphate, β-Ca$_3$(PO$_4$)$_2$ (β-TCP), cannot be obtained from synthetic aqueous systems and it is therefore not surprising that it does not occur in biologic systems. Pure β-TCP can only be prepared by solid state reactions or by sintering calcium-deficient apatite (Ca/P molar ratio, about 1.5) at temperatures 800 °C and above.

The presence of $Mg^{2=}$ ions in solution allows the formation of biologic and synthetic Mg-substituted tricalcium phosphate (β-TCMP or Mg-TCP) [57,64,77, 113]. Other ions that allows the formation of substituted TCP from solution includes: zinc, nickel, cobalt [91]. β-TCMP can form at low or high pH (pH 5 or 9) and temperatures 25 °C to 95 °C. Larger crystals are favored at low pH [64,71].

β-TCMP or Mg-TCP heated at the same temperature as that used in the preparation of unsubstituted β-TCP is less soluble than the pure β-TCP [38,64,71].

Zn-substituted TCP (Zn-TCP) is less soluble than Zn-free TCP [42].

2.4.5 Tetracalcium Phosphates (TTCP)

TTCP is prepared by solid state reactions (e.g., $CaHPO_4$ + $CaCO_3$) at high temperatures. TTCP is very reactive and can rapidly convert to apatite in a wet atmosphere.

2.5 BIOLOGIC APATITES AND RELATED CALCIUM PHOSPHATES

Biologic apatites (mineral phases of calcified tissues), idealized as calcium hydroxyapatite, $Ca_{10}(PO_4)_6(OH)_2$ [50], are associated with minor but important components such as CO_3 and Mg and are more accurately described as carbonate apatite with Type B carbonate substitution (CO_3-for-PO_4 coupled with Na-for-Ca) [57,59,64,107]. Biologic apatites differ from synthetic ceramic HA used as bone graft materials in composition, in crystal size (Figure 2.13), in lattice parameters (Table 2.2) and in dissolution properties [6,59,64]. The larger a-axis dimension of human enamel apatite compared to pure HA was first believed to be due to the CO_3-for-OH substitution [21]. However, since it has been demonstrated that carbonate substitution in biologic apatite, like human enamel apatite, is predominantly CO_3-for-PO_4 coupled with Na-for-Ca substitution [57,59], the larger a-axis of human enamel compared to pure HA may be attributed to other types of substitution, such as HPO_4-for-PO_4, partial Cl-for-OH, or partial substitution for Ca of larger cations (e.g., Sr^{2+}) [57,59,64].

Biologic apatites differ in crystallite size (enamel $\gg$ dentin or bone) and also differ in the concentrations of Mg^{2+} and CO_3^{2-} ions (bone > dentin $\gg$ enamel) [6,57,59,64,89]. In synthetic systems, presence of Mg^{2+} or CO_3^{2-} ions causes the formation of smaller and more soluble crystals and when simultaneously, present, exert a synergistic effect on the properties of the apatite crystals [57,59,64, 73,89,92,103]. The larger size and lower solubility of enamel apatite compared to either dentin or bone apatite may be attributed to the difference in their composition [57,59,64]. Biologic apatites are usually calcium deficient (Ca/P molar ratio <1.67). Upon ignition at 700 °C and above, Mg-TCP and HA are obtained [57,59,64].

While only one type (i.e., CHA or CFA) of calcium phosphate is present in normal calcifications (enamel, dentin, cementum, bone), different types of calcium phosphates co-exist in some pathologic calcifications or diseased states as shown in Table 2.1 [57,59,64]. For example, in dental calculus, simultaneous presence of DCPD, OCP, Mg-βTCP and CHA have been observed [59,64,112].

2.6 CALCIUM PHOSPHATE-BASED BIOMATERIALS

The first successful application of a calcium phosphate reagent for bone repair was reported in 1920 [1]. It was not until more than 50 years later that calcium phosphate materials were developed for medical and dental applications [2,18,46]. Commercial calcium phosphate ceramics used currently as biomaterials for bone repair, augmentation, substitution include: HA, calcium-deficient apatite (CDA), β-TCP, BCP (intimate mixture of HA and β-TCP of varying HA/β-TCP ratios), listed in Table 2.6 [2,12,15,18,46,62,64,70,75,84]. Commercial HA is either of biologic (e.g., coral, bovine bone, marine algae) or synthetic origin [16,35, 62,64,120].

HA ceramic (used as biomaterials) and biologic apatite (e.g., bone mineral) differ in the following properties (Figure 2.11) [6,64]: (a) crystal size, (b) composition, and (c) solubility. HA and biologic apatite also differs in their manner of dissolution: biologic apatite shows preferential dissolution of the core, while HA has non-preferential dissolution [14].

HA bioceramics (commercial) are usually prepared by preparation at high pH (e.g., pH 10) then sintering between 950 °C and 1100 °C [18,46,64].

TABLE 2.6. Clinical Applications of Commercial Calcium Phosphate (CaP) Biomaterials

CaP Biomaterials	Applications	Ref
HA (ceramic, bovine-bone derived, coral derived)	bone graft substitute, sinus grafting, periodontal defects, bone augmentation, orthopedic, scaffold, drug delivery	[2,15,16, 18,20,23, 35,46,54,62,64,70, 75,120]
HA (ceramic)	abrasive, source for plasma-sprayed coating on orthopedic and dental implants	[18,30,37,46,55]
β-TCP	bone graft substitute, fractures, spinal fusion, dental, orthopedic	[62,64,75]
BCP (HA + β-TCP)	spine fusion, revision surgery, fractures, bone graft substitute, trauma surgery, opthalmic implant, scaffold	[12,75 96,119]
HA/polyethylene, BCP/silicon	middle ear prostheses	[8,75]
Calcium phosphate cement, CPC	bone filler bone tumor, bone cyst, periodontal defects, fracture	[101]

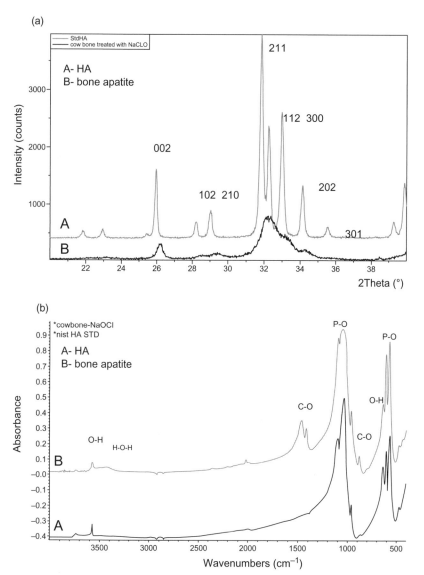

Figure 2.11. Comparative x-ray diffraction profile (11A) and FT-IR spectra (11B) of ceramic HA and bovine bone showing difference in crystal size (HA ≫ bone) and in composition (B), primarily in the presence of CO₃ in bone apatite (11B).

HA is also used as a source material for depositing coating on commercial orthopedic and dental implants by plasma-spray method [30,82] and as an alternative abrasive material for implant surface modification [37,55]. Composite biomaterials made with calcium phosphates include polyethylene/HA, silicon/BCP, and collagen/CHA [8,43,75,93].

Carbonate substituted apatites for use as bone substitute material has been prepared from biologic materials. For example, commercial coralline HA (Prosteon® < Interpore Co, Irvine, California) is prepared by the hydrothermal conversion of coral, *Porites* ($CaCO_3$ in aragonite form) in the presence of ammonium phosphate [15,35,110]. Bovine bone-derived commercial products are prepared by special treatment of bovine bone such as removal of organic phase without sintering (BioOss®, Geitslich, Switzerland) or by special treatment including sintering at 900 °C or above (Endobon®, Darmstad, Germany) [16]. Experimental CHA for bone repair were prepared by hydrolysis method [111] and by hydrothermal conversion. Carbonate apatite (CHA) blocks can be prepared by the hydrothermal conversion of calcite or gypsum blocks in the presence of $(NH_4)_2HPO_4$ or Na_2HPO_4 [117,118] or hydrothermal conversion of α-TCP in the presence of carbonate-containing solutions [121]. Conversion of calcite block to carbonate apatite block is time dependent (Figure 2.12) and also dependent on the concentration of the phosphate solution.

Commercial calcium phosphate cements consist of a powder and liquid component. The powder component is usually a mixture of two or more kinds of calcium phosphates (e.g., α-TCP, TTCP, DCPD, ACP) that when mixed with the liquid component sets into a product consisting of CDA, CHA or DCPD [11,48,51,74,101].

Experimental calcium phosphates recommended as biomaterials or as coatings on implants include: CHA, CFA, OCP, Mg-TCP, Zn-TCP, calcium phosphate glass, etc [4,39,68,71,99,111].

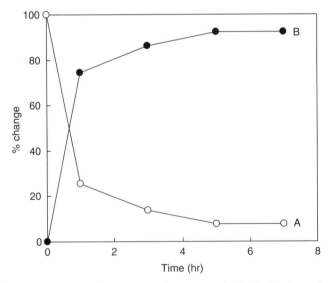

Figure 2.12. Transformation of calcite to carbonate apatite by hydrothermal conversion of calcite in the presence of 1 mol/L Na_2HPO_4, 60 °C. The amount of calcite decreased while the amount of carbonate apatite increased with time.

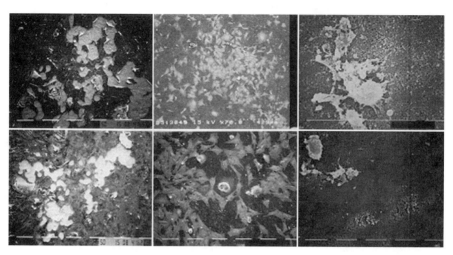

Figure 2.13. SEM images showing the osteoclastic resorption of HAP, CHA and CFA showing that apatite containing F (CFA) had the least number and smallest size of osteoclastic resorption pits.

Composites consisting of polymer and HA, BCP and other calcium phosphates are also being used as scaffolds for bone regeneration by tissue engineering [96,119]. The polymers used are either natural (e.g., collagen, chitosan) or synthetic (e.g., PLA, PLGA).

Reactivity of apatites and related calcium phosphates considered as potential candidates for biomaterials are usually evaluated *in vitro* by the cell response. Different substitutions in the apatite elicit different cell responses [29,36,122,123]. For example, osteoclasts (bone-resorbing cells) were shown to have greater activity (greater number and larger resorption pits) on carbonate-substituted apatites compared to F-substituted apatites, as shown in Figure 2.13 [29]. Osteoblasts (bone-forming cells) were shown to have greater activity on F-containing apatites compared to F-free apatites, *in vitro* [28,36].

In vivo, the amount of bone formation or type of bone (lamellar or woven) also depends on the composition [111]. Figure 2.14 shows histological pictures of similar size granules of carbonate apatite and HA implanted in bone defect in rat cranium after 12 weeks. The size of the HA granule was not changed significantly, while the size of the CHA granule was greatly reduced. In addition, greater amount of new bone surrounded the CHA granule compared to that around HA granule.

The properties of calcium phosphate based biomaterials that make them superior materials include: similarity in composition to the bone mineral, bioactivity, and osteoconductivity [65]. Bioactivity is the ability to directly bond with bone thus forming a uniquely strong interface [104]. *In vitro*, bioactivity is usually determined by the formation of carbonate apatite on the material surface after immersion in "simulated biologic fluid" (SBF) with electrolyte composition

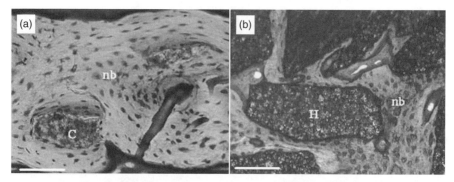

Figure 2.14. Histological micrographs showing carbonate apatite granule (A) and sintered hydroxyapatite (HAP) granule (B) 12 weeks after implantation in rat calvaria (toluidine blue staining). Bar = 100 μm. C: carbonate apatite; H: sintered HAP; nb: new bone; pb: parietal bone. The sizes of the carbonate apatite and HAP granules before implantation were similar. (See color insert.)

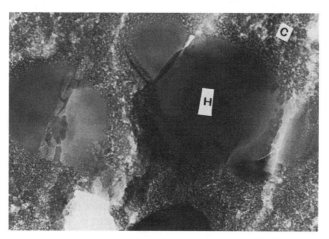

Figure 2.15. *In vivo* transformation of calcium phosphate ceramic (H) to carbonate apatite nanocrystals (c) similar to bone apatite [64,67,88].

similar to that of serum [54]. *In vivo*, bioactivity is characterized by the formation of carbonate apatite on the surface of the material resulting from the partial dissolution of the calcium phosphate ceramic (Figure 2.15), reacting with the electrolytes in the biological fluid and forming carbonate apatite similar to bone apatite [33,67,88]. Osteoconductive property is the ability of the calcium phosphate material to act as a template guiding the growth of the new bone (Figure 2.14). Appropriate geometry and combination of interconnecting macroporosity and microporosity, apatite (Figure 2.16) can impart osteoinductive (ability to induce *de novo* bone formation) properties [53]. However, the exact geometry and appropriate combination of macro- and microporosities are yet to be established.

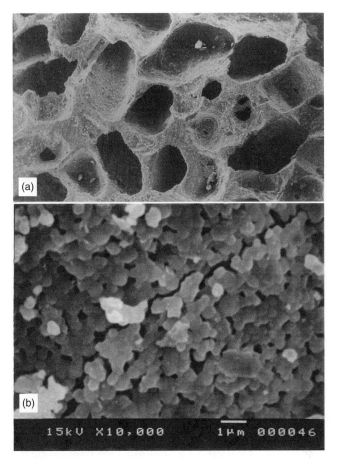

Figure 2.16. SEM images showing macroporosity (A) and microporosity (B) in sintered cow bone.

Medical and dental applications of calcium phosphate biomaterials include: repair of bone defects, bone fracture repair, alveolar ridge augmentation, ear implants, spine fusion, etc. (Table 2.6) HA has been demonstrated to be an efficient carrier for bone growth factors [53] or for drug delivery [23]. More recently, synthetic bone mineral was demonstrated to prevent bone loss induced either by mineral deficiency or estrogen deficiency in rats [85,105].

ACKNOWLEDGMENTS

Support of research grants from the National Institutes of Health for some of the author's work presented here are gratefully acknowledged. Special thanks to Gary Cantig and Fang Yao for the preparation of some of the figures included in this chapter.

REFERENCES

1. Albee FH. Studies in bone growth: triple calcium phosphate as a stimulus to osteogenesis. Ann Surg 1920;71:32–36.

2. Aoki H. *Medical Applications of Hydroxyapatite*. Ishiyaku EuroAmerica, Inc: Tokyo, 1994.

3. Arends J, Shuthof J, Van der Linden WH, Bennema P, Van Den Berg, PJ. Preparation of pure hydroxyapatite single crystals by hydrothermal recrystallization. J Crystal Growth 1979;46:213–220.

4. Barrere F, vander Valk Cm, Dalmeijer RAJ, Meijer G, Van Blitterswijk CA, De Groot K, Layrolle P. Osteogenicity of octacalcium phosphate coatings applied on porous metal implants. J Biomed Mater Res A 2003;66:770–788.

5. Beevers CA, McIntyre DB. The atomic structure of fluorapatite and its relation to that of tooth and bone mineral. Miner Mat 1956;27:254–259.

6. Ben-Nissam B, LeGeros RZ. Biologic and synthetic apatite. In: Bowlin GL, Wnek G (Ed). *The encyclopedia of Bioamterials and Biomedical Engineering*. Volume 2. Taylor and Francis Book, Dekker: New York (in press).

7. Bonel G, Montel G. Sur une nouvelle apatite carbonate synthetique. CR Seance Acad Sci Paris 1964;258:923–926.

8. Bonfield W, Grynpas MD, Tully AE, Bowman J, Abram J. Hydroxyapatite reinforced polyethylene—a mechanically compatible implant material for bone replacement. Biomaterials 1981;2:186–186.

9. Botelho CM, Brooks RA, Best SM, Lopez MA, Santos JD, Rushton N, Bonfield W. Human osteoblast response to silicon-substituted hydroxyapatite. Biomed Mater Res 2006;79A:723–730.

10. Brown W, Smith J, Lehr J, Frazier A. Crystallographic and chemical relations between octacalcium phosphate and hydroxyapatite. Nature 1962;196:1050–1055.

11. Brown WE, Chow LC. Dental restorative cement pastes. US Pat No. 4,518,430 (1988).

12. Daculsi G, Laboux O, Marad O, Weiss P. Current state of the art of biphasic calcium phosphate ceramics. J Mater Sci Mater Med 2003;14:195–200.

13. Daculsi G, LeGeros RZ, Jean A, Kerebel L-M, Kerebel B. Possible physico-chemical processes in human dentin caries. J Dent Res 66:1356–1359.

14. Daculsi G, LeGeros RZ, Mitre D. Crystal dissolution of biological and ceramic apatites. Calcif Tiss Int 1989;45:95–103.

15. Damien E, Revell PA. Coralline hydroxyapatite bone graft substitute: A review of experimental studies and biomedical applications. J Appl Biomat Biomech 2004;2:65–75.

16. Dard M, Bauer A, Liebendorgen A, Wahlig H, Dingeldein E. Preparation physicochemical and biological evaluation of a hydroxyapatite ceramic from bovine spongiosa. Acta Odonto Stom 1994;185:61–69.

17. Deer WA, Howie RA, Zussman J. *An Introduction to Rock-forming Minerals*. Longman: Hong Kong, 1985; pp. 504–509.

18. deGroot K. Ceramics of calcium phosphates: Preparation and properties. In: deGroot K (Ed). Bioceramics of Calcium Phosphate. CRC Press: Boca Raton, 1983; pp. 100–114.

19. DeJong WF. La substance minerale dans les os. Res Trav Chim 1926;45:445–448.

20. Denissen H, deGroot K. Immediate dental root implants from synthetic dense calcium hydroxyapatite. J Prost Dent 1979;42:551.

21. Elliott JC. *The Crystallographic Structure of Dental Enamel and Related Apatites.* PhD Thesis, University of London, 1964.

22. Ellliott JC. *Structure and Chemistry of Apatites and other Calcium Orthophosphates.* Elsevier: The Netherlands, 1994; pp. 137–138.

23. Ferraz MP, Mateus AY, Sousa JC, Monteiro FJ. Nanohydroxyapatite microspheres as delivery system for antibiotics: Release kinetics, antimicrobial activity and interaction with osteoblasts. J Biomed Mater Res 2007;81A:994–1004.

24. Fleet ME, Liu X, King PL. Accommodation of the carbonate ion in apatite: an FTIR and X-ray structure study of crystal synthesized at 2–4 GPa. Am Miner 2004;89:1422–1432.

25. Fleet ME, Liu X. Location of type B carbonate ion in type A-B carbonate apatite synthesized at high pressure. J Solid State Chem 2004;177:3174–3182.

26. Fleet ME, Liu X. Coupled substitution of type A and B carbonate in sodium-bearing apatite. Biomaterials 2007;28:916–926.

27. Fowler BO. Infrared studies of apatites. II. Preparation of normal and isotopically substituted calcium, strontium and barium hydroxyapatites and spectra-structure-composition correlations. Inorg Chem 1974;13:207–214.

28. Frondoza C, LeGeros RZ, Hungerford DS. Effect of bovine bone-derived materials on human osteoblast-like cells in vitro. Bioceramics 1998;11:289–291.

29. Fujimori Y, Mishima H, Sugaya K Sakae T, LeGeros RZ, Kozawa Y, Nagura H. In vitro interactions of osteoclast-like cells and hydroxyapatite ceramics. Bioceramics 1998;11:335–338.

30. Geesink RGT, Manley MT (eds). Hydroxylapatite Coatings in Orthopaedic Surgery. Raven Press: New York, 1993.

31. Gibson IR, Best SM, Bonfield W. Chemical characterization of silicon-substituted hydroxyapatite. J Biomed Mater Res 1999;44:422–428.

32. Hattori T, Iwadate Y. Hydrothermal preparation of calcium hydroxyapatite powders. J Am Ceram Soc 1990;73:1803–1805.

33. Heughebaert M, LeGeros RZ, Gineste M, Guilhem A, Bonel G. Physico-chemical characterization of deposits associated with HA ceramics implanted in non-osseous sites. J Biomed Mater Res 1988;22:254–268.

34. Heughebaert JC, Zawacki SJ, Nancollas GH. The growth of nonstoichiometric apatite from aqueous solution at 37 °C. I. Methodology and growth at pH 7.4. J Coll Inter Sci 1990;135:20–32.

35. Holmes RE, Hagler HK. Porous hydroxylapatite as a bone graft substitute in mandibular contour augmentation. J Oral Maxillofac Surg 1987;45:421–426.

36. Inoue M, LeGeros RZ, Inoue M, Tsujigiwa H, Nagatsuka H, Yamamoto T, Nagai N. In vitro response of osteoblast-like and odontoblast-like cells to unsubstituted and substituted apatites. J Biomed Mater Res 2004;70A:585–593.

37. Ishikawa K, Miyamoto Y, Nagayama M, Asaoka K. Blast coating method: New method of coating titanium surface with hydroxyapatite at room temperature. J Biomed Mater Res (Appl Biomater) 1997;38:129–134.

38. Ito A, Hita T, Sogo Y, Ichinose N, LeGeros RZ. Solubility of magnesium-containing ß-tricalcium phosphate: Comparison with that of zinc-containing ß-tricalcium phosphate. Key Engineer Mat 2006;309–311:239–242.

39. Ito A, Kawamura H, Otsuka M, Ikeuchi M, Ohgushi H, Ishikawa K, Onuma K, Kanzaki N, Sogo Y, Ichinose N. Zinc releasing calcium phosphate for stimulating bone formation. Mater Sci Eng 2002;C22:21–25.

40. Ito A, Maekawa K, Tsutsumi S, Ikazaki F, Tateishi T. Solubility product of OH-carbonated hydroxyapatite single crystals. J Biomed Mater Res 1997;34:269–272.

41. Ito A, Nakamura S, Aoki H, Akao M, Traoka K, Tsutsumi S, Onuma K, Tateishi T. Hydrothermal growth of carbonate-containing hydroxyapatite single crystals. J Crystal Growth 1996;163:311–317.

42. Ito A, Senda K, Sogo Y, Oyane A, Yamazaki A, LeGeros RZ. Dissolution rate of zinc-containing β-tricalcium phosphate ceramics. Biomed Mater 2006;1:134–139.

43. Itoh M, Shimazy A, Hirata I, Yoshida Y, Shintani H, Okazaki M. Characterization of CO3AP-collagen sponges using X-ray high-resolution microtomography. Biomaterials 2002;25:2577–2583.

44. Ivanova TI, Frank-Kamenetskaya OV, Kol'tsov AB. Synthesis, crystal structure and thermal decomposition of potassium-doped carbonate hydroxyapatite. Zeit Kristallogr 2004;219:479–486.

45. Jahnke RA. The synthesis and solubility of carbonate fluorapatite. J Ci 1984;284:58–78.

46. Jarcho M. Calcium phosphate ceramics as hard tissue prosthetics. Clin Orthopaed 1981;157:259–278.

47. Jean A, Kerebel B, Kerebel LM, LeGeros RZ, Hamel H. Effects of various calcium phosphate biomaterials on reparative dentine bridge formation. J Endo 1988;14:83–87.

48. Julien M, Khairoun I, LeGeros RZ, Delplace S, Pilet P, Weiss P, Daculsi G, Bouler J-M, Guicheux J. Physico-chemical-mechanical and in vitro biological properties of calcium phosphate cements with doped amorphous calcium phosphates. Biomaerials 2007;28:956–965.

49. Kamakura S, Sasano Y, Homma H, Suzuki O, Kagayama M, Motegi K. Implantation of octacalcium phosphate (OCP) in rat skull defects enhances bone repair. J Dent Res 1999;78:1682–1687.

50. Kay M, Young RA, Posner AS. The crystal structure of hydroxyapatite. Nature 1964;204:1050–1052.

51. Khairoun I, LeGeros RZ, Daculsi G, et al. Macroporous resorbable and injectible calcium phosphate based cements (MCPC). Provisional patent application no. PCT/US2005/004084 (2005).

52. Kijkowska R, Lin S, LeGeros RZ. Physico-chemical and thermal properties of chlor-, fluor- and hydroxyapatites. Key Engineer Mat 2002;218–220:41–34.

53. Kuboki Y, Takita H, Kobayashi D. BMP-induced osteogenesis on the surface of hydroxyapatite with geometrically feasible and non-feasible structures: Topology of osteogenesis. J Biomed Mater Res 1998;39:190–199.

54. Kokubo T. Formation of biologically active bone-like apatite on metals and polymers by a biomimetic process. Thermochim Acta 1996;280:479–490.

55. LeGeros JP, Daculsi G, LeGeros RZ. Tissue response to grit-blasted Ti alloy. Proc. 25thAnnual International Soc of Biomaterials, 1998.

56. LeGeros JP, Lin S, Mijares D, Dimaano F, LeGeros RZ. Electrochemicaly deposited calcium phosphate coating on titanium alloy substrates. Key Engineer Mat 2005;284–286:247–250.

57. LeGeros RZ. *Crystallographic Studies of the Carbonate Substitution in the Apatite Structure*. PhD Thesis, New York University 1967.

58. LeGeros RZ. Apatites from aqueous and non-aqueous systems.: Relation to biological apatites. Proc 1st Int Congr on Phophorous Compounds (IMPHOS), Rabat Morocco, 1977; pp. 347–360.

59. LeGeros RZ. Apatites in biological systems. Prog Crystal Growth Charact 1981;4: 1–45.

60. LeGeros RZ. Incorporation of magnesium in synthetic and in biological apatites. In: *Tooth Enamel IV*. Fearnhead RW, Suga S (eds). Elsevier Science Publishers, Amsterdam 1984;169–174.

61. LeGeros RZ. Preparation of octacalcium phosphate (OCP): A direct fast method. Calcif Tissue Int 1985;37:194–197.

62. LeGeros RZ. Calcium phosphate materials in restorative dentistry: A. review. Adv Dent Res 1988;2:164–183.

63. LeGeros RZ. Chemical and crystallographic events in the caries process. J Dent Res 1990;69 (Spec Iss):567–574.

64. LeGeros RZ. *Calcium Phosphates in Oral Biology and Medicine*. Monographs in Oral Sciences. Vol 15. Myers H (Ed). 1991. Karger: Basel.

65. LeGeros RZ. Properties of osteoconductive biomaterials: Calcium phosphates. Clin Orthopaed Rel Res 2002;395:81–98.

66. LeGeros RZ. Biodegradation and bioresorption of calcium phosphate ceramics. Clin Mat 1993;14:65–88.

67. LeGeros RZ, Daculsi G. In vivo transformation of biphasic calcium phosphate ceramics: Histological ultrastructural and physico-chemical characterization. In: *Handbook in Bioactive Ceramics*. Vol 2. Yamamuro T, Hench L, Wison-Hench J (Eds). CRC Press: Boca Raton 1990;17–28.

68. LeGeros RZ, Lee Y-K. Synthesis of amorphous calcium phosphates for hard tissue repair using conventional melting technique. J Mat Sci 2004;39:5577–5579. LeGeros RZ, LeGeros JP. Dense hydroxyapatite. In: Hench LL, Wilson J (Eds). *An Introduction to Bioceramics*. World Scientific: Singapore, 1993; pp. 139–180.

69. LeGeros RZ, LeGeros JP. Brushite crystals grown by diffusion. J Crystal Growth 1972;13:4767–480.

70. LeGeros RZ, LeGeros JP. Hydroxyapatite. In: Kokubo T (Ed). *Handbook of Biocramics and their Applications*. Woodhead Publishing Ltd: London (in press).

71. LeGeros RZ, Gatti AM, Kijkowska R, Mijares DQ, LeGeros JP. Mg-substituted tricalcium phosphates: formation and properties. Key Engineer Mater 2004;254–256:127–130.

72. LeGeros RZ, Suga S. Crystallographic nature of fluoride in the enameloids of fish. Calcif Tiss Int 1980;32:169–174.

73. LeGeros RZ, Tung MS. Chemical stability of carbonate- and fluoride-containing apatites. Caries Res 1983;17:419–429.

74. LeGeros RZ, Chohayeb A, Shulman A. Apatitic calcium phosphate: Possible restorative materials. J Dent Res 1982;61:343.

75. LeGeros RZ, Daculsi G, LeGeros JP. Bioactive bioceramics. In: Pietrzak WS, Eppley BL (Eds). *Muskuloskeletal Tissue Regeneration: Biological materials and Methods.* Humana Press Inc: New Jersey (in press).

76. LeGeros RZ, Bleiwas CB, Retino M, Rohanizadeh R, LeGeros JP. Zinc effect on the in vitro formation of calcium phosphates: relevance to clinical inhibition of calculus formation. Am J Dent 1999;12:65–70.

77. LeGeros RZ, Daculsi G, Kijkowska R, Kerebel B. The effect of magnesium on the formation of apatites and whitlockites. In: Itokawa Y, Durlach J (eds). *Proc Magnesium Symposium 1988: Magnesium in Health and Disease.* New York, Libbey, 1989; pp. 11–19.

78. LeGeros RZ, Go PP, Vandemaele KH, LeGeros DJ. Transformation of calcium carbonates and calcium phosphates to carbonate apatites: Possible mechanism for phosphorite formation. Proc 2nd Int Conger on Phosphorous Compounds. Boston 1980; pp. 41–53.

79. LeGeros RZ, Kijkowska R, Jia WT, LeGeros JP. Fluoride-cation interaction in the formation and stability of apatites. J Fluor Chem 1988;41:53–64.

80. LeGeros RZ, Kijkowska R, Tung M, LeGeros JP. Effect of strontium on some properties of apatites. In: Fearnhead RW, Suga S (eds). *Enamel Symposium V.* Amsterdam, Elsevier, 1990.

81. LeGeros RZ, LeGeros JP, Trautz OR, Shirra WP. Conversion of monetite, $CaHPO_4$, to apatites: effect of carbonate on the crystallinity and morphology of apatite crystallites. Adv X-ray Anal 1971;14:57–66.

82. LeGeros RZ, LeGeros JP, Kim Y, Kijkowska R, Zheng R, Bautista C, Wong JL. Calcium phosphates in plasma-sprayed HA coatings. Ceramic Trans 48: 173–189.

83. LeGeros RZ, LeGeros JP, Trautz OR, Klein E. Spectral properties of carbonate in carbonate-containing apatites. Dev Appl spectrosc 1970;7B:3–12.

84. LeGeros RZ, Lin S, Rohanizadeh R, Mijares D, LeGeros JP. Biphasic calcium phosphate bioceramics: Preparation, properties and applications. J Mater Sci Mater in Med 2003;13:201–210.

85. LeGeros RZ, Mijares D, Yao F, Xi Q, Ricci J, LeGeros JP. Synthetic bone mineral (SBM) for osteoporosis therapy. Part I. Prevention of bone loss induced by mineral deficiency. Bioceramics 20 (in press).

86. LeGeros RZ, Pan CM, Suga S, Watabe N. Crystallo-chemical properties of apatite in atremate brachiopod shells. Calcif Tiss Int 1985;98–100.

87. LeGeros RZ, Trautz OR, LeGeros JP, Klein E. Carbonate substitution in the apatite structure. Bull Soc chim 1968:1712–1718.

88. LeGeros RZ, Orly I, Gregoire M, Daculsi G. Substrate surface dissolution and interfacial biological mineralization. In: *The Bone-Biomaterial Interface.* Davies JE (ed). Univ of Toronto Press 1991;76–86.

89. LeGeros RZ, Sakae T, Bautista C, Retino M, LeGeros JP. Magnesium and carbonate in enamel and synthetic apatites. Adv Dent Res 1996;19:225–231.

90. LeGeros RZ, Shirra WP, Miravite MA, LeGeros JP. Amorphous calcium phosphates: Synthetic and biological. *Coll Int CNRS No. 230: Physico-chimie et cristallographie des apatites d'interet biologique.* Paris, CNRS 1973; pp 105–115.

91. LeGeros RZ, Taheri MH, Quirolgico G, LeGeros JP. Formation and stability of apatites: Effects of some cationic substituents. Proc. 2nd Int Congr on Phosphorous Compounds. Boston 1980; pp. 89–103.

92. LeGeros RZ, Trautz OR, LeGeros JP. Apatite crystallites: Effect of carbonate on morphology. Science 1967;155:1409–1411.

93. Lickorish D, Ramshaw JAM, Werkmeister JA, Glattauer V, Howlett CR. Collagen-hydroxyapatite composite prepared by biomimetic process. J Biomed Mater Res 2004;68A:19–27.

94. Lin S, LeGeros RZ, LeGeros JP. Adherent octacalcium phosphate coating on titanium alloy using modulated electrochemical deposition method. J Biomed Mater Res 2003;66A:810–828.

95. Linton JL, Sohn B-V, Yook J-I, LeGeros RZ. Effects of calcium phosphate ceramic bone graft materials on permanent teeth eruption in beagles. Cleft Palate-Craniofacial J 2002;39:197–2007.

96. Livingstone TL, Daculsi G. Mesenchymal stem cells combined with biphasic calcium phosphate ceramics promote bone regeneration. J Mater Sci Mat Med 2003:13:211–218.

97. Margolis HC, Moreno EC. Kinetic and thermodynamic aspects of enamel demineralization. Caries Res 1985;19:22–35.

98. McConnell D. The crystal chemistry of carbonate apatites and their relationship to the composition of calcified tissue. J Dent Res 1952;31:53–63.

99. Moon H-J, Kim N-H, Kim N-M, Choi S-H, Kim K-D, LeGeros RZ, Lee Y-K. Bone formation in calvaria defects of Sprague-Dawley rat by transplantation of calcium phosphate glass. J Biomed Mater Res 2005;74A:497–502.

100. Moreno EC, Kresak M, Zahradnik RT. Physicochemical aspects of fluoride-apatite systems relevant to the study of dental caries. Caires Res (Suppl 1)1977;11:142–177.

101. Niwa S, LeGeros RZ. Injectable calcium phosphate cements for repair of bone defects. In: *Tissue Engineering and Biodegradable Equivalents: Scientific and Clinical Applications*. Lewandrowski K-U, Wise DL, Trantolo DJ, Gresser JD (Eds). Marcel Dekker Inc: New York 2002;385–500.

102. Obadia L, Rouillon T, Buhjoli B, Daculsi G, Bouler JM. Calcium deficient apatite synthesized by ammonia hydrolysis of dicalcium phosphate dihydrate: Influence of temperature, time and pressure. J Biomed Mater Res 2007;80B:32–42.

103. Okazaki M, LeGeros RZ. Properties of heterogeneous apatites containing magnesium, fluoride and carbonate. Adv Dent Res 1996;10:252–259.

104. Osborn JF, Newesely H. The material science of calcium phosphate ceramic. Biomaterials 1980;1:108–111.

105. Otsuka M, Oshinbe A, LeGeros RZ, Tokudome Y, Ito A, Otsuka K, Higuchi WI. Efficacy of a new injectable calcium phosphate ceramic suspension on improving bone properties of ovariectomized rats. J Pharm Sci (in press).

106. Prener JS. The growth and crystallographic properties of calcium fluor- and chlorapatite crystals. J Electrochem Soc 1967;114:77–83.

107. Rey C, Renugoplakrishan V, Collins B. Fourier transform infrared spectroscopic study of the carbonate ions in bone mineral during aging. Calcif Tissue Int 1991;49: 251–258.

108. Rohanizadeh R, LeGeros RZ, Harsono M, Bendavid A. Adherent apatite coating on titanium substrate using chemical deposition. J Biomed Mater Res 2005;72A:428–438.

109. Rokbani R, LeGeros RZ, Ariguib NK, Ayeti T, LeGeros JP. Formation of apatites in the system. KCl-$CaCl_2$-$Ca_3(PO_4)_2$-K_3PO_4-H_2O at 25 °C. Bioceramics 1998;11:747–750.

110. Roy DM, Linnehan SA. Hydroxyapatite formed from coral skeleton carbonate by hydrothermic exchange. Nature 1973;247:220–227.

111. Sakae T, Ookubo A, LeGeros RZ, Shimogoryou R, Sato Y, Yamamoto H, Kozawa Y. Bone formation induced by several carbonate- and fluoride-containing apatites implanted in dog mandible. Key Engineer Mater 2003;240–242:395–398.

112. Schroeder HE. *Formation and Inhbition of Dental Calculus*. Vienna: Hubert, 1969.

113. Schroeder LW, Dickens B, Brown WE. Crystalllographic studies of the role of Mg as a stabilizing impurity in β-$Ca_3(PO_4)_2$. II. Refinement of Mg-containing β-$Ca_3(PO_4)_2$. J Solid State Chem 1977;22:253–262.

114. Sogo Y, Itro A, Yokoyama D, Yamazaki A, LeGeros RZ. Synhtesis of fluoride-releasing carbonate apatite for bone substitutes. J Mater Sci: Mater Med 2007;18:1001–1007.

115. Suetsugu Y, Takahashi Y, Okamura FP, Tanaka J. Structure analysis of A-type carbonate apatite by a single-crystal spray diffraction method. J Solid State Chem 2000;155:292–297.

116. Suetsugu Y, Tanaka J. Crystal growth of carbonate apatite using a $CaCO_3$ flux. J Mater Sci Mater in Med 1999;10:561–566.

117. Suzuki Y, Matsuya S, Udoh K, Nakagawa M, Tsukiyama Y, Koyano K, Ishikawa K. Fabrication of hydroxyapatite block from gypsum block based on $(NH_4)_2HPO_4$ treatment. Dent Mater J 2005;24:515–521.

118. Takeuchi A, Maruta M, Matsuya S, Nakagawa M, Ishikawa K. Preparation of carbonate apatite block from gypsum by hydrothermal treatment. Arch BioCeram Res 2006;6:99–102.

119. Texiera C, Karkia C, Neweliksky U, LeGeros RZ. Biphasic calcium phosphate: a scaffold for growth plate chondrocytes. Tissue Eng 2006;12:2283–2289.

120. Valentini P, Abensur D, Wenz B. Sinus grafting with porous bone mineral (Bio-Oss) for implant placement: a 5-year study on 15 patients. J Periodontol Restor Dent 2000;20:245–254.

121. Wakae H, Takeuchi A, Matsuya S, Munar M, Nakagawa M, Udoh K, Ishikawa K. Preparation of carbonate apatite foam by hydrothermal treatment of a-TCP foam in carbonate salt solutions. Arch Bioceram Res 2006;6:103–105.

122. Webster TJ, Ergun C, Doremus R, Bizios R. Hydroxylapatite with substituted magnesium, zinc, cadmium and yttrium. II. Mechanisms of osteoblast adhesion. J Biomed Mater Res 2002;59;312–317.

123. Winters J, Kleckner A, LeGeros RZ. Fluoride inhibits osteoclastic bone resorption in vitro. J Dent Res 1989;68:353.

124. Young RA, Elliott JC. Atomic scale bases for several properties of apatites. Arch Oral Biol 1966;11:699–707.

125. Young EJ, Sherida DM, Munson EL. Manganese and strontium-bearing fluoapatite from the Peerless Pegmatite South Dakota. Am Mineral 1966;51:1516–1524.

126. Zapanta-LeGeros R. Effect of carbonate on the lattice parameters of apatite. Nature 1965;206:403–405.

3

MATERIALS FOR ORTHOPEDIC APPLICATIONS

Shekhar Nath and Bikramjit Basu

Department of Materials and Metallurgical Engineering, Indian Institute of Technology Kanpur, Kanpur, India

Contents

	Abbreviations	54
3.1	Overview	54
3.2	Introduction	55
3.3	Structure and Properties of Hard Tissues	57
3.4	Processing and Properties of Bioceramics and Bioceramic Composites	59
	3.4.1 Calcium Phosphate Based Biomaterials	59
	3.4.2 Hydroxyapatite-Ceramic Composites	62
	3.4.3 Hydroxyapatite-Titanium Composites	63
	3.4.4 Glass-Ceramics Based Biomaterials	66
	3.4.4.1 Mica Based Glass Ceramics	66
	3.4.4.2 Other Bioglass-Ceramics	69
	3.4.5 Bioinert Ceramics	70
3.5	Polymeric Biomaterials	72
	3.5.1 Polymer-Polymer Composites	73
	3.5.2 Polymer-Ceramic Composites	74
	3.5.2.1 HDPE-HAp-Al_2O_3 Hybrid Composites	76
3.6	Metals and Alloys in Biomedical Applications	79
	3.6.1 Issues Limiting Performance of Metallic Biomaterials	81
	3.6.1.1 Wear of Implants	81

Advanced Biomaterials: Fundamentals, Processing, and Applications, Edited by Bikramjit Basu, Dhirendra S. Katti, and Ashok Kumar

     3.6.1.2 Corrosion of Metallic Implants   81
  3.6.2 Ti-Based Alloys   83
  3.6.3 Co-Cr-Mo, Ni or Ta–Based Alloys   85
  3.6.4 Other Non-Ferrous Metals and Their Alloys   86
3.7 Coating on Metals   86
3.8 Outlook and Recommendations for Future Work   91
  Acknowledgments   93
  References   93

Abbreviations

AS: Artificial Saliva
BCP: Biphasic Calcium Phosphate
BG: Bio Glass
BMO: Bone Marrow Cells
CaP: Calcium Phosphate
CF: Carbon Fiber
CP: Commercially Pure
CT: Computer Tomography
CTE: Coefficient of Thermal Expansion
DLC: Diamond Like Carbon
DLF: Direct Laser Forming
DSC: Differential Scanning Calorimetry
EDS: Energy Dispersive Spectroscopy
EVA: Ethyl Vinyl Alcohol
FGM: Functionally Graded Materials
FHA: Flurohydroxyapatite
FSZ: Fully Stabilized Zirconia
HAp: Hydroxyapatite
HDPE: High Density Polyethylene
HIP: Hot Isostatic Pressing
KF: Kevler Fiber
MRI: Magnetic Resonance Imaging
MW: Microwave
OCP: Octa Calcium Phosphate
PDMS: Poly Di-methyl Sulphonate
PE: Polyethylene
PEEK: Polyethylene Ether Ketone

PEMF: Pulse electromagnetic fields
PET: Polyethylenetelephthalate
PLA: Poly Lactic Acid
PLLA: Poly-L-Lactide Acid
PLDA: Polylactideglycolide Acid
PMMA: Polymethylmethacrylate
PS: Poly Sialane
PSZ: Partially stabilized Zirconia
PTFE: Ploy tetrafluro ethylene
PU: Poly Urethane
SBF: Simulated Body Fluid
SEM: Scanning Electron Microscopy
SPS: Spark Plasma Sintering
SR: Silicone Rubber
SS: Stainless Steel
TCP: Tricalcium Phosphate
TEM: Transmission Electron Microscopy
THR: Total Hip Replacement
TTCP: Tetracalcium Phosphate
UHMWPE: Ultra High Molecular Weight
   Polyethylene
XRD: X-Ray Diffraction
Y-TZP: Yttria doped Tetragonal Zirconia
   Polycrystal
ZCP: Zero Current Potential
ZTA: Zirconia Toughened Alumina

3.1 OVERVIEW

This chapter reviews various materials and their properties that are relevant in biomedical applications, such as hard tissue replacement. A major emphasize has been placed on presenting various design aspects, in terms of materials processing of ceramics and polymer based biocomposites. Among the bioceramic composites, the research results obtained with hydroxyapatite (HAp)-based biomaterials with metallic (Ti) or ceramic (Mullite) reinforcements as well as SiO_2-MgO-

Al_2O_3-K_2O-B_2O_3-F glass ceramics and stabilized ZrO_2 based bioinert ceramics are summarized. The physical as well as tribological properties of polyethylene (PE) based hybrid biocomposites are discussed to illustrate the concept of how physical/wear properties can be enhanced along with biocompatibility due to combined addition of bioinert and bioactive ceramic to a bioinert polymeric matrix. The tribological and corrosion properties of some important orthopedic metallic alloys based on Ti or Co-Cr-Mo are also illustrated. Finally, a summary presents the future perspective on orthopedic biomaterials development and some unresolved issues.

3.2 INTRODUCTION

The recent development in scientific understanding, particularly in the area of material science and biological science, has enabled an impressive progress in developing new biomaterials. In the last few decades, materials for biomedical applications have received greater attention in the scientific community, primarily due to the fact that suitably designed biomaterials are capable of replacing, reconstructing and regenerating human and animal body tissues for long term use, without much toxic or inflammation effects. In specific applications, such as hard tissue replacements, materials are being developed to maintain a balance between the mechanical properties of the replaced tissues and the biochemical effects of the material on the tissue. Both areas are of great importance as far as the clinical success of materials is concerned. However, in most (if not all) biological systems, a range of properties is required, such as biological activity, mechanical strength, chemical durability, and so on. Therefore, often a clinical need can only be fulfilled by a designed material, which exhibits a complex combination of properties.

Various examples of current usage of orthopedic biomaterials include joints (knee, hip, ankle, and so on), bone filling materials or bone spacers. The development of new biomaterials not only extends toward monolithic bulk materials but also composites of different classes of materials along with coating. The major issues in the development of biocompatible coatings are the coating/bio interface adhesion as well as lifetime of coatings, being limited by factors like non-uniform coating thickness, delamination due to mismatching of co-efficient of thermal expansion (CTE) and weak interface bonding between metal substrate and phosphate coatings[1]. Among different kinds of biomaterials, ceramics are used as bone-filling material and load-bearing components in various orthopedic joint replacements. To achieve better chemical resistance and mechanical strength, various composites, such as metal-ceramic, ceramic-polymer and ceramic-ceramic, are being developed. In designing composites, it is important to optimize composite composition as well as microstructure/phase assemblage for a specific tissue replacement application. Among various bioceramic materials, HAp, having similar mineral composition to bone and teeth, is widely studied for various applications requiring good bioactive property[2]. Although HAp is a highly

TABLE 3.1. Mechanical Properties of Bioactive Glass/Ceramic/Ceramic Composites

Materials	Strength (MPa)		Elastic modulus, E (GPa)	Fracture toughness, KIC (MPa m$^{1/2}$)
	Compressive	Bending		
Bioglasss (45S5)	—	42	35	—
HAp	500–1000	115–200	80–110	<1
20 vol% Y-TZP- HAp composite	700–800	180	160	1.5
20 vol% Al$_2$O$_3$- HAp composite	600–700	200	175	1.25
Glass-ceramic A-W	1080	220	118	2

[7,23,136].

biocompatible and bioactive material, it has poor mechanical properties (see Table 3.1), which limit its load bearing applications as bulk monolithic material. To this end, hydroxyapatite could be used in combination with another metal/ceramic phase, which can improve the mechanical properties of HAp without deteriorating its biocompatibility. The motivation for developing HAp-based composites stems from the requirement to fabricate materials with improved strength and toughness properties with the least amount of reaction phases. A popular application of HAp or in general, calcium phosphate (CaP) based bioceramics, includes coatings on orthopedic and dental implants of metals and their alloys[3,4]. All the above aspects are discussed in this chapter with the use of experimental results on HAp-Ti or HAp-mullite composites. Also discussed are the properties or performance of HAp coatings on metallic substrates (e.g., Co-Cr-Mo).

Among metals, titanium and its alloys have been extensively used as an implant material in different medical applications for more than 30 years. This has been facilitated by their excellent mechanical properties and high corrosion resistance[5]. One of the primary advantages, originally cited for the titanium implant, was its osseous integration[6] with the bone of the jaw. In recent years, however, this attachment has been more accurately described as a tight apposition or mechanical fit and not true bonding[7]. Besides discussion on Ti alloys, particularly their corrosion/wear properties, this chapter briefly discusses the potential of some metals, like Mg in biomedical applications.

Among various biopolymers (High Density Polyethylene (HDPE), Poly Tetrafluro Ethylene (PTFE), Polymethylmethacrylate (PMMA) etc.), are widely used in biomedical applications, because of its excellent biocompatible property along with better mouldability, availability as well as for its low cost[8]. In the last few decades, substantial research efforts were invested to develop bioactive composites as bone analogue replacement by reinforcing bioinert high density polyethylene matrix with bioactive HAp ceramic particulates. As mentioned earlier, the physical tribological and biocompatibility properties of HDPE-based biocomposites will be discussed to a larger extent. While this chapter has attempted to cover various materials from the perspective of biomedical applications, the following aspects are not covered in any detailed manner: a) synthesis of hydroxyapatite powders, and b) processing of porous bioactive coatings or porous bulk biomaterials.

Section 3.2 emphasizes the chemistry and properties of natural hard tissues. In discussing different materials system and their applications, the discussion starts with hydroxyapatite based composite biomaterials.

Section 3.3 provides examples of different HAp based composites, which are well characterized and reported in the existing literature. In addition to the literature summary, the research results from the authors' group have been incorporated. In a subsection, different bioinert ceramics have been presented with examples from the literature. The experimental results from the authors' group on bioinert ceramics are also included and discussed elaborately. The next subsection describes the possibility of using glass-ceramic materials for orthopedic or dental applications along with authors' recent research results. In some specific implant applications, the importance of using bioinert material cannot be ignored.

Section 3.4 deals with polymeric biomaterials and their possible composites in combination with other materials. In sections 3.4.1 and 3.4.2, the earlier works on polymer–polymer and polymer–ceramic composite materials are discussed.

Section 3.5 critically assesses various examples of metallic biomaterials, as well as the wear and corrosion properties of different metallic implants.

Section 3.6 deals with coating on metallic implants including their *in vivo* functionality.

Finally, section 3.7 closes the chapter with an outlook on the present work and the future perspective.

3.3   STRUCTURE AND PROPERTIES OF HARD TISSUES

As mentioned in the previous section, the focus of this review is on hard tissue replacement materials and therefore, it is important, in the first place, to discuss the structure and properties of the natural hard tissues, that is, bone and teeth. Based on its physical appearance, bone can be classified as cancellous and cortical bones. Cancellous bone (also called trabecular or spongy bone) has porous structure and behaves like an isotropic material under mechanical loading. On the other hand, cortical bone has highly anisotropic microstructure, which leads to higher strength in the direction of the loading axis[9]. Table 3.2 summarizes the mechanical properties of bone and teeth.

Structurally, all hard tissues are formed from the four phases: collagen fibers, Ca-P rich mineral, organic substances, and water. The relative fractions of each phase vary between bone types/teeth as well as on age/sex and anatomical location within living body. Some related data for a typical cortical bone are included in Table 3.3. In the case of teeth enamel, the mineral (HAp) content is as high as 95%. For the same reason, enamel is the hardest material in the human body. Excluding organic mass and water, bone can be described as a natural nanocomposite, containing HAp nano-particles and collagen fiber. The collagen fibers pro-

TABLE 3.2. Mechanical Properties of Different Hard Tissues of Human System

Tissues	Elastic modulus (GPa)	Tensile strength (MPa)
Cortical bone	17.7	133
Cancellous bone	0.30	15
Enamel	85	11.5 transverse, 42.2 parallel
Dentine	32.4	44.4

[137,138,139,140].

TABLE 3.3. Composition of Bone

Organic—Collagen Fibres (Type 1)	16%
Mineral—Hydroxyapatite [Hap- Ca10(PO4)6(OH)2]	60%
Ground Substance	2%
Water	23%

[7].

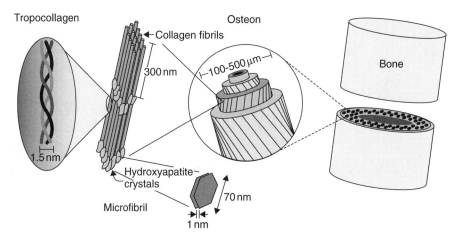

Figure 3.1. Schematic representation of a bone structure, showing the complexity of bone structure. (Reproduced from ref.[141])

vide the framework and architecture of bone, with HAp particles located between the fibers. The ground substance is formed from proteins, polysaccharides and mucopolysaccharides, which together act as cement. Except for these, the living portion, i.e., osteoblast, osteoclast and osteocytes, are present in the structure and such cells actually influence biological properties to a great extent. The detailed structure of a cortical bone is shown schematically in Figure 3.1. At the nano level structure, HAp nanoparticles (20–40 nm) are shown to be adhered and dispersed in the collagen matrix. At top level structure hierarchy, the three dimensional schematic of bone structure is also shown (Figure 3.1). It is quite evident that the synthetic materials cannot mimic such extremely complex structural hierarchy of bone. However, they can provide the bone's external properties to some extent. Another limitation of synthetic materials is that they can not repair themselves (wound healing) as living bone does.

Nevertheless, extensive efforts are still underway to develop and explore various material combinations in the attempt to develop biocompatible materials. The following sections present the structure and properties of Ca-P based materials.

3.4 PROCESSING AND PROPERTIES OF BIOCERAMICS AND BIOCERAMIC COMPOSITES

3.4.1 Calcium Phosphate Based Biomaterials

Calcium phosphate (CaP)-based ceramics offer great potential in many applications requiring bonding with the bone. The most popular bioactive calcium phosphate material is hydroxyapatite [with chemical composition of $Ca_{10}(PO_4)_6(OH)_2$], having similar mineral composition of bone and teeth. In Figure 3.2, the stability region of HAp in $CaO-P_2O_5-H_2O$ ternary system has been shown. A number of compounds with varying Ca/P ratio, belonging to CaP family, are of relevance to biomedical applications. These include octacalcium phosphate (OCP, Ca/P = 1.33), tricalcium phosphate (TCP, Ca/P = 1.5), HAp (Ca/P = 1.67) and tetracalcium phosphate (TTCP, Ca/P = 2). TCP can also exist in two polymorphs: α-TCP and β-TCP. While TCP and HAp are the commonly reported phases in CaP-based materials, *in vitro* or *in vivo* formation of OCP or other phases are also reported to a limited extent[10,11]. Between these two, α-TCP formation is favored at high

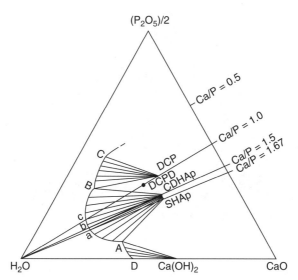

Figure 3.2. Ternary Phase diagram of $CaO-P_2O_5-H_2O$ ternary system showing the stability region of different CaP phases along with hydroxyapatite.

temperature. Also, Ca/P ratio of less than 1.0 is not biomedically important. It needs to be pointed out here that a number of literature reports has emphasized that nonstoichiometric HAp promotes better osteoconduction property[12].

Various attempts have been made to experimentally assess the cytocompatibility of CaP-based materials. For example, Suzuki et al.[13] showed that serum protein adsorbed on the surface of TCP-HAp ceramics appears to be effective in preventing cell rupture by functioning as an intermediate layer that prevents direct contact between cells and the unstable surface of the materials.

Chen et al.[14] investigated the bone bonding mechanism of crystalline HAp *in vivo*. It is reported that initially, a layer of amorphous HAp was formed on the HAp implant surface and a bone like apatite layer formed after three months, in between the implant and bone tissue. At a later stage (after six months), direct bone-HAp implant contact is established and collagen fiber enters inside the implant material. Therefore, the interface region shows good mechanical strength with the new bone apposition.

Xin et al.[15] compared the CaP formation behavior of few bioceramics *in vitro* (simulated body fluid) and *in vivo*. The investigated bioceramics include sintered porous solids, including bioglass, glass-ceramics, hydroxyapatite, α-tricalcium phosphate and β-tricalcium phosphate. The presence of octacalcium phosphate was observed on all types of bioceramic surfaces *in vitro* and *in vivo*, except on β-TCP. They concluded that Ca-P formation on bioceramic surfaces is more difficult *in vivo* than *in vitro*.

In an interesting study, Dong et al.[16] investigated the effect of low pressure during culture on the bone formation of osteoblast/porous hydroxyapatite composite *in vivo*. Scanning electron microscopy (SEM) observations (Figure 3.3)

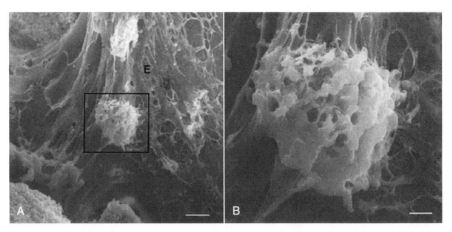

Figure 3.3. A) SEM images of cross-sections of osteoblast-HAp composites after two weeks of implantation. The pore surface is covered by round cells as well as collagenous extracellular matrix. E indicates collagenous extracellular matrix. Bar = 37.5 mm. B) Higher magnification of the large rectangular area in A. Round cells of active osteoblast, can be seen on the surface of HAp. Bar = 5 μm[16].

indicate the formation of mineralized collagenous extracellular matrix as well as active osteoblast in HAp/BMO composite at two weeks after implantation. It was concluded that the application of low-pressure system to subculture of bone cells to porous HAp blocks is beneficial to increase bone tissue formation *in vivo*.

Gatti et al.[17] compared the bone in growth on implantation of HAp and TCP granules. They claimed that the TCP granules induce total bone growth after four months of implantation, whereas HAp granules crumbled and no new bone induction was seen even 12 months after implantation. Such observation with HAp granules in the biological fluid was attributed to the scant cohesive strength among the particles.

Blacik et al.[18] conducted the weight bearing study of porous HAp/TCP (60/40) ceramics, implanted as intramedullary fixation in segmental bone defects in rabbit bone. They found that these ceramics are limited in their ability to treat load-bearing segmental bone defects, but no failure was observed at the early stages of implantation. However, additional internal fixation should be used when immediate mobilization and load bearing is required.

Fini et al.[19] studied the effect of pulse electromagnetic fields (PEMF) on the osteointegration of hydroxyapatite implants in cancellous bone. They found that PEMFs enhanced early HAp osteointegration in the trabecular bone of healthy rabbits and were associated with a higher degree of bone mineralization and maturation, which was also maintained for six week and three week periods of non-stimulation.

It is known that microstructure plays an important role in mechanical properties, and therefore a study was conducted to assess such effect in the implanted material *in vivo*. Okuda et al.[20] observed the effect of the microstructure of β-tricalcium phosphate on the metabolism of subsequently formed bone tissue. Comparing rod shaped and globular shaped particles, it was argued that rod shaped β-TCP possibly helped to stimulate osteoblastic activity. There have been some reports, mostly from the research group of Webster, that the presence of increased grain boundaries enhances osteoblast cell adhesion. However, the authors' recent study on thermally etched surfaces of sintered HAp shows that L929 fibroblast cells spread across the grains in a significant manner (see Figure 3.4). Such aspect requires further study in this direction to confirm the microstructural aspect on cell adhesion.

From the preceding discussion, it is clear that HAp is a highly biocompatible and bioactive material the dissociation of HAp to TCP has been a major processing challenge. Nevertheless, an optimal presence of TCP, in particular 60:40 ratio of HAp:TCP is an ideal example of biphasic calcium phosphate (BCP) ceramics, which can exhibit good combination of controlled biodegradation and bioactivity. A subsequent chapter by Daculsi and co-workers introduces the concept of the development of BCP ceramics as well as their processing and properties.

Despite good biocompatibility property, pure HAp has very poor mechanical properties (Table 3.1) and therefore cannot be used in load bearing applications. The use of HAp is limited by bone filler application, mostly as porous HAp block. Consequently, hydroxyapatite needs to be used in combination with

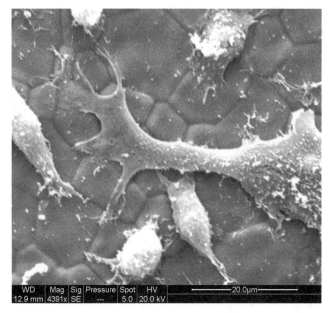

Figure 3.4. Mouse fibroblast (L929) cell adhesion on thermally etched hydroxyapatite surface showing no such difference in cell adhesion on grain and grain boundary region.

another material to develop bulk composite material with good mechanical properties (see Table 3.1) or used as a coating on biomaterial. Some examples are hydroxyapatite coating on metal[21,22], alumina-hydroxyapatite composite[23,24], zirconia hydroxyapatite[25,26] composite. In the last decade, researchers have attempted to develop biocomposites by combining bioactive HAp with bioinert ceramic phase, like Al_2O_3 or ZrO_2.

3.4.2 Hydroxyapatite-Ceramic Composites

Zirconia, irrespective of its morphology and phase composition, did not induce the decomposition of hydroxyapatite matrix in the hot pressed HAp–ZrO_2 composites[27]. Improvements in toughness and strength achieved for HAp–ZrO_2 composites were not accompanied by an increase in the Weibull modulus (an indicator of strength reliability for brittle ceramics). In a different study, HAp–Al_2O_3 composites of functionally graded structure can be fabricated by the underwater-shock compaction technique without the use of any sintering-aid[28]. The composite showed continuous compositional variation after heat treatment up to 1200 °C. Hill and Clifford observed that HAp decomposes at 950 °C[29] and accordingly, sintering experiments were carried out using flurohydroxyapatite (FHA), while replacing HAp. It was found that FHA has better thermal stability than HAp and it can be sintered at 1400 °C[30] with 40% ZrO_2 without dissociation. Also, the biocompatibility of FHA is comparable with pure HAp.

Another study[31] revealed that HAp in HAp-ZrO_2-Al_2O_3 nano-composites formed biphasic calcium phosphate (BCP) when hot pressed at 1400 °C. BCP is reported to have high biocompatibility. Recently, BCP ceramics have received increased attention as an ideal bone substitute due to its controlled degradability[32]. Any composite that shows superior mechanical and physical properties and is also biodegradable would be the material of choice in near future. The literature report indicates that it is possible to alter HAp:TCP ratio to form BCP of desired properties[32]. In one of the earlier studies, it was observed that 10 wt% phosphate glass additions to HAp-composites leads to partial dissociation of HAp to TCP[33]. By varying the glass addition, the resorption of TCP can be controlled. Suchanek and co-workers[34] developed HAp-HAp_w (whisker) composite, which was hot pressed at 1000–1100 °C. Despite the use of whiskers as a toughening agent, the toughness of HAp-HAp_w (10% addition) could be increased to 1.1 MPa$m^{0.5}$ under optimal processing conditions. It is, however, possible that toughness could be further improved with increase in whisker addition, but such experiments are not conducted as yet.

The following discusses the processing-property results, obtained with several CaP-based biocomposites. In the authors' recent investigation[35], they synthesized HAp-Mullite composite, which was densified successfully by pressureless sintering and without any sintering additives. Detailed analysis revealed that dissociation of HAp to TCP depends on sintering temperature as well as mullite content. Higher mullite containing (>20 wt%) samples are more prone towards dissociation. β and α-TCP are the main phases along with mullite for higher mullite content samples. Both solid state and liquid phase sintering guided the densification mechanism towards dense, crack, pore free body. Limited reaction between Mullite and CaO produce grain boundary alumino-silicate phases. Mullite grains grow anistropically (needle shaped) because of liquid phase sintering. The transmission electron microscopy (TEM) images in Figure 3.5, show the presence of mullite needle in HAp/TCP matrix. X-ray diffraction (XRD) patterns of HAp-30 wt% mullite and HAp-10 wt% mullite, sintered at 1350 °C along with ball-milled powder are shown in Figure 3.6, which shows that HAp is predominantly present along with α-TCP in case HAp-10 wt% mullite. In contrast, in case of 30 wt% mullite, the major phase is β-TCP. This newly developed material could be appropriate for bone replacement material.

3.4.3 Hydroxyapatite-Titanium Composites

Besides the development of HAp-based bioceramic composites, efforts have been put forward to fabricate a HAp-metal particulate composite with better mechanical properties. Wataria et al.[36] fabricated Ti/HAp functionally-graded materials (FGM) specimens using Spark Plasma Sintering (SPS). The optimization of both mechanical and biological properties was also pursued. SPS processed Ti/HAp FGM showed that the maturation of newly formed bone was preceded in the HAp-rich region. The gradient functions in the biochemical affinity to osteogenesis and the mechanical properties with stress relaxation in

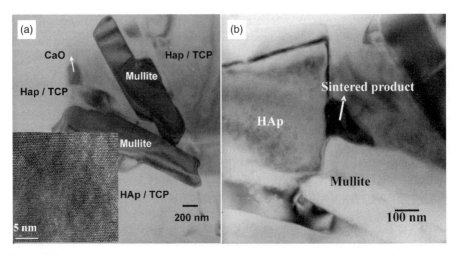

<u>Figure 3.5.</u> (a) Low magnification bright field TEM image of HAp-10 wt% mullite, sintered at 1350 °C, showing typical mullite needle along with HAp phase. (b) Higher magnification image, showing the presence of sintered product at the mullite–HAp interface[35].

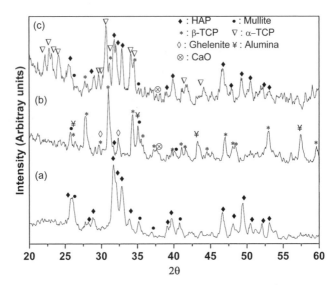

<u>Figure 3.6.</u> X-ray diffraction pattern of (a) ball milled powder of HAp-30 wt% mullite composite mixture, (b) HAp-30 wt% mullite composite (sintered at 1350 °C for 2 hrs in air) and (c) HAp-10 wt% mullite composite (sintered at 1350 °C for 2 hrs in air)[35].

Ti/HAp FGM could attain the efficient biocompatibility for implant. The study demonstrated that the tissue reaction changes gradually in response to the gradient composition or structure of materials. This study thus implies the possibility to control the tissue response by functionally graded structure of biomaterials.

Ning et al.[37] showed that the biocomposite, fabricated from HAp and Ti powders by powder metallurgy technique, has the ability to induce apatite nucleation and growth on its surface when immersed in SBF solution. Among all the crystal phases in the as-fabricated composite, Ti_2O has the ability to induce apatite formation. Furthermore, the dissolved CaO phase also provides favorable conditions for the apatite nucleation and growth.

In a recent study on HAp-Ti system (sinter at 1200 °C), the composite with a lower initial Ti content contains major crystalline phases of $CaTiO_3$, CaO and Ti_xP_y. On increasing the initial Ti content to 50 vol%, Ti_2O and residual α-Ti were also observed. Further increase in initial Ti content resulted in a composite with only α-Ti as main crystalline phase. TCP-TiO_2 biocomposites[38], with a controlled α: β-TCP ratio, can be obtained by varying the heat-treatment conditions.

In order to make a comprehensive study on processing-microstructure-physical and biological property correlationship, HAp-Ti composites are sintered at different temperature (1000–1400 °C) in different atmospheres like argon, hydrogen and air[39]. The sintering reactions of air sintered samples were analyzed by thermodynamic consideration, which successfully describe the oxidation of Ti (TiO_2 formation), followed by dissociation of HAp and the formation of $CaTiO_3$. The experimental results clearly reveal that sintering of various HAp-Ti compositions leads to TCP/HAp-TiO_2 microstructure with little traces of $CaTiO_3$ and CaO in some of the sintered samples. The microstructural analysis indicated abnormal grain growth of monolithic HAp, when sintered at a temperature higher than 1200 °C.

For various HAp-Ti compositions, the characteristic presence of a larger TiO_2 lump, surrounded by coarser TCP phase, is also recorded. In case of samples, sintered in argon atmosphere, HAp-5 wt% Ti exhibits better results in terms of densification and mechanical properties. The hardness values were in the range of 4–6 GPa, which is better than air sintered samples (2–4 GPa). Also, in argon atmosphere, retention of Ti is possible along with undissociated HAp phase (up to 10 wt% Ti addition to HAp). In contrast, sintering in H_2 atmosphere could not prevent the oxidation of Ti and HAp dissociation. For example, HAp-40 wt% Ti sample, sintered at 1400 °C in H_2 atmosphere, contain only single phase $CaTiO_3$. Even the densification process was hindered by high temperature chemical reactions and the formation of gaseous reaction products.

Cell culture experiments on air sintered samples using L929 fibroblast cells provide clear evidences of cell adhesion and cell proliferation on HAp-Ti composites. The general observation has been that the cells are attached closely with neighboring cells, and thereby, form a cellular network (characteristic of fibroblast type cells) on the composite surface (Figure 3.7). The observation of cellular bridges i.e., cell-cell interaction as well as flattening of the cells indicate good cytocompatibility property of the developed composite (see Figure 3.7). Importantly, the addition of bioinert Ti (up to 30 wt%) does not show any degradation in cell adhesion properties.

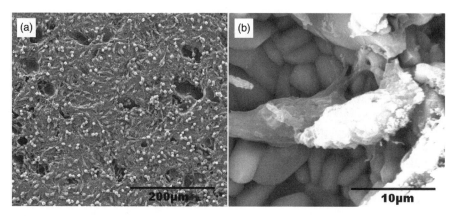

Figure 3.7. SEM images, revealing the adherence of L929 mouse fibroblast cells seeded for 24 hours on HAp-20Ti (a) & (b)[39].

3.4.4   Glass-Ceramics Based Biomaterials

Glass ceramics are the polycrystalline materials, which are formed during prolonged heat treatment of glass at elevated temperature (above glass transition temperature (T_g)). This is an alternative route for synthesizing polycrystalline ceramics. The amount of crystalline ceramic phase may vary between 50–99 vol%. The important advantage of this route is that an almost pore-free body can be fabricated, which is otherwise difficult to produce by sintering route.

In the last decade, a number of glass-ceramic systems are being researched for their biomedical, in particular, dental restoration applications. It can be recalled here that human teeth act as a mechanical device during masticatory processes such as cutting, tearing, and grinding of food particles. Teeth get damaged or worn away with age and therefore, partial or total replacement of human teeth with a suitable biocompatible material is required.

3.4.4.1   Mica Based Glass Ceramics. In recent times, the research on the development of new dental restoratives has attracted wider attention, both in the materials community as well as among dentists. It was also recognized that bioceramic materials with enhanced mechanical, chemical, and tribological properties are believed to be a potential material for dental restoration purposes if their machinability problem can be countered. In this context, machinable mica-based glass ceramics appear to be a feasible solution to fabricate an all-ceramic dental implant. The researchers in the authors' group[40] carried out a systematic study to understand the influence of varying heat treatment conditions on SiO_2-MgO-Al_2O_3-K_2O-B_2O_3-F (46SiO_2, 16MgO, 17Al_2O_3, 10K_2O, 7B_2O_3, 4F) glass-ceramic system by adopting two sets of heat treatment experiments. In this study, critical single stage heat treatment experiments were performed at 1000 °C for varying soaking time of 8–24 hours with 4 hours time interval and as a function of temperature for 4 hours in the temperature range of 1000–1120 °C

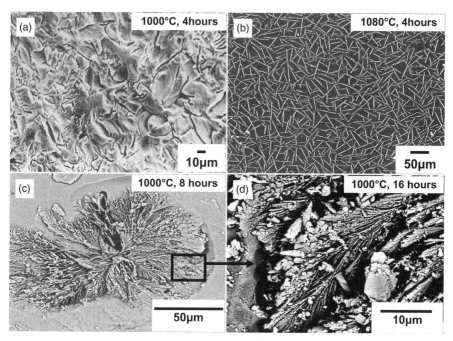

Figure 3.8. SEM mages of glass ceramics samples (SiO$_2$-MgO-Al$_2$O$_3$-K$_2$O-B$_2$O$_3$-F) heat treated at (a) 1000 °C, 4 hours, showing no sign of crystallinity, (d) 1120 °C, 4 hours showing usual randomly oriented interlocked mica flakes. (c) SEM images of time variation samples (heat treated at 1000 °C), showing single "Butterfly" shaped crystals (soaking time 8 hours) (d) "Tree leave" structure at the end of each mica rod (soaking time 16 hours)[40].

with 40 °C temperature interval with heating rate of 10 °C/min for both sets of experiments.

The results of critical heat treatment experiments have revealed scientifically interesting information about the crystal growth mechanisms. Figure 3.8 shows the microstructures of glass and glass ceramic, heat treated at different temperatures of up to 1120 °C for four hours. The microstructure is characterized by interlocked, randomly oriented mica plates when heat treated at different temperature. When the base glass is heat treated for longer time period, such as more than four hours, a new type of crystal morphology appears, whose growth pattern can be approximately described by spherulitic-dendritic like crystallization habit. Image "c" and "d" in Figures 3.8 represent the morphology of a novel shaped crystal, which has a "butterfly" like pattern with mica rods radiating from a central nucleus.

The possible mechanism for the development of this unusual microstructure is discussed with reference to a nucleation-growth kinetics based model. The activation energy for crystal nucleation and Avrami index are computed to be 388 KJ/mol and 1.3 respectively, assuming Johnson-Mehl-Avrami model of crystallization. Another important result is that a maximum of around 70% crystalline phase ("butterfly" morphology) can be obtained after heat treatment at 1000 °C for 24 hours, while a lower amount (~58%) of interlocked plate like mica crystals is formed after heat treatment at 1040 °C for four hours. Also, the glass ceramics with plate-like crystals exhibited the highest hardness of 5.5 GPa. In a recent study[41] on slightly different compositions (48.94SiO_2, 17.45MgO, 16.29Al_2O_3, 7.15K_2O, 5.25B_2O_3, and 3.85F) of same glass ceramics with suitable heat treatment schedule showed much improved hardness (~8 GPa).

The chemical durability of dental ceramics is an important property that affects their clinical performances. This is due to the fact that they are constantly exposed to various aqueous environments. The *in vitro* dissolution tests of similar glass composition were carried out by immersing the selected glass ceramic samples in artificial saliva (AS) for various time periods of up to six weeks. SEM images and SEM-EDS analysis of the surface of the sample immersed in AS for different time periods of two, three and six weeks were taken in order to assess the extent of Ca-P layer formation on the surface. Figure 3.9 shows the spherical particles of diameter 2–3 μm on the surface after six weeks of immersion in AS. EDS analysis of spherical particles indicates the strong peaks of Ca, P and O, thereby confirming the formation of Ca-P compounds. Further, the analysis of EDS data indicate that the composition of those spherical brighter contrasting particles, which cover the majority of surface area, can be characterized by Ca-P ratio of 1.57 (average). Ca-P is a highly bioactive material and therefore the formation of these layers on the glass ceramics sample will increase its bioactivity.

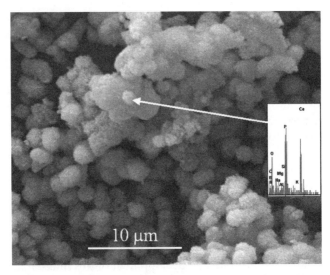

Figure 3.9. SEM observation of glass-ceramic surface (SiO_2-MgO-Al_2O_3-K_2O-B_2O_3-F, heat treated at 1040 °C for 12 hours), after immersing in AS solution for 6 weeks. EDS analysis of the spherical particles is shown inset[41].

3.4.4.2 *Other Bioglass-Ceramics.*

Besides Macor-based glass ceramics, several other glass ceramics were developed in the last few decades. Among various glass ceramic materials, 45S5 glass, originally invented by Hench & co-workers, is known to be the best bioactive glass material[42]. Its typical composition[43] is SiO_2: 46.1, P_2O_5: 2.6, CaO: 26.9, Na_2O: 24.4. A recent study by Chevalier & co-workers[44] report crystallization kinetics of 45S5 glass. It is known that 45S5 glass undergoes a series of structural transformations, leading to the formation of $Na_2CaSi_2O_6$ crystals at 610 °C. However, poor mechanical properties and lack of machinability has been a major concern for 45S5 glass. Therefore, these materials cannot be used for dental applications or any biomedical applications requiring the complex shape.

Besides 45S5 glass, Bioverit® I base glass has wider clinical applications including the possibility of using Bioverit II base glass as a matrix for Ti particle reinforced composite coatings[45]. The coatings were prepared by a single step vacuum plasma spray method on Ti-6Al-4V substrates. The mechanical characterization showed a good adherence of the coatings to the substrate and the toughening effect of the dispersed Ti particles.

In another study, Bioverit® III base glass- and glass-ceramic matrix/Ti particles composites were prepared by means of a simple pressureless sintering method[46]. The sintering process was carefully optimized by means of differential scanning calorimetry (DSC) and hot stage microscopy. The optimized sintering conditions were accomplished by a viscous flow process, obtaining nearly full density amorphous matrix composites that were subsequently ceramised to obtain glass-ceramic matrix composites. Better mechanical properties were exhibited by both the glass- and glass-ceramic matrix composites when compared with the corresponding pure matrices. Such a comparison was also found true for the glass-ceramic matrix composite, when compared with the glass-matrix. The cell growth of fibroblasts on the surface of the glass-ceramic matrix composites confirms their biocompatibility.

In a different system, complex reactions between Ti and hydroxyapatite occurred during the sintering of Ti/HAp/BG composites[47]. Moreover, the addition of bioactive glass to Ti/HAp showed little effect on the phase components of the composites. Bioverit®III glass-ceramic matrix/Y-PSZ particulate composites, successfully prepared by means of pressureless sintering, also confirmed the toughening effect of the Y-PSZ particles[48].

A different study reported that highly dense (>98% of relative density) Si_3N_4–bioglass composite[49] has potential advantage of each constituent, that is, the high fracture toughness of Si_3N_4 with the bioactivity of a bioglass. The most significant feature concerning the mechanical properties of this new biomaterial composite is the improvement in fracture toughness (4.4 MPam$^{1/2}$) and bending strength (383 ± 47 MPa) with respect to currently used mechanical bioceramics, glasses and glass ceramics for load bearing applications. However, a detailed biocompatibility study on Si_3N_4/bioglass composite is yet to be carried out. Barrors et al.[50] investigated the *in vivo* bone tissue response of another fluoride containing canasite glass-ceramic ($0.47K_2O$ $0.94Na_2O$ $1.42CaO$ $5.67SiO_2$ $1.5CaF_2$).

Hydroxyapatite was used as control sample for this experiment. The canasite formulation evaluated was not osteoconductive and appeared to degrade in the biological environment. It was therefore concluded that the canasite formulation used was unsuitable for use as implant.

3.4.5 Bioinert Ceramics

This section discusses, bioinert materials and their application areas. The use of carbon and inert glass fibers have important applications[51] for their typical anisotropic properties. These engineering fibers have been mainly used as a reinforcement for orthopaedic devices, such as femoral hip stems, knee prosthesis and fracture fixation plates. Because of the inability of carbon and inert glass to form any bioactive bonds, they have not been used in bone analogue materials. Also, the carbon-based composites, used for articulating surfaces, are reported to have a tendency to cause inflammatory problems due to the loss of carbon particles[52].

One potential bioinert ceramic, that is, Al_2O_3, showed good performance *in vivo*, although the low fracture toughness (3–4 MPam$^{1/2}$) typically restricts its use in demanding applications. On the other hand, tetragonal zirconia ceramic (8–11 MPam$^{1/2}$) has a better edge over alumina. Various attempts have however been made to toughen Al_2O_3 by adding monoclinic ZrO_2, partially stabilized ZrO_2 (PSZ), and so on. This leads to the development of zirconia-toughened alumina[53]. Dense ZTA has considerably better toughness[54] and wear resistance[55,56] than monolithic alumina. Although ceramic composite materials have potential use in load-bearing orthopedic applications, very few materials have been tested clinically so far.

In an important investigation, Hayashi et al.[57] studied the *in vivo* response of bioinert ceramics such as alumina ceramic (99.5% purity Al_2O_3), zirconia ceramic (5 wt% Y_2O_3 stabilized ZrO_2), SUS316L stainless steel (Fe: 65%: Cr: 18%; Ni: 13%; Mo: 2%; Mn: 2%). The results were compared with dense sintered hydroxyapatite (HAp). The push out test results revealed the bone-implant interface shear strength for alumina, zirconia, steel and HAp as ~0.8, 0.9, 0.5, 12.1 MPa, respectively. It was concluded that the bioinert ceramics should not be used as a bone bonding material, but as the material for the articulating surface.

Colon et al.[58] described the function of osteoblast and staphylococcus epidermidis on nanophase ZnO and TiO_2 inert bioceramics. It was evident from their result that nanophase ceramics (ZnO, TiO_2) had decreased staphylococcus epidermidis adhesion and increased osteoblast adhesion in comparison to macropahse materials.

Among the stabilized zirconia ceramics, Y-TZP (yttria doped tetragonal zirconia polycrystal) has been the most attractive material in terms of toughness and structural properties. However, the leaching of yttria in humid environments and related degradation in properties have been a major bottleneck for wider applications of Y-TZP. To this end, PSZ (Mg, Ca-doped) has several advantages and such systems offer opportunities to control microstructure by tailoring a combination of sintering and subsequent annealing conditions. The authors' recent investigation[59,60] on Ca and Mg-doped zirconia reveals that 8 mol% CaO-doped PSZ ceramics possess 97.5% ρ_{th} and 16 mol% CaO-doped FSZ possess only 91.6% ρ_{th}, whereas more than 95% ρ_{th} in both Mg-PSZ and Mg-FSZ can be obtained, when all are microwave (MW) sintered at 1585 °C for one hour. The microstructure of Ca-PSZ ceramic is characterized by bimodal grain size distribution of coarser m-ZrO_2 grains, embedded in cubic matrix. The optimized microstructure of both Mg-PSZ and Mg-FSZ samples are characterized by the presence of coarser grains with size in the range of 5–10 μm. The obtained microstructure is superior compared to conventional sintering route, which normally results in grain sizes of 20–50 μm.

SEM investigation also shows the presence of microporosity (<10 μm), trapped at both intragranular as well as intergranular regions. XRD analysis reveals that MW sintered Ca-FSZ contains predominantly c-ZrO_2 phase, whereas the presence of monoclinic zirconia was recorded as a predominant phase in Mg-PSZ samples. Although for FSZ samples, the predominant phase is cubic, except for samples sintered at 1500 °C, for which the major phase is m-ZrO_2. The optimized Ca-PSZ and Ca-FSZ ceramics exhibit Vickers hardness of around 10 GPa and 9 GPa, respectively; whereas the toughness was measured for Ca-PSZ as 6 MPam$^{0.5}$. Similarly, Mg-PSZ ceramics, sintered at 1585 °C possess a better combination of hardness (10.6 GPa) and fracture toughness (6.8 MPa m$^{0.5}$).

Apart from microstructural investigation and mechanical property measurement, the tribological properties in dry and simulated body fluid were also evaluated. For both Mg and Ca-doped ZrO_2, a steady state COF of ~0.5 against bearing steel ball is measured in dry condition and shows lower values (~0.35–0.4) in SBF lubrication contact. The wear mechanism is dominated by the formation of Fe_xO_y-rich tribochemical layer, which was in contact with steel counterbody after the steady state was attained. In the case of SBF medium, such tribochemical layer additionally contains chloride compound. SEM images of the worn surfaces on CaO doped zirconia are shown in Figure 3.10 and the formation of a tribochemical layer is evident.

The investigated CaO/MgO doped materials experience wear rate in the order of 10^{-5} mm^3/Nm (in air) and 10^{-6} to 10^{-7} mm^3/Nm (in SBF) with the lowest wear rate recorded with FSZ materials in SBF solution. The tribochemical layers appear to form on abraded surface and thereby, reduce the material damage from continued wear process. From the above, it should be clear that the optimized MgO-doped or CaO-doped ZrO_2 exhibit much better combination of mechanical properties, when compared to bioinert Al_2O_3 or majority of the glass ceramics and their composites. However, further experiments to study cytotoxicity property and clinical trials need to be conducted on these materials to assess their potential for biomedical applications. The above results also demonstrate the efficacy of MW sintering as a processing tool to fabricate bioceramics with comparable or better processed materials (pressureless sintering and post fabrication annealing).

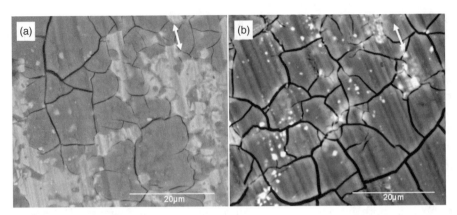

Figure 3.10. SEM images of worn surfaces of Ca-FSZ ceramics (MW, 1585 °C) (a) and that on Ca-PSZ ceramic (b) after testing against steel in SBF. The double pointed arrow indicates fretting direction. Fretting conditions: 10^5 cycles, 10 Hz frequency, 10 N load and 80 μm stroke length. Counterbody: 6 mm diameter steel ball[59].

In their recent work, González et al.[61] described the method of synthesizing bio-silicon carbide (SiC) from plants and also proved the biocompatibility of this new generation of biomaterials by *in vitro* and *in vivo* experiments. For their work, they chose specific plant species as templates whose chemical composition can be changed by some specific transformation method while maintaining the original biostructure. By this method, it is possible to develop lightweight and high-strength scaffolds for bone substitution. Their *in vitro* and *in vivo* experiments demonstrated how the plant species became colonized by the hosting bone tissue due to its unique interconnected hierarchic porosity.

3.5 POLYMERIC BIOMATERIALS

Polymers are useful in different engineering applications due to their light weight, low COF ductility and easy formability/moldability. However, polymers lack high E-modulus, hardness and strength compared to ceramics and metals. Few of the polymers possess good biocompatible properties that could be exploited in designing several biomaterials. The following overview reviews selected polymers and their composites that were extensively used and investigated as hard tissue biomaterials over the last few decades.

Major advantages of polymers are their attractive properties and availability in a wide variety of composition, and forms (solid, fibers, fabrics, films and gels). Polymeric materials can be broadly classified as thermoplastics and thermosets. For example, HDPE and PEEK are examples of thermoplastics, while SR, PDMS, PMMA are examples of thermosets[62]. Despite their good biocompatibility, many of the polymeric materials are mainly used for soft tissue replacement (such as skin, blood vessel, cartilage, ligament replacement etc).

TABLE 3.4. Mechanical Properties of Different Synthetic Biopolymers which could be Used as Hard Tissue Replacement

Materials	Elastic modulus (GPa)	Tensile strength (MPa)
HDPE	0.88	35
PTFE	0.5	27.5
PA	2.1	67
PMMA	2.55	59
PET	2.85	61
PEEK	8.3	139
PS	2.65	75

The combination of modulus and strength properties of most of the polymers, as summarized in Table 3.4, do not meet the lower bound requirement of natural cortical bone (Table 3.2).

Low stiffness (E-modulus) and high wear rate does not permit their use as load-bearing hard tissue applications (such as bone, teeth, joint, and so on). Hence, a new approach to the design of implanted biomaterials with tailor-made properties is attempted for various polymer biocomposite materials[63]. The polymer biocomposite materials consist of one or more reinforcing phases (ceramics, metals and polymers) in a polymer matrix. These composites are considered as an alternative choice to overcome various shortcomings of homogeneous polymers. Besides significant improvement in creep, fatigue resistance and other mechanical properties, one major advantage of polymer biocomposites[64] is their radio transparency and non-magnetic features. Such combinations of properties allows them to be scanned by various modern imaging and modern diagnostic methods, like computer tomography (CT) and magnetic resonance imaging (MRI). This feature has broadened the application area of polymeric materials to cranial implants as well.

3.5.1 Polymer-Polymer Composites

Polymer–polymer composite has important commercial implications, as new materials are being developed for various hard tissue replacements (acetabular cup, knee replacement). Examples of few new polymer–polymer composites include CF/UHMWPE, PET/PU, CF/C, CF/PEEK, CF/PMMA, PS/CF, etc[65]. One attractive aspect of the composite approach is the ability to control properties via several variables. Important variables that can be adjusted to control properties include:

a) type of continuous phase matrix,
b) type of polymer particles,
c) particle size distribution and
d) number of reinforcing phases[66].

The fabrication of synthetic analogues of bone is a great challenge to material scientists. As mentioned in section 3.3, bone itself is a composite material in nature with a polymeric phase collagen.

In THR applications, one of the major problems arises with the mismatching of stiffness of the prosthesis and the femur bone. The metal stem has five to six times higher stiffness than host bones, which causes stress shielding problem[67,68,69]. As a solution, some researchers introduced CF/PS[70] and CF/C[71] polymer composites to replace the metal stem. Improved creep property, more strength, and moderate stiffness are the major characteristics of this type of polymer composites. To mimic the mechanical properties of the femur bone, the use of another polymer composite, such as CF/PEEK stem prosthesis, are successfully achieved[72,73,74]. A few examples of other polymers for THR application include CF/Epoxy, CF/C, and CF/PE, and so on. However, lower stiffness, E-modulus, and poor mechanical strength associated with polymer composites implants limits their long-term use as suitable bone replacement materials. To overcome this problem, ceramic–polymer composites have been developed as hard tissue replacement materials[75].

3.5.2   Polymer-Ceramic Composites

Major advantages of the ceramic materials are their good biocompatibility, high hardness and improved corrosion and wear-resistance properties. However, a large mismatch in E modulus (stiffness) between the hard tissue and ceramic implant materials effectively caused stress shielding or stress protection problems, as the bone is insufficiently loaded compared to the implanted materials[76]. Also, the stress shielding affects the healing and remodeling process, leading to a decrease in bone density. This is because of the fact that bone growing cells (osteoblast) progressively become less productive and form a lower strength porous bone, which is called trabecular or cancellous bone.

Another major shortcoming of ceramic biomaterials is their lower fracture toughness value, which limits their use as load-bearing implant materials. In this case, low modulus materials, such as polymers could be combined with ceramic to obtain combination of desired material properties. Building on several years of research, HAp/HDPE, SiO_2/silicone rubber, HAp/EVA, BCP/PMMA, HAp/PLA, HAp/PEEK, bioactive glass/PMMA, nano-HAp/Poly (hexamethylene adipamide) composite materials are being developed[77].

Among various ceramic containing polymer biocomposites, hydroxyapatite reinforced HDPE composites are extensively studied for their potential use as hard tissue replacement materials and has been successfully used in orbital surgery and developed as an analogue material for bone replacement. The closer property matching of HAp/HDPE composite (E Modulus: 2–5 GPa, Tensile strength: 18–25 MPa) to bone, reduces the problem of bone resorption, which is associated with the use of metal/ceramic implants.

Bonfield et al.[78] was the first to develop hydroxyapatite reinforced high density polyethylene (HDPE) biomaterial for skeletal applications and coined a trade name HAPEX™ for HAp/HDPE composite. In a refined processing route,

Bonfield used coupling agents, such as 3-trimethoxysiyl propylmethacrylate for HAp and acrylic acid for HDPE, to improve bonding (by both chemical adhesion and mechanical coupling) between HAp and HDPE. The improvement in bonding resulted in enhanced ductility and tensile strength. In the case of untreated composite, only mechanical bonding exists at the filler-matrix interface, which resulted from the shrinkage of HDPE around individual HAp particles during thermal processing.

Bonfield et al.[79] also reported an optimum combination of mechanical and biological performance with HAp/HDPE composite containing 40 vol% of HAp. An *in vitro* cell culture study showed that 40 vol% HAp/HDPE composite enhanced cellular activity by increasing proliferation rate and differentiation compared to the 20 vol% HAp/HDPE composite[80]. The extensive mechanical measurements reveal the tensile strength, E-modulus and strain-to-failure for surface-treated composite to be 23.2 MPa, 3.9 GPa and 6.8%, while that of untreated composite to be 20.7 MPa, 4.3 GPa and 2.6%, respectively[81].

In a subsequent work, *in vitro* study revealed that HAPEX™ attached directly to a bone by chemical bonding (bioactive fixation), rather than forming fibrous encapsulation (morphological fixation). The effect of HAp particle size on the polymer-ceramic composite properties was also investigated by various researchers[82]. It was found that HAp particles (finer) reinforced HDPE exhibited higher E-modulus and hardness. It has been observed that the mechanical properties were significantly increased with an increase in HAp volume fraction, while fracture strain decreased. The tribological properties (that is, wear rate and coefficient of friction) of unfilled HDPE and HAp/HDPE composites were investigated[83] against duplex stainless steel on a tri-pin-on-disc tribometer under dry and lubricated conditions using distilled water, aqueous solution of protein (egg albumen) and glucose as lubricants. In general, HAp/HDPE composite exhibited a lower COF (~0.02–0.04) compared to unfilled HDPE (~0.035–0.045). The composite with 10 vol% of HAp was found to exhibit improved friction and wear behavior.

Recently, many researchers are attempting to improve the mechanical properties of the HDPE-based composites with minimal compromise on the biocompatibility component, by incorporating other ceramic phases into the polymer matrix[84]. The partial replacement of HAp filler particles with PSZ particles led to an increase in the strength and fracture toughness of HAp/HDPE composites. The compressive stress, set up by the volume expansion associated with tetragonal to monoclinic phase transformation of PSZ, inhibits or retards the crack propagation within the composite. This results in an enhanced fracture toughness of the HAp/ZrO$_2$/HDPE composite[85].

In another study, Al$_2$O$_3$, a bioinert material, has been investigated to replace ZrO$_2$ in the HAp/ZrO$_2$/HDPE composite. The excellent mechanical properties and chemical properties of Al$_2$O$_3$ with respect to HAp are considered as a new trend in designing a polymer-ceramic biocomposite[86]. Other HAp-polymer composites used in hard tissue replacements are HAp/PEEK[87,88,89], HAp/EVA[90], and nano HAp/poly (hexamethylene adipamide)[91] composite.

Hasegawa et al.[92] studied *in vivo*, spanning over a period of 5–7 years, high-strength HAp/poly(L-lactide) composite rods for the internal fixation of bone fractures. In this work, uncalcined HAp (u-HAp) and calcined HAp (c-HAp) were used as reinforcing phases in PLLA matrix. The u-HAp and c-HAP rods were implanted in the femurs of 25 rabbits. The samples were collected after the natural death of the rabbits. It was found that the implanted materials were re-sorbed after six years of implantation. The presence of remodeled bone and tra-becular bone bonding were the significant outcome. Osteolytic and osteoarthritis problem was not observed.

Another possible application of polymer matrix composite could be cranial implants. Itokawa et al.[93] reported the results of an *in vivo* study (spanning over a year) on the response of bone to a hydroxyapatite–polymethylmethacrylate cra-nioplasty composite. New bone formation was observed after 12 and 24 weeks of implantation. After one year, the presence of new bone formation was seen at the interface region.

3.5.2.1 *HDPE-HAp-Al₂O₃ Hybrid Composites.*

3.5.2.1 *HDPE-HAp-Al₂O₃ Hybrid Composites.* In a recent approach by Basu and his coworkers[94], HDPE-HAp-Al$_2$O$_3$ composites were developed and the mechanical, tribological and cell adhesion properties evaluated. This work demonstrated how the stiffness and hardness as well as the biocompatibility prop-erty of bioinert High density Polyethylene (HDPE) can be significantly improved by the combined addition of both bioinert and bioactive ceramic fillers. In the work of Basu et al., HDPE/HAp/Al$_2$O$_3$ biocomposites with various compositions were processed at the optimized compression molding condition (130 °C, 0.5 h, 92 MPa pressure). The microstructural analysis confirms homogeneous distribu-tion of finer ceramic fillers (2–5 μm) in HDPE matrix.

Importantly, higher elastic modulus (6.2 GPa) and improved hardness (226.5 MPa) were obtained with the HDPE/20 vol% HAp/20 vol% Al$_2$O$_3$ com-posite. The simultaneous addition of Al$_2$O$_3$ and HAp leads to an improvement in mechanical properties, when compared to that of HDPE-20 vol% Al$_2$O$_3$ (H$_v$-131.1 MPa, E-modulus-2.7 GPa) or HDPE/20 vol% HAp (H$_v$-129.5 MPa, E-modulus-2.4 GPa).

Another important result was that the maximum hardness (252 MPa) and elastic modulus (7.1 GPa) have been attained in case of 40 vol% Al$_2$O$_3$ reinforced HDPE composite (without any HAp).

The above experimental results also required an assessment as to whether or not good tribological properties of HDPE are compromised due to HAp/Al$_2$O$_3$ addition. Therefore, a series of wear experiments were conducted. The fretting testing parameters included a normal load of 10 N, relative displacement of 80 μm, frequency of 10 Hz and testing duration of 100,000 cycles. The accuracy of the temperature and humidity maintained in this investigation was 35 ± 2 °C and 45 ± 5 %, respectively.

The results of a number of a fretting tests on developed biocomposites against steel/Al$_2$O$_3$/ZrO$_2$ reveal that the addition of HAp and/or Al$_2$O$_3$ (up to a maxi-mum of 40 vol%) to HDPE still allow to retain favorable friction properties, as a lower steady state of 0.12 or lower has been achieved for optimized HDPE-20 vol% Al_2O_3-20 vol% HAp materials.

Under the investigated fretting conditions, HDPE/20 vol% HAp/20 vol% Al_2O_3 composite showed enhanced wear resistance against both zirconia[95] (wear rate ~1.08 × 10^{-6} and 1.787 × 10^{-6} mm^3/Nm in SBF and atmospheric condition, respectively) and steel counterface[96] (wear rate ~2.3 × 10^{-6} and 3.87 × 10^{-6} mm^3/Nm in SBF and air, respectively) in comparison to unreinforced HDPE (wear rate ~ order of 10^{-5} mm^3/Nm). Overall, the lowest wear rate is recorded against alumina counter-body[97], irrespective of fretting environment and composite composition. Table 3.5, summarizes COF and wear rate of different composites against different counterbodies and fretting mediums.

In general, a decrease in wear rate in SBF condition is observed for all the tested materials. Importantly, the present investigation reveals that partial replacement of HAp by 20 vol% Al_2O_3 in the HAPEX™ (40 vol% HAp-HDPE composite) composition improves the wear properties of the developed composites. Figure 3.11 shows the fretted zone of this composite and emphasized the hindrance in material removal by addition of hard ceramic particulates.

Cell culture experiments for 24 hours, involving L929 fibroblast cells, clearly reveal the favorable cell adhesion property of the newly developed HDPE/20 vol% HAp/20 vol% Al_2O_3 biocomposite. To provide evidence, SEM images are acquired and presented in Figure 3.12.

In addition to results obtained with HDPE-20HAp-20Al_2O_3 and HDPE-40HAp composite, cell attachment on the standard biocompatible disc (poly-L-lysine-coated glass coverslips, negative control sample) is also shown. Figures 3.12e and 3.12f clearly show that fibroblast cells proliferated to a considerable extent on the control sample surface. Importantly, cells are also proliferated to a greater extent on the HDPE-20HAp-20Al_2O_3 composite as well as on the HDPE-40HAp sample. At many of the investigated regions, the general observation has been that the cells are attached closely with neighboring cells, and thereby form a cellular network (characteristic of fibroblast type cells) on the composite surface.

Closer observations of SEM images reveals that in the case of control disc, the cells are more round-shaped; whereas in the case of developed composites, cells are flattened with cell filapodia extending sideways in order to increase contact with the underlying substrate (composite).

In many investigated regions, such phenomenon resulted in enhanced cell–cell interactions, leading to formation of cellular bridges (see Figures 3.12b, 3.12d, and 3.12f).

The above observations are clear indicators of good biocompatibility property. It can be inferred that the HAp containing composite is as biocompatible as the control disc. However, pure HDPE (unreinforced) is essentially bioinert polymer and the addition of ceramic fillers (HAp), in the present case, clearly enhanced the cell adhesion property, even when a large amount of Al_2O_3 filler was added.

The above observations also confirm favorable cell adhesion properties of HDPE-20HAp-20Al_2O_3 composite, which would encourage tissue formation/

TABLE 3.5. Friction and Wear Properties of Investigated Biocomposites Compression Moulded Under Optimized Processing Conditions (130 °C, 0.5 h, 5 ton load). The Details of the Tribological Properties Can be Found Elsewhere

Sample Designation	Steady state COF						Wear rate ($\times 10^{-6}$ mm^3/Nm)					
Counterbodies	Zirconia		Steel		Alumina		Zirconia		Steel		Alumina	
Environment	Air	SBF	Air	SBF	Air	SBF	Air	SBF	Air	SBF	Air	SBF
HDPE	0.05	0.04	0.09	0.07	0.07	0.05	13.8 ± 0.5	8.1 ± 0.2	25.2 ± 0.5	11.5 ± 0.2	8.9 ± 0.3	8.3 ± 0.3
HDPE-HAp (20 vol%)	0.08	0.07	0.09	0.08	0.08	0.05	7.1 ± 0.4	4.9 ± 0.4	9.5 ± 0.4	7.8 ± 0.4	4.9 ± 0.2	4.6 ± 0.2
HDPE-Al$_2$O$_3$ (20 vol%)	0.12	0.06	0.13	0.09	0.13	0.07	4.3 ± 0.6	2.3 ± 0.3	8.7 ± 0.6	4.6 ± 0.3	4.2 ± 0.2	3.3 ± 0.2
HDPE-HAp (20 vol%)-Al$_2$O$_3$ (20 vol%)	0.11	0.05	0.13	0.09	0.12	0.11	1.8 ± 0.4	1.1 ± 0.7	3.9 ± 0.4	2.3 ± 0.7	0.7 ± 0.1	0.6 ± 0.1
HDPE-Al$_2$O$_3$ (40 vol%)	0.15	0.07	0.15	0.11	0.16	0.12	0.9 ± 0.5	0.2 ± 0.4	2.8 ± 0.5	1.8 ± 0.4	0.3 ± 0.1	0.1 ± 0.1
HDPE-HAp (40 vol%)	0.09	0.07	0.11	0.09	0.09	0.11	3.9 ± 0.3	3.4 ± 0.6	6.6 ± 0.3	4.9 ± 0.6	2.5 ± 0.2	3.0 ± 0.2

[94].

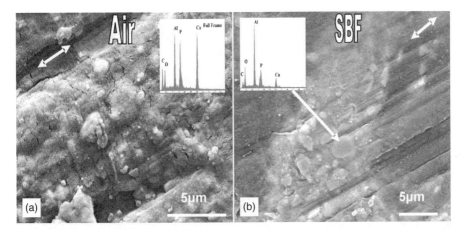

Figure 3.11. SEM images revealing evidence of abrasion on as-fretted/worn surface of HDPE-20 vol% HAp-20 vol% Al$_2$O$_3$ in two different environments: air (a) and SBF (b). Fretting conditions: 100,000 cycles, 10 Hz frequency, 10 N load and 80 μm stroke length. counterbody: 10 mm diameter zirconia ball. EDS results of the noticeable tribological features are depicted as inserts in the corresponding micrographs[95].

growth on the implanted surface. The mechanism of fibroblast cell attachment to the sample surface is guided by the interaction of protein receptors in cell membrane with cell adhesion proteins. Also, cell adhesion protein originates from the plasma and physiological fluid. Protein receptors on the cell surface enhance cell attachment to the biocompatible sample surface. These receptors transduce biochemical signals to the nucleus by activating the same intercellular signaling pathways used by growth factor receptors. The more rapid the cells spread, the higher their rate of proliferation[98]. The presence of hydroxyapatite or similar biocompatible materials stimulates the above cell growth functions, culminating in cell proliferation throughout the sample surface.

3.6 METALS AND ALLOYS IN BIOMEDICAL APPLICATIONS

Because of better physical properties such as strength, toughness, or ductility, some biocompatible metals and their alloys are often used for joint and bone implants. The applications of metals include bone replacement, bone repair, metal plates for fractures, dental implants (fillings and posts), screws and staples, parts of other devices like artificial hearts, pacemakers and catheters. The major issues for metallic implants are biocompatibility, wear resistance and corrosion resistance in body fluid. In the following sections, such issues will be discussed first, followed by a discussion on the properties and applications of various implant metals and alloys in reference to literature discussed earlier.

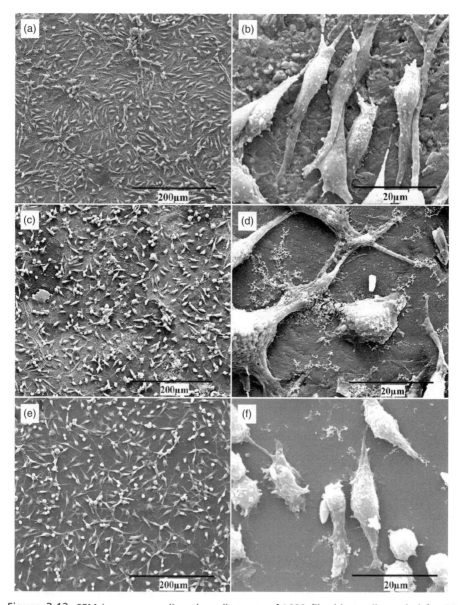

Figure 3.12. SEM images, revealing the adherence of L929 fibroblast cells seeded for 24 hours on HDPE-20HAp-20Al (S4) (a) & (b), HDPE-40HAp (S6) sample (c) & (d) and control disc (e) & (f). The culture medium was DMEM[94].

3.6.1 Issues Limiting Performance of Metallic Biomaterials

3.6.1.1 Wear of Implants. For implant applications, wear of metallic implants is a serious concern for various biomaterials. The examples are different joints of the human body, where two similar or dissimilar materials come in contact. In a typical HIP prosthesis, a metallic stint is attached to a ceramic ball, and the ceramic ball moves inside the polymeric acetabular cup. At the joint of the metal–ceramic interface, fretting fatigue could be responsible for loosening of the implant. On the other hand, the ceramic ball–polymer cup interface experiences sliding wear. The presence of body fluid and different types of proteins may trigger the wear rate *in vivo*.

Pazzaglia et al.[99] investigated the reason behind the loosening of metal-plastic total hip prosthesis. Metal-on-plastic total hip prostheses liberate metal particles due to wear of the femoral stem. Such relative movement between two surfaces presumably aids the passage of metal particles from the cement–metal interface to the cement–tissue interface in the absence of direct contact via fissures in the cement. Metallic wear debris may also be shed from the femoral head articulating in the cup if the latter is contaminated with an abrasive, such as bone cement; however, this was not noticed. Irrespective of the mechanism of their production and release, particles of stainless steel and Co-Cr-Mo alloy at the bone–cement interface encourage macrophage-related bone resorption[99]. It was suggested that this aspect represents a contributing and in some cases not inconsiderable factor in loosening of metal-plastic total hip prostheses.

In their work on tribological behavior of Ti based alloys, Choubey et al.[100] conducted fretting wear experiments on a number of Ti-alloys, in simulated body fluid environment. Their results revealed that the COF of Ti-6Al-4V alloy lies between 0.46–0.50 and COF of Ti–5Al–2.5Fe alloys is 0.3 (see Figure 3.13). The major wear mechanism was found to be tribomechanical abrasion, transfer layer formation, and cracking.

3.6.1.2 Corrosion of Metallic Implants. Most of the metallic implants corrode in contact with body fluid. Sometimes, these corrosion products are harmful to the human body and in most of the cases, the mammalian cells cannot metabolize these corroded waste. Therefore, it is important to study the corrosion behavior of metallic implants *in vitro*, that is, prior to *in vivo* application.

Steel is well known for its excellent strength properties and has been used as implant materials for a long time. Sivakumar et al.[101] compared the corrosion behavior of super-ferritic steel, duplex steel and 316 stainless steel (SS) and found that super-ferritic and duplex stainless steels can be adopted as implant materials due to their higher pitting and crevice corrosion resistance. Different alloying elements in stainless steel may have allergic and carcinogenic effect. To prove this characteristic, Hierholzer et al.[102] studied the corrosion behavior of SS in infected plated fractures. They observed that both the absolute concentration of the ions

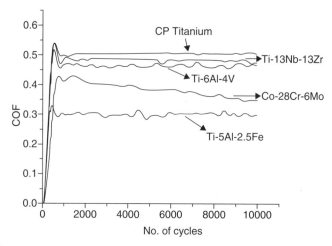

Figure 3.13. Comparative plot, showing the evolution of coefficient of friction (COF) with number of fretting cycles for potential orthopedic implant materials against steel at 10 N load, 10 Hz frequency, and 80 μm displacement stroke[100].

and the Ni:Cr ratio in the tissues adjacent to stainless steel implants is greater in infected cases than that in non-infected cases. Thus, infection as a cause of allergy has to be considered.

As a result, using a different alloy (other than steel) for metal implants was tested. Williams and Clark[103] compared the corrosion of cobalt in aqueous media both with and without the presence of the protein serum albumin, using a number of experimental techniques. The corrosion rate was found to increase significantly in the presence of albumin. Although the effect was related to albumin concentration to a certain extent, there was no equivalence between the metal ions released and the albumin present. It was believed that the effect was due to a catalytic process, where the albumin reversibly bound cobalt during the corrosion process.

Spriano et al.[104] characterized the samples of Ti-6Al-7Nb alloy with surfaces presenting a different chemical and mechanical state. Their results show that the Ti-6Al-7Nb alloy presents bioactive ability and good corrosion resistance after an appropriate surface treatment, which consists of a two-step chemical etching and heat treatment.

In evaluating the corrosion behavior of Ti based alloys in Hank's solution, Choubey et al.[105] compared electrochemical and corrosion behavior results for four different types of alloys: Ti-6Al-4V, Ti-6Al-4Nb, Ti-6Al-4Fe and Ti–5Al–2.5Fe. The passivation parameters of breakdown potential (E_b), passive current density (i_{pass}), and the passive range (E_b–ZCP) were estimated from the polarization curves; these are tabulated in Table 3.6.

The zero current potential (ZCP) of all Ti-alloys was in the range of –276 to –585 mV vs. SCE. The passive current densities were obtained around the middle of the passive range (Table 3.6). The passive current densities of the alloys inves-

TABLE 3.6. Passivation Parameters Obtained from Potentiodynamic Polarization Curves in Hank's Solution at 37 °C. The Passivation Parameters are Zero Current Potential: ZCP, Breakdown Potential: E_b, Passive Current Density: i_{pass} and the Passivation Range (E_b-ZCP)

Sample	ZCP (mV vs. SCE)	E_b (mV vs. SCE)	i_{pass} (μA/cm^2)	E_b-ZCP (mV)
Ti-6Al-4V	−276	1277	3.0	1553
Ti-6Al-4Nb	−170	1182	1.4	1352
Ti-6Al-4Fe	−257	1152	1.3	1409
Ti-5Al-2.5Fe	−461	1244	1.2	1705

[105].

TABLE 3.7. Corrosion Rates of the Ti Alloys Determined by Tafel Extrapolation Method in Hank's Solution at 37 °C and pH of 7.4. The Parameters are, Zero Current Potential: ZCP, Zero Current Potential: The Cathodic (β_c) and Anodic (β_a), The Corrosion Current Densities (i_{corr})

Sample	ZCP (mV vs. SCE)	β_c (mV/ decade)	β_a (mV/ decade)	i_{corr} (μA/ cm^2)	Corrosion rate (μm/year)
Ti-6Al-4V	−231	−176	168	0.16	1.39
Ti-6Al-4Nb	−596	−158	185	0.10	0.86
Ti-6Al-4Fe	−390	−122	181	0.04	0.35
Ti-5Al-2.5Fe	−588	−102	175	0.13	1.13

[105].

tigated were of the same order of magnitude. The highest breakdown potential (w) was exhibited by Ti-6Al-4V. The passive range in the case of materials exhibiting stable passive behavior is provided by the difference between breakdown and zero current potential. The addition of aluminum decreased the passive range significantly, as can be noted from the data for Ti-15Al.

On the other hand, Nb addition increased the passive range but not as much as that for Ti-6Al-4V (Table 3.6). The zero current potential, the cathodic (β_c) and anodic (β_a) Tafel slopes, the estimated corrosion current densities (i_{corr}) and corrosion rates are tabulated in Table 3.7. Considering the maximum corrosion rate determined for each alloy (a conservative estimate), it is noted that the corrosion rates of Ti–5Al–2.5Fe, Ti–6Al–4V, Ti–6Al–4Fe and Ti–6Al–4Nb are comparable. Importantly, the corrosion rate is not drastically affected by the amount of Fe substitution. The results of Choubey et al. clearly revealed that all the alloys exhibited stable passive polarization behavior.

3.6.2 Ti-Based Alloys

Titanium and its alloys are being developed largely for different implant applications. They encompass mechanical properties that are suitable for the applications. Due to their excellent corrosion resistance in body fluid, they are the most accepted metallic materials for clinical applications. The interactions between titanium and the body tissues, which allow osseointegration in contact with bone, produce a strong attachment to epithelial and connective tissues. The cementless fixation of hip prosthesis components and the retention of dentures by oral implants are two exciting examples of the clinical application of titanium. Yoshiki Oshida describes the science and technology of integrated Ti implant in a separate chapter of this book.

Vannoort[106] assessed the different possible application of Ti in human body. The two most popular applications of Ti and its alloy include dental inserts and THR application. He showed that Ti had good biocompatibility property in both the applications.

Gordin et al.[107] developed a new Ti-based alloy that combined Ti with the non-toxic elements, like Ta and Mo. This newly developed titanium alloys exhibited spontaneous passivity and high corrosion resistance in Ringer's solution (SBF).

In another study[108], novel TiZr alloy foams with relative densities of approximately 30% ρ_{th} were fabricated by a powder metallurgical process. The TiZr alloy foams displayed an interconnected porous structure resembling bone and the pore size ranged from 200-to-500 μm. The compressive plateau stress and the E-modulus of the TiZr foam were 78.4 MPa and 15.3 GPa, respectively. Both the porous structure and the mechanical properties of the TiZr foam were very close to those of natural bone.

Hollander et al.[109] tested DLF-produced (Direct Laser Forming) Ti6Al4V material for hard tissue applications. The cells spread and proliferated on DLF-processed Ti6Al4V over a culture time of 14 days. On porous specimens, osteoblasts grew along the rims of the pores and formed circle-shaped structures.

Matter and Burch[110] illustrated their experience with titanium implants, especially with the limited contact dynamic compression plate system. They confirmed the outstanding biocompatibility of Ti metal.

Johansson and co-workers[111] demonstrated that commercially pure (cp) Ti and cp Zirconium can be well accepted for tibia implants. After implantation in an animal or human body, the interface between metallic implant and bone plays an important role towards the curing of patients. Good chemical bonding or mechanical interlocking is desired for long term implantation.

Sennerby et al.[112] analyzed the interface zone between cortical bone and threaded non-alloyed titanium implant, which was inserted in the rabbit tibia for 12 months. Their observations suggested that mineralized bone reached close to the surface of titanium implants inserted in the rabbit tibia for 12 months; however, a direct contact was not established.

Muster et al.[113] observed the growth process of two different metals, that is Ti and gold. They showed that in the case of a bone–titanium interface, an intermediate compound is built which definitely contributes to its stability. In gold–bone interfaces, such a compound has not been observed, and growth seems less regular. In the case of the bone–titanium interfaces, a partial substitution of Ca with Ti occurs in the hydroxyapatite. This intermediate compound may be considered as a factor of stability and tolerance.

3.6.3 Co-Cr-Mo, Ni or Ta–Based Alloys

In an interesting study, Plotz et al.[114] described the technique of cementless prosthesis using spongy metal surface. The shaft and metal cup of the prosthesis are made of a Co-Cr-Mo alloy and are completely covered by spongy metal surface. They summarized the results, after implanting this type of metal on 100 patients. After one year, 82% of patients were pain-free with the prosthesis fixed by bony ingrowth, 8% were pain-free with the prosthesis fixed by dense fibrous tissue, and 10% were not pain-free, but did not desire revision surgery. Ni and Ni-based alloys are widely used in different medical treatments and devices. Also, it can be present as a contaminant in fluids for intravenous administration or released from surgical implants and other medical devices.

Fell[115] described the risk of intravenous injection of human albumin solutions contaminated with Ni causing Ni-sensitive subjects and patients to have impaired renal function. This investigation showed that the concentration of Ni in human albumin solutions, recently produced in two European countries (the United Kingdom and Italy), is substantially reduced in comparison with previous reports.

Tantalum is highly resistant to chemical attack and shows little adverse biological response. Metals coated with tantalum and tantalum itself does not degrade in extraction media during exposure to body fluid media. Tantalum has been widely used in clinical applications for more than 50 years in the following areas[116]:

a) radiographic marker for diagnostic purposes, due its high density,

b) material of choice for permanent implantation in bone,

c) vascular clips, with the particular advantage, that since tantalum, being anti-ferromagnetic, is highly suited to MRI scanning,

d) for repair of cranial defects,

e) flexible stent to prevent arterial collapse,

f) stent to treat biliary and arteriovenous (haemodialyzer) fistular stenosis,

g) for fracture repair and

h) for dental applications.

Aronson et al.[117] undertook a specific study of tantalum markers in radiography with pin and spherical markers, being implanted into bony and soft tissues of rabbits and children. No significant macroscopic and microscopic reaction was noted around the markers and those implanted into bone were firmly fixed, exhibiting close contact with adjacent bone lamellae.

In a review article, Semlitsch and Willert[118] reported various applications of metals and metallic alloys in THR prosthesis. The ball head of THR can be made either of Fe-18Cr-14Ni-3Mo, Fe-20Cr-10Ni-4Mn-3Mo-Nb-N, or Co-28Cr-6Mo-0.2C, Co-28Cr-6Mo-0,08C, Ti-6Al-7Nb/TiN, Ti-6Al-7Nb/ODH, or Co-28Cr-6Mo-0.2C; whereas the cup can be made of UHMW-polyethylene, Al_2O_3, and

Co-28Cr-6Mo-0.2C. The above described alloys for ball application are also useful for stem application. The implant alloys composition of Fe-18Cr-14Ni-3Mo and Fe-20Cr-10Ni-4Mn-3Mo-Nb-N can be fixed for cementless prosthesis. No systematic evaluation of corrosion and wear study of these implant alloys in SBF solution has yet been carried out.

3.6.4   Other Non-Ferrous Metals and Their Alloys

In a review article, Staiger et al.[119] first reported magnesium as a light weight metal with mechanical properties similar to natural bone. The *in vivo* degradation of Mg occurred via corrosion in the electrolytic physiological environment. The experimental results implicate the potential of magnesium-based implants to serve as biocompatible, osteoconductive, degradable implants for load-bearing applications. The development, performance and integration with bone tissue of porous magnesium-based implants required further investigation as well as clinical trials.

Among metals, aluminum is, however, considered as a potentially hazardous agent. The pathological findings in different organs illustrate that Al-metal can accumulate in brain, muscle, liver and bone. Dittert and co-workers[120] scrutinized whether patients with cementless total hip endoprostheses made out of titanium alloys containing aluminum are at risk and reported that Al containing biomaterials can be regarded as safe as far as the risk of aluminum release *in vivo* is concerned. Histological studies of bone from the bone–metal interface also showed no local deposits of released aluminum, in cases in which Ti alloys with Al as a minor element.

3.7   COATING ON METALS

As mentioned earlier, an alternative approach to use biomaterials is in the form of coatings. An impetus for developing various coatings is that the properties of coated bioimplants will combine advantageous properties of both coating and substrate materials. For example, bioactive ceramic coatings on metallic implant exhibit good strength (due to metal) as well as good bioactivity (due to ceramic coating).

The coating/substrate adhesion or deposition route also influences the physical properties of coatings. For example, HAp containing glass coating on Ti dental implants is reported to have better adhesion than the flame-sprayed HAp coatings. HAp containing glass coatings have specific advantageous properties, which includes increased abrasion resistance, improved aesthetics (color, and so on) and enhanced bioactivity.

An *in vitro* study was used to investigate the biological response of HAp/Ti-6Al-4V composite[121] coatings in SBF solutions. The coatings were found to undergo two biointegration processes, such as dissolution during the initial four weeks soaking in SBF and the subsequent bonelike apatite crystal precipitation. These coatings showed superior mechanical stability to the pure HAp coatings, indicating much better long-term stability of the composite coatings in physiological environment. With the interposition of a composite bond coat composed of 50 vol% HAp and 50 vol% TiO_2, a composite coating on titanium substrate[122] was fabricated by plasma spraying and no chemical reaction was observed between HAp and TiO_2. Toughness increases with the addition of TiO_2.

Godley and co-workers[123] argued that the essential condition for a biomaterial to bond with living bone is the formation of a biologically active bonelike apatite on its surface. In their work, it was demonstrated that chemical treatment can be used to create a calcium phosphate (CaP) surface layer, which might provide the alkali-treated Nb metal with bone-bonding capability. The formation of a similar CaP layer upon implantation of alkali-treated Nb into the human body should promote the bonding of the implant to the surrounding bone. This bone bonding capability could make Nb metal an attractive material for hard tissue replacements. This possibility requires further investigation.

Pajamaki et al.[124] studied the effect of glass-ceramics coating on Titanium implants. They exhibited the results with uncoated Ti, and showed that after 52 weeks, the coated metal showed 78% bone ingrowth, whereas in the case of uncoated metal, the bone coverage was only 37%.

Munting[125] explained the merit and demerit of HAp coating on metal implants. The limitation of hydroxyapatite coatings to implant fixation were discussed following a five-year histomorphological study of the bony incorporation of macroporous stemless hemiarthroplasties in dogs. The results, obtained with implants without coating, with a pure titanium coating and with a hydroxyapatite coating were compared. Munting showed that HAp coating suffers from limited strength and poor fatigue strength[125]. Also, HAp can be dissolved *in vivo* in an acidic environment, created by macrophages. Bone ingrowths can be observed in contact with resection surface. To this end, the coating thickness is the most important parameter as thicker coating has a chance to delaminate and thinner coating has a shorter life. A coating with thickness of 40–60 μm has been reported to be ideal one.

Wang et al.[126] compared the *in vivo* bone apposition on plasma-sprayed and electrochemically deposited hydroxyapatite coatings on Ti6Al4V alloy with uncoated Ti6Al4V alloy. It was revealed that plasma-sprayed HAp coatings had a higher bone apposition ratio than those exhibited by bare Ti-6Al-4V and electrochemically deposited HAp coatings after seven days. However, after 14 days of implantation, both the coated materials exhibited similar bone apposition ratios, much higher than that for uncoated Ti-6Al-4V. Figure 3.14 shows the interaction of tissue with plasma-sprayed (3.14a) and electrochemically deposited (3.14b) coatings.

In their work, Chen et al.[127] converted the surface of bioinert NiTi shape memory alloy into a bioactive surface by immersing the implant alloy into simu-

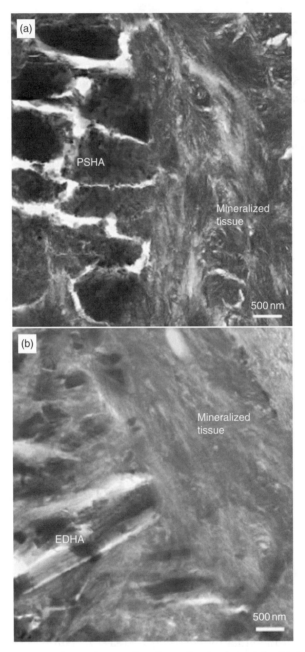

Figure 3.14. Crosssection TEM micrographs of samples, implanted for 14 day in rabbits for different materials. (a) Plasma Sprayed HAp, and (b) Electrochemically Deposited HAp coatings, Thin sections were stained with uranyl acetate and lead citrate[126].

lated body fluid. The alloy compounds were surface treated by HNO_3 and NaOH aqueous solutions, prior to immersing in SBF. It was found that an HAp layer formed on the surface of the NiTi alloy after immersing 48 hours inside SBF. The surface modified and as received NiTi cylindrical implants were bilaterally implanted into the femurs of rabbits. It was observed that HAp coating can facilitate fast proliferation of osteoblasts. Direct bony coverage of the surface-modified NiTi implants at six weeks of implantation was monitored. After 13 weeks of implantation, the interface between the coated implant and the bone shows the nature of osteo-bonding. On the other hand, the interface between the uncoated implant and the bone has gaps, showing a weak bone–implant interface (Figure 3.15).

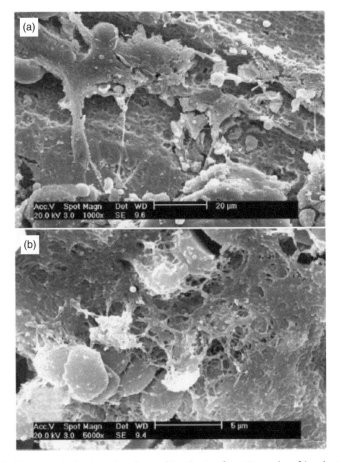

Figure 3.15. The morphologies of surface of implants after 13 weeks of implantation. (a) A little bulged cell and collagen fibrous on uncoated NiTi implant. (b) A large number of bone cells and collagen fibrous networks on coated NiTi implant[127].

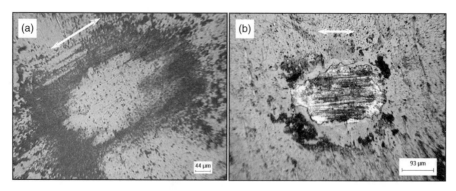

Figure 3.16. Optical microscopy images of the worn surface on DLC coated Co-Cr-Mo surface illustrating: the mild wear after fretting at 10 N load for 10,000 cycles (a) and the severe wear after fretting at 10 N load after 100,000 cycles (b). Arrows indicate fretting directions. The counterbody is bearing steel and the double pointed arrows indicate the fretting. DLC coating is worn through as seen by the white contrast in (b)[128].

In a different work, Choubey et al.[128] explored the tribological behavior of CVD-DLC coated Co-Cr-Mo alloys under fretting contacts. They conducted the wear experiments on coated materials in Hank's balanced salt solution to assess the *in vitro* performance in simulated body fluid (physiological) solution. In SBF solution, DLC-coated Co-Cr-Mo alloys exhibited low COF of 0.07–0.10, whereas high COF (0.4) was experienced by uncoated Co-Cr-Mo, under identical fretting conditions. The wear mechanism was mainly governed by the mild wear with no significant change in surface morphology in DLC-coated flat material. The uncoated Co-Cr-Mo exhibited extensive plastic deformation and delamination induced grain pull out at higher load of 10 N after 10,000 cycles (see Figure 3.16). The obtained research results indicated the superior tribological performance of DLC coatings as compared to uncoated Co-Cr-Mo alloys.

In a review article, Hanawa[129] summarized the effect of metal ion release from the metallic implants *in vivo*. The oxide films, formed on the surface of metallic materials, play an important role and protect the surface to release ions. Low concentration of dissolved oxygen, inorganic ions, proteins, and cells may accelerate the metal ion release. Also, the formation and breakdown as well as regeneration time of oxide layer on metallic implant surface may control the release rate.

In some specific applications, ions/debris can be released from the implants due to some mechanical actions, like wear and fretting. The behavior of metal ion release into biofluid is governed by the electrochemical rule. The released metal ions do not always combine with biomolecules to casue toxicity, because an active ion immediately combine with a water molecule or an anion near the ion to form an oxide, hydroxide, or inorganic salt. It was concluded[129] that there is little chance that the metal ions can combine with biomolecules to cause cytotoxicity, allergy, and other biological influences.

3.8　OUTLOOK AND RECOMMENDATIONS FOR FUTURE WORK

After reviewing the existing literature on synthesis, properties and different applications, it is quite clear that the appropriate material for each specific biomedical application is still to be discovered.

In the case of ceramic-based monolithic and composite biomaterials, the major concern is low fracture toughness in spite of having excellent biocompatibility. A vast research initiative is needed to increase the fracture toughness values of ceramic-based biomaterials up to the safe limit of use, by manipulating microstructure and other structural parameters. An alternative route to developing biocompatible as well as mechanically-strong material is to develop ceramic coatings on metal, which provide the biocompatibility of ceramics as well as the mechanical strength of substrate metal. The properties of such ceramic coatings depend on the coatings' thickness, deposition condition and the coating-substrate interface properties. In both coating and bulk applications, the bioactive CaP based ceramics are the most important implant materials due to their excellent response inside human body. The fracture toughness of CaP based materials should lie between 3–5 MPa m$^{0.5}$.

The strategy to provide effective tools for bone replacement and repair would be the use of Ca/P based biomaterials assisted osseointegration involving an appropriate choice of the structure, microstructure, and chemical compositions. This approach would, in principle, allow the production of bioactive materials available "off-the-shelf" and with known predictable properties. At this stage, microporosity has been suggested as one of the principal factors determining the osteoinductive properties of an implant[130]. However, mineral crystals, morphologies, chemical composition and mechanical behaviour could also play a major role in biological response and in the relative and/or combined importance of these parameters in the manifestation of the osteoinductive response. To this end, its duration and persistence have not yet been clearly determined.

One of the key perspectives in orthopedic implants is the use of nanosized Ca-phosphate particles. Both stoichiometric as well as non-stoichiometric HAp powders would be used in producing nanobiocomposites of desired composition. The interest for nanocrystalline apatite has grown since last few years. Apatite nanocrystals are the main component of hard biological tissues such as bone and dentine[131] and they play a major role in the biological activity of orthopedic biomaterials[132,133,134] However, these reactive nanocrystals are difficult to shape into available carriers without altering their nanocrystalline nature and their biological properties are not yet totally understood to optimize their shape/function properties.

Most of the polymers are currently used in soft tissue replacement such as tendon, cartilage, skin, and so on. Except these, few polymers could be suitable in load-bearing applications due to their lightweight, excellent corrosion resistance in body fluid and low COF. However, the major concerns for such applications are low E-modulus and hardness values of polymeric materials. As mentioned in Table 3.2 the E-modulus of cortical bone is in the range of ~17 GPa. Efforts should be made to develop polymer matrix composite materials, whose E-modulus and hardness can be raised to more than 8 GPa and 0.5 GPa, respectively. The maximum hardness of cortical bone is nearly ~0.5 GPa. With an increase of E-modulus and hardness, the wear resistance of polymer is expected to be improved. The development of nanobiocomposites could be useful for such applications.

Considering their high fracture toughness/strength, metals are an excellent choice in load-bearing applications. The development of newer alloys will definitely broaden the area of materials selection. However, many aspects of *in vitro* and *in vivo* evaluation need to be carried out for newer alloys (such as Ti-5Al-2.5 Fe). More research efforts need to be invested to improve the corrosion and wear resistance of metallic biomaterials inside the human body. The required properties for hard tissue replacement biomaterials (ceramics, metals and polymers and their composites) are from a literature review and shown summarized in a schematic diagram in Figure 3.17.

Future efforts in the development[135] of biocompatibility methodology will probably be directed towards the development of materials, which will allow normal differentiation and function of tissues into which the materials are placed. In predicting areas in which new research will probably occur, two areas should be mentioned: molecular biology of host tissue in response to materials; and molecular interactions between biological molecules and synthetic materials or tissue-material combinations.

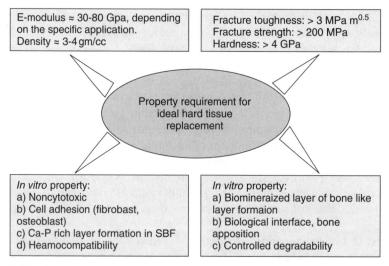

Figure 3.17. The properties of an ideal hard tissue replacement biomaterial are showing in block diagrams.

ACKNOWLEDGMENTS

The authors wish to thank Department of Biotechnology, India; Department of Science and Technology, India; Council of Scientific and Industrial Research, India for financial supports in various projects. The authors would like to thank S. Ganesh of Biological Sciences and Bioengineering Department, IIT-Kanpur for helping us in cell experiments.

REFERENCES

1. J.-A. Epinette and M. T. Manley, Fifteen years of clinical experience with hydroxy-apatite coatings in joint arthroplasty, Springer Verlag (2004).
2. L. L. Hench, "Bioceramics," J. Am. Ceram. Soc., **81 [7]** 1705–28 (1998).
3. R. M. Souto, M. M. Laz and R. L. Reis, Biomaterials, **24 [23]** 4213–21 (2003).
4. I. Knets, M. Dobelis, J. Laizans, R. Cimdins and V. Vitins, Journal of Biomechanics, **31** [Suppl. **1**] 166 (1998).
5. H. J. Rack and J. I. Qazi, "Titanium alloys for biomedical applications," Mat. Sci. Engg. C., **26** 1269 (2006).
6. L. Jimguo, "Behaviour of titanium and titania-based ceramics *in vitro* and *in vivo*," Biomaterials, **14** 229 (1993).
7. B. D. Ratner, A. S. Hoffman, F. J. Schoen and J. E. Lemons, Biomaterials Science: An Introduction to Materials in Medicine, San Diego, CA: Academic Press (1996).
8. S. Ramakrishna, J. Mayer, E. Wintermantel and K. W. Leong, "Biomedical applications of polymer-composite materials: a review," Comp. Sc. Tech., **61** 1189–1124 (2001).
9. J. Black, Orthopaedic Biomaterials: Research and Practice, Churchill Livingstone (1988).
10. R. Z. LeGeros, "Preparation of Octacalcium Phosphate (OCP): A Direct Fast Method," Calcif. Tiss. Int., **37** 194–7 (1985).
11. W. E. Brown, N. Eidelman and B. Tomazic, "Octacalcium Phosphate as a Precursor in Biomineral Formation," Adv. Dent. Res., **1 [2]** 306–13 (1987).
12. F. Betts, N. C. Blumenthal and A. S. Posner, "Bone Mineralization," J. Crys. Grow., **53** 63–73 (1981).
13. T. Suzuki, R. Ohashi, Y. Yokogawa, K. Nishizawa, F. Nagata, Y. Kawamoto, T. Kameyama and M. Toriyama, "Initial Anchoring and Proliferation of Fibroblast L-929 Cells on Unstable Surface of Calcium Phosphate Ceramics," J. Biosc. Bioengg., **87 [3]** 320–327 (1999).
14. Q. Z. Chen, C. T. Wong, W. W. Lu, K. M. C. Cheung, J. C. Y. Leong and K. D. K. Luk, "Strengthening mechanisms of bone bonding to crystalline hydroxyapatite *in vivo*," Biomaterials, **25** 4243–4254 (2004).
15. R. Xin, Y. Leng, J. Chen and Q. Zhang, "A comparative study of calcium phosphate formation on bioceramics *in vitro* and *in vivo*," Biomaterials, **26** 6477–86 (2005).
16. J. Dong, T. Uemura, H. Kojima, M. Kikuchi, J. Tanaka and T. Tateishi, "Application of low-pressure system to sustain *in vivo* bone formation in osteoblast-porous hydroxyapatite composite," Mat. Sc. Engg. C, **17** 37–43 (2001).

17. A. M. Gatti, D. Zaffe and G. P. Poli, "Behaviour of tricalcium phosphate and hydroxyapatite granules in sheep bone defects," Biomaterials, **11** 513–17 (1990).

18. C. Balcik, T. Tokdemir, A. Senkoylu, N. Koc, M. Timucin, S. Akin, P. Korkusuz and F. Korkusuz, "Early weight bearing of porous HA/TCP (60/40) ceramics *in vivo*: A longitudinal study in a segmental bone defect model of rabbit," Acta Biomat., **3** 985–996 (2007).

19. M. Fini, R. Cadossi, V. Cane, F. Cavani, G. Giavaresi, A. Krajewski, L. Martini, N. N. Aldin, A. Ravaglioli, L. Rimondini, P. Torricelli and R. Giardino, "The effect of pulsed electromagnetic fields on the osteointegration of hydroxyapatite implants in cancellous bone: a morphologic and microstructural *in vivo* study," J. Ortho. Res., **20** 756–63 (2002).

20. T. Okuda, K. Ioku, I. Yonezawa, H. Minagi, G. Kawachic, Y. Gonda, H. Murayama, Y. Shibata, S. Minami, S. Kamihira, H. Kurosawa and T. Ikeda, "The effect of the microstructure of β tricalcium phosphate on the metabolism of subsequently formed bone tissue," Biomaterials, **28** 2612–21 (2007).

21. R. M. Souto, M. M. Laz and R. L. Reis, "Degradation characteristics of hydroxyapatite coatings on orthopaedic TiAlV in simulated physiological media investigated by electrochemical impedance spectroscopy," Biomaterials, **24 [23]** 4213–21 (2003).

22. I. Knets, M. Dobelis, J. Laizans, R. Cimdins and V. Vitins, "Glass and hydroxyapatite coating on titanium implant," J. Biomech., **31 [1]** 166 (1998).

23. S. Gautier, E. Champion and D. Bernache-Assollant, "Processing, Microstructure and Toughness of Al₂O₃ Platelet-Reinforced Hydroxyapatite," J. Euro. Ceram. Soc., **17 [11]** 1361–69 (1997).

24. J. Li, B. Fartash and L. Hermansson, "Hydroxyapatite—alumina composites and bone-bonding," Biomaterials, **16 [5]** 417–22 (1995).

25. R. R. Rao and T. S. Kannan, "Synthesis and sintering of hydroxyapatite–zirconia composites," Mater. Sci. Engg. C, **20 [1–2]** 187–93 (2002).

26. V. V. Silva, F. S. Lameiras and R. Z. Domínguez, "Microstructural and mechanical study of zirconia-hydroxyapatite (ZH) composite ceramics for biomedical applications," Comp. Sci. Tech., **61 [2]** 301–310 (2001).

27. A. Rapacz-Kmita, A. Slosarczyk and Z. Paszkiewicz, "Mechanical properties of HAp–ZrO₂ composites," J. Euro. Cera. Soc., **26 [8]** 1481–88 (2006).

28. A. Chiba, S. Kimura, K. Raghukandan and Y. Morizono, "Effect of alumina addition on hydroxyapatite biocomposites fabricated by underwater-shock compaction," Mat. Sc. Engg. A, **350** 179–83 (2003).

29. R. Hill and A. Clifford, "Apatite-mullite glass-ceramics," J. Non-Cryst. Sol., **196** 346–51 (1996).

30. C. M. Gorman and R. G. Hill, "Heat-pressed ionomer glass-ceramics. Part I: an investigation of flow and microstructure," Dent. Mat., **19 [4]** 320–26 (2003).

31. Y. M. Kong, C. J. Bae, S. H. Lee, H. W. Kim and H. E. Kim, "Improvement in biocompatibility of ZrO₂–Al₂O₃ nano-composite by addition of HA," Biomaterials, **26 [5]** 509–17 (2005).

32. I. Manjubala and M. Sivakumar, "In-situ synthesis of biphasic calcium phosphate Ceramics using microwave irradiation," Mat. Chem. Phys., **71** 272–8 (2001).

33. D. C. Tancred, B. A. O. McCormack and A. J. Carr, "A quantitative study of the sintering and mechanical properties of hydroxyapatite/phosphate glass composites," Biomaterials, **19 [19]** 1735–43 (1998).

34. W. Suchanek, M. Yashima, M. Kakihana and M. Yoshimura, "Hydroxyapatite/Hydroxyapatite-Whisker Composites without Sintering Additives: Mechanical Properties and Microstructural Evolution," J. Am. Ceram. Soc., **80 [11]** 2805–13 (1997).

35. S. Nath, K. Biswas and B. Basu, "Processing and Phase formation and microstructure studies of novel HAp-Mullite composites," Scripta Materialia, **58 [12]** 1054–7 (2008).

36. F. Wataria, A. Yokoyamaa, M. Omorib, T. Hiraic, H. Kondoa, M. Uoa and T. Kawasakia, "Biocompatibility of materials and development to functionally graded implant for bio-medical application," Compo. Sc. Tech., **64** 893–908 (2004).

37. C. Q. Ning and Y. Zhou, "*In vitro* bioactivity of a biocomposite fabricated from HA and Ti powders by powder metallurgy method," Biomaterials, **23** 2909–15 (2002).

38. F. Caro, K. S. Oh, R. Fameryl and P. Boch, "Sintering of TCP-TiO$_2$ biocomposites: inßuence of secondary phases," Biomaterials, **19** 1451–4 (1998).

39. S. Nath, R. Tripathi and B. Basu, "Understanding Phase Stability, Microstructure Development and Biocompatibility in Calcium Phosphate-titania Composites, Synthesized from Hydroxyapatite and Titanium Powder Mix," Materials Science and Engineering C, **29** 97–107 (2009).

40. S. Roy, "*Mica based machineable glass ceramics, (in Ind.)*," in M. Tech Thesis, Indian Institute of Technology Kanpur, Kanpur (2005).

41. A. R. Molla, "*Mica based machineable glass ceramics with different fluoride content, (in Ind.)*," in M. Tech Thesis, Indian Institute of Technology Kanpur, Kanpur (2007).

42. D. C. Clupper, J. E. Gough, P. M. Embanga, I. Notingher, L. L. Hench and M. M. Hall, "Bioactive evaluation of 45S5 bioactive glass fibres and preliminary study of human osteoblast attachment," J. Mater. Sci. Mater. Med., **15 [7]** 803–8 (2004).

43. K. D. Lobel and L. L. Hench, "*In Vitro* Protein Interactions with a Bioactive Gel-Glass," J. Sol-Gel Sci. Tech., **7** 69–76 (1996).

44. L. Lefebvre, J. Chevalier, L. Gremillard, R. Zenati, G. Thollet, D. Bernache-Assolant and A. Govin, "Structural transformations of bioactive glass 45S5 with thermal treatments," Acta. Materialia, **55** 3305–13 (2007).

45. E. VerneÂ, M. Ferraris, C. Jana and L. Paracchini, "Bioverit1 I base glass/Ti particulate biocomposite: 'in situ' vacuum plasma spray deposition," J. Euro. Cera. Soc., **20** 473–9 (2000).

46. E. VerneÂ, M. Ferraris and C. Jana, "Pressureless Sintering of Bioverit1 III/Ti Particle Biocomposites," J. Euro. Cera. Soc., **19** 2039–47 (1999).

47. C. Q. Ninga and Y. Zhoub, "On the microstructure of biocomposites sintered from Ti,HA and bioactive glass," Biomaterials, **25** 3379–87 (2004).

48. C. Fernandeza, E. Verne, J. Vogel and G. Carlb, "Optimisation of the synthesis of glass-ceramic matrix biocomposites by the 'response surface methodology'," J. Euro. Cera. Soc., **23** 1031–38 (2003).

49. M. Amarala, M. A. Lopesb, R. F. Silva and J. D. Santos, "Densification route and mechanical properties of Si$_3$N$_4$–bioglass biocomposites," Biomaterials, **23** 857–62 (2002).

50. V. M. da R. Barros, L. A. Salata, C. E. Sverzut, S. P. Xavier, R. van Noort, A. Johnson and P. V. Hatton, "*In vivo* bone tissue response to a canasite glass-ceramic," Biomaterials, **23** 2895–2900 (2002).

51. G. Zhang, R. A. Latour, Jr., J. M. Kennedy, H. D. Schutte, Jr. and R. J. Friedman, "Long-term compressive property durability of carbon fibre-reinforced polyetheretherketone composite in physiological saline," Biomaterials, **17 [8]** 781–9 (1996).

52. T. R. Martin, S. W. Meyer and D. R. Luchtel, "An Evaluation of the Toxicity of Carbon Fiber Composites for Lung Cells *in vitro* and *in vivo*," Environ. Res., **49** 246–61 (1989).

53. J. Wang and R. Stevens, "Zirconia-toughened alumina (ZTA) ceramics," J. Mater. Sci., **24** 3421–40 (1989).

54. A. H. D. Aza, J. Chevalier, G. Fantozzi, M. Schehl and R. Torrecillas, "Crack growth resistance of alumina, zirconia and zirconia toughened alumina ceramics for joint prostheses," Biomaterials, **23 [3]** 937–45 (2002).

55. B. Kerkwijk, L. Winnubst, E. J. Mulder and H. Verweij, "Processing of homogeneous zirconia-toughened alumina ceramics with high dry-sliding wear resistance," J. Am. Ceram. Soc., **82 [8]** 2087–93 (1999).

56. C. He, Y. S. Wang, J. S. Wallace and S. M. Hsu, "Effect of microstructure on the wear transition of zirconia-toughened alumina," Wear, **162–164** A314–A321 (1993).

57. K. Hayashi, T. Inadome, H. Tsumura, T. Mashima and Y. Sugioka, "Bone-implant interface mechanics of in tivo bio-inert ceramics," Biomaterials, **14** 1173–9 (1993).

58. G. Colon, B. C. Ward and T. J. Webster, "Increased osteoblast and decreased Staphylococcus epidermidis functions on nanophase ZnO and TiO_2," J. Biomed. Mat. Res. Part A, **78A [3]** 595–604 (2006).

59. S. Nath, N. Sinha and B. Basu, "Microstructure, Mechanical and Tribological Properties of Microwave Sintered Ca-stabilized Zirconia for Biomedical Applications," Ceram. Inter., **34** 1509–1520 (2008).

60. S. Nath, S. Bajaj and B. Basu, "Microstructure, Mechanical and Tribological Properties of Microwave Sintered Mg-doped Zirconia," Int. J. App. Ceram. Tech., **5 [1]** 49–62 (2008).

61. P. González, J. P. Borrajo, J. Serra, S. Chiussi, B. León, J. Martínez-Fernández, F. M. Varela-Feria, A. R. de Arellano-López, A. de Carlos, F. M. Muñoz, M. López and M. Singh, "A New Generation of Bio-derived Ceramic Materials for Medical Applications," J. Biomed. Mat. Res. A, **88A** 807–813 (2009).

62. S. Ramakrishna, J. Mayer, E. Wintermantel and K. W. Leong, "Biomedical applications of polymer-composite materials: a review," Comp. Sc. Tech., **61** 1189 (2001).

63. S. M. Lee, "Orthopedic Composites, International Encyclopedia of Composites, New York," **4** 74 (1991).

64. B. Harris, "The mechanical behavior of composite materials," Symp. Soc. Exp. Biol., **34** 37–74 (1980).

65. P. Christel, L. Claes and S. A. Brown, "Carbon reinforced composites in orthopedic surgery," in M. Szycher, A comprehensive guide to medical and pharmaceutical application, CRC Press, Lancaster, USA, 499 (1991).

66. B. D. Bauman, "Polymer-Polymer composites made with surface modified particles and fibers, K Plast 2001 Düsseldorf Germany," October (2001). http://inhanceproducts.com/tech_lit/CRM-18034.pdf.

67. H. Amstutz, "Mechanism and clinical significance of wear debris-induced osteolysis," Clinic. Ortho. Rel. Res., **276** 7 (1992).

68. N. Blumenthal, "A new technique for quantitation of metal particualates and metal reaction products in tissue near implants," J. App. Biomater., **5** 191 (1994).

69. E. Schneider, "Comperativestudy of the initial stability of cementless hip prostheses," Clin. Othop., **248** 200 (1989).

70. K. St. John, "Applications of advanced composites in orthopedic implants," in M. Szycher, Biocompatible polymers, metals and composites. Lancaster: Technomic Publishing, 861 (1983).

71. P. Christel, A. Meunier, S. Leclercq, P. Bouquet and B. Buttazzoni, "Devolopement of carbon-carbon hip prostheses," J. Biomed. Mater. Res. Appl. Biomet., **21** 191 (1987).

72. M. Akay and N. Aslan, "Numerical and experimental stress analysis of a polymeric composite hip joint prostheses," J. Biomed. Mater. Res., **31** 167 (1996).

73. T. Peter, R. Tognini, J. Mayer and E. Wintermantel, "Homoelastic, anisotropic osteosynthesis system by net-shape processing of endless carbon fiber reinforced polyetheretherketone (PEEK)," in J. Goh, A. Nather, Proc. of 9th conference on biomedical engineering, Singapore, National University of Singapore, 317 (1997).

74. E. Wintermantel, A. Bruinink, K. Ruffiex, M. Petitmermet and J. Mayer, "Tissue engineering supported with structured biocompatible materials: goals and achievements," in M. Speidal, Uggowitzer, Materials in medicine, Switzerland: ETH zurich, 1 (1998).

75. W. Bonefield, "Composites for bone replacement," J. Biomed. Eng., **10** 522 (1998).

76. B. Moyen, P. Lahey, E. Weinberg and W. Harris, "Effects on intact femora of dogs of the application and removal of metal plates," J. Bone Joint Sur., **60A [7]** 940 (1978).

77. S. Ramakrishna, J. Mayer, E. Wintermantel and K. W. Leong, "Biomedical applications of polymer-composite materials: a review," Compos. Sci. Technol., **61 [9]** 1189–224 (2001).

78. M. Wang, S. Deb and W. Bonfield, "Chemically coupled hydroxyapatite-polyethylene composites: processing and characterization," Mat. Letters, **44 [2]** 119–24 (2000).

79. M. Wang and W. Bonefield, "Chemically coupled hydroxyapatite-polyethylene composite: structure and properties," Biomaterials, **22** 1311 (2001).

80. L. D. Silvio, M. J. Dalby and W. Bonfield, "Osteoblast behaviour on HA/PE composite surfaces with different HA volumes," Biomaterials, **23 [1]** 101–7 (2002).

81. W. Bonefield, "Hydroxyapatite reinforced polyethylene as an analogous material for bone replacement," Am. Acad. Sci., **523** 173 (1988).

82. M. Wang, R. Joseph and W. Bonefield, "Hydroxyapatite-polyethylene composites for bone substitution: effects of ceramic particle size and morphology," Biomaterials, **19** 2357 (1998).

83. M. Wang, M. Chandrasekaran and W. Bonefeild, "Friction and wear of hydroxyapatite reinforced high density polyethylene against the stainless steel counterface," J. Mater. Sc. Mater. Med., **13** 607 (2004).

84. R. Rothon, Particulate-filled polymer composites, Longman Scientific and Technical, New Work, 294 (1995).

85. A. Y. Sadi, S. S. Homaeigohar, A. R. Khavandi and J. Javadpour, "The effect of partially stabilized zirconia on the mechanical properties of the hydroxyapatite-polyethylene composites," J. Mater. Sc. Mater. Med., **15** 853 (2004).

86. Y. M. Kong, S. Kim and H. E. Kim, "Reinforcement of hydroxyapatite bioceramic by addition of ZrO_2 coated with Al_2O_3," J. Am. Ceram. Soc., **82 [11]** 2963 (1999).

87. J. R. Sarasua and P. M. Remiru, "The mechanical behaviour of PEEK short fiber composites," J. Mater. Sci., **30** 3501–8 (1995).

88. M. S. A. Bakar, P. Cheang and K. A. Khor, "Mechanical properties of injection molded hydroxyapatite–Polyetheretherketone biocomposites," Compo. Sci. Technol., **63** 421–5 (2003).

89. M. S. A. Bakar, M. H. W. Cheng, S. M. Tang, S. C. Yu, K. Liao, C. T. Tan, K. A. Khor and P. Cheang, "Tensile properties, tension–tension fatigue and biological response of polyetheretherketone–hydroxyapatite composites for load-bearing orthopedic implants," Biomaterials, **24** 2245–50 (2003).

90. S. Yu, K. P. Hariram, R. Kumar, P. Cheang and K. K. Aik, "*In vitro* apatite formation and its growth kinetics on Hydroxyapatite/polyetheretherketone biocomposites," Biomaterials, **26** 2343–52 (2005).

91. X. Wang, Y. Li, J. Wei and K. Groot, "Devolopement of biomimetic nano-hydroxyapatite/poly (hexamethylene adipamide) composites," Biomaterials, **23 [9]** 4787 (2002).

92. S. Hasegawaa, S. Ishii, J. Tamura, T. Furukawa, M. Neo, Y. Matsusueb, Y. Shikinami, M. Okuno and T. Nakamura, "A 5–7 year *in vivo* study of high-strength hydroxyapatite/poly (L-lactide) composite rods for the internal fixation of bone fractures," Biomaterials, **27** 1327–32 (2006).

93. H. Itokawa, T. Hiraide, M. Moriya, M. Fujimoto, G. Nagashima, R. Suzuki and T. Fujimoto, "A 12 month *in vivo* study on the response of bone to a hydroxyapatite–polymethylmethacrylate cranioplasty composite," Biomaterials, **28** 4922–27 (2007).

94. S. Nath, S. Bodhak and B. Basu, "HDPE-Al₂O₃-HAp Composites for Biomedical Applications: Processing and Characterization," J. Biomed. Mat. Res. Part B, Appl. Biomat., **88B [1]** 1–11 (2009).

95. S. Bodhak, S. Nath and B. Basu, "Understanding the Fretting Wear Properties of HAp, Al₂O₃ containing HDPE Biocomposites against ZrO₂," J. Biomed. Mater. Res. Part A, **85A [1]** 83–98 (2008).

96. S. Nath, S. Bodhak and B. Basu, "Tribological investigation of Novel HDPE-HAp-Al₂O₃ hybrid biocomposites against Steel under Dry and Simulated Body Fluid Condition," J. Biomed. Mater.Res. Part A, **83A [1]** 191–208 (2007).

97. S. Bodhak, S. Nath and B. Basu, "Friction and Wear Properties of Novel HDPE-HAp-Al₂O₃ Composites against Alumina counterface," J. Biomat. Appl., **23** 407–433 (2009).

98. B. D. Ratner, A. S. Hoffman, F. J. Schoen and J. E. Lemons, Biomaterials Science: An Introduction to Materials in Medicine, Elsevier Academic Press, London (2004).

99. U. E. Pazzaglia, L. Ceciliani, M. J. Wilkinson and C. Dell'Orbo, "Involvement of Metal Particles in Loosening of Metal-Plastic Total Hip Prostheses," Arch. Orthop. Trauma Surg., **104** 164–74 (1985).

100. A. Choubey, B. Basu and R. Balasubramaniam, "Tribological behavior of Ti-based alloys in simulated body fluid solution at fretting contacts," Mater. Sci. Engg. A, **379** 234–9 (2004).

101. M. Sivakumar, U. K. Mudali and S. Rajeswari, "Compatibility of ferritic and duplex stainless steels as implant materials: *in vitro* corrosion performance," J. Mater. Sci., **28** 6081–6 (1993).

102. S. Hierholzer, G. Hierholzer, K. H. Sauer and R. S. Paterson, "Increased Corrosion of Stainless Steel Implants in Infected Plated Fractures," Arch. Orthop. Trauma Surg., **102** 198–200 (1984).

103. D. F. Wllliams and G. C. F. Clark, "The corrosion of pure cobalt in physiological media," J. Mater. Sci., **17** 1675–82 (1982).

104. S. Spriano, M. Bronzoni, F. Rosalbino and E. Vern, "New chemical treatment for bioactive titanium alloy with high corrosion resistance," J. Mater. Sci. Mater. Medi., **16** 203–11 (2005).

105. A. Choubey, R. Balasubramaniam and B. Basu, "Effect of replacement of V by Nb and Fe on the electrochemical and corrosion behavior of Ti–6Al–4V in simulated physiological environment," J. All. Compo., **381** 288–94 (2004).

106. R. V. Noort, "Review Titanium: the implant material of today," J. Mater. Sci., **22** 3801–81 (1987).

107. D. M. Gordina, T. Glorianta, G. Nemtoi, R. Chelariuc, N. Aeleneid, A. Guilloua and D. Ansela, "Synthesis, structure and electrochemical behavior of a beta Ti-12Mo-5Ta alloy as new biomaterial," Mater. Lett., **59** 2936–41 (2005).

108. C. E. Wen, Y. Yamada and P. D. Hodgson, "Fabrication of novel TiZr alloy foams for biomedical applications," Mat. Sci. Engg. C, **26 [8]** 1439–44 (2006).

109. D. A. Hollander, M. von Walter, T. Wirtz, R. Sellei, B. S. Rohlfing, O. Paar and H.-J. Erli, "Structural, mechanical and *in vitro* characterization of individually structured Ti–6Al–4V produced by direct laser forming," Biomaterials, **27** 955–63 (2006).

110. P. Matter and H. B. Burch, "Clinical experience with titanium implants, especially with the limited contact dynamic compression plate system," Arch. Orthop. Trauma Surg., **109** 311–13 (1990).

111. C. B. Johansson, A. Wennerberg and T. Albrektsson, "Quantitative comparison of screw-shaped commercially pure titanium and zirconium implants in rabbit tibia," J. Mater. Sci. Mater. Medi., **5** 340–4 (1994).

112. L. Sennerby, P. Thomsen and L. E. Ericson, "Ultrastructure of the bone-titanium interface in rabbits," J. Mater. Sci. Mater. Medi., **3** 262–71 (1992).

113. D Muster, J. H. Jaeger, M. Bouzouita, C. Burggraf and C. Baltzinger, "Application of Physical Surface Methods to the Study of the Stability and Structure of Bone-Metal Interfaces," Anat. Clin., **4** 183–8 (1982).

114. W. Plotz, R. Gradinger, H. Rechl, R. Ascherl, S. Wicke-Wittenius and E. Hipp, "Cementless prosthesis of the hip joint with 'spongy metal' surface A prospective study," Arch. Orthop. Trauma Surg., **111** 102–9 (1992).

115. M. Patriarca and G. S. Fell, "Monitoring of Sources of Clinical Exposure to Nickel," Mikrochim Acta., **123** 261–9 (1996).

116. http://www.tantalum-coating.com/Literatur.htm

117. A. S. Aronson, N. Jonsson and P. Alberius, "Tantalum markers in radiography," Sleletal Radiol., **14** 207–11 (1985).

118. M. Semlitsch and H. G. Willert, "Implant materials for hip endoprostheses: old proofs and new trends," Arch. Orthop. Trauma Surg., **114** 61–7 (1995).

119. M. P. Staigera, A. M. Pietaka and J. Huadmaia, "George Dias Magnesium and its alloys as orthopedic biomaterials: A review," Biomaterials, **27** 1728–34 (2006).

120. D. D. Dittert, G. Wamecke and H. G. Willert, "Aluminum levels and stores in patients with total hip endoprostheses from TiAlV or TiAlNb alloys," Arch. Orthop. Trauma Surg., **114** 133–136 (1995).

121. Y. W. Gua, K. A. Khora and P. Cheang, "*In vitro* studies of plasma-sprayed hydroxyapatite/Ti-6Al-4V composite coatings in simulated body fluid (SBF)," Biomaterials, **24** 1603–11 (2003).

122. Y. PengLu, M. S. Li, S. T. Li, Z. G. Wang and R. F. Zhu, "Plasma sprayed hydroxyapatite+titania composite bond coat for hydroxyapatite coating on titanium substrate," Biomaterials, **25** 4393–403 (2004).

123. R. Godley, D. Starosvetsky and I. Gotman, "Bonelike apatite formation on niobium metal treated in aqueous NaOH," J. Mater. Sci. Mater. Medi., **15** 1073–77 (2004).

124. J. Pajamaki, S. Lindholm, O. Andersson, K. Karlsson, A. Yli-Urpo and R. R. Happonen, "Glass-ceramic-coated titanium hip endoprosthesis Experimental study in rabbits," Arch. Orthop. Trauma Surg., **114** 119–22 (1995).

125. E. Munting, "The contributions and limitations of hydroxyapatite coatings to implant fixation: A histomorphometric study of load bearing implants in dogs," Inter. Ortho. (SICOT), **20** 1–6 (1996).

126. H. Wang, N. Eliaz, Z. Xiang, H. P. Hsu, M. Spector and L. W. Hobbs, "Early bone apposition *in vivo* on plasma-sprayed and electrochemically deposited hydroxyapatite coatings on titanium alloy," Biomaterials, **27 [23]** 4192–203 (2006).

127. M. F. Chen, X. J. Yang, R. X. Hu, Z. D. Cui and H. C. Man, "Bioactive NiTi shape memory alloy used as bone bonding implants," Mater. Sci. Engg. C, **24** 497–502 (2004).

128. A Choubey, A Dorner-Reisel and B. Basu, "Friction and Wear Behaviour of DLC Coated Biomaterials in Simulated Body Fluid Solution at Fretting Contacts," Key Engg. Mat., **264–268 [3]** 2115–18 (2004).

129. T. Hanawa, "Metal ion release from metal implants," Mater. Sci. Engg. C, **24** 745–52 (2004).

130. P. Habibovic, T. M. Sees, M. A. van den Doel, C. A. Van Blitterswijk and K. de Groot, "Osteoinduction by biomaterials-Physicochemical and structural influences," J. Biomed. Mater. Res. A., **77A [4]** 747–62 (2006).

131. J. C. Elliott, Structure and Chemistry of the Apatites and Other calcium Orthophosphates, Amsterdam: Elsevier (1994).

132. T. Kokubo, S. Ito, Z. T. Huang, T. Hayashi, S. Sakka, T. Kitsugi and T. Yamamuro, "Ca-P rich layer formed on high strength bioactive glass-ceramics A-W," J. Biomed. Mater. Res., **24** 331–43 (1990).

133. M. M. Peireira, A. E. Clark and L. L. Hench, "Calcium phosphate formation on sol-gel-derived bioactive glasses *in vitro*," J. Biomed. Mater. Res., **28 [6]** 693–8 (1994).

134. G. Daculsi, R. Z. LeGeros, M. M. Heughebaert and I. Barbieux, "Formation of carbonate apatite crystals after implantation of calcium phosphate ceramics," Calcif. Tissue Int., **46** 20–7 (1990).

135. C. T. Hanks, J. C. Watahaz and Z. Suni, "*In vitro* models of biocompatibility: A review," Dent. Mater., **12** 186–93 (1996).

136. H. W. Kim, Y. H. Koh, S. B. Seo and H. E. Kim, "Properties of fluoridated hydroxyapatite–alumina biological composites densified with addition of CaF_2," Mater. Sci. Engg. C, **23** 515–21 (2003).

137. R. L. Reis and T. S. Román, Biodegradable systems in tissue engineering and regenerative medicine, United States of America, CRC Press (2005).

138. B. Ivanov, A. M. Hakimian, G. M. Peavy and R. F. Haglund, Jr, "Mid-infrared laser ablation of a hard biocomposite material: mechanistic studies of pulse duration and interface effects," Applied Surface Science, **208–209** 77–84 (2003).

139. K. O'Kelly, D. Tancred, B. McCormack and A. Carr, "A quantitative technique for comparing synthetic porous hydroxyapatite structure and cancellous bone," J. Mater. Sci. Mater. Med., **7** 207–213 (1996).

140. M. Giannini, C. J. Soares and R. M. de Carvalho, "Ultimate tensile strength of tooth structures," Dental Materials **20** 322–329 (2004).

141. M. A. Meyers, P.-Y. Chen, A. Y.-M. Lin and Y. Seki, "Biological materials: Structure and mechanical properties," Progress in Materials Science **53** 1–206 (2008).

4

THE MICRO MACROPOROUS BIPHASIC CALCIUM PHOSPHATE CONCEPT FOR BONE RECONSTRUCTION AND TISSUE ENGINEERING

Guy Daculsi[1,2], Franck Jegoux[1,3], and Pierre Layrolle[1]

[1]*INSERM, Université de Nantes, UMR U791, Faculté de Chirurgie Dentaire, Place Alexis Ricordeau, 44042 Nantes Cedex 01, France*
[2]*CHU de Bordeaux/INSERM, CIC-Innovations Technologiques Biomatériaux, Bordeaux France*
[3]*CHU Pontchaillou Service ORL et chirurgie maxillofaciale, Rennes France*

Contents

4.1	Overview	102
4.2	Introduction	103
4.3	The Fundamental Physical, Chemical and Biological Properties of Biphasic Calcium Phosphate Bioceramics	104
	4.3.1 Introduction to Macroporosity and Microporosity	104
	4.3.2 Physical and Chemical Properties	106
	4.3.3 Mechanical Properties	107
	4.3.4 Bioactivity, Osteogenic Properties	107
	4.3.4.1 Composition	109
	4.3.4.2 Dissolution Properties	109
	4.3.4.3 Cell Proliferation and Colonization	109
	4.3.4.4 *In Vivo* Experiment	109
4.4	Bioceramics: New Developments	113
	4.4.1 Microstructure Improvement	113
	4.4.2 BCP-Based Macroporous Cements	114

Advanced Biomaterials: Fundamentals, Processing, and Applications, Edited by Bikramjit Basu, Dhirendra S. Katti, and Ashok Kumar
Copyright © 2009 The American Ceramic Society

4.4.3   How to Improve the Radiopacity of Bioactive Injectable
        Bone Substitutes   115
4.4.4   BCP for Resorbable Osteosynthesis   118
4.4.5   BCP Scaffolds for Bone Tissue Engineering   120
4.4.6   BCP Scaffolds with Mesenchymal Stem Cells (MSC)   124
4.4.7   BCP Scaffolds for Growth Plate Chondrocyte Maturation   125
4.4.8   BCP Granules and Polymers for Injectable Bioceramics   125
        4.4.8.1 Suspension   125
        4.4.8.2 Self-Hardening Injectible-Mouldable Composite   126
4.4.9   BCP/Fibrin Glue   127
4.4.10 BCP Granules for Drug Delivery   128
4.5 Clinical Applications   129
   4.5.1   Applications in Dentistry   129
           4.5.1.1 Prevention of Bone Resorption   129
           4.5.1.2 Sinus Lift Augmentation   130
   4.5.2   Applications in Orthopedics   130
           4.5.2.1 Cervical Spine Arthrodesis   131
           4.5.2.2 Anterior Cervical Fusion with PEEK Cage   131
           4.5.2.3 High Tibial Valgisation Osteotomy (HTO)   131
4.6 Conclusion   132
     Acknowledgments   133
     References   133

4.1   OVERVIEW

Developing calcium phosphate ceramics and other related biomaterials for bone grafts requires better control of biomaterial resorption and bone substitution processes. The biphasic calcium phosphate ceramics (BCP) concept is determined by an optimum balance between the more stable HA phase and the more soluble TCP. The material is soluble and gradually dissolves in the body, seeding new bone formation as it releases calcium and phosphate ions into the biological medium.

The main attractive feature of BCP ceramic is its ability to form direct bone bonding with host bone, resulting in a strong interface. The formation of this dynamic interface is the result of a sequence of events involving interaction between biological fluid and cells, as well as the formation of carbonated hydroxyapatite (CHA), which is similar to bone mineral, by means of dissolution/precipitation processes. Associating micro and macroporosity with the BCP chemical concept resulted in high osteogenicity and osteoinductive properties. At the present time, micro macroporous scaffolds are commercially available in blocks, particulates and customised designs, and specific matrices have been developed for combination with bone marrow or mesenchymal stem cells for tissue engineering (hybrid bone). The search for the ideal scaffold for tissue egineering and bone reconstruction in low trophic areas or large bone reconstruction remains a challenge, as those currently available are not appropriate.

In addition, the need for material for Minimally Invasive Surgery (MIS) has led to the development of a concept combining specific granules with polymer or self-setting calcium phosphate cement for injectable/mouldable bone substitutes. Different types of injectable/mouldable bone substitutes have been developed:

a) injectable biomaterial without initial hardening, where BCP granules are associated with a hydrosoluble polymer;
b) the association of MBCP and fibrin sealant,
c) the association of synthetic self hardening polymers and
d) new generation macroporous calcium phosphate cements.

The purpose of this chapter is to review the fundamental properties of biphasic calcium phosphate bioceramics, their biological properties, the development of new technologies for tissue engineering, and examples of clinical applications.

4.2 INTRODUCTION

In 1920, Albee reported the first successful application of a calcium phosphate reagent for the repair of a bone defect in humans [1]. More than 50 years later, clinical use of a "tricalcium phosphate" preparation in surgically-created periodontal defects in animals was reported by Nery et al. [2] and the use of dense hydroxyapatite HA as an immediate replacement for tooth root was reported by Dennnissen [3]. Largely through the separate efforts of Jarcho, de Groot and Aoki in the early 1980s [4–7], synthetic hydroxyapatite (HA) and β-tricalcium phosphate (β-TCP), became commercially available as bone substitute materials for dental and medical applications. The BCP concept has been widely developed by Daculsi and Legeros since the 1990s [8–11].

Developing BCP ceramics and other related biomaterials for bone grafts required controlling the processes of bioceramic resorption and bone formation at the expense of the biomaterial [12–15]. Synthetic bone graft materials are available as alternatives to autogeneous bone for repair, substitution or augmentation.

The BCP concept [10] is based on an optimum balance between the more stable phase (HA) and the more soluble phase (β-TCP). BCP bioceramics are soluble and gradually dissolve *in vivo*, seeding new bone formation as it releases calcium and phosphate ions into the biological medium. Commercial BCP bioceramics consist of a mixture of hydroxyapatite (HA), $Ca_{10}(PO_4)_6(OH)_2$ and beta-tricalcium phosphate (β-TCP), $Ca_3(PO_4)_2$ of varying HA/β-TCP ratios (Table 4.1).

At the present time, commercial BCPs are sold in Europe, U.S., Brazil, Japan, Korea, Taiwan and China as bone-graft or bone substitute materials for orthopedic and dental applications under various trade marks. Currently, BCP bioceramics are recommended for use as an alternative or additive to autogeneous bone for orthopedic and dental applications.

TABLE 4.1. Commercial BCP and BCP Composites

HA/β-TCP ratio	
60/40	MBCP® (Biomatlante, France)
20/80	MBCP2000® (Biomatante France)
20/80	Tribone 80® (Strycker Europe)
55/45	Eurocer 400® (FH France)
60/40	Osteosynt® (Einco Ltd, Brazil)
60/40	Triosite® (Zimmer, IND)
60/40	4Bone® (MIS Israel)
60/40	SBS® (Expanscience France)l)
60/40	4Bone® (MIS Israel)
60/40	Kainos +® (Signus Germay)
60/40	Hatric® (Arthrex Germany, US)
60/40	OptiMX® (Exactech USA)
65/35	BCP® (Medtronic)
65/35	Eurocer 200® (FH France)
BCP cement	MCPC™ (Biomatlante France)
Composites	
BCP/Collagen	Allograft (Zimmer, IN)
BCP/HPMC	MBCP Gel ® (Biomatlante France)
BCP/Fibrin	Tricos® (Baxter BioSciences BioSurgery)
BCP/Silicon	FlexHA (Xomed, FL)

Exploratory studies have demonstrated the potential uses for BCP ceramic as a scaffold for tissue engineering in bone regeneration, gene therapy, and drug delivery. More recently, the BCP granule concept has been applied to the development of a new generation of injectable, mouldable bone substitutes [16,17]. BCP granules are combined with various polymers, natural (e.g., fibrin sealant) or synthetic (e.g., hydrosoluble polymer), to develop an injectable bone substitute, IBS [17], or calcium phosphate cement to improve macroporosity and provide greater osteoconduction [18].

The present review focuses on the main physical and chemical properties of various BCP bioceramics such as micro and macrostructure, role and performance of different HA/TCP ratios, new developments in bioceramics for injectable, mouldable BCP bioceramics and the clinical relevance of such bioceramics.

4.3   THE FUNDAMENTAL PHYSICAL, CHEMICAL AND BIOLOGICAL PROPERTIES OF BIPHASIC CALCIUM PHOSPHATE BIOCERAMICS

4.3.1   Introduction to Macroporosity and Microporosity

Two physical properties of bioceramics were considered to be very important for optimum biological performance in bioceramic-cell interaction, bioceramic resorption, bioceramic-tissue interface and new bone formation. These fundamental physical properties are interconnecting macroporosity and appropriate microporosity [19,20].

Macroporosity in BCP ceramic is introduced by incorporating volatile materials (e.g., naphthalene, hydrogen peroxide or other porogens), heating at temperatures of less than 200 °C and subsequent sintering at higher temperatures [19,21–25]. Macroporosity is formed as a result of the release of the volatile materials (Figure 4.1). Microporosity is a consequence of the temperature and duration of sintering [20]: the higher the temperature, the lower the microporosity content and the lower the specific surface area (Figure 4.2).

At present, commercial BCP products of different or similar HA/β-TCP ratios are manufactured in many parts of the world and their successful use in medicine and dentistry has been reported [11,26–31]. The total porosity (macroporosity plus microporosity) of these products is reported to be about 70% of the bioceramic volume. Current BCP commercial products with HA/β-TCP ratios

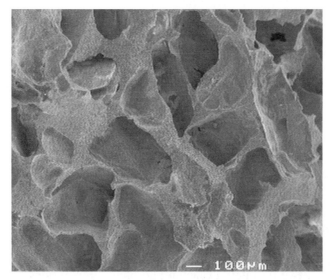

Figure 4.1. Macroporosity of MBCP observed with SEM.

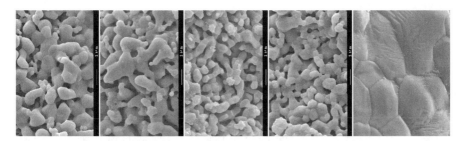

Figure 4.2. SEM of discs sintered at 1050 °C (D1, D2, and D3) and at 1200 °C (D4, D5).

ranging from 60/40 to 75/25 (Table 4.1), present similar macroporosity percentages (50 to 60%), but microporosity percentages are very different, varying from 3% to 25%.

A low microporosity percentage and low surface area can result in lower bioactivity and lower dissolution properties. Microporosity of at least 20% with a specific surface area of more than $2 m^2/g$ is required for optimal BCP efficacy.

Ideally, pore size for a bioceramic material should be similar to that of bone. It has been demonstrated that microporosity (diameter <10 μm) allows body fluid circulation whereas macroporosity (diameter >100 μm) provides a scaffold for bone-cell colonisation.

Significant improvements in the method for introducing macroporosity/microporosity have recently been developed in the production of micro-macroporous BCP (MBCP2000®, Biomatlante, France) [32]. In this method, CDA is mixed with a combination of selected particles of naphthalene and sugar. After isostatic compaction, the CDA block is subjected to a specific process of sublimation/calcination. The BCP obtained using the classic naphthalene porogen (MBCP) compared to that using a mixture of porogens, naphthalene and sugar (MBCP2000), resulted in differences in density, Specific Surface Area (SSA) of the crystal, compression strength and total porosity (Table 4.2). The permeability after incubation in bovine serum of MBCP2000 was twice as high as that of MBCP, and MBCP2000 showed a 30% increase in absorption compared to MBCP. The considerably higher permeability of MBCP2000 compared to MBCP cannot be explained by any difference in total porosity but may be attributed to differences in pore size, particularly mesopores.

4.3.2 Physical and Chemical Properties

As β-TCP is more soluble than HA [33], the extent of dissolution of BCP ceramics of comparable macroporosity and particle size will depend on the HA/β-TCP ratio: the higher the ratio, the lower the extent of dissolution [8,10,13]. The dissolution properties are also affected by the methods used in producing the BCPs: whether from a single calcium–deficient apatite phase (BCP1) or from a mechanical mixture of two unsintered calcium phosphate preparations (BCP2): BCP2

TABLE 4.2.

	Temperature sintering	Duration	Temperature step control
D1	1050	5	none
D2	1050	5	900 °C, 3H
D3	1050	5	900 °C, 3H
D4	1200	5	900 °C, 12H
D5	1200	5	900 °C, 12H

(Temperature rise, 5 °C/min; cooling rate; 1 °C/min). Continuous heating for BCP specimens D1 and D5; programmed heating for D2, D3, and D4).

has a higher extent of dissolution than BCP1 [33]. In some cases, BCP ceramic with similar HA/β-TCP ratios could present different dissolution rates [34]. This phenomenon may be caused by processing variables (sintering time and temperature) that may affect total macroporosity and microporosity: the greater the macroporosity and microporosity, the greater the extent of dissolution. *In vivo*, dissolution of BCP ceramics is manifested by a decrease in crystal size and an increase in macro- and microporosity [9–12].

4.3.3 Mechanical Properties

It is logical for the pore size and percentage of macroporosity of the BCP ceramic to affect the mechanical properties [22]. The preparation method has also been found to have a significant influence on compressive strength. BCP ceramic prepared from a single calcium-deficient apatite phase is reported to have higher compressive strength (2 to 12 MPa) than BCP ceramic prepared by mixing two unsintered calcium phosphate preparations (2MPa): one which, after sintering at 1200 °C, results in only HA and the other which results in only β-TCP [34]. Initial mechanical property is not the best criterion for evaluating the efficacy of bone ingrowth. For example, BCP with high mechanical properties because of low microporosity (as a result of a high sintering temperature) may have reduced bioresorption and bioactivity. On the contrary, it has been demonstrated that the initial mechanical property of BCP increased two or three times (2 to 6 MPa) in a few weeks after implantation thanks to the physical and chemical events of dissolution and biological precipitation into the micropores [12].

4.3.4 Bioactivity, Osteogenic Properties

The main attractive feature of bioactive bone graft materials such as BCP ceramic is its ability to form a strong direct bond with host bone resulting in a strong interface compared to bioinert or biotolerant materials which form a fibrous interface [9–15]. The formation of the dynamic interface between bioactive materials and host bone is believed to be the result of a sequence of events involving interaction with cells and the formation of carbonate hydroxyapatite (CHA), which is similar to bone mineral, by means of dissolution/precipitation processes [12,15].

Bioactivity is described as the property of a material to form carbonate hydroxyapatite (CHA) on its surface *in vitro* [15,35,36] or *in vivo* [9,37–39]. Osteoinductivity or osteogenic property is the property of the material to induce bone formation *de novo* or ectopically (in non-bone forming sites). Bioceramics (calcium phosphates, bioactive glass) do not usually have osteoinductive properties [19]. However, several reports have shown the osteoinductive properties of certain calcium phosphate bioceramics such as coralline HA (derived from coral) or those observed in certain studies using BCP [40–41]. Reddi [42] explains these apparent osteoinductive properties as the ability of particular ceramics to concentrate bone growth factors that are circulating in the biological fluids, and these growth factors induce bone formation. Ripamonti [43] and Kuboki [44] independently postulated that the geometry of the material is a critical parameter in bone induction. Others have speculated that low oxygen tension in the central region of implants might provoke a dedifferentiation of pericytes from blood microvessels into osteoblasts [45]. It has been also postulated that the nanostructured rough surface or the surface charge of implants might cause the asymmetrical division of stem cells into osteoblasts [46].

Surface microstructure appears to be a common property of the materials that induce ectopic bone formation. Recent studies have indicated the critical role played by micropores on ceramic-induced osteogenesis. For example, it has been reported that bone formation occurred in dog muscle inside porous calcium phosphate ceramics with surface microporosity but bone was not observed inside the dense surface of macroporous ceramics [47]. It has also been reported that metal implants coated with a microporous layer of octacalcium phosphate could induce ectopic bone in goat muscle, while a smooth layer of carbonated apatite on these porous metal implants was not able to induce bone formation [48]. In all the previous experiments, ectopic bone formation occurred inside the macroporous ceramic blocks.

It has been demonstrated that sintering temperature has a drastic effect on the microporosity of calcium phosphate ceramics: the higher the sintering temperature, the denser the ceramic surface. To evaluate microporosity, how it is produced and the role it plays, the authors precipitated calcium-deficient apatite (CDA) prepared to provide BCP with an HA/β-TCP ratio of 60/40 + 2, then sintered between 1000 °C and 1200 °C; discs (25 mm diameter) were prepared for an *in vitro* test and machined into implants (3 mm diameter) for *in vivo* implantation. The discs were distributed into five groups: D1, D2, D3, D4 and D5, and sintered using various conditions (heating rate and temperature) (Figure 4.2) (Table 4.2). All groups were subjected to the same rate of temperature rise (5 °C/min), cooling rate (1 °C/min) and total sintering period (5 h). The discs in groups D2, D3 and D4 were heated to 900 °C then allowed to remain at this temperature for 3 h (D2) or 12 h (D3 and D4). The final temperature was 1050 °C for groups D1, D2 and D3, and 1200 °C for groups D4 and D5. XRD and FTIR analyses of the sintered discs showed only the BCP phase with an HA/β-TCP ratio of 60/40. Surface area, microporosity percent, cell coverage are summarized in Table 4.3.

TABLE 4.3.

	SSA m^2/g ± 0.01	% micropores	% cell coverage	dissolution ppm Ca, 60 min
D1	3.5	80	35 ± 1.2	7.8
D2	3.2	60	35 ± 1.0	7.9
D3	3.1	50	28 ± 1.5	6.9
D4	0.3	10	20 ± 2.0	3.8
D5	0.8	10	16 ± 2.0	3.1

4.3.4.1 Composition. XRD analysis showed the final HA/βTCP ratios for all BCP specimens to be 60/40 ± 2, independent of the sintering conditions. No differences in relative intensities or broadening of the diffraction peaks were observed in any of the BCP specimens. In the FTIR spectra, only absorption bands attributed to the OH group for the HA and to the PO_4 groups for the HA and the β-TCP were observed. An apparent decrease in the intensity of the OH absorption bands, loss of resolution and broadening of the OH and PO_4 absorption bands were observed in the FTIR spectra of BCP specimens D4 and D5 compared to those of D1, D2, and D3.

4.3.4.2 Dissolution Properties. Dissolution experiments in an acidic buffer (0.1 M KAc, pH 6, 37 °C) showed differences in the extent of dissolution as reflected by the concentration of Ca ions released into the acidic buffer over time. Maximum dissolution (maximum change in Ca concentration in the buffer) was observed in the first ten minutes after exposing the BCP discs to the acidic buffer, and no significant change in Ca concentration was observed after 60 minutes. The BCP discs in groups D1 and D2 behaved almost identically followed by D3, indicating greater solubility than the BCP discs in groups D4 and D5.

4.3.4.3 Cell Proliferation and Colonization. An established mouse fibroblast cell line L929 was used. After seven days of culture, it was observed that percentage cell coverage on the BCP disc surfaces differed: much higher percentage coverage was observed on the surfaces of D1 and D2 discs (80 and 60%, respectively) than on the surfaces of D3, and even lower for surfaces of D4 and D5 discs (about 10 to 20%), as shown in Table 4.3. The cells on BCP discs D1 and D2 were observed to have proliferated and to be present all over the surface of the discs while the cells on the D4 and D5 discs showed much less proliferation and were observed only on the areas where they were originally deposited. The cells on the surface of the D1 and D2 discs had polygonal shapes while the cells on D4 and D5 appeared to be more rounded and contracted. Furthermore, the cells on D5 were characterised by long filopodia. The surfaces of the D1 and D2 discs appeared grainy and rougher while the surfaces of the D5 discs appeared smooth and similar to the surface as it was before the *in vitro* experiment.

4.3.4.4 In Vivo Experiment. The right and left epiphyses of rabbits were implanted, and two defects created, one in the upper part (cancellous bone) and one in the diaphysis (no bone trabeculae, only bone marrow). After three weeks, the implants were processed for histology. All the implanted BCP discs showed good biocompatibility. However, bone growth and bone contact were very different for the discs implanted in the cancellous bone of the epiphysis compared to those in bone marrow: the higher the density, the lower the osteogenicity, particularly for the discs implanted in the bone marrow site. Moreover, the higher the density (D5 discs), the lower the amount of newly-formed bone in direct contact with the implant surface (Figures 4.3, 4.4 and 4.5).

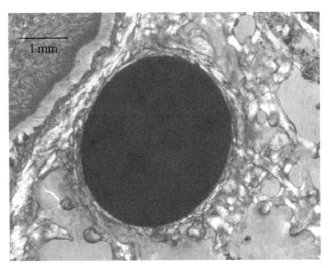

Figure 4.3. Disc D3 implanted in rabbit epiphysis cancellous bone, polarised light microscopy.

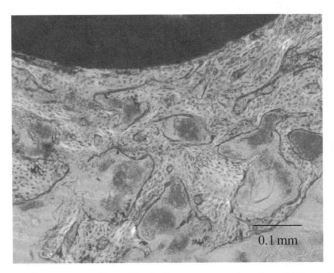

Figure 4.4. Disc D1 implanted in the bone marrow site of a rabbit epiphysis.

Current FDA and/or CE-approved commercial BCP products (e.g., *MBCP®, Biosel®, TCH®, Calciresorb®, Triosite®, Tribone® 80, OpteMix®, Hatric®*, etc) with similar HA/βTCP ratios and similar percentage macroporosity (60 to 70%) can vary in the interconnectivity of their macroporosity and in their percentage microporosity. Differences in the porogens used to provide the macroporosity, plus differences in sintering temperature and conditions, all affect percentage

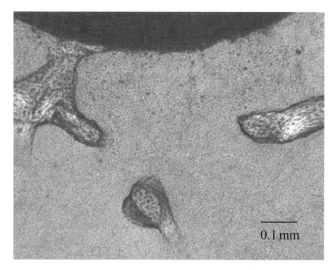

Figure 4.5. Disc D5 implanted in the bone marrow site of a rabbit epiphysis.

microporosity. It is therefore not surprising that these products may show different *in vivo* performances. For the BCP bioceramic to have osteogenic/osteoinductive properties, high percentage microporosity and macroporosity are required. These data showed that higher osteogenic properties were observed with BCP discs with lower density (produced at a lower sintering temperature). These results confirm that microporosity promotes osteogenic/osteoinductive properties in BCP bioceramics.

The properties of ceramic, such as composition, geometry, porosity, size and microstructure, should be considered as critical parameters for bone induction. These properties play a more important role in bone induction than in mechanical stability [49].

Such osteogenic/osteoinductive properties for BCP ceramics can be explained by the formation of microcrystals with Ca/P ratios similar to those of the bone apatite crystals observed after implantation of MBCP. The abundance of these crystals was directly related to the initial β-TCP/HA ratio in the BCP: the higher the ratio the greater the abundance of the microcrystals associated with the BCP crystals. Using high resolution TEM, the authors demonstrated that the formation of these bone apatite-like microcrystals after implantation of calcium phosphates (HA, BCP) was non-specific, that is, not related to implantation site (osseous or non-osseous sites), subject of implantation, or type of CaP ceramics.

The coalescing interfacial zone of biological apatite and residual BCP ceramic crystals (mostly HA), provides a scaffold for further bone-cell adhesion and stem cell differentiation into osteogenic lines, and further bone ingrowth. The bone repair or bone regeneration process involves dissolution of calcium phosphate crystals and then a precipitation of needle-like carbonate hydroxyapatite

(CHA) crystallites in micropores close to the dissolving crystals. The coalescing zone forms the new biomaterial/bone interface, which includes the participation of proteins and CHA crystals originating from the BCP ceramic crystals. This has been described as a coalescing zone and dynamic interface (50).

If the coalescing zone (chemical bonding) caused by precipitation of the biological apatites can be considered to be related to dissolution of the calcium phosphate (higher for β TCP) [10,15], then it can be suspected that the kinetics of bone ingrowth at the expense of the bioceramics is directly related to the HA/TCP ratio of the biphasic calcium phosphate. In 1998, the authors reported using TEM the difference at the crystal level between HA, TCP and various types of BCP, have never published data at the bony tissue level. To determine the influence of ratio on tissue ingrowth and bioceramic resorption, the authors used different types of BCP (pure HA, pure β-TCP, HA/TCP 27/75, 50/50 and 75/25) for filling maxillofacial defects in dog mandibulars (only granules with micropore content), and critical size defects in dog femoral epiphyses (6 mm in diameter filled with a cylindrical implant that was both micro and macroporous). The implantation period was four, six or twelve weeks. From the two studies it appears that no statistical difference was measured for either bone ingrowth or bioceramic resorption in the BCP samples. Large bone remodelling appears in both BCP samples (Figure 4.6) with well-architectured bone (lamellar bone), and osteoconduction was evidenced. For the pure HA and pure β-TCP, significant differences were measured for bioceramic resorption, the higher resorption over time from four to twelve weeks was reported for TCP. However, in spite of the considerable resorption for TCP, there was no more bone ingrowth than for HA, the TCP appeared to have been resorbed without osteoconduction, and cells and unmineralised tissue had taken the place of the TCP (Figure 4.7). For HA, as there was no apparent resorption, the space for bone ingrowth was still limited. On the contrary, for both types of BCP an equilibrium was observed between bioceramic resorbtion and bone ingrowth. At 12 weeks, no significant difference was measured in the three types of BCP tested, in spite of what appeared to be a slight increase in bioceramic resorption for the higher HA/TCP ratio (75/25).

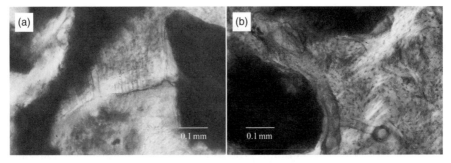

Figure 4.6. (a) BCP in mandibular area with HA/TCP ratio of 20/80 and (b) ratio of 80/20.

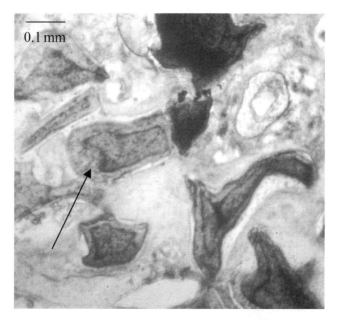

Figure 4.7. Pure β-TCP implanted in a dog mandibular defect showing no bone contact with the granules and extensive resorption at the surface of the grain (arrow).

4.4 BIOCERAMICS: NEW DEVELOPMENTS

4.4.1 Microstructure Improvement

At present, granules and particles are used increasingly in mouldable, injectable or resorbable composites. However, the biological behaviour of the particles can be influenced not only by chemical composition and crystalinity, but by several other parameters such as granulometry and microporosity. The influence of microporosity on new-bone formation, though apparently one of the more complicated variables, has rarely been studied, unlike macroporosity. A recent study by O. Malard et al. [51] is reported. Two different porosities of biphasic calcium phosphate granules were prepared (20% and 40% porosity) and evaluated in rat critical size defects. This study sought to specify the role of microporosity in an *in vivo* experiment, as well as examine the amount and kinetics of newly-formed bone ingrowth, and the biodegradation of BCP ceramic. LP (20%) and HP (40%) microporous granules were prepared from calcium-deficient apatite (CDA) sintered at 1050 °C which resulted in a biphasic calcium phosphate BCP of 60% HA and 40% β-TCP. XRD showed BCP content without trace of carbonate, with an HA/β-TCP ratio of 60/40. No difference was observed between the HP and LP granules. SEM image analysis showed that porosity was 17.6% ± 3.6 for LP granules and 39.7% ± 10.3 for HP granules (p < 0.001). LP granules were regular rounded granules and HP granules were more irregular in shape, with a sharper surface.

Density of the LP was 3.096 gram per cm 3 ± 0.003 and was 3.093 gram per cm 3 ± 0.002 for the HP (no significant difference, $p = 0.18$). SEM image analysis showed that the LP granules had a mean diameter granulometry of $780\,\mu m \pm 148$ and the HP samples of $814\,\mu m \pm 207$ (no significant difference, $p = 0.13$).

After three and six weeks of implantation, newly-formed bone was observed in both samples. Bone ingrowth was less apparent at three weeks than at six weeks and seemed to develop faster after implantation of high porosity granules. In the early stages, it consisted of woven bone containing many osteocytes. Newly-formed bone was observed mainly in the deep zones of the implanted defects from the surface to the core, initially in close contact with the BCP particles (without fibrous interposition) but always close to the bordering bone. Osteoid appeared around the ceramic particles and was observed at the early time of three weeks. Using SEM, bone ingrowth at three weeks in the LP group was $5\% \pm 0.3$ of the implanted defect, and was greater than in the HP group ($1.6\% \pm 0.4$, $p < 0.0001$). At six weeks, in the LP group, the amount of newly-formed bone was $4.3\% \pm 0.5$ of the implanted defect, and was lower than in the HP group ($8.6\% \pm 1.6$, $p = 0.044$). Between three and six weeks, the amount of newly-formed bone increased in the HP group ($p < 0.0001$).

During the same interval, the amount of newly-formed bone did not significantly increase in the LP group ($p = 0.25$). The BCP surface area in the implanted bone defects at three weeks was not statistically different between the two groups ($p = 0.1$), and no more significant at six weeks ($p = 0.8$). The decrease in the BCP surface area was not significant between three to six weeks in the LP group ($p = 0.4$) or in the HP group ($p = 0.3$). With the LP granules, new bone formation was significantly greater at three weeks than with HP. This could be related to higher macrophagous activity with regard to the release of large particles (as confirmed by histological examination), in addition to the release of Ca and P ions. Between three and six weeks, newly-formed bone did not significantly increase in the LP granules, whereas it did with the HP (5-fold increase), confirming previous studies about high initial inflammation, and macrophagous activity acting as a booster for osteogenic cell differentiation [52].

At the later time of six weeks, there was an inversion in the amount of newly-formed bone, with more newly-formed bone in the HP implants confirming the osteo-inductive property of the micropores as described in other animal models. The reason why granules that are less porous can induce faster bone ingrowth is not clear and needs further experiments. It has not been clearly elucidated why higher porosity is related to a huge increase in new bone formation after three weeks.

4.4.2   BCP-Based Macroporous Cements

The need for a material for Minimally Invasive Surgery (MIS) prompted the development of a concept for injectable, mouldable calcium phosphate cement (CPC) as bone substitutes. Currently, several calcium phosphate bone cements are commercially available and more are being investigated. The concept was first introduced by LeGeros et al. in 1982 [53] and the first patent was obtained by Brown and Chow [54] in 1986. All the current CPCs are reported to have good mechanical properties and reasonable setting times. However, after setting, these materials remain dense and do not provide rapid bone substitution because of the lack of macroporosity. Numerous studies have reported the applications of currently available commercial calcium phosphate cements [55]. New BCP-based calcium phosphate cement has recently been developed (patent) [56]. The MCPC consists of multiphasic calcium phosphate phases, including BCP, and *in vivo*, the components of the cement resorb at different rates allowing the formation of interconnecting macroporosity, thus facilitating bone ingrowth and substitution of the cement with the newly-forming bone [18].

The powder component is essentially made of a settable and resorbable matrix (which includes alpha-TCP, stabilised amorphous calcium phosphate (s-ACP) and monocalcium phosphate monohydrate, MCPM). A sieved fraction of macroporous biphasic calcium phosphate (BCP) granules ranging between 80 and 200 µm in diameter are incorporated into the matrix. The cement liquid is an aqueous solution of Na_2HPO_4.

After setting MCPC in distilled water at 20 °C, the mechanical properties in compression of such materials were 10 Mpa ± 2 at 24 h and 15 MPa ± 2 after 48 h. The cohesion time for injectability was reached after 20 minutes. Animal models using critical size defects in rabbit epiphyses or goat vertebral bodies demonstrate the performance and efficacy of this concept of calcium phosphate cement. MBCP granules act as a scaffold for bone osteoconduction, and resorption of the ACP content of the cement allowed macroporosity and bone ingrowth between and at the surface of the BCP granules, extending to the core of the implanted site. The cement matrix dissolved as was expected, forming an open structure and interconnecting porosity.

SEM analyses showed that organised bone trabeculae were well differentiated from the residual granules. After 12 weeks, few granules were fully integrated into the new cortical bone and deeper into the core, spongious bone was formed. Bone remodelling was in evidence at both six and twelve weeks in rabbits and less extensively in the goat model, in spite of six months of implantation (Figure 4.8). These differences could be explained by the mechanical strain and the osteogneic properties of the implantation sites. X-ray microtomography (microCT) demonstrated bone ingrowth at the expense of the cement and surrounding the residual BCP granules. Bone trabeculae were observed coming from the spongious bone to the implant site. Resorption of the BCP granules was evident from six to twelve weeks.

4.4.3 How to Improve the Radiopacity of Bioactive Injectable Bone Substitutes

In the context of bone healing, biomaterials need to have certain specific characteristics: providing bone regeneration, being resorbable, having mechanical or rheological properties [57]. Currently, for Minimally Invasive Surgery (MIS),

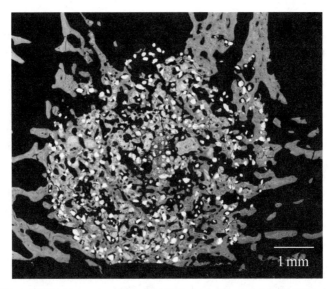

<u>Figure 4.8.</u> MCPC implantation in a rabbit epiphysis femoral defect, SEM observation.

X-ray contrast performance also provides important data, as the radiopacity of materials is required during the implantation process to ensure the location of the filled material [58]. Various radiopaque agents (RA) such as barium sulfate, zirconium oxide or iodine have been tested (mechanical properties, cytotoxicity effects) [59]. In vertebroplasty, the non resorbable acrylic bone cements (poly-methyl methacrylate, PMMA) contain barium sulphate [60]. To obtain a resorbable injectable bone substitute with rheological properties and x-ray contrast characteristics, Serge Baroth et al. [61] have developed "rounded" calcium phosphate granules loaded with an RA such as barium salt or with rare earth elements containing bismuth, lutetium and gadolinium. The four RA produced were: barium sulphate ($BaSO_4$), lutetium oxide (Lu_2O_3), bismuth oxide (Bi_2O_3) and gadolinium phosphate ($GdPO_4$). CDA (BCP 60-40) were mixed with RA (20% w/w) to obtain radiopaque calcium phosphate composites. The composites were shaped in 80–200 µm "rounded" granules or pellets (ten mm in diameter, one mm thickness). The materials were sintered according to specific processes. Steam sterilisation (121 °C, 30 minutes for pellets) or dry sterilization (180 °C, four hours for granules) were used for *in vitro* and *in vivo* tests.

X-ray diffraction (XRD) and infra-red spectroscopy (FTIR) showed integration of the Ba into the CaP crystal lattice, while no substitution was noticed for the other RA used. SEM observation of the composite surfaces showed that the addition of our RA to the calcium phosphate matrix had an influence on crystal shape, crystal size and microporosity. With the addition of $BaSO_4$, large crystals were obtained with low microporosity and a smooth surface. With the addition of Bi_2O_3, crystals grew in needle shapes with significant microporosity. With Lu_2O_3 and $GdPO_4$, the microporosity was significant with small crystals and a number of fragments present on the BCP/Lu_2O_3 matrix.

TABLE 4.4.

	density	crystal size	SSA	compression strength	Total porosity
MBCP	0.83 g/cc	1.5 μm	1.7 m^2/g	6 MPa	69%
MBCP2000	0.75 g/cc	0.5 μm	1.6 m^2/g	4 MPa	73%

TABLE 4.6.

Materials	Plastic control	Act D	BCP/Ba	BCP/Bi	BCP/Lu
MTS activity (%) at 72 h	100	10	100	98	55

(SSA: specific surface area).

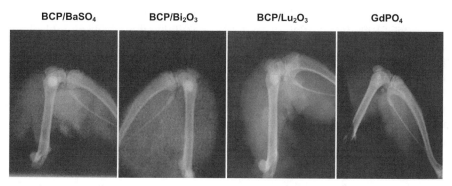

BCP/BaSO$_4$ **BCP/Bi$_2$O$_3$** **BCP/Lu$_2$O$_3$** **GdPO$_4$**

Figure 4.9. Radiographies of rat femoral epiphyses containing radiopaque granules after three weeks of implantation.

RA cytotoxicity was quantified *in vitro* according to ISO 10993-5 on extracted using osteoblastic cells MC3T3-E1. The RA cytotoxicity test showed no adverse effect (when MTS activity decreased more than 20%) on BaSO$_4$ and Bi$_2$O$_3$, whereas Lu$_2$O$_3$ was cytotoxic for osteoblastic cells (Table 4.4).

Whatever the matrix type (chemical composition or surface topography), it had an influence on cell behaviour. The MC3T3-E1 had classic osteoblastic morphology (long pseudopodia with good spreading), except for the Bi$_2$O$_3$ matrix, where the cell morphology and spreading were modified. Proliferation was the parameter most affected by the different types of pellet, it was greater with BCP/Ba, lower but equal with BCP/Lu and Gd, and lower still with BCP/Bi.

In situ radiopaque evaluation of our different materials showed that the BCP/Ba and BCP/Bi had the best contrast intensity when compared to the bone environment (Figure 4.9).

Histological results after *in vivo* implantation in rat epiphyses revealed newly-formed bone and granule resorption, and the quality of the bone ingrowth in contact with the materials. BCP/Ba and BCP/Gd materials had the most bone ingrowth quantitatively and qualitatively speaking, when compared to the BCP/Bi and BCP/Lu implanted materials [61].

Improved visualisation is necessary when bone defects are filled. The BCP/Ba composite has given promising results for developping a radiopaque, resorbable, injectable bone substitute designed for MIS, particularly in spine surgery for vertebroplasty.

4.4.4   BCP for Resorbable Osteosynthesis

Following a loss of osseous substance of tumoral or traumatic origin, it is often necessary to restore the osseous structure associating osteosynthesis and bone substitute. However a second operation is required to remove the osteosynthesis after wound healing, otherwise the osteosynthesis (such as titanium or Peek) will remain in place definitively. Resorbable osteosynthesis has been developed using resorbable polymers for many years [62–64]. Resorption control and higher osteogenic properties have improved using a combination of calcium phosphate granules, generally b-Tricalcium phosphate. PL DLLA polymers are resorbable by means of hydrolysis but are not well controlled over time. After six months, the hydrolysis appears in all the samples and suddenly the mechanical properties disappear. This uncontrolled process can appear in six or twelve months, often before bone ingrowth healing and mechanical stability have been attained. For osteosynthesis, better control of mechanical stability is required and thus promote bone ingrowth at the expense of the implant.

The advantage of a composite with PL DLLA and PCa is that it is possible to control the hydrolysis over time, to maintain the initial mechanical properties during bone ingrowth and then have long term mechanical properties from bone ingrowth at the expense of the implant. The development of composites combining PL DLLA and PCa have proved from the use of interference screws that the hydrolysis is controlled and delayed over time until wound healing. A recent study [65,66] reported the resorption kinetics of a composite using PL DLLA (Poly [L-Lactide-co-D, L-Lactide] acid) charged with PCa granules and the interaction with an injectable substitute such as MBCP gel. The injectable biomaterial was non self hardening, the biomaterial consists of BCP granules associated with a hydrosoluble polymer. The material was shown to be perfectly biocompatible and potentially resorbable and, thanks to its initial plasticity, it assumes the shape of the bone defects very easily, eliminating the need to shape the material to adjust it to the implantation site. MBCP gel has no mechanical properties and must be associated with osteosynthesis during the bone ingrowth process. However, bone cells are able to invade the spaces liberated by the disappearance of the polymer carrier. Bone ingrowth takes place all around the granules and at the expense of the resorption of the BCP granules. In time, mechanical properties could be observed due to the presence of the newly-formed bone [17,67–69]. Moreover, the three-dimensional structure of the network favourably influenced recruitment, cellular differentiation, angiogenesis and the formation of bone tissue.

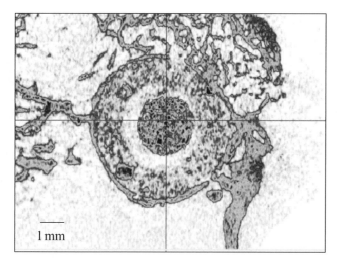

Figure 4.10. MicroCT image analysis showing the bone ingrowth architecture at the expense of both the composite and MBCP gel.

PL DLLA tubes charged with 20% BCP granules (six mm in diameter and eight mm in length with an open internal channel of four mm) were sterilised by irradiation at 25 KGrays. The tubes were implanted in rabbit femoral epiphyses. Some implants were kept empty, and others were filled with MBCP gel®. After six months, both samples were well-integrated into newly-formed bone. The composite showed considerable resorption on the surface and bone ingrowth into the implant with osteoconduction at the surface of the BCP granules (Figure 4.10). The shape of the implant was significantly changed by bone ingrowth at the expense of the implant. As a result, secondary mechanical properties appeared thanks to bone ingrowth at the expense of the composite, contrary to the pure polymer. In the hole of the defect, large bone ingrowth was observed at the expense of the MBCP gel.

Bone trabeculae and direct bone formation were observed between and at the surface of the BCP granules of the MBCP gel. The thickness of the newly-formed bone at the surface was around 300 µm. Bone architecture and bone remodelling were observed only after six months of implantation. The bone trabeculae were perpendicular to the shell of the newly-formed bone directly in contact with the composite. All the surfaces evidenced by the 3D reconstruction were osteoconductive and supported bone formation (Figure 4.11).

Resorbable polymers such as PLLA (poly lactide acid) and poly DL lactide co-glycolide (PDLG) have been used in clinical applications for many years [70]. It is often reported that such polymers cannot have bioabsorption kinetics that are adapted to bone reconstruction. The addition of a calcium phosphate like β-TCP, or calcium carbonate, improves resorption control, probably thanks to the release of Ca and PO_4 ions, neutralising the acid released as a result of the hydrolysis of the polymer. In the composite using biphasic calcium phosphate granules,

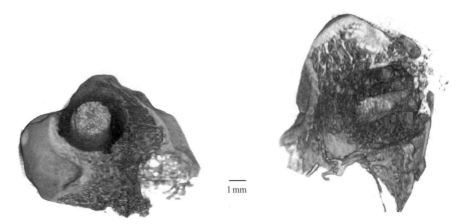

1 mm

<u>Figure 4.11.</u> MicroCT 3D reconstruction showing the hollow implant filled with MBCP Gel and bone trabeculae forming a shell at the surface of the implant with bone bridges perpendicular to the implant surface.

we obtained bone growth at the expense of the composite. Histology and micro CT were performed to examine the bone ingrowth and the interaction with the injectable bone substitute. The cooperation of the two materials for the mechanical performance of the composite and high osteogenic bone substitute can promote new surgical technology.

The hydrolysis of the PL DLLA/CaP composite had no incidence on the bone ingrowth at the expense of the MBCP gel. It appears that the lactic acid released by the hydrolysis had no effect on the osteogenic properties of the MBCP Gel. After 26 weeks, the composite was not fully substituted, only the surface at 200 to 300 μm appeared to have been transformed and invaded by newly-formed bone. The surface of the composite was osteoconductive without fibrous encapsulation.

This efficiency can be attributed to the calcium phosphate granules integrated into the PL DLLA. Certain authors attribute this process to a buffered effect of the calcium salts particles [71]. PL DLLA/CaP composites will provide suitable resorbable osteosynthesis associated with a non hardening injectable bone substitute. The PL DLLA/CaP composite can play a part in developing a concept for resorbable osteosynthesis and dedicated bone substitutes such as MBCP gel. The synergy of the two medical devices can contribute to new, less invasive, surgical technology, suppressing the need for a second operation to remove the osteosynthesis. Initial mechanical stability will be attained thanks to the PL DLLA/CaP composite and major bone ingrowth with secondary mechanical properties similar to those of natural bone will be achieved over time.

4.4.5   BCP Scaffolds for Bone Tissue Engineering

Reconstruction of large segmental bone defects is still a challenge in either orthopedics or oral oncology situations. Ceramics alone have failed to provide enough

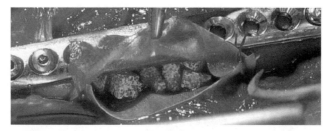

Figure 4.12. Collagen membrane containing MBCP® granules in the defect area.

new bone formation. Most models associate isolation from whole bone marrow aspirates, *ex vivo* expansion and then an attachment of mesenchymal stem cells to the biomaterial. However there are several critical questions regarding the quality of cell population isolation, the preservation of stem cell properties after expansion, and, given the complexity of the model, its reproducibility in clinical and surgical applications [72]. Moreover it is still a challenge in tumoral therapy, and few studies have focused on the use of ceramics in irradiated bone. The authors have previously reported good results for bone substitution with BCP and bone marrow grafts in pre-radiation or post-radiation conditions in animal studies [73,74]. Recently Jegoux et al. [75] reported the association of MBCP® granules with a 20/80 HA/TCP ratio, a porcine collagen membrane, and bone marrow for reconstruction in an irradiatepreclinical model.

Bone implantations were performed in rabbits. Segmental defects two cm in length were surgically removed from the middle height of the femur. Osteosyntheses were performed by two superposed steel plates. A 30×40 mm resorbable porcine collagen membrane was placed around the defect and then completely filled with MBCP® granules (Figure 4.12).

External fractionated radiation delivery was initiated two weeks after implantation and performed at ONCOVET (59650 Villeneuve d'Ascq, France). The delivered doses were calculated to be equivalent to those used in the treatment of squamous cell carcinoma in rabbits. Irradiation was strictly localised on the hind legs. Irradiation was delivered by low-energy photons from an X-ray source with energy of 300KVp (PANTAK, THERAPAX DXT 300, Gulmay Medical, UK). A total cumulative dose of 32 Gy was delivered at a rate of two Gy per day, four days per week, for four weeks. One week after radiation, an autologous BM graft was injected into the implanted site. One ml of BM was removed from the right humeral epiphysis with an 18 G needle previously heparinated (50 mg of heparin in 1000 ml of physiologic serum dilution) and were then immediately injected transcutaneously into the centre of the implants under radioscopic control.

Eighteen weeks after the BM injection, the implants were analysed. Ilium aspirate was technically more difficult to perform than in other sites in both species, owing to the orientation of the cortical surface that was also covered in thick muscles. Physiological bone marrow cells were found in all samples and cell counts confirmed that the grafts enclosed the physiological bone marrow without blood recovery. The global abundance of haematopoietic cells was significantly

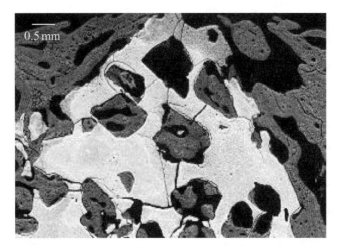

Figure 4.13. SEM observations showing the newly-formed bone in close contact with MBCP macropores.

lower in tibial sites than in the ilium or humeral sites in dogs ($p < 0.05$), whereas no difference was observed between any sites in rabbits. No difference was found between the ilium or humerus with respect to global haematopoietic cell abundance and count for every lineage. The overall quantity of haematopoietic cells was significantly lower in dogs than in rabbits for all sites ($p < 0.05$).

Three-dimensional imaging made possible an overall examination of the implants and showed a bony formation bridging the whole length of the defect in all implants. 2D imaging showed that newly-formed bone repartition was homogeneous in three implants and relatively heterogeneous in others. In the latter, new bone was observed essentially around the implant at the initial collagen membrane location. The new bone formation was observed both around the MBCP® granules and in the macropores with direct contact (Figure 4.13).

With both polarised light microscopy and SEM using BSE, the bone appeared well-mineralised and organised. Lamellar bone was observed directly in contact with the MBCP granules without fibrous interposition. From each host bone, the new bone formation had developed bone extremities from the defect to the core with osseous continuity. However, the bone ingrowth was not homogeneous according to the repartition in the axial section. In three implants, new bone was formed both in the centre and the periphery of the implant, and the MBCP granules appeared totally integrated. In the other three, newly-formed bone was observed mainly on the periphery of the osseous defects. The border of the defect was filled with compact bone with dense, lamellar structures with few spaces for vessels and soft tissue. The center of the defect for these three implants was filled with few osseous trabeculae, but large amounts of haematopoietic precursors and blood cells were observed. Some granules had no close contact with new bone formation but were associated with the considerable cellular content of the haematopoietic cells. This trend for peripheral trabecular bone formation was also observed in the first three implants in which the MBCP granules were filled with both compact bone at the border, and trabecular bone within the granules. Neither acellular, avascular areas nor fibrous encapsulation was observed in either sample. No statistical difference was observed between the centre and the quarters of the length defect according to the ceramic and newly-formed bone calculated with SEM image analysis.

As autologous bone grafts or biomaterial alone have failed to reconstruct large defects, BM cells have been proposed in this indication. BM is composed of haematopoietic cells and mesenchymal stem cells (MSC). The latter are multi-potent and can differentiate, among others, into an osteoblastic lineage. BM has been reported to contain almost one-to-two percent of cells with the potential for osteoblastic differentiation [76] and MSC osteoinduction properties have been well demonstrated [77,78]. Some studies have reported several differences in the quantity and quality of bone marrow MSC depending on the location of the bone, especially between orofacial and long bone. There are also limitations for collecting sufficient BM samples because of the limited size or inaccessibility of certain bones. Therefore, determining an appropriate technique and most favorable site for BM collecting could be critical for completing experimental models. This study revealed that BM samples are significantly less rich in the tibia than in the humerus and ilium in dogs while no significant difference was observed in rabbits. BM samples are significantly less rich in dogs than in rabbits ($p < 0.05$). The humerus collecting technique appeared to be more reproducible than that of the ilium, essentially because it was relatively easier to approach. These significant differences in relation to bone location and species are consistent with the need to better define experimental models in BM-based tissue engineering. Moreover, comparisons of studies conducted in different animal models should be made with caution.

Few studies have focused on large segmental defects in high weight bearing bones. The viability of a critical size segmental defect in a rabbit femur is a challenge in itself as osteosynthesis must support physiological loading and the defect should not heal spontaneously until the end of the implantation delay. Two cm defects in rabbit femurs have been described as critical size defects at 16 weeks [79,80]. The presented defect was considered to be critical and for ethical reasons no control group was constituted. Potential use of faster resorbable ceramics in bone tissue engineering have been suggested [81] and the authors chose a bio-ceramic with a 20/80 HA/TCP ratio for this study. As periosteum was removed, a porcine collagen membrane was used to maintain the granules in the defect.

External radiotherapy after major bone removal and reconstruction is a common situation either in orthopedic and orofacial oncology. The effects of radiation on normal bone are well known: BM is deprived, and there is less vascularisation, bone ingrowth and bone remodeling [82–86]. The adjunction of an osteogenic component to the ceramic thus appears to be necessary when bone formation limitation factors (large and segmental defect, maximal biomechanical stimulation, radiation) are cumulated. Although MSC adjunction has proved its efficacy in improving bone ingrowth in these critical conditions, there are still several questions regarding donor site, isolation and expansion methods, and stem cell behaviour. Moreover, such demanding protocols are less likely to be reproducible in tumoral surgery owing to waiting times and high costs. The experimental results indicated successful bone ingrowth of the composite associating MBCP® + collagen membrane+ post radiation total BM graft in a critical size defect in rabbit femurs. Bridging of the defect with lamellar and well-organised bone was achieved in all animals. These observations are consistent with a biomechanical stimulated implant due to chosen osteosynthesis. The quantities of bone and ceramic were identical at the different levels of the implant, which is unusual in macroporous calcium phosphate bioceramics where centripetal bone colonisation is classic. These observations suggest that bone marrow grafts in the centre of a defect may have osteoinductive properties. Although the whole axial plane of the defect was not completely filled with newly-formed bone, a tendency for periosteum-like formation was observed in most animals. The collagen membrane is a biocompatible barrier that also acts as a resorbable healing scaffold that can lead to periosteum-like tissue formation on the external bony surface [87].

This study allowed the authors to better define bone tissue engineering models by determining the most favorable donor site—which is the humeral site in both dog and rabbit models—and to achieve optimal outcomes in further irradiated bone regeneration studies. These findings show that a composite associating a collagen membrane filled with MBCP® granules with a total autologous bone marrow graft injection can successfully repair a critical segmental defect in irradiated bone. This has significant implications for the bone tissue engineering approach to patients with cancer-related segmental bone defects.

Tissue engineering for bone regeneration involves the seeding of osteogenic cells (that is, mesynchymal stem cells, MSC) on to appropriate scaffolds and subsequent implantation of the seeded scaffolds into the bone defect. Bone marrow-derived mesenchymal stem cells (MSCs) are multipotential cells that are capable of differentiating into, at the very least, osteoblasts, chondrocytes, adipocytes, tenocytes, and myoblasts [88–90]. From a small volume of bone marrow, MSCs can be isolated and culture-expanded into large numbers due to their proliferative capacity, and they maintain their functionality after culture expansion and cryopreservation [91]. MSCs are thus thought to be a readily available and abundant source of cells for tissue engineering applications. Several reports have shown the efficiency of BCP scaffolds of different HA/β-TCP ratios [92,93].

4.4.6 BCP Scaffolds with Mesenchymal Stem Cells (MSC)

Arinzeh et al. [93] reported a comparative study of BCP with different HA/β-TCP ratios as scaffolds for human mesenchymal stem cells (hMSC) used to induce bone formation. The study was designed to determine the optimum HA/β-TCP ratio in BCP in combination with MSCs that would promote rapid and uniform bone formation *in vivo*. Their study demonstrated that the BCP scaffold with the lower HA/β-TCP ratio (20/80) loaded with hMSCs promoted the greatest amount of bone and the new bone formed was uniformly distributed throughout the porous structure of the BCP scaffold. Scaffolds made from 100% HA, higher HA/β-TCP ratios and 100% TCP stimulated lesser amounts of bone formation at six weeks post-implantation. In this *in vitro* study of hMSC differentiation on 60/40 HA/β-TCP versus 20/80 HA/β-TCP, hMSCs had expressed osteocalcin, a specific bone marker, when grown on the 20/80 HA/TCP, without the presence of the osteoinductive media, by four weeks. The enhanced amount of bone formation for hMSC-loaded 20/80 HA/TCP *in vivo* and apparent differentiation into the bone cell phenotype, as characterised by the expression of osteocalcin *in vitro* under normal culture conditions, may be due in part to the rate of degradation, the degradation products, and surface chemistry of 20/80 HA/β-TCP in relation to the other BCP compositions. The concentration of degradation products and hMSC interaction with the surface and its varying chemistries may be responsible for the optimal bone formation exhibited by the 20/80 formulation.

The rate of degradation or resorption of HA/β-TCP ceramics *in vivo* can be accelerated by increasing the amount of the more soluble phase, TCP. In order to design a scaffold that supports bone formation while gradually being replaced by bone, an optimum balance between the more stable HA phase and the more soluble β-TCP phase must be achieved.

4.4.7   BCP Scaffolds for Growth Plate Chondrocyte Maturation

Recently, Teixera et al. [46] reported the efficiency of an MBCP scaffold for cartilage regeneration. The purpose of the study was to create an *in vitro* cartilage template as the transient model for *in vivo* endochondral bone formation. This study reported successful growth and maturation of chondrocytes (isolated from chick embryonic tibia on macroporous BCP (MBCP®). The thickness of the chondrocyte and extracellular matrix layer increased in the presence of retinoic acid. Alkaline phosphatase activity and expression, proteoglycan synthesis, cbfa1 and type one collagen mRNA levels also increased in the presence of retinoic acid. This study demonstrated for the first time the proliferation and maturation of chondrocytes, and matrix depositing on MBCP, suggesting the potential for such scaffolds in tissue engineering via the endochondral bone formation mechanism.

4.4.8   BCP Granules and Polymers for Injectable Bioceramics

The need of a material for minimally invasive surgery (MIS) has led to the development of BCP granules combined with polymers, producing injectable/mouldable bone substitutes. Three types of injectable/mouldable bone substitutes have been developed.

4.4.8.1   Suspension. MBCP Gel™ is a non self-hardening injectable biomaterial. It is composed of BCP granules associated with a hydrosoluble polymer. These materials have been shown to be perfectly biocompatible and potentially resorbable and, thanks to their initial plasticity, they assume the shape of

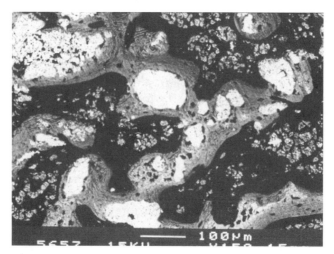

Figure 4.14. MBCP Gel after four weeks of implantation in rabbit femoral epiphyses, SEM using BSE showing the BCP particles (white) closely associated with bone trabeculae.

bone defects very easily, eliminating the need to shape the material to adjust it to the implantation site. MBCP gel does not have the mechanical properties of hydraulic bone cements. However, bone cells are able to invade the spaces created by the disappearance of the polymer carrier (Figure 4.14). Bone ingrowth takes place all around the granules at the expense of the resorption of the BCP granules. In time, the mechanical properties are increased due to the presence of the newly-formed bone [95–98]. Numerous reports both *in vitro* and *in vivo* have confirmed the efficacy and performance of this concept for an injectable bone substitute used in bone reconstruction [99–103].

4.4.8.2 Self-Hardening Injectable-Mouldable Composite. IBS 2 [104, 105] is a self-hardening composite. The BCP granules are associated with silanised hydrogel HPMC-Si. The guiding principle of silanised hydrogel HPMC-Si is its hydrophilic and liquid property (it is viscous before being mixed with the calcium phosphate load and injection) and its pH-controlled reticulation process. The silanized hydrogel/calcium phosphate composite presented self reticulation obtained by the change in pH as a catalyst and with an exothermic effect. Once in the implantation site, in contact with the biological buffer liquids, a chemical reaction without additive and without any catalyst allows bridging and reticulation between the various macromolecular chains. This reaction is triggered by the change in pH.

The advantage of ready-to-use mixtures is their easiness of use and the reproducibility of the final material. Their kinetics for osseous reconstruction can be fast because of the many inter-granular paths. These materials have relatively few intrinsic primary mechanical properties, even if the vehicles used harden by reticulation. Achieving mechanical properties is secondary as it is obtained, thanks to rapid, physiological bone ingrowth. The use of active substances or growth promoters locally released by these mixtures will make possible fast, biological secondary hardening.

4.4.9 BCP/Fibrin Glue

The association of bioceramics (Tricos®) and fibrin sealants may develop the clinical applications of composite bone substitutes [106]. As far as the calcium phosphate granules are concerned, they are not easy to handle. They are limited to filling bone cavities and are not available for bone apposition. In addition, improved performances of bioceramics can be made by adding bioactive factors. In this context, the adjunction of a binding agent such as fibrin glue facilitates the stability of the granules at the site of implantation and provides the scaffold effect of bioceramics with additional osteogenic property. Fibrin-calcium phosphate composite was obtained by mixing Baxter's fibrinogen, the thrombin components of fibrin sealant (Tisseel® Baxter BioSciences BioSurgery) and TricOs® granules. Macroporous Biphasic Calcium Phosphate TricOs® is a mixture of HA/β-TCP in a 60/40 ratio. Granules of one to two mm in diameter presenting both macroporosity (50–55%) and microporosity (30–35%) were used. To enhance the working time, a low thrombin concentration (four U) was used. The Tisseel/TricOs volume ratio was one for two. Numerous preclinical studies have been performed in rabbits and goats, both for biocompatibility and biofonctionality using, for example, sinus lift augmentation, and bone filling in long bone. Histology, histomorphometry and X-ray microtomography have shown the osteogenic properties of the composite [106,107] (Figure 4.15).

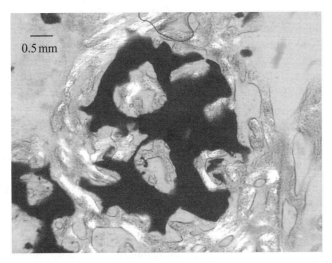

Figure 4.15. Polarized light microscopy of the Tricos granules combined with fibrin glue Tisseel in a rabbit femoral epiphysis defect showing large bone ingrowth into the macropores surrounding the not yet resorbed granules.

4.4.10 BCP Granules for Drug Delivery

Calcium phosphate bioceramics have frequently been proposed for the adsorption of bioactive factors and Drug Delivery Systems. However recently, Smucker et al. [108] reported for the first time a study demonstrating enhanced posterolateral spinal fusion rates in rabbits using a synthetic peptide (B2A2-K-NS) coated on to microporous granules of BCP with a 60/40 HA/TCP ratio. Different concentrations of the peptide (a synthetic receptor-targeted peptide that appears to amplify the biological response to *rh*BMP-2) were tested. This study provided more evidence of mature/immature bone ingrowth across the inter-transverse process spaces than did the controls. Microporous macroporous biphasic calcium phosphate granule bioceramics for peptide adsorption and local delivery seem to be a good compromise for future associations of osteoconductive/osteogenic properties for such bioceramics and the osteoinductive properties of peptides and growth factors.

Other kinds of drug which can be delivered are antibiotics. It is common practice for surgeons to mix antibiotics with bone grafts when treating infected bone defects or for preventing infection after surgery [109]. Local delivery of antibiotics is both pharmacologically more effective and safe. Bioactive cements have been shown to be an ideal carrier for antibiotics for local delivery if properly formulated [110,111]. New calcium phosphate cement has been specifically engineered to have micro-porosity, macro-porosity and resorbability for optimal cell adhesion, cell migration, and bone formation. Recently, the MCPC® reported in this paper was associated with gentamycin [112].

The gentamycin release profiles from the cement samples with different setting times were quite similar. Both cement groups showed an initial burst of gentamycin release in the first 24-hours. After the initial burst, the release rate slowed significantly, and stayed relatively constant after day seven up to the day 28 endpoint. The amount and rate of the initial burst release was affected by the cement setting time. The release of gentamycin from the cement set for one hour showed greater variation than the cement allowed to set for 24 hours. Within the first 24 hours, approximately 72% of the gentamycin was released from the cement with a one hour set time, compared to slower release of approximately 51% of the gentamycin from the cement with a 24 hour set time. By 28 days, around 87% and 76% of the gentamycin had been released from the cements that had set for either one hour or 24 hours, respectively. The gentamycin release rates from both the one hour and 24 hour set-time samples were almost constant after day seven, averaging $59\,\mu g$/day for the cement with a one hour set time, and $87\,\mu g$/day for the 24 hour set time. In our release system, therefore, these constructs are capable of producing gentamycin concentrations of $12\,\mu g$/ml and $17\,\mu g$/ml on a daily basis for the one hour and 24 set–time cement samples, respectively. This is more than one order of magnitude greater than the Minimum Inhibitory Concentration (MIC) for reference strains of S. aureus, which is in the range of 0.12–$0.25\,\mu g$/ml [113].

It was interesting to note that the cement without gentamycin showed a decrease in ultimate compressive strength during setting from 24 to 48 hours in phosphate buffered saline at 37 °C. The ultimate compressive strength dropped from 5.5 MPa, to 3.87 MPa, indicating that the cement had probably dissolved. When the gentamycin was present, the cement showed an increase in both the strength and modulus when the set time was extended from 24 to 48 hours. It appeared that the addition of gentamycin may have delayed the dissolution of the cement, while allowing it to continue to set, to further increase the mechanical properties.

Owing to its unique preparation method and bioresorbability, the bioactive cement employed in this study may be effective as both a bone graft substitute and as a carrier for the local delivery of antibiotics to prevent or treat infections. An ideal bioactive cement can release a clinically effective amount of antibiotics initially, maintain a steady release of a safe dose over an extended period, and retain no residual amount of antibiotics after the desired treatment time is over. As demonstrated in this study, the MCPC™ bioactive cement released over 50% of the loaded gentamycin per cylinder, that is, 7.5 mg, in the first 24 hours. A steady release of a therapeutically significant amount of gentamycin, that is, about 60 to 90 µg of gentamycin per day, was maintained up to 28 days. As the MCPC™ is engineered to bioresorb and quickly develop a macroporous structure, the remaining amount of two-to-four mg of gentamycin per set-time sample is expected to discharge completely as the bioactive cement resorbs. The MCPC™ resorbable bone substitute has demonstrated its potential to be used as a carrier for the local delivery system for gentamycin. Future studies will expand the investigation to evaluate the release profile and mechanical properties of this bioactive cement when loaded with other antibiotics such as tobramycin and vancomycin.

4.5 CLINICAL APPLICATIONS

BCP bioceramics of various sizes and shapes are widely used all over the world in maxillofacial surgery, dentistry, ENT surgery, and orthopedics. Here, the authors report some examples of clinical applications for MBCP.

4.5.1 Applications in Dentistry

Dental applications for BCP include prevention of bone loss after tooth extraction, repair of periodontal defects, and sinus lift augmentation [114–116].

4.5.1.1 Prevention of Bone Resorption. Bone loss occurs after tooth extraction, causing reduction of alveolar ridge height and width resulting in difficulty in fitting dentures or placing dental implants. BCP granules with an HA/TCP ratio of 60/40 or 20/80 (MBCP® and Tribone 80®, respectively) were placed in the alveolar cavity immediately after tooth extraction and followed up radiographically from zero to five years, with biopsies taken at different time periods from six months to five years [116]. The radiographs revealed newly-formed bone with higher density and residual BCP granules. After six months, a lesser amount of BCP granules with 20HA/80TCP were observed compared to 50HA/40TCP. In addition, during drilling, clinicians reported higher bone density without interference from residual granules. Organised and well-mineralised bone ingrowth was observed using micro CT and light microscopy. In all cases, the radiopacity of the implantation sites decreased with time indicating that resorption and bone ingrowth proceeded at the expense of the BCP granules. Observation after one and five years showed that alveolar ridge height had been maintained, compared to the control (no BCP) which showed a decrease in alveolar ridge height of two to five mm. Five years after implantation, the resorption of the BCP was 78% for the 60/40 and 87% for the 20/80, and bone ingrowth 38% and 32%, respectively. Resorption and bone ingrowth were not significantly different for the BCP of different HA/TCP ratios.

4.5.1.2 Sinus Lift Augmentation. The problems involved in delivering MBCP granules into tooth sockets has discouraged many dental surgeons. A recently developed product composed of MBCP granules in a polymer carrier provides a ready-to-use injectable bone substitute (MBCP Gel™) [95]. The osteoconductive potential of this innovative biomaterial has already been demonstrated for clinical applications in an animal model with the quantification of each component, BCP, bone and soft tissue [17]. Macroporous BCP in a polymer carrier has been shown to be effective in filling dental sockets after tooth extraction because it maintained the alveolar bone crest, supported bone healing and was gradually substituted by bone tissue.

In vivo resorption, just like *in vitro* dissolution, depends on chemical composition and particle size [117]. MBCP Gel™ with 40 to 80 µm BCP granules was used for bone regeneration around dental implants placed in fresh extraction sockets in a dog model [101]. Three months after implantation, the BCP granules were no longer visible using SEM. In the same animal model and after the same implantation time, most of the BCP granules (200 to 500 µm granules) were still present. In the case of nanoparticles (BCP particle size smaller than ten µm), complete and fast resorption of the BCP granules was observed, but so was significant inflammation [51]. The particle size of the BCP (or any resorbable biomaterials) should thus be adapted to the clinical situation. For pre-prosthetic surgery large granule size compatible with injection should be used out of preference and for pre-implantation surgery, small granule size compatible with acceptable levels of inflammation is recommended.

4.5.2 Applications in Orthopedics

BCP has been used in orthopedic applications for the last 20 years. Its efficacy has been demonstrated in numerous preclinical and clinical studies [26–31,118–120]. Below are brief descriptions of selected clinical situations using specific shaped blocks (custom-designed) for spine arthrodesis (cage insert) and wedges for tibial valgisation osteotomy.

4.5.2.1 Cervical Spine Arthrodesis. Several studies have been published using bioceramic inserts for filling cage fusion [121–124]. Mousselard [125] recently reported a clinical study of a prospective, comparative, multicentre and randomized study comparing iliac grafts and a macroporous BCP.

4.5.2.2 Anterior Cervical Fusion with PEEK Cage. Peek cervical radiolucent fusion cages provide immediate mechanical support after anterior cervical discectomy. The aim of this study was to compare the clinical efficiency and quality of the fusion after reconstruction with an anatomically-shaped PEEK cage associated with an iliac crest autograft or with MBCP in the surgery of cervical disc. The addition of an iliac autograft makes possible an excellent fusion rate, but is associated with increased morbidity and persistent pain at the donor site. Clinical reports by Scareo prospectively comparing the two techniques has shown the clinical advantage of using MBCP and avoiding bone graft harvesting. Fifty-eight patients were selected in a multicentre, comparative and prospective study with 24-month follow-up. The patients undergoing anterior cervical decompression and fusion were randomised for autologous graft or MBCP. After 24 months, cervical X rays showed 87% complete fusion, 13% uncertain fusion and 0% real pseudarthrosis in the autograft group versus 86%, 10% and 4%, respectively, in the MBCP group. No implant failures were recorded. These results suggest that the use of an insert associated with an anterior cage allows better recovery for patients while achieving a fusion rate similar to that of ACDF with a tricortical graft, and does not have the associated complications. Using an MBCP insert is safe and avoids potential graft site morbidity and pain in comparison with an autologous graft procedure.

4.5.2.3 High Tibial Valgisation Osteotomy (HTO). Many surgical procedures have been described for high tibial valgisation osteotomy (HTO) as a treatment for medial femorotibial arthritis with genu varum deformity. Filling the cavity created by the opening has remained a problem, although various osteosynthetic solutions have been proposed. Bone substitutes have been used in a number of different cases [126–128].

A single centre prospective study [129] from December 1999 to December 2002 was completed involving 42 patients (13 females and 29 males, average age 46 years) who underwent HTVO with medial addition for various types of deformity using custom-designed wedges made of micro-macroporous biphasic calcium phosphate bioceramic bone substitute and an orientable locking screw plate (Numelock II®, Stryker). After one year, correction was unchanged in 99.5% of the cases. Histological analysis showed MBCP resorption and bone ingrowth into the pores and at the expense of the bioceramic. Residual MBCP fragments showed ingrowth of trabecular and/or dense lamellar bone both on the surface and in the macropores. X-ray radiography and microCT revealed a well-organised and mineralised structure of newly-formed bone. In spite of a certain number of fractures in the MBCP wedges during implantation, or proximal screws fractured without compromising the stability or post-operative correction angles, high bone ingrowth was reported. This study indicated that MBCP wedges in combination with orientable locking screws and plates are a simple, safe, and fast surgical technique for HTO.

4.6   CONCLUSION

The concept of biphasic calcium phosphate ceramics (BCP) is determined by an optimum balance between the more stable HA phase and the more soluble TCP. The material is soluble and gradually dissolves in the body, seeding new bone formation as it releases calcium and phosphate ions into the biological medium. As a means of promoting these events, and in order to develop calcium phosphate ceramics and other related biomaterials for bone grafts, a better control of the biomaterials resorption and bone substitution processes is needed.

The main attractive feature of BCP ceramic is its ability to form a direct bond with the host bone, resulting in a strong interface. The formation of this dynamic interface is the result of a sequence of events involving interaction with cells and the formation of carbonate hydroxyapatite CHA (similar to bone mineral) by means of the dissolution/precipitation processes. Associating micro and macroprosity with the BCP concept has resulted in high osteogenicity and osteoinductive properties. At the present time, MBCP is commercially available in blocks, particulates and customised designs. Specific matrices have been developed for combination with bone marrow or mesenchymal stem cells for tissue engineering (hybrid bone). The need for a material for Minimally Invasive Surgery (MIS) has led to the development of a concept for BCP granules combined with a polymer or calcium phosphate cement to create an injectable/mouldable bone substitute.

The challenge today will be to improve technologies for large bone defect reconstruction or for bone reconstruction in osteo radionecrosis, combining tissue engineering and scaffold. To support this challenge, studies will have to increase the capacity of osteogenic and hematopietic cell growth into large samples (colonization), and to promote angiogenesis for living bone.

The second evolution of BCP concept will be the association with resorbable osteosynthesis for "orthobiologic system," to avoid second surgery, time to remove the metal osteosynthesis after bone healing at the expense of the bioceramics, or to maintain on time unresorbable bioinert materials as PEEK or titanium.

The third is the development of Minimal Invasive Surgery that required specific injectible bone substitute with or without self hardening; the combination with Hydrogels is the main research and development in the field of bone substitute and tissue engineering.

ACKNOWLEDGMENTS

The collaboration of the following clinicians is gratefully acknowledged: Prof. Jean-Louis Rouvillain (CHU Fort de France Martinique), Dr Hugues Mousselard (CHU Pitié Salpétrière Paris France), Dr Nicolas Mailhac (Tours France), Dr Clemencia Rodriguez (Bogota University, Colombia), Said Khimacke (Dental Faculty of Nantes) and all the others clinicans contributions.

The authors also gratefully acknowledge their colleagues from Nantes University and INSERM EMI 99 03, Nantes Hospital, (O. Malard, S. Barroth, P. Weiss, et all the others), Nantes Microscopy SC3M department (Paul Pilet), and the Calcium Phosphate Research Lab at New York University College of Dentistry (Racquel Legeros and John Legeros) and Biomtlante SAS France (Xavier Bourges, Françoise Moreau) and Nantes Veterinary School (Eric Aguado and Eric Goyenvalle).

Parts of this work were supported by CPER Pays de Loire, RNTS 2002 form French Ministry of research, INSERM EMI 9903, and National Agency for Research ANR Biorimp 2005.

REFERENCES

1. Albee FH (1920). Studies in bone growth: Triple calcium phosphate as a stimulus to osteogenesis. Ann Surg 71:32–36.
2. Nery EB, Lynch KL, Hirthe WM, Mueller KH (1975). Bioceramic implants in surgically produced infraboney defects. J Periodontol 63:729–735.
3. Denissen HW (1979). Dental root implant of apatite ceramic, experimental investigations and clinical use of dental root apatite ceramics, PhD Thesis, Amsterdam, Vrije Universiteit.
4. Jarcho M (1981). Calcium phosphate ceramics as hard tissue prosthetics. Clin Orthop 157:259–278.
5. De Groot K (1983). Ceramics of calcium phosphate: preparation and properties, In: Bioceramics of Calcium Phosphates. CRC Press, Boca Raton, 100–114.
6. Metsger SD, Driskell TD, Paulsrud JR (1982). Tricalcium phosphate ceramic: a resorbable bone implant: Review and current uses. J Am Dent Assoc 105:1035–1048.
7. Aoki H, Kato K (1975). Study on the application of apatite to dental materials. Jpn Ceram Soc 10:469.
8. Daculsi G (1998). Biphasic calcium phosphate concept applied to artificial bone, implant coating and injectable bone substitute. Biomaterials 19:1473–1478.
9. LeGeros RZ, Nery E, Daculsi G, Lynch K, Kerebel B (1988). In vivo transformation of biphasic calcium phosphate of varying β-TCP/HA ratios: ultrastructural characterization. Third World Biomaterials Congress (abstract no. 35).
10. Daculsi G, LeGeros RZ, Nery E, Lynch K, Kerebel B (1989). Transformation of biphasic calcium phosphate ceramics: ultrastructural and physico-chemical characterization. J Biomed Mat Res 23:883–894.

11. Daculsi G, Passuti N (1990). Effect of macroporosity for osseous substitution of calcium phosphate ceramic. Biomaterials 11:86–87.

12. Trecant M, Delecrin J, Royer J, Goyenvalle E, Daculsi G (1994). Mechanical changes in macroporous calcium phosphate ceramics after implantation in bone. Clin Mater 15:233–240.

13. LeGeros RZ, Lin S, Rohanizadeh R, Mijares D, LeGeros JP (2003). Biphasic calcium phosphates: Preparation and properties. J Mater Sci: Mat in Med 14:201–210.

14. Hench LL, Splinter RJ, Allen WC, Greelee TK (1978). Bonding mechanisms at the interface of ceramic prosthetic materials. J Biomed Mater Res 2:117–141.

15. Daculsi G, LeGeros RZ, Heugheaert M, Barbieux I (1990). Formation of carbonate apatite crystals after implantation of calcium phosphate ceramics. Calcif Tissue Int 46:20–27.

16. Daculsi G (2006). Biphasic calcium phosphate Granules concept for Injectable and Mouldable Bone Substitute. Advances in Science and Technology Volume 49, Trans Tech Publications, Switzerland, pp 9–13.

17. Daculsi G, Weiss P, Bouler JM, Gauthier O, Aguado E (1999). Bcp/hpmc composite: a new concept for bone and dental substitution biomaterials. Bone 25:59–61.

18. Daculsi G, Khairoun I, LeGeros RZ, Moreau F, Pilet P, Bourges·X, Weiss P, Gauthier O (2006). Key Engineering Materials 330–332:811–814.

19. LeGeros RZ (2002). Properties of osteoconductive biomaterials: calcium phosphates. Clin Orthopaed Rel Res 395:81.

20. Goyenvalle E, Aguado E, Legeros R, Daculsi G (2007). Effect of Sintering Process on Microporosity, and bone growth on Biphasic Calcium Phosphate Ceramics. Key Engineering Materials vols 333–334, in press, Trans Tech Publication Switzerland.

21. Bouler JM, Trécant M, Delécrin J, Royer J, Passuti N, Daculsi G (1996). Macroporous Biphasic Calcium Phosphate Ceramics: Influence of Five Synthesis Parameters on Compressive Strength. J Biomed Mater Res 32:603–609.

22. LeGeros RZ (2002). Properties of osteoconductive biomaterials: calcium phosphates. Clin Orthopaed Rel Res 395:81.

23. Goyenvalle E, Aguado E, Legeros R, Daculsi G (2007). Effect of Sintering Process on Microporosity, and bone growth on Biphasic Calcium Phosphate Ceramics. Key Engineering Materials vols 333–334, in press, Trans Tech Publication Switzerland.

24. Hubbard WG (1974). PhD Thesis, Physiological calcium phosphate as orthopedic biomaterials Milwaukee Wisconsin, Marquette University.

25. Schmitt M (2000). «Contribution à l'élaboration de nouveaux matériaux biphasés en phosphate de calcium». Thèse de doctorat, Université de Nantes.

26. Daculsi G, Bagot D'arc M, Corlieu P, Gersdorff M (1992). Macroporous Biphasic Calcium Phosphate efficiency in mastoid cavity obliteration. Ann Orol Rhinol Laryngol 101:669–674.

27. Gouin F, Delecrin J, Passuti N, Touchais S, Poirier P, Bainvel JV (1995). Comblement osseux par céramique phosphocalcique biphasée macroporeuse: A propos de 23 cas. Rev Chir Orthop 81:59–65.

28. Ransford AO, Morley T, Edgar MA, Webb P, Passuti N, Chopin D, Morin C, Michel F, Garin C, Pries D (1998). Synthetic porous ceramic compared with autograft in scoliosis surgery. A prospective, randomized study of 341 patients. J Bone Joint Surg Br 80(1):13–18.

29. Cavagna R, Daculsi G, Bouler J-M (1999). Macroporous biphasic calcium phosphate: a prospective study of 106 cases in lumbar spine fusion. Long term Effects Med Impl 9:403–412.

30. Soares EJC, Franca VP, Wykrota L, Stumpf S (1998). Clinical evaluation of a new bioaceramic opthalmic implant. In LeGeros RZ, LeGeros JP (Eds) Bioceramics 11, Singapore, World Scientific, pp 633–636.

31. Bagot d'Arc M, Daculsi G, Emam N (Sep 2004). Biphasic ceramics and fibrin sealant for bone reconstruction in ear surgery. Ann Otol Rhinol Laryngol 113(9):711–720.

32. Daculsi G (2006). High performance of new interconnected MicroMacroporous Biphasic Calcium Phosphate matrices MBCP2000 for bone tissue engineering. Proceedings 20th European Conference on Biomaterials, Nantes France.

33. Bouler JM, Trécant M, Delécrin J, Royer J, Passuti N, Daculsi G (1996). Macroporous Biphasic Calcium Phosphate Ceramics: Influence of Five Synthesis Parameters on Compressive Strength. J Biomed Mater Res 32:603–609.

34. LeGeros RZ, Lin S, Rohanizadeh R, Mijares D, LeGeros JP (2003). Biphasic calcium phosphates: Preparation and properties. J Mater Sci: Mat in Med 14:201–210.

35. Daculsi G, Laboux O, Malard O, Weiss P (2003). Current state of the art of biphasic calcium phosphate bioceramics. J Mater Sci Mater Med 14:195–200.

36. Hench LL (1994). Bioceramics: From concept to clinic. J Am Ceram Soc 74:1487–1510.

37. Basle MF, Chappard D, Grizon F, Filmon R, Delecrin J, Daculsi G, Rebel A (1993). Osteoclastic Resorption of CaP biomaterials implanted in rabbit bone. Calcif Tiss Int 53: 348–356.

38. Gauthier O, BoulerJ-M, Aguado E, Pilet P, Daculsi G (1998 Jan–Feb). Macroporous biphasic calcium phosphate ceramics: influence of macropore diameter and macroporosity percentage on bone ingrowth. Biomaterials 19(1–3):133–139.

39. Kokubo T, Takadama H (2006 May). How useful is SBF in predicting in vivo bone bioactivity? Biomaterials 27(15):2907–2915.

40. LeGeros RZ (2002). Properties of osteoconductive biomaterials: calcium phosphates. Clin Orthopaed Rel Res 395:81.

41. Le Nihouannen D, Daculsi G, Saffarzadeh A, Gauthier O, Delplace S, Pilet P, Layrolle P (2005 June). Ectopic bone formation by microporous calcium phosphate ceramic particles in sheep muscles. Bone 36(6):1086–1093.

42. Reddi AH (2000). Morphogenesis and tissue engineering of bone and cartilage: Inductive signals, stem cells and biomimetic biomaterials. Tissue Eng 6:351–359.

43. Ripamonti U (1991). The morphogenesis of bone in replicas of porous hydroxyapatite obtained by conversion of calcium carbonate exosk eletons of coral. J Bone Joint Surg Am 73:692–703.

44. Kuboki Y, Takita H, Kobayashi D (1998). BMP-induced osteogenesis on the surface of hydroxyapatite with geometrically feasible and nonfeasible structures: topology of osteogenesis. J Biomed Mater Res 39:190–199.

45. Diaz-Flores L, Gutierrez R, Lopez-Alonso A, Gonzalez R, Varela H (1992 Feb). Pericytes as a supplementary source of osteoblasts in periosteal osteogenesis. Clin Orthop Relat Res (275):280–286.

46. Habibovic P, Yuan H, van der Valk CM, Meijer G, van Blitterswijk CA, De Groot K (2005). Microenvironment as essential element for osteoinduction by biomaterials. Biomaterials 26:3565–3575.

47. Yuan H, Kurashina K, Joost de Bruijn D, Li Y, de Groot K, Zhang X (1999). A preliminary study of osteoinduction of two kinds of calcium phosphate bioceramics. Biomaterials 20:1799–1806.

48. Barrere F, van der Valk CM, Dalmeijer RA, Meijer G, van Blitterswijk CA, de Groot K, Layrolle P (2003). Osteogenicity of octacalcium phosphate coatings applied on porous titanium. J Biomed Mater Res 66A:779.

49. Daculsi G, LeGeros RZ, Grimandi G, Soueidan A, LeGeros J (2008). Effect of Sintering Process of HA/TCP (BCP) Bioceramics on Microstructure, Dissolution and Cell Proliferation. Key Engineering Materials vols 361–363: 1139–1142, Trans Tech Publication Switzerland.

50. Daculsi G, Dard M (1994). Bone-Calcium-Phosphate ceramic interface Osteosynthese International 2:153–156.

51. Malard O, Gautier H, Daculsi G (2008). In vivo demonstration of 2 types of Microporosity on the kinetic of bone ingrowth and biphasic calcium phosphate bioceramics resorption, Key Engineering Materials vols 361–363, 1233–1236, Trans Tech Publication Switzerland.

52. Malard O, Bouler JM, Guicheux J, Heymann D, Pilet P, Coquard C, Daculsi G (1999). Influence of biphasic calcium phosphate granulometry on bone ingrowth, ceramic resorption, and inflammatory reactions: preliminary *in vitro* and *in vivo* study. J Biomed Mater Res 46(1):103–111.

53. LeGeros RZ, Chohayeb A, Shulman A (1982). Apatitic calcium phosphates: possible restorative materials. J Dent Rs 61 (spec issue):343.

54. Brown WE, Chow LC (1987). "A new calcium phosphate water-setting cement" in Brown PW (ed). Cement Research Progress 1986. Americin Ceramic Society, Westerville, OH pp. 352–379.

55. Niwa S, LeGeros RZ (2002). "Injectable calcium phosphate cements for repair of bone defects". In: Lewandrowski K-U, Wise DL, Trantolo DJ, Gresser JD. Tissue Engineering and Biodegradable Equivalents. Scientific and Clinical Applications. Marcel Dekker, New York, pp. 385–400.

56. Khairoun I, LeGeros RZ, Daculsi G, Bouler JM, Guicheux J, Gauthier O (2004). Macroporous, resorbable and injectable calcium phosphate-based cements (MCPC) for bone repair, augmentation, regeneration and osteoporosis treatment. Provisional patent no. 11/054,623.

57. Gauthier O, Muller R, von Stechow D, Lamy B, Weiss P, Bouler J-M, et al. (2005). In vivo bone regeneration with injectable calcium phosphate biomaterial: a three-dimensional micro-computed tomographic, biomechanical and SEM study. Biomaterials 2005/9;26(27):5444–5453.

58. Ginebra MP, Albuixech L, Fernández-Barragán E, Aparicio C, Gil FJ, San Román J, Vázquez B, Planell JA (2002). Mechanical performance of acrylic bone cements containing different radiopacifying agents. Biomaterials, Volume 23, Issue 8, April 2002, Pages 1873–1882.

59. van Hooy-Corstjens CSJ, Govaert LE, Spoelstra AB, Bulstra SK, Wetzels GMR, Koole LH (2004). Mechanical behaviour of a new acrylic radiopaque iodine-containing bone cement. Biomaterials, Volume 25, Issue 13, June 2004, Pages 2657–2667.

60. Kurtz SM, Villarraga ML, Zhao K, Ediin AA (2005). Static and fatigue mechanical behavior of bone cement with elevated barium sulfate content for treatment of vertebral compression fractures Biomaterials, Volume 26, Issue 17, Pages 3699–3712.

61. Baroth S, Bourges X, Fellah B, Daculsi G (2008). Radioopaque strategy for bone injectable substitute, Key Engineering Materials 361–363:39–42.

62. Lajtai G, Schmiedhuber G, Unger F, Aitzetmüller G, Klein M, Noszian I, Orthn E (2001). Bone tunnel remodeling at the site of biodegradable interference screws used for anterior cruciate ligament reconstruction. Arthroscopy: The J. Arthros. Rel. Surg. Volume 17, Issue 6, Pages 597–602.

63. Barber FA, Boothby MH (2007). Bilok Interference Screws for Anterior Cruciate Ligament Reconstruction: Clinical and Radiographic Outcomes. Arthroscopy: The Journal of Arthroscopic & Related Surgery, Volume 23, Issue 5, Pages 476–481.

64. Rotunda AM, Narins RS (2007). Poly-L-lactic acid: a new dimension in soft tissue augmentation. Dermatol Ther 19(3):151–158.

65. Jouan G, Goyenvalle E, Aguado E, Cognet R, Moreau F, Bourges X, Daculsi G (2008). PL DLLA calcium phosphate composite combined with MBCP gel® for new surgical technologies: Resorbable Osteo Synthesis and Bone Substitute. Key Engineering Materials vols 361–363, 571–574, Trans Tech Publication Switzerland.

66. Jouan G, Goyenvalle E, Aguado E, Cognet R, Moreau F, Bourges X, Daculsi G (2008). PL DLLA calcium phosphate composite combined with Macroporous Calcium Phosphate Cement MCPC® for new surgical technologies combining Resorbable Osteo Synthesis and Injectable Bone Substitute. Key Engineering Materials vols 361–363, 411–414, Trans Tech Publication Switzerland.

67. Gauthier O, Bouler Jm, Aguado E, Legeros Rz, Pilet P, Daculsi G (1999). Elaboration conditions influence physicochemical properties and in vivo bioactivity of macroporous biphasic calcium phosphate ceramics. J of Mater Sc: Mat in Med 10:199–204.

68. Gauthier O, Bouler Jm, Weiss P, Bosco J, Daculsi G, Aguado E (1999). Kinetic study of bone ingrowth and ceramic resorption associated with the implantation of different injectable calcium-phosphate bone substitutes. J Biomed Mater Res 47(1):28–35.

69. Gauthier O, Bouler JM, Weiss P, Bosco J, Aguado E, Daculsi G (1999 Aug). Short-term effects of mineral particle sizes on cellular degradation activity after implantation of injectable calcium phosphate biomaterials and the consequences for bone substitution. Bone 25(2 Suppl):71S–74S.

70. Magarelli N, Savastano MA, Palmieri D, ZAppacosta R, Lattanzio G, Salini V, Orso CA, Guglielmi G, Colosimo C (2007). Poly-L-lactic acid beta-tricalcium phosphate screws: a preliminary in vivo biocompatibility stud. Int J Immunopathol Pharmacol 20:207–211.

71. Cotton NJ, Egan MJ, Brunelle JE (2008 Apr). Composites of poly(DL-lactide-co-glycolide) and calcium carbonate: In vitro evaluation for use in orthopedic applications. J Biomed Mater Res A 85(1):195–205.

72. Miura M, Miura Y, Sonoyama W, Yamaza T, Gronthos S, Shi S (2006). Bone marrow-derived mesenchymal stem cells for regenerative medicine in craniofacial region. Oral Dis 12(6):514–522.

73. Lerouxel E, Weiss P, Giumelli B, Moreau A, Pilet P, Guicheux J, Corre P, Bouler JM, Daculsi G, Malard O (2006 Sep). Injectable calcium phosphate scaffold and bone marrow graft for bone reconstruction in irradiated areas: an experimental study in rats. Biomaterials 27(26):4566–4572.

74. Malard O, Guicheux J, Bouler J-M, Gauthier O, de Montreuil CB, Aguado E, Daculsi G (2005). Calcium phosphate scaffold and bone marrow for bone reconstruction in irradiated area: a dog study. Bone 2005/2;36(2):323–330.

75. Jegoux F, Aguado E, Cognet R, Malard O, Moreau F, Daculsi G, et al. (2008). Repairing segmental defect with a composite associating collagen membrane and MBCP® combined with total bone marrow graft in irradiated bone defect: an experimental study in rabbit. Key Engineering Materials 333–334.

76. Olmsted-Davis EA, Gugala Z, Camargo F, Gannon FH, Jackson K, Kienstra KA, et al. (2003). Primitive adult hematopoietic stem cells can function as osteoblast precursors. Proc Natl Acad Sci U S A 100(26):15877–15882.

77. Ohgushi H, Kitamura S, Kotobuki N, Hirose M, Machida H, Muraki K, et al. (2004). Clinical application of marrow mesenchymal stem cells for hard tissue repair. Yonsei Med J 45 (Suppl):61–67.

78. Ohgushi H, Miyake J, Tateishi T (2003). Mesenchymal stem cells and bioceramics: strategies to regenerate the skeleton. Novartis Found Symp 249:118–127; discussion 27–32, 70–74, 239–241.

79. Crigel MH, Balligand M (2002). Critical size defect model on the femur in rabbits. Vet Comp Orthop traumatol 15:158–163.

80. Hollinger JO, Kleinschmidt JC (1990). The critical size defect as an experimental model to test bone repair materials. J Craniofac Surg 1(1):60–68.

81. Livingston TL, Gordon S, Archambault M, Kadiyala S, McIntosh K, Smith A, et al. (2003). Mesenchymal stem cells combined with biphasic calcium phosphate ceramics promote bone regeneration. J Mater Sci Mater Med 14(3):211–218.

82. Dudziak ME, Saadeh PB, Mehrara BJ, Steinbrech DS, Greenwald JA, Gittes GK, et al. (2000). The effects of ionizing radiation on osteoblast-like cells in vitro. Plast Reconstr Surg 106(5):1049–1061.

83. Matsumura S, Jikko A, Hiranuma H, Deguchi A, Fuchihata H (1996). Effect of X-ray irradiation on proliferation and differentiation of osteoblast. Calcif Tissue Int 59(4): 307–308.

84. Nathanson A, Backstrom A (1978). Effects of 60Co-gamma-irradiation on teeth and jaw bone in the rabbit. Scand J Plast Reconstr Surg 12(1):1–17.

85. Nussenbaum B, Rutherford RB, Krebsbach PH (2005). Bone regeneration in cranial defects previously treated with radiation. Laryngoscope 115(7):1170–1177.

86. Sabo D, Brocai DR, Eble M, Wannenmacher M, Ewerbeck V (2000). Influence of extracorporeal irradiation on the reintegration of autologous grafts of bone and joint. Study in a canine model. J Bone Joint Surg Br 82(2):276–282.

87. von Arx T, Broggini N, Jensen SS, Bornstein MM, Schenk RK, Buser D (2005). Membrane durability and tissue response of different bioresorbable barrier membranes: a histologic study in the rabbit calvarium. Int J Oral Maxillofac Implants 20(6):843–853.

88. Pittenger MF, Mackay AM, Beck SC, Jaiswal RK, Douglas R, Mosca JD, Moorman MA, Simonetti DW, Craig S, Marshak DR (1999) Multilineage potential of adult human mesenchymal stem cells. Science 284:143–147.

89. Caplan AI, Fink DJ, Goto T, Linton AE, Young RG, Wakitani S, Goldberg V, Haynesworth SE (1993). In Jackson DW et al. (ed), The Anterior Cruciate Ligament: Current and Future Concepts, New York, Raven Press, 405–417.

90. Jaiswal N, Haynesworth SE, Caplan AI, Bruder SP (1997). Osteogenic differentiation of purified culture-expanded human mesenchymal stem cells in vitro. J Cell Biochem 64:295–312.

91. Bruder SP, Jaiswal N, Haynesworth SE (1997). Growth kinetics, self-renewal, and the osteogenic potential of purified human mesenchymal stem cells during extensive subcultivation and following cryopreservation. J Cell Biochem 64:278–294.

92. Kadiyala S, Jaiswal N, Bruder SP (1997). Culture-expanded, bone marrow-derived mesenchymal stem cells can regenerate a critical-sized segmental bone defect. Tissue Engineering 3:173–185.

93. Livingston Arinzeh T, Peter S, Archambault M, Van Den Bos C, Gordon S, Kraus K, Smith A, Kadiyala S (2003). Allogeneic mesenchymal stem cells regenerate bone in a critical-sized canine segmental defect. Journal of Bone and Joint Surgery American 85-A:1927–1935.

94. Teixeira CC, Nemelivsky Y, Karkia C, LeGeros RZ (2006). Biphasic calcium phosphate: a scaffold for growth plate chondrocytes. Tissue Engineering 12:2283–2289.

95. Daculsi G, Weiss P, Bouler JM, Gauthier O, Aguado E (1999). Biphasic Calcium Phosphate hydrosoluble polymer composites: A new concept for Bone and dental substitution Biomaterials, Bone 25:59–61.

96. Gauthier O, Bouler JM, Aguado E, Legeros Rz, Pilet P, Daculsi G (1999). Elaboration conditions influence physicochemical properties and in vivo bioactivity of macroporous biphasic calcium phosphate ceramics. J of Mater Sc: Mat in Med 10:199–204.

97. Gauthier O, Bouler Jm, Weiss P, Bosco J, Daculsi G, Aguado E (1999). Kinetic study of bone ingrowth and ceramic resorption associated with the implantation of different injectable calcium-phosphate bone substitutes. J Biomed Mater Res 47(1):28–35.

98. Gauthier O, Bouler JM, Weiss P, Bosco J, Aguado E, Daculsi G (1999). Short-term effects of mineral particle sizes on cellular degradation activity after implantation of injectable calcium phosphate biomaterials and consequences for bone substitution. Bone 25:71–74.

99. Millot F, Grimandi G, Weiss P, Daculsi G (1999). Preliminary in vivo studies of a new injectable bone substitute. Cells and Mat 9:21–30.

100. Dupraz A, Nguyen TP, Richard M, Daculsi G, Passuti N (1999). Influence of a cellulosic ether carrier on the structure of biphasic calcium phosphate ceramic particles in an injectable composite material. Biomaterials 20:663–673.

101. Gauthier O, Boix D, Grimandi G, Aguado E, Bouler Jm, Weiss P, Daculsi G (1999) A new injectable calcium phosphate for immediate bone filling of extraction sockets: a preliminary study in dogs. J Periodontol 70:375–383.

102. Gauthier O, Bouler Jm, Weiss P, Bosco J, Daculsi G, Aguado E (1999). Kinetic study of bone ingrowth and ceramic resorption associated with the implantation of different injectable calcium-phosphate bone substitutes. J Biomed Mater Res 47(1):28–35.

103. Gauthier O, Bouler JM, Weiss P, Bosco J, Aguado E, Daculsi G (1999). Short-term effects of mineral particle sizes on cellular degradation activity after implantation of injectable calcium phosphate biomaterials and consequences for bone substitution. Bone 25:71–74.

104. Lapkowski M, Weiss P, Daculsi G, Et Dupraz A (1997). Patent WO 97/05911 Déposant: CNRS, Composition pour biomatériau, procédé de préparation II Date de dépôt: 20 Février.

105. Fellah BH, Weiss P, Gauthier O, Rouillon T, Pilet P, Daculsi G, Layrolle P (2006 Apr). Bone repair using a new injectable self-crosslinkable bone substitute, J Orthop Res 24(4):628–635.

106. Le Guehennec L, Layrolle P, Daculsi G (2004 Sep). A review of bioceramics and fibrin sealant. Eur Cell Mater 13(8):1–11.

107. LeNihouannen DL, Saffarzadeh A, Aguado E, Goyenvalle E, Gauthier O, Moreau F, Pilet P, Spaethe R, Daculsi G, Layrolle PJ (2007 Feb). Osteogenic properties of calcium phosphate ceramics and fibrin glue based composites. J Mater Sci Mater Med 18(2):225–235.

108. Smucker JD, Aggarwal D, Zamora PO, Atkinson BL, Bobst JA, Nepola JV, Fredericks DC (2007). Assessment of B2A2-K-NS peptide coated on an osteoconductive granule in a rabbit postrolateral fusion model, proceedings AAOS, 12–14 February San Diego USA.

109. Hanssen AD (2005 Aug). Local antibiotic delivery vehicles in the treatment of musculoskeletal infection. Clin Orthop Relat Res (437):91–96. Review.

110. Sasaki T, Ishibashi Y, Katano H, Nagumo A, Toh S (2005). J Arthroplasty 20:1055–1059.

111. Frutos P, Torrado S, Perez-Lorenzo ME, Frutos G (2000). A validated quantitative colorimetric assay for gentamicin. J Pharm Biomed Anal 21:1149–1159.

112. McNally A, Sly K, Lin S, Bourges X, Daculsi G (2008). Release of Antibiotics from Macroporous Injectable Calcium Phosphate Cement. Key Engineering Materials vols 361–363, 359–362, Trans Tech Publication Switzerland.

113. Andrews JM (2001 Jul). Determination of minimum inhibitory concentrations. J Antimicrob Chemother 48 (Suppl 1):5–16. Erratum in: J Antimicrob Chemother 2002 Jun;49(6):1049.

114. Nery EB, Lynch KL, Hirthe WM, Mueller KH (1975). Bioceramic implants in surgically produced infraboney defects. J Periodontol 63:729–735.

115. Clemencia Rodríguez M, Jean A, Kimakhe S, Sylvia Mitja S, Daculsi G (2007). Five years clinical follow up bone rgeneration with CaP Bioceramics. Proceedings IADR, New Orleans.

116. Clemencia Rodríguez M, Jean A, Kimakhe S, Sylvia Mitja S, Daculsi G (2008). Five Years Clinical Follow up Bone Regeneration with CaP Bioceramics Key Engineering Materials vols 361–363, 1339–1342, Trans Tech Publication Switzerland.

117. LeGeros RZ (1993). Biodegradation and bioresorption of calcium phosphate ceramics. Clin Mater 14:65–88.

118. Daculsi G, Passuti N, Martin S, Deudon C, LeGeros RZ (1990). Macroporous calcium phosphate ceramic for long bone surgery in human and dogs. J Biomed Mater Res 24:379–396.

119. Delecrin J, Takahashi S, Gouin F, Passuti N (2000). A synthetic porous ceramic as a bone graft substitute in the surgical management of scoliosis: a prospective, randomized study. Spine 25:563–569.

120. Wykrota LL, Garrido CA, Wykrota FHI (1998). Clinical evaluation of biphasic calcium phosphate ceramic use in orthopedic lesions. In LeGeros RZ, LeGeros JP (Eds) Bioceramics 11, Singapore, World Scientific, pp 641–644.

121. Shima T, Keller JT, Alvira MM, Mayfield FH, Dunker SB (1979). Anterior cervical discectomy and interbody fusion. An experimental study using a synthetic tricalcium phosphate. J Neurosurg 51:533–538.

122. Toth JM, An HS, Lim TH, Ran Y, Weiss NG, Lundberg WR, Xu RM, Lynch KL (1995). Evaluation of porous biphasic calcium phosphate ceramics for anterior cervical interbody fusion in a caprine model. Spine 20(20):2203–2210.

123. Zdeblick TA, Cooke ME, Wilson D, Kunz DN, McCabe R (1993). Anterior cervical dissectomy, fusion and plating. A comparative animal study. Spine 18(14):1974–1983.

124. Zdeblick TA, Ghanayem AJ, Rapoff AJ, Swain C, Basset T, Cooke ME, Markel M (1998). Cervical interbody fusion. An animal model with and without bone morphogenetic protein. Spine 23:758–765.

125. Pascal-Moussellard H, Catonné Y, Robert R, Daculsi G (2007). Anterior cervical fusion with PEEK cages: clinical results of a prospective, comparative, multicenter and randomized study comparing iliac graft and a Macroporous Biphasic Calcium Phosphate. Proceedings ESB 20, Nantes France.

126. Lascart T, Favard L, Burdin P, Traoré O (1998). Utilisation du phosphate tricalcique dans les ostéotomies tibiales de valgisation par addition interne. Ann Orthop Ouest 30:137–141.

127. Bonnevialle P, Abid A, Mansat P, Verhaeghe L, Clement D, Mansat M (2002). Ostéotomie tibiale de valgisation par addition médiale d'un coin de phosphate tricalcique. Rev Chir Orthop 88:486–492.

128. Koshino T, Murase T, Saito T (2003). Medial opening-wedge high tibial osteotomy with use of porous hydroxyapatite to treat medial compartment osteoarthritis of the knee. J Bone Joint Surg [Am] 85-A:78–85.

129. Rouvillain JL (2007). MBCP™ Wedges Performance During Open Medial Tibial Osteotomy. Proceedings ESB 20, Nantes France.

5

SCIENCE AND TECHNOLOGY INTEGRATED TITANIUM DENTAL IMPLANT SYSTEMS

Yoshiki Oshida[1] and Elif Bahar Tuna[2]

[1]*Indiana University School of Dentistry, Professor Emeritus, Syracuse University College of Engineering, Research Professor, Smith College of Engineering, Department of Mechanical and Aerospace Engineering, Syracuse University, Syracuse, New York, USA*
[2]*Istanbul University Faculty of Dentistry, Department of Pediatric Dentistry, Capa Istanbul, Turkey*

Contents

5.1 Overview	143
5.2 Introduction	144
5.3 Requirements for Successful Implant Systems	146
5.3.1 Biological Compatibility	146
5.3.2 Mechanical Compatibility	151
5.3.3 Morphological Compatibility	153
5.4 Osseointegration and Bone/Implant Interface	157
5.5 Integrated Implant System	163
5.6 Conclusions	167
References	167

5.1 OVERVIEW

At the interface of placed implant surface receiving vital tissue, there are interactions between the *foreign* material and the surrounding *host* living tissue, fluid,

Advanced Biomaterials: Fundamentals, Processing, and Applications, Edited by Bikramjit Basu, Dhirendra S. Katti, and Ashok Kumar

and blood elements. Some of these are simply adaptive. Others are hazardous, both in the short and long terms, to the survival of the living system. For placed implants to exhibit biointegration to receiving hard tissue and biofunctionality thereafter, there are at least three major required compatibilities. They include biological compatibility, mechanical compatibility, and morphological compatibility to receiving host tissues. In this chapter, these three compatibilities will be reviewed and discussed. If any surface layer of implant systems possesses all three required characteristics, expected outcome should be achieved with so-called integrated implant system. For such systems, a gradient function concept should be introduced, and surface layer should be fabricated with gradient functional material system(s). This chapter proposes a novel, integrated implant system.

5.2   INTRODUCTION

Dental implants are an ideal option for people in good general oral health who have lost a tooth (or teeth) due to periodontal disease, an injury, or some other reason. Dental implants—as an artificial tooth root and usually made from commercially-pure titanium ASTM Grades 1 through 4 or Ti-based alloys—are biocompatible metal anchors surgically positioned in the jaw bone (in other words, surgically traumatized bone) underneath the gums to support an artificial crown where natural teeth are missing. Using the root form implants, the closest in shape and size to the natural tooth root, the non-union (due to tramatization) bone healing period usually varies from as few as three months to six or more. During this time, osseointegration occurs. The bone grows in and around the implant, creating a strong structural support, to which a superstructure will be later attached by either cemetation or a screw-tightening retaining technique.

Today, titanium and some of its alloys are considered to be among the most biocompatible materials. Titanium's superiority is indicated by its preferential use in many recent applications in maxillofacial, oral, neuro and cardiovascular-surgery, as well as its increased preference in orthopedics. Moreover, titanium and its alloys have been successfully used for orthopedic and dental implants. Direct bony interface promised more predictability and longevity than previously used systems; hence, oral implantology gained significant additional momentum. A carefully planned full rehabilitation of the mouth using state-of-the-art methods can free the patient of dental problems for decades. However, this can only be achieved with the complete cooperation of the patient, accompanied by regular supervision and care by the dental surgeon and the dental hygienist.

According to Binon, there are about 25 dental implants manufacturing companies, producing approximately 100 different titanium dental implant systems with a variety of diameters, lengths, surfaces, platforms, interfaces, and body designs. The most logical differentiation and distinctions are based on the implant/abutment interface, the body shape, and the implant-to-bone surface [Binon, 2000].

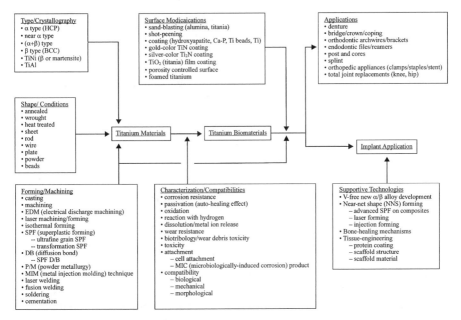

Figure 5.1. Interacting map of various disciplines involved in titanium materials.

Why do titanium and its alloys show such good biocompatibility compared with other alloys? The answer to this question is generally that titanium is passive in aqueous solutions, and the passive film that forms on titanium is stable, even in a biological system including chemical and mechanical environments. Such an interpretation is true in many cases. However, the presence of the passive film is only part of the answer, considering the complex interfacial phenomena found between titanium and a biological system, in both biological and biomechanical environments.

Figure 5.1 [Oshida, 2007a] demonstrates the uniqueness of titanium materials. Along with stainless steels, titanium materials are only two types of materials which are widely and equally used in both engineering and medical/dental fields. From this figure, several important and interesting points can be derived; there are:

1. more than three different matrix phases available, depending on amount of alloying elements as α-stabilizer or β-stabilizer;
2. a variety of primary products available;
3. all kinds of forming technology applicable;
4. if required characteristics and compatibilities are satisfied, titanium materials can be considered as titanium biomaterials for various medical/dental applications, and furthermore;
5. with supportive technologies, successful implants can be fabricated.

This chapter discusses several important points related to successful implantology and surface interactions with biological environments.

5.3 REQUIREMENTS FOR SUCCESSFUL IMPLANT SYSTEMS

The implantation of devices for the maintenance or restoration of a body function imposes extraordinary requirements on the materials of construction. Foremost among these is an issue of biocompatibility. There are interactions between the *foreign* material and the surrounding *host* living tissue, fluid and blood elements. Some of these are simply adaptive. Others constitute a hazard, both short and long term, to the survival of the living system [Long et al., 1998; Brunski et al., 2000]. There are mechanical and physical properties which the material must provide, and a structural nature which the system should exhibit. Some of these govern the ability of the device to provide its intended function from a purely engineering viewpoint.

Others—such as tribology (specifically friction and wear), corrosion and mechanical compliance—significantly relate to biocompatibility concerns. Human implantation applications impose more stringent requirements on reliability than does any other engineering task. In most applications, an implanted device is expected to function for the life of the patient. As the medical profession becomes more emboldened, the device lifetime must stretch to more than 30 years, if follow-up maintenance is carefully and thoroughly performed. Yet, there are very few engineering devices which have been designed to function for more than 30 years. It is necessary to think in terms of reliability of performance of thousands of devices for the lifetime of a patient and a tolerable expectation of failure of perhaps no more than one in one thousand [Bannon et al., 1983; Brunski et al., 2000].

One of many universal requirements of implants, wherever they are used in the body, is the ability to form a suitably stable mechanical unit with the neighboring hard or soft tissues. A loose (or unstable) implant may function less efficiently or cease functioning completely, or it may induce an excessive tissue response. In either case, it may cause the patient discomfort and pain. In several situations, a loose implant was deemed to have failed and needed to be surgically removed. For a long time it has been recognized that any types of implants (for both dental implants and orthopedic implants), should possess a biological compatibility against an implant receiving surrounding hard/soft tissues.

There are at three least major required compatibilities for placed implants to exhibit biointegration to receiving hard tissue and biofunctionality thereafter. They include biological compatibility, mechanical compatibility, and morphological compatibility to receiving host tissues [Oshida et al., 1994; Oshida, 2000].

5.3.1 Biological Compatibility

Corrosion is one of the major processes that cause problems when metals are used as implants in the body. Their proper application to minimize such problems requires that one has an understanding of principles underlying the important degradative process of corrosion. Such an understanding results in proper application, better design, choice of appropriate test methods to develop better designs, and the possibility of determining the origin of failures encountered in practice [Kruger, 1979; Greene, 1983].

Titanium is a highly reactive metal and will react within microseconds to form an oxide layer when exposed to the atmosphere [Kasemo, 1983]. Although the standard electrode potential was reported in a range from -1.2 to -2.0 volts for the Ti $\leftrightarrow$ Ti^{+3} electrode reaction [Tomashov, 1966; CRC Handbook, 1966], due to strong chemical affinity to oxygen, it easily produces a compact oxide film, ensuring high corrosion resistance of the metal. This oxide, which is primarily TiO$_2$, forms readily because it has one of the highest heats of reaction known ($\Delta H = -915$ kJ/mole) (for $298.16°\sim2000°K$) [American Society for Metals, 1991; Ashby et al., 1980]. It is also quite impenetrable to oxygen (since the atomic diameter of Ti is 0.29 nm, the primary protecting layer is only about five to 20 atoms thick) [Lautenschlager et al., 1993]. The formed oxide layer adheres strongly to the titanium substrate surface. The average single-bond strength of the TiO$_2$ to Ti substrate was reported to be about 300 kcal/mol, while it is 180 kcal/mol for Cr$_2$O$_3$/Cr, 320 kcal/mol for Al$_2$O$_3$/Al, and 420 kcal/mol for both Ta$_2$O$_5$/Ta and Nb$_2$O$_5$/Nb [Douglass, 1995]. Adhesion and adhesive strength of Ti oxide to substrates are controlled by oxidation temperature and thickness of the oxide layer, as well as the significant influence of nitrogen on oxidation in air. In addition, adhesion is greater for oxidation in air than in pure oxygen [Coddet et al., 1987], suggesting that the influence of nitrogen on the oxidation process is significant.

The service conditions in the mouth are hostile, both corrosively and mechanically. All intraorally placed parts are continuously bathed in saliva, an aerated aqueous solution of about 0.1 N chlorides, with varying amounts of Na, K, Ca, PO$_4$, CO$_2$, sulphur compounds and mucin. The pH value is normally in the range of 5.5 to 7.5, but under plaque deposits it can be as low as 2.0. Temperatures can vary $\pm36.5°C$, and a variety of food and drink concentrations apply for short periods. Loads may be up to 1000 N (with normal masticatory force ranging from 150 N to 250 N), sometimes at impact speeds. Trapped food debris may decompose to create sulphur compounds, causing placed devices's discoloration [Brockhurst, 1980]. With such hostile conditions, biocompatibility (biological compatibility) of metallic materials essentially equates to corrosion resistance because it is thought that alloying elements can only enter the surrounding organic system and develop toxic effects by conversion to ions through chemical or electrochemical processes. After implant placement, initial healing of the bony compartment is characterized by the formation of blood clots at the traumatized wound site, protein adsorption and adherence of polymorphonuclear leukocyte. Then approximately two days after placement of the implant, fibroblasts proliferate into the blood clot, organization begins, and an extracellular matrix is produced. Approximately one week after the implant is placed, appearance of osteblast-like cells and new bone is seen. New bone reaches the implant surface by osseoconduction, through growth of bone over the surface and migration of bone cells over the implant surfaces [Steinmann, 1980].

During implantation, titanium releases corrosion products—mainly titanium oxide or titanium hydro-oxide—into the surrounding tissue and fluids even though it is covered by a thermodynamically stable oxide film [Ferguson et al., 1962; Meachim et al., 1973; Ducheyne et al., 1984]. An increase in oxide thickness, as well as incorporation of elements from the extra-cellular fluid (P, Ca, and S) into the oxide, has been observed as a function of implantation time [Sundgren et al., 1986]. Moreover, changes in the oxide stoichiometry, composition, and thickness have been associated with the release of titanium corrosion products *in vitro* [Ducheyne et al., 1988]. Properties of the oxide, such as stoichiometry, defect density, crystal structure and orientation, surface defects, and impurities were suggested as factors determining biological performance [Fraker et al., 1973; Albrektsson et al., 1983; Albrektsson et al., 1986].

The performance of titanium and its alloys in surgical implant applications can be evaluated with respect to their biocompatibility and capability to withstand the corrosive species involved in fluids within the human body [Solar, 1979]. This may be considered as an electrolyte in an electrochemical reaction. It is well documented that the excellent corrosion resistance of titanium materials is due to the formation of a dense, protective, and strongly-adhered film, called a passive film. Such a surface situation is referred to as passivity or a passivation state. The exact composition and structure of the passive film covering titanium and its alloys is controversial. This is the case not only for the "natural" air oxide, but also for films formed during exposure to various solutions, as well as those formed anodically. The "natural" oxide film on titanium ranges in thickness from 2-to-7 nm, depending on such parameters as the composition of the metal and surrounding medium, the maximum temperature reached during the working of the metal, the surface finish, and so on.

The excellent corrosion resistance associated with titanium materials is due to the stability of surface titanium oxide films. If such oxide films possess protectiveness against the hostile environments, strong adherence to the Ti substrate, and dense structure, they are said to be passive film. To form such passive films, chemical or electrochemical treatment is normally conducted. Oxides formed on Ti materials are varied with a general form; TiO_x ($1 < x < 2$). Depending on x values, there are five different crystalline oxides, including:

(1) cubic TiO ($a_o = 4.24 \text{Å}$),
(2) hexagonal Ti_2O_3 ($a_o = 5.37 \text{Å}$, ($= 56°48'$),
(3) tetragonal TiO_2 (anatase) ($a_o = 3.78 \text{Å}$, $c_o = 9.50 \text{Å}$),
(4) tetragonal TiO_2 (rutile) ($a_o = 4.58 \text{Å}$, $c_o = 2.98 \text{Å}$), and
(5) orthorhombic TiO_2 (brookite) ($a_o = 9.17 \text{Å}$, $b_o = 5.43 \text{Å}$, $c_o = 5.13 \text{Å}$).

Besides these, there are non-stoichiometric oxide (when x is not integral) and amorphous oxides. It is widely believed that, among these oxides, only rutile

Condition	Type of crystalline structure of formed titanium oxide		
Physical depositon			**Anatase**
Dry oxidation	**Rutile**		
Wet oxidation	**Rutile**	**R + A**	**Anatase**
Solution pH	Low pH (acid)	————————————————→	High pH (alkaline)

<u>Figure 5.2.</u> Types and stabilities of oxides formed on titanium materials.

and anatase type oxides are stable at normal conditions. Figure 5.2 summarizes the formation of these oxides under various forming processes [Oshida, 2007a]. It is of interest to note that choice for rutile formation or anatase formation depends on the acidity of used electrolyte.

Mechanically polished (with SiC paper grit #600) commercially pure titanium (ASTM CpTi Grade 4) plates (10 × 30 × 2 mm) were variously chemical-treated:

(1) AC: acid-treated (HF/HNO$_3$/H$_2$O) at room temperature for five seconds,
(2) AK: alkaline-treated (5 mol NaOH) at 70 °C for 24 hours, and
(3) HP: hydrogen peroxide-treated (50%) at room temperature for ten seconds.

Such chemically-treated surfaces were examined for surface roughness and surface contact angle measurements. Figure 5.3 shows their relationship, where mark "4" represents AC-treated surface, while marks "5" and "7" represent AK-treated and HP-treated surfaces, respectively.

It was observed that AC-treated surface shows the hydrophobic nature, while AK- and HP-treated surfaces show hydrophilic character. After chemical stripping surface oxide films from titanium substrate, the thus isolated oxide films were subjected to TEM (transmission electron microscopy) to identify the crystalline structure(s). It was also found that AC-treated hydrophobic surface oxide was made of only rutile type TiO$_2$, while AK- and HP-treated surfaces consisted of a mixture of rutile and anatase type oxides [Lim et al., 2001; Oshida, 2007b].

The level of neutrophil priming and activation following implant placement may be linked to the development and maintenance of long-term stability and osseointegration [Gaydos et al., 2000]. Bisphosphonate effect on neutrophil activation was furthermore examined on these differently treated surfaces. Neutrophils were isolated from whole blood collected from healthy human donors, on a double dextran gradient. Treated surfaces were incubated with 5 × 10^5 neutrophils per curette. Luminol-dependent CL (chemiluminescence) was recorded for 60 minutes (priming or inflammatory phase), followed by secondary stimulation with 10^{-7} M phorbol myristate acetate at 60 minutes (activation phase) for a

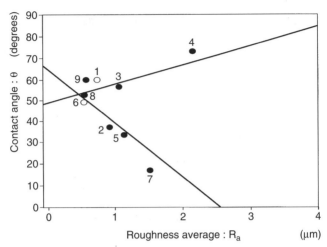

Figure 5.3. Relationhsip between surface roughness and surface contact angle of variously treated commercially-pure titanium (ASTM CpT Grade 4).

continuous CL measurement over 120 minutes. SEM evaluation was preformed. Results indicated that: AK- and HP-treated surfaces produced significantly higher CL responses than cells for AC-treated surface ($p < 0.001$); SEM evaluation revealed some neutrophil attachment onto the AK- and HP-treated substrate, suggesting that cells were viable with normal function, and; these results indicate that both AK- and HP-treated surfaces (which were covered with a mixture of rutile and anatase type TiO_2 oxide films) are capable of priming neutrophils, when compared to AC-treated surface which was covered only with rutile oxide [Oshida, 2007c].

Using Auger Electron Spectroscopy (AES) to study the change in the composition of the titanium surface during implantation in human bone, it was observed that the oxide formed on titanium implants grows and takes up minerals during the implantation [McQueen et al., 1982; Sundgren et al., 1986]. The growth and uptake occur even though the adsorbed layer of protein is present on the oxide, indicating that mineral ions pass through the adsorbed protein. It was shown that, using Fourier Transform Infrared Reflection Absorption Spectroscopy (FTIR-RAS), phosphate ions are adsorbed by the titanium surface after the protein has been adsorbed. Using x-ray photoelectron spectroscopy (XPS) [Liedberg et al., 1984], it was demonstrated that oxides on commercially-pure titanium and titanium alloys (Ti-6Al-4V) change into complex phosphates of titanium and calcium containing hydroxyl groups which bind water on immersion in artificial saliva (pH: 5.2) [Hanawa, 1991]. All these studies indicate that the surface oxide on titanium materials reacts with mineral ions, water, and other constituents of biofluids, and that these reactions in turn cause a remodeling of the surface.

It was shown that titanium is in almost direct contact to bone tissue, separated only by an extremely thin cell-free non-calcified tissue layer. Transmission electron microscopy revealed an interfacial hierarchy that consisted of a 20–40 nm thick proteoglycan layer within four nm of the titanium oxide, followed by collagen bundles as close as 100 nm and Ca deposits within five nm of the surface [Healy et al., 1992a]. To reach the steady-state interface described, both the oxide on titanium and the adjacent tissue undergo various reactions. The physiochemical properties of titanium have been associated with the unique tissue response to the materials; these include the biochemistry of released corrosion products, kinetics of release and the oxide stoichiometry, crystal defect density, thickness and surface chemistry [Healy et al., 1992b].

As seen above, in general, the titanium passivating layer not only produces good corrosion resistance, but it seems also to allow physiological fluids, proteins, and hard and soft tissue to come very close and/or deposit on it directly. Reasons for this are still largely unknown, but may have something to do with factors such as the high dielectric constant for TiO_2 (50 to 170 vs. 4–10 for alumina and dental porcelain), which should result in considerably stronger van der Waal's bonds on TiO_2 than other oxides; TiO_2 may be catalytically active for a number of organic and inorganic chemical interactions influencing biological processes at the implant interface. The TiO_2 oxide film may permit a compatible layer of biomolecule to attach [Brånemark, 1985; Kasemo et al., 1985].

5.3.2 Mechanical Compatibility

Biomechanics involved in implantology should at least include the nature of the biting forces on the implants, transferring of the biting forces to the interfacial tissues, and the interfacial tissues reaction, biologically, to stress transfer conditions. Interfacial stress transfer and interfacial biology represent more difficult, interrelated problems. While many engineering studies have shown that variables such as implant shape, elastic modulus, extent of bonding between implant and bone, and so on, can affect the stress transfer conditions, the unresolved question is whether there is any biological significance to such differences.

The successful clinical results achieved with osseointegrated dental implants underscore the fact that such implants easily withstand considerable masticatory loads. In fact, one study showed that bite forces in patients with these implants were comparable to those in patients with natural dentitions. A critical aspect affecting the success or failure of an implant is the manner in which mechanical stresses are transferred smoothly from the implant to bone. It is essential that neither implant nor bone be stressed beyond the long-term fatigue capacity. It is also necessary to avoid any relative motion that can produce abrasion of the bone or progressive loosening of the implants. An osseointegrated implant provides a direct and relatively rigid connection of the implant to the bone.

This is an advantage because it provides a durable interface without any substantial change in form or duration. There is a mismatch of the mechanical properties and mechanical impedance at the interface of Ti and bone. It is interesting to observe that from a mechanical standpoint, the shock-absorbing action would be the same if the soft layer were between the metal implant and the bone.

In the natural tooth, the periodontum, which forms a shock-absorbing layer, is in this position between the tooth and jaw bone [Skalak, 1983]. Natural teeth and implants have different force transmission characteristics to bone.

Compressive strains were induced around natural teeth and implants as a result of static axial loading, whereas combinations of compressive and tensile strains were observed during lateral dynamic loading [Oshida, 2007a]. Magnitude of strain around the natural tooth is significantly lower than the opposing implant and occluding implants in the contra-lateral side for most regions under all loading conditions. It was reported that there was a general tendency for increased strains around the implant opposing natural tooth under higher loads and particularly under lateral dynamic loads [Hekimoglu et al., 2004].

By means of finite element (FEM) analysis, stress-distribution in bone around implants was calculated with and without stress-absorbing element [van Rossen et al., 1990]. A freestanding implant and an implant connected with a natural tooth were simulated. For the freestanding implant, it was concluded that the variation in the modulus of elasticity of the stress-absorbing element had no effect on the stresses in bone. Changing the shape of the stress-absorbing element had little effect on the stresses in cortical bone. For the implant connected with a natural tooth, it was concluded that a more uniform stress was obtained around the implant with a low modulus of elasticity of the stress-absorbing element. It was also concluded that the bone surrounding the natural tooth showed a decrease in the height of the peak stresses.

The dental or orthopedic prostheses, particularly the surface zone thereof, should respond to the loading transmitting function. The placed implant and receiving tissues establish a unique stress-strain field. Between them, there should be an interfacial layer. During the loading, the strain-field continuity should be held, although the stress-field is obviously in a discrete manner due to different values of modulus of elasticity between host tissue and foreign implant material. If the magnitude of the difference in modulus of elasticity is large, then the interfacial stress, accordingly, could become so large that the placed implant system will face a risky failure or detachment situation. Therefore, materials for implant or surface zone of implants should be mechanically compatible to mechanical properties of receiving tissues to minimize the interfacial discrete stress. This is the second compatibility and is called as the mechanical compatibility.

Figure 5.4 [Oshida, 2007a] compares yield strengths and modulus of elasticity of various biomaterials in log-log plot, where P: polymeric materials, B: bone, HSP: high strength polymers (such as Kevlar, Kapton, PEEK, etc.), D: dentin, TCP: tricalcium phosphate, HAP: hydroxyapatite, E: enamel, TI: commercially pure titanium (all unalloyed grades), TA: titanium alloys (e.g., Ti-6Al-4V), S: steels (e.g., 304 and 316 stainless steels), A: alumina, PSZ: partially stabilized zirconia, and CF: carbon fiber, respectively.

From the figure, it is greatly surprising to note the large differences in both yield strength and modulus of elasticity between TI as a foreign implant material and B as a receiving hard tissue. Even depositing HAP onto TI surface would

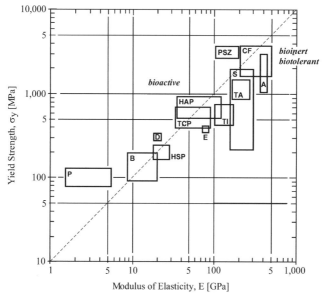

Figure 5.4. Yield strength versus modulus of elasticity of various biomaterials.

not be a great help in terms of filling this large gap between two inorganic and organic materials. Accordingly, even the post-operation osseointegration has been successfully achieved; the stress field in the TI-B system should be discrete, due to a great difference in modulus of elasticity between TI and B materials. This presents the challenging problem of how to fill such a great gap which will be discussed later in this chapter.

5.3.3 Morphological Compatibility

In a scientific article [Oshida et al., 1994], it was found that the surface morphology of successful implants has an upper and lower limitations in average roughness (1~50μm) and average particle size (10~500μm), regardless of types of implant materials (either metallic, ceramics, or polymeric materials), as seen in Figure 5.5. If a particle size is smaller than 10μm, the surface will be more toxic to fibroblastic cells and have an adverse influence on cells due to their physical presence independent of any chemical toxic effects. If the pore is larger than 500μm, the surface does not maintain sufficient structural integrity because it is too coarse. This is the third compatibility—morphological compatibility [Oshida et al., 1994; Oshida, 2000].

It has been shown that methods of implant surface preparation can significantly affect the resultant properties of the surface and subsequently the biological responses that occur at the surface [Keller et al., 1989a; Keller et al., 1989b; Keller et al., 1990]. Recent efforts have shown that the success or failure of dental implants can be related not only to the chemical properties of the implant surface,

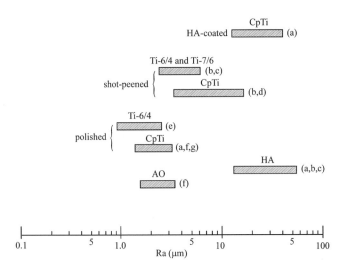

References
(a) Buser D, Schenk RK, Steinemann SG, Fiorellini JP, Fox CH, Stich H. Influence of surface characteristics on bone integration of titanium implants; A histomorphometric study in miniature pigs. Biomed Mater Res 1991;25:889-902.
(b) Jamsen JA, van der Waerden JPCM, Wolke JGC. Histologic investigation of the biologic behavior of different hydroxyapatite plasma-coatings in rabbits. Biomed Mater Res 1993;27:603-610.
(c) Wang BC, Lee TM, Chang E, Yang CY. The shear strength and the failure mode of plasma-sprayed hydroxyapatite coating to bone: The effect of coating thickness. Biomed Mater Res 1993;27:1315-1327.
(d) Steinemann SG, Eulenberger J, Maeusli PA, Schoeder A. Biological and biomechanical performances of biomaterials. Amsterdam: Elsevier Science, 1986. p.409-414.
(e) Hayashi K, Inadome T, Mashima T, Sugioka Y. Comparison of bone-implant interface shear strength of solid hydroxyapatite and hydroxyapatite-coated titanium implants. Biomed Mater Res 1993;27:557-563.
(f) Thomas KA, Cook SD. Am evaluation of variable influencing implant fixation by direct bone apposition. Biomed Mater Res 1985;19:875-901.
(g) Li J. Behavior of titanium and titanium-based ceramics in vitro and in vivo. Biomater 1993;14:229-232.

Figure 5.5. Distribution of surface roughness of successfully implanted and clinically biofunctioning materials.

but also to its macromorphologic nature [Schroeder et al., 1981; Rich et al., 1981; Buser et al., 1991].

From an *in vitro* standpoint, the response of cells and tissues at implant interfaces can be affected by surface topography or geometry on a macroscopic basis [Schroeder et al., 1981; Buser et al., 1991], as well as by surface morphology or roughness on a microscopic level [Rich et al., 1981; Murray et al., 1989]. These characteristics undoubtly affect how cells and tissues respond to various types of biomaterials. Of all the cellular responses, it has been suggested that cellular adhesion is considered the most important response necessary for developing a rigid structural and functional integrity at the bone/implant interface [Cherhoudi et al., 1988]. Cellular adhesion alters the entire tissue response to biomaterials [von Recum, 1990].

The effect of surface roughness (Ra: 0.320, 0.490, and 0.874 μm) of the titanium alloy Ti-6Al-4V on the short- and long-term response of human bone marrow cells *in vitro* and on protein adsorption was investigated. Cell attachment, cell proliferation, and differentiation (alkaline phosphatase specific activity) were determined. The protein adsorption of bovine serum albumin and fibronectin, from single protein solutions on rough and smooth Ti-6Al-4V surfaces was examined with XPS and radio labeling. It was found that:

1. cell attachment and proliferation were surface roughness sensitive, and increased as the roughness of Ti-6Al-4V increased,
2. human albumin was adsorbed preferentially onto the smooth substratum, and
3. the rough substratum bound a higher amount of total protein (from culture medium supplied with 15% serum) and fibronectin (10-fold) than did the smooth one [Deligianni et al., 2001].

Events leading to integration of an implant into bone, and hence determining the long-time performance of the device, take place largely at the interface formed between the tissue and the implant [Yang et al., 2003]. The development of this interface is complex and is influenced by numerous factors, including surface chemistry and surface topography of the foreign material [Albrektsson et al., 1983; Kasemo et al., 1986; Schenk et al., 1998; Masuda et al., 1998; Larsson et al., 2001]. For example, Oshida et al. treated NiTi by acid-pickling in $HF:HNO_3:H_2O$ (1:1:5 by volume) at room temperature for 30 seconds to control the surface topology and selectively dissolve Ni, resulting in a Ti-enriched surface layer [Oshida et al., 1992], demonstrating that surface topology can be relatively easily controlled.

The role of surface roughness on the interaction of cells with titanium model surfaces of well-defined topography was investigated using human bone-derived cells (MG63 cells). The early phase of interactions was studied using a kinetic morphological analysis of adhesion, spreading, and proliferation of the cells. SEM and double immunofluorescent labeling of vinculin and actin revealed that the cells responded to nanoscale roughness with a higher cell thickness and a delayed apparition of the focal contacts. A singular behavior was observed on nanoporous oxide surfaces, where the cells were more spread and displayed longer and more numerous filopods. On electrochemically microstructured surfaces, the MG63 cells were able to go inside, adhere, and proliferate in cavities of 30 or 100μm in diameter, whereas they did not recognize the 10μm diameter cavities. Cells adopted a three-dimensional shape when attaching inside the 30μm diameter cavities. It was concluded that nanotopography on surfaces with 30μm diameter cavities had little effect on cell morphology compared to flat surfaces with the same nanostructure, but cell proliferation exhibited a marked synergistic effect of microscale and nanoscale topography [Zinger et al., 2004].

It was pointed out that surface topography played an importance on cellular reactions [Eriksson et al., 2001]. Surface plays a crucial role in biological interactions for four reasons. First, the surface of a biomaterial is the only part in contact with the bioenvironment. Second, the surface region of a biomaterial is almost always different in morphology and composition from the bulk. Differences arise from molecular rearrangement, surface reaction, and contamination. Third, for biomaterials that do not release nor leak biologically active or toxic substances, the characteristics of the surface govern the biological response. And fourth, some surface properties, such as topography, affect the mechanical stability of the implant/tissue interface [Wen et al., 1996].

On a macroscopic level (roughness > 10µm) roughness influences the mechanical properties of the titanium/bone interface, the mechanical interlocking of the interface, and the biocompatibility of the material [Ratner, 1983; Baro et al., 1986]. Surface roughness in the range from 10nm to 10µm may also influence the interfacial biology, since it is the same order as the size of the cells and large biomolecules [Kasemo, 1983]. Microroughness at this level includes material defects, such as grain boundaries, steps and kinks, and vacancies that are active sites for adsorption, and therefore influence the bonding of biomolecules to the implant surface [Moroni et al., 1994]. Microrough surfaces promote significantly better bone apposition than smooth surfaces, resulting in a higher percentage of bone in contact with the implant. Microrough surfaces may influence the mechanical properties of the interface, stress distribution, and bone remodeling [Keller et al., 1987]. Increased contact area and mechanical interlocking of bone to a microrough surface can decrease stress concentrations resulting in decreased bone resorption. Bone resorption takes place shortly after loading smooth surfaced implants [Pilliar et al., 1991], resulting in a fibrous connective tissue layer, whereas remodeling occurs on rough surfaces [Gilbert et al., 1995].

Successful clinical performance of machine/turned CpTi implants has resulted in a wide-spread usage of them. However, in bone of poor quality and quantity, the results have not always been good, motivating the development of novel types of osseointegrated implants. The development of Ti implants has depended on new surface-processing technologies. Recently developed clinical oral implants have been focused on topographical changes of implant surfaces, rather than alterations of chemical properties [Deporter et al., 1999; Buser et al., 1999; Plamer et al., 2000; Testori et al., 2001; Sul, 2003]. These attempts may have been based on the concept that mechanical interlocking between tissue and implant materials relies on surface irregularities in the nanometer to micron level. Recently published *in vivo* investigations have shown significantly improved bone tissue reactions by modification of the surface oxide properties of Ti implants [Ishizawa et al., 1995; Larsson et al., 1997; Skripitz et al., 1998; Fini et al., 1999; Henry et al., 2000; Sul et al., 2001; Sul et al., 2002a; Sul et al., 2002b].

It was found that in animal studies, bone tissue reactions were strongly reinforced with oxidized titanium implants, characterized by a titanium oxide layer thicker than 600nm, a porous surface structure, and an anatase type of Ti oxide with large surface roughness compared with turned implants [Sul et al., 2001; Sul et al., 2002a]. This was later supported by work done by Lim et al. [Lim et al., 2001] and [Oshida, 2007b], who found that the alkali-treated CpTi surface was covered mainly with anatase type TiO_2, and exhibited hydrophilicity, whereas the acid-treated CpTi was covered with rutile type TiO_2 with hydrophobicity. Besides this characteristic crystalline structure of TiO_2, it was mentioned that good osseo-integration, bony apposition, and cell attachment of Ti implant systems [Meachim et al., 1973; Albrektsson et al., 1987] are partially due to the fact that the oxide layer, with unusually high dielectric constant of 50–117, depending on the TiO_2 concentration, may be the responsible feature [Kasemo, 1983; Lausmaa, 1986].

5.4 OSSEOINTEGRATION AND BONE/IMPLANT INTERFACE

Broadly speaking, two types of anchorage mechanisms have been described: biomechanical and biochemical. Biomechanical binding is when bone in-growth occurs into micrometer sized surface irregularities. Realistically, the term osseo-integration probably best describes this biomechanical phenomenon. Biochemi-cal bonding may occur with certain bioactive materials where there is primarily a chemical bonding, with possible supplemental biomechanical interlocking. The distinct advantage with the biochemical bonding is that the anchorage is accom-plished within a relatively short period of time, while biomechanical anchorage takes weeks to develop. This would clinically translate into the possibility of earlier restorative loading of implants. Most commercially available implants depend on biomechanical interlocking for anchorage. All implants must exhibit biomechanical as well as morphological compatibility [Albrektsson, 1983; Oshida et al., 1994].

Defining the nature of biomaterial surfaces is crucial for understanding inter-actions with biological systems. Surface analysis requires special techniques and instruments considering the analysis of a 50 Å thick region in one mm, two areas on the surface of a specimen that is one mm in total thickness. Devices intended to be implanted or interfaced intimately with living tissue may be composed of a variety of materials. Understanding the biological performance and efficacy of these biomaterials requires a thorough knowledge of the nature of their surfaces. The nature of the surface can be described in terms of surface chemistry, surface energy, and morphology [Ratner et al., 1987].

The biological events occurring at the bone–implant interface are influenced by the topography, chemistry, and wettability of the implant surface, as seen in the above. A goal of biomaterials research has been, and continues to be, the development of implant materials which are predictable, controlled, guided, with rapid healing of the interfacial tissues, both hard and soft. The performance of biomaterials can be classified in terms of the response of the host to the implant, and of the behavior of the material in the host. This is actually related to which side is being observed at the host (vital tissue)/foreign materials (implant) interface.

The event that occurs almost immediately upon implantation of metals, as with other biomaterials, is adsorption of proteins. These proteins come first from blood and tissue fluids at the wound site, and later from cellular activity in the interfacial region. Once on the surface, proteins can desorb (undenatured or denatured, intact or fragment), remain, or mediate tissue-implant interaction

[Bruck, 1991]. The host response to implants placed in bone involves a series of cell and matrix events, ideally culminating in tissue healing that is as normal as possible, and that ultimately leads to intimate apposition of bone to the biomaterials, that is, the operative definition of osseointegration.

For this intimate contact to occur, gaps that initially exist between the bone and implant at surgery must be filled initially by a blood clot, and bone damaged during preparation of the implant site must be repaired. During this time, unfavorable conditions, such as, micromotion (a biomechanical factor) will disrupt the newly forming tissue, leading to formation a fibrous capsule [Bannon et al., 1983]. The criteria for clinical success of osseointegration are based on functionality and compatibility, which depend on the control of several factors including:

(1) biocompatible implant material using commercially pure titanium,
(2) design of the fixture; a threaded design is advocated creating a larger surface per unit volume as well as evenly distribution loading forces,
(3) the provision of optimal prosthodontic design and implant maintenance to achieve ongoing osseointegration,
(4) specific aseptic surgical techniques and a subsequent healing protocol which are reconcilable with the principles of bone physiology; this would incorporate a low heat/low trauma regimen, a precise fit, and the two-stage surgery program,
(5) a favorable status of host-implant site from a health and morphologic standpoint,
(6) non-loading of the implant during healing is a basic tenet of osseointegration, and
(7) the defined macro-microscopic surface of the implant as it relates to the host tissue [Adell et al., 1981].

The implantation of any foreign material in soft tissue initiates an inflammatory response. The cellular intensity and duration of the response is controlled by a variety of mediators and determined by the size and nature of the implanted material, site of implantation, and reactive capacity of the host [Marchant, 1986]. Dental implants vary markedly in the topography of the surfaces that contact cells. Four principles of cell behavior first observed in cell culture explain to some extent the interactions of cells and implants:

(1) contact guidance aligns cells and collagen fibers with fine grooves, such as those produced by machining,
(2) rugophilia describes the tendency of macrophages to prefer rough surfaces,
(3) the two-center effect can explain the orientation of soft connective tissue cells and fibers attached to porous surfaces, and
(4) haptotaxis may be involved in the formation of capsules around implants with low-energy surfaces [Brunette, 1988].

Surface roughness has been shown to be an influencing parameter for cell response. Bigerele et al. [Bigerele et al., 2002] compared the effect of roughness organization of Ti-6Al-4V or CpTi on human osteoblast response (proliferation and adhesion). Surface roughness is extensively analyzed at scales above the cell size (macro-roughness) or below the cell size (micro-roughness) by calculation of relevant classic amplitude parameters and original frequency parameters. It was found that the human osteoblast response on electro-erosion Ti-6Al-4V surfaces or CpTi surface was largely increased when compared to polished or machine-tooled surfaces after 21 days or culture, and that the polygonal morphology of human osteoblast on these electro-erosion surfaces was very close to the aspects of human osteoblast *in vivo* on human bone trabeculae. It was concluded that electro-erosion (creating a rough surface) is a promising method for preparation of bone implant surfaces, as it could be applied to the preparation of most biomaterials with complex geometries.

Ti oxide films were synthesized on Ti, Co alloy, and low-temperature isotropic pyrolytic carbon by the ion beam enhanced deposition technique [Pan et al., 1997]. The amorphous non-stoichiometrical Ti oxide films (TiO_{2-x}) were obtained. Blood compatibility of the films was evaluated by clotting time measurement, platelet adhesion investigation, and hemoplysis analysis. It was found that the blood compatibility of the material was improved by the coating of Ti oxide films. The non-stoichiometric TiO_{2-x} has n-type semiconductive properties because very few cavities exist in the valence band of TiO_{2-x}; charge transfer is difficult from the valence band of fibrinogen into the material. On the other hand, the n-type semiconductive TiO_{2-x} with a higher Fermi level can decrease the work function of the film, which makes electrons move out from the film easily. As a result, it was concluded that the deposition of fibrinogen can be inhibited and blood compatibility improved.

Favorable wound healing responses around metallic implants depend on critical control of the surgical and restorative approaches used in dental implant treatments. One critical parameter that has not been biologically studied is the role of a clean, sterile oxide surface on an implant. This oxide surface can alter the cellular healing responses, and potentially the bone remodeling process, depending on the history of how that surface was milled, cleaned, and sterilized prior to placement. Phenotypic responses of rat calvarial osteoblast-like cells were evaluated on CpTi surfaces. These surfaces were prepared to three different clinically relevant surface preparations (1 μm, 600 grit, and 50 μm grit sand blast), followed by sterilization with either ultraviolet light, ethylene oxide, argon plasma-cleaning, or routine clinical autoclaving. It was found that osteocalcin and alkaline phosphatase, but not collagen expression, were significantly affected by surface roughness when these surfaces were altered by argon plasma-cleaning, and that on a per-cell basis, levels of the bone-specific protein, ostocalcin, and enzymatic activity of alkaline phosphatase were highest on the smooth 1 μm polished surface, and lowest on the roughest surface for the plasma-cleaned CpTi [Stanford et al., 1994].

Buser et al. [Buser et al., 1991] treated CpTi surface by blasting, acid-treatment in HCl/H_2SO_4, and the HA-coating. It was reported that rough implant surfaces generally demonstrated an increase in bone apposition compared to polished or fine structured surfaces; the acid treated CpTi implants had an additional stimulating influence on bone apposition; the HA-coated implants showed the highest extent of bone-implant interface, and; the HA coating consistently revealed signs of resorption.

Generally, roughened surfaces have been used as the endosseous area of a dental implant in order to increase the total area available for osseo-apposition. However, there is still considerable controversy concerning the optimal surface geometry and physicochemical properties for the ideal endosseous portion of a dental implant. Knabe et al. [Knabe et al., 2002] used rat bone marrow cells (RBM) to evaluate different Ti and HA dental implant surfaces. The implant surfaces were a Ti surface having a porous Ti plasma-sprayed coating (Ti-TPS), a Ti surface with a deep profile structure (Ti-DPS), an uncoated Ti substrate with a machined surface (Ti-ma), and a machined Ti substrate with a porous HA plasma-sprayed coating (Ti-HA). RSM cells were cultured on the disc-shaped test substrates for 14 days. The culture medium was changed daily and examined for Ca and P concentration. It was reported that: all tested substrates facilitated rat bone marrow cell growth of extra cellular matrix formation; Ti-DPS and Ti-TPS to the highest degree, followed by Ti-ma and Ti-HA; Ti-DPS and Ti-TPS displayed the highest cell density, and thus seems to be well suited for the endosseous portion of dental implants, and; the rat bone marrow cells cultured on Ti-HA showed a delayed growth pattern due to high phosphate ion release.

The modern range of medical devices presents contrasting requirements for adhesion in biological environments. For artificial blood vessels, the minimum adhesion of blood is mandatory, whereas the maximum blood cell adhesion is required at placed implant surfaces. Strong bio-adhesion is desired in many circumstances to assure device retention and immobility. Minimal adhesion is absolutely essential in others, where thrombosis or bacteria adhesion would destroy the utility of the implants. In every case, primary attention must be given to the qualities of the first interfacial conditioning films of bio-macromolecules deposited from the living systems. For instance, fibrinogen deposits from blood may assume different configurations on surfaces of different initial energies, and thus trigger different physiological events [Baier, 1986; Glantz et al., 1986].

Sunny et al. [Sunny et al., 1991] showed that the Ti oxide film on Ti significantly affects the adsorption rate of albumin/fibrinogen. Multinucleated giant cells have been observed at interfaces between bone marrow and Ti implants in mouse femurs, suggesting that macrophage-derived factors might perturb local lymphopoesis, possibly even predisposing to neoplasia in the B lymphocyte lineage. It has been found that an implant-marrow interface with associated giant cells persists for at least 15 years, and that precursor B cells show early increase in number and proliferative activity; however, at later intervals they do not differ significantly from controls. Rahal mentioned, in mice study, that following initial marrow regeneration and fluctuating precursor B cell activity, and despite the presence of giant cells, Ti implants apparently become well-tolerated by directly apposed bone marrow cells in a lasting state of the so-called myelointegration [Rahal et al., 2000].

Sukenik et al. [Sukenik et al., 1990] modified the surface of Ti by covalent attachment of organic monolayers anchored by a siloxane network. This coating completely covers the metal and allows controlled modifications of surface properties by the exposed chemical end-groups of the monolayer forming surfactant. The attachment of such a film allows different bulk materials (e.g., glass and Ti) to have identical surface characteristics, and this can be used in regulating cell adhesion responses. It was found that this control over surface functionality can modulate the functions of fibronectin in regulating attachment and neurite formation by neuronal cells, and that the effect on bacteria adherence is achieved by using such monolayers to vary surface hydrophilicity is also assessed.

Cell adhesion is involved in various natural phenomena such as embryogenesis, maintenance of tissue structure, wound healing, immune response, and metastasis, as well as tissue integration of biomaterial [Anselme, 2000]. The biocompatibility of biomaterials is very closely related to cell behavior on contact with them, and particularly to cell adhesion to their surface. Surface characteristics of materials (topography, chemistry or surface energy) play an essential part in osteoblast adhesion on biomaterials. Thus attachment, adhesion, and spreading belong to the first phase of cell/material interactions, and the quality of this first phase will influence the cell's capacity to proliferate and to differentiate itself on contact with the implant. It is essential for the efficacy of orthopedic or dental implants to establish a mechanically solid interface with complete fusion between the material's surface and the bone tissue with no fibrous interface. Moreover, the recent development of tissue engineering in the field of orthopedic research makes it possible to envisage the association of autologous cells and/or proteins that promote cell adhesion with osteoconductive material to create osteoinductive materials or hybrid materials.

Thus, a complete understanding of cell adhesion, and particularly osteoblast adhesion, on materials is now essential to optimize the bone/biomaterial interface at the heart of these hybrid materials. This includes an understanding of the molecules involved in bone cell adhesion, particularly regarding interaction with the materials, but also the need to take into account osteoblastic reaction to the mechanical constraints, which will be applied to implanted materials *in vivo*. The application of non-destructive *in vivo* mechanical constraints to the cell/biomaterial interface permits understanding of the effects of mechanical stimulation on the synthesis of adhesion proteins, cell growth, and cell differentiation, and provides essential information for the development of hybrid materials.

To investigate the roles of compositions and properties of Ti surface oxides in cellular behavior of osteoblasts, the surface oxides of Ti were modified in compositions and topography by anodic oxidation in two kinds of electrolytes, $0.1\,m$ H_3PO_4 and a mixture of $0.03\,M$ calcium glycerophosphate and $0.15\,M$ calcium acetate. It was found that phosphorous (P: about 10 at%) or both Ca (1–6 at%) and P (3–6 at%) were incorporated into the anodized surfaces in the form of phosphate and calcium phosphate, and that contact angles of all the anodized oxides were in the range of 60–90 degrees, suggesting relatively high hydrophobicity. It was also mentioned that cell culture experiments demonstrated absence of cytotoxicity and an increase of osteoblast adhesion and proliferation by the anodic oxides [Zhu et al., 2004].

Characteristics of the porous surfaces may be important in improving the bone in-growth into the porous coatings. Quicker and more mature interstitial bone formation was obtained using a porous rather than a solid structure, due to differences of penetration by some growth factors and bone marrow cells [Jasty et al., 1993; Simske et al., 1995; Chang et al., 1996]. Li et al. [1997] examined the effect of the surface macrostructure of a dimpled CpTi implant on bone in-growth *in vivo* by means of histological examination and a push-out test. Dimples had diameters of 100, 140, and 160 μm, and distance between dimple centers of about 400 μm. Cylindrical implants were inserted in one of each rabbit for one-and-a-half, three, and 13 months. The femur with the implant of each animal was then examined in a push-out test. It was found that the dimpled CpTi surface results in an increased retention of the implant in bone due to interlocking between vital bone and the dimples.

Nishiguchi et al. [Nishiguchi et al., 1999] evaluated the bone-bonding ability of three differently treated samples of CpTi: as a smooth surface control; treated in 5 M NaOH solution for 24 hr at 60 °C, and; plus-heated at 600 °C for one hour. The plates were inserted transcortically into the proximal metaphyses of bilateral rabbit tibiae. The tensile failure loads between implants and bones were measured at two intervals using a detaching test. It was reported that the tensile failure loads of the alkali- and alkali-heat treated group were 27 and 40 MPa, at 8 and 16 weeks, and significantly higher than those of the other Ti groups, and that histological examination revealed that alkali- and heat-treated Ti was in direct contact with bone, but the other Ti groups had a thin intervening fibrous tissue. It was concluded that the alkali-treated Ti without heat treatment had no bone-bonding ability due to the unstable reactive surface layer of alkali-treated Ti, and that both alkali and heat treatment are essential for preparing bioactive Ti. This bioactive Ti is thought to be useful for orthopedic implants with cementless fixation.

There is increasing attention given to the influence of surface condition, in particular, on methods to control. Strain hardening [Montero-Ocampo et al., 1996], laser-surface treatment [Villermaux et al., 1997], and chemical passivation methods [Trépanier et al., 1998] are all well known. From histological examinations, it has been found that implant loosening is generally associated with the formation of fibrous tissue at the bone-implant interface. To improve implant biocompatibility and osseointegrtaion, Ti-6Al-4V alloy was treated by passivation by immersion in 30% HNO_3 for 1 hr, or passivation in boiling distilled water for 10 hr [Ku et al., 2002], allowing an increase in the oxide layer thickness of Ti-6Al-4V alloy used in orthopedic implants. The kinetics of gene expression over 120 hours was followed for 58 genes to quantify the effect of the developed surface treatment. Twenty-eight genes were further selected to compare the effects of surface treatments on osteoblasts. Based on the genes studied, a general pathway for the cell reaction was proposed according to the surface treatment used:

(1) metal ion release changes the time course of gene expression in the focal adhesion kinase pathway;

(2) once the accumulation of metal ions released from the Ti surface exceeds a threshold value, cell growth is diminished and apoptosis may be activated;

(3) protein tyrosine kinase up-regulation is also induced by metal ion release;

(4) expression of the Bc1-2 family and Bax may suggest that metal ions induce apoptosis.

5.5 INTEGRATED IMPLANT SYSTEM

In order to achieve the aforementioned three requirements for successful implants [Oshida et al., 1994] titanium implant surfaces need to be modified. They can be treated by additive methods (to form surface convex texturing), such as the titanium beads plasma spray procedure, to increase effective surface area. They have also been modified by subtractive methods (to form surface concave texturing) such as acid pickling, acid etching, sandblasting, and other small particle-blasting to change the texture, as well as to increase the surface area. The development and use of these surface modifications have been based on the fact that an improved osseointegration can be achieved by increasing the topography or roughness of the implant surface [Klokkevold et al., 1997]. Mechanical and morphological compatibilities can be achieved by surface texturing by means of chemical, physical, mechanical or combined processes. Ti materials have modulus of elasticity value of about 150–250 GPa while bone structure has only 10–20 GPa, as seen in Figure 5.4. Also it is already known that successful implant systems possess optimum surface roughness (see Figure 5.5), ranging from 1 μm to 50 μm. To achieve both mechanical and morphological compatibilities, new concept such as GAF-C/D (gradually altering function concept and design) should be taken into serious consideration [Jetro, 1994; Bogdanski et al., 2002; Oshida, 2007d].

Technologies supportive to the implant developments have been well advanced. They should include:

(1) coating (such as sol-gel coating [Kim et al., 2004], plasma immersion ion implantation method [Maitz et al., 2005], etc.),

(2) laser surface engineering, including amorphous phase formation [Agarwal et al., 2000], laser alloying [Draper et al., 1985; Galerie et al., 1992], and direct laser forming [Hollander et al., 2006],

(3) near net shape forming (NNS) [Ringeisen et al., 2001; Finke et al., 2002; Klug et al., 2004] and nanotechnology [Frosch et al., 2004; Macak et al., 2005; Oh et al., 2005],

(4) surface texturing and porous/foamed structure, including texturing process [NASA, 1997; Banks, 1997], macroporous Ti structure formation [Fujibayashi et al., 2004], and

(5) tissue engineering and scaffold structures and materials, including film and 3-D structure [Li and Chang, 2004; Taira et al., 2005; Burgess, 2005; Lee et al., 2005; Walboomers et al., 2005; Ni et al., 2006; Wu et al., 2006], and elecrospinning [Hohman et al., 2001; Li et al., 2005; Buttafoco et al., 2006].

With the aforementioned supportive technologies, surfaces of dental and orthopaedic implants have been remarkably advanced. These applications can include not only ordinal implant system but also miniaturized implants, as well as customized implants.

There were two ways of implant anchorage or retention: mechanical and bioactive [De Putter et al., 1986; Albrektsson et al., 2004]. Mechanical retention basically refers to the metallic substrate systems such as titanium materials. The retention is based on undercut forms such as vents, slots, dimples, screws, and so on, and involves direct contact between bone and implant with no chemical bonding. The osseointegration depends on biomechanical bonding. The potentially negative aspect with biomechanical bonding is that it is time consuming. Bioactive retention is achieved with bioactive materials such as HA or bioglass, which bond directly to bone, similar to ankylosis of natural teeth. The bioactivity is the characteristic of an important material which allows it to form a bond with living tissues. It is important to understand that bioactive implants may, in addition to chemical bonding, show biomechanical anchorage; hence a given implant may be anchored through both mechanisms. Bone matrix is deposited on the HA layer because of some type of physiochemical interaction between bone collagen and the HA crystals of the implant [Denissen et al., 1986]. Recent research has further redefined the retention means of dental implants into the terminology of osseointegration versus biointegration. When examining the interface at a higher magnification level, Sundgren et al. [Sundgren et al., 1986] showed that unimplanted Ti surfaces have a surface oxide (TiO_2) with a thickness of about 35 nm. During an implantation period of eight years, the thickness of this layer was reported to increase by a factor of ten. Furthermore, calcium, phosphorous, and carbon were identified as components of the oxide layer, with the phosphorous strongly bound to oxygen, indicating the presence of phosphorous groups in the metal oxide layer. Many retrospective studies on retrieved implants, as well as clinical reports, confirm the aforementioned important evidence that surface titanium oxide film grows during the implantation period, and that calcium, phosphorous, carbon, hydroxyl ions, proteins, and so on, are incorporated in an ever-growing surface oxide even inside the human biological environments [Ellingsen, 1991; Albrektsson et al., 2004].

Numerous *in vitro* studies on treated or untreated titanium surfaces were covered and to some extent were incorporated with Ca and P ions when such surfaces were immersed in SBF (simulated body fluid). Additionally, since bone and blood cells are rugophilia, to accommodate for the bone growth, but also to facilitate such cells adhesion and spreading, titanium surfaces need to be textured to accomplish and show appropriate roughness. Furthermore, gradient functional concept (GFC) on materials and structures has been receiving special attention not only in industrial applications, but in dental as well as medical fields. Particularly, when such structures and concepts are about to be applied to implants, its importance becomes more clinically crucial.

For example, the majority of implant mass should be strong and tough, so that occlusal force can be smoothly transferred from the placed implant to the receiving hard tissue. However, the surface needs to be engineered to exhibit some extent of roughness. From such macro-structural changes from bulk core to the porous case, again the structural integrity should be maintained. The GFC can also be applied for the purpose of having a chemical (compositional) gradient. Ca, P-enrichment is not needed in the interior materials of the implants. Some other modifications related to chemical dressing or conditioning can also be utilized for achieving gradient functionality on chemical alternations on surfaces as well as near-surface zones.

To summarize this chapter, the author proposes an ideal implant structure which is integrated by bioengineering and biomaterials science. Oshida previously proposed the four important factors and requirements for successful and biofunctional implant systems: biological compatibility (or, biocompatibility) mechanical compatibility (or mechanocompatibility), morphological compatibility, and crystallographic compatibility (or micro-morphological compatibility) [Oshida, 2000].

Figure 5.6 illustrates a schematic and conceptual Ti implant which possesses a gradual function of mechanical and biological behaviors, so that mechanical

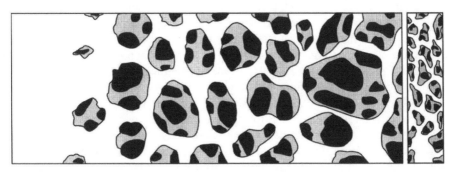

Ti implant					bone
body	sub-surface zone	surface layer		bony growth zone	
strong	←	Biomechanical strength		←	weak
Modulus of Elasticity [GPa]					
250~200	← 150~100 ←	100~50	←	50~20	← 20~10
weak	→	Biological and Biochemical reactions		→	strong

Figure 5.6. Schematic and conceptual Ti implant with gradient mechanical and biological functions.

compatibility and biological compatibility can be realized. Since microtextured Ti surfaces [Masuda et al., 1998; Zinger et al., 2004; Leven et al., 2004] and/or porous Ti surfaces [Jasty et al., 1993; Simske et al., 1995; Chang et al., 1996] promote fibroblast apposition and bone ingrowth, the extreme left side representing the solid Ti implant body should have gradually increased internal porosities towards the right side which is in contact with vital hard/soft tissue. Accordingly, mechanical strength of this implant system decreases gradually from left to right, whereas biological activity increases from left to right. Therefore, the mechanical compatibility can be completely achieved, and it can be easily understood by referring to Figure 5.4. Porosity-controlled surface zones can be fabricated by an electrochemical technique [Aziz-Kerrzo et al., 2001], polymeric sponge replication method [Larsson et al., 2001], powder metallurgy technique, superplastic diffusion bonding method [Cook et al., 1988], or foamed metal structure technique [Kohn et al., 1990].

Once the Ti implant is placed in hard tissue, TiO_2 grows and increases its thickness [Kubaschewski et al., 1962; Drath et al., 1975; Root et al., 1977; Tummler et al., 1986; Sundgren et al., 1986; Lausmaa et al., 1990; Wisbey et al., 1991; Healy et al., 1992b; Sutherland et al., 1993; Eliades, 1997], due to more oxygen availability inside the body fluid, as well as the co-existence of superoxidant. It is very important to mention here that Ti is not in contact with the biological environment, but rather there is a gradual transition from the bulk Ti material, stoichiometric oxide (i.e., TiO_2), hydrated polarized oxide, adsorbed lipoproteins and glycolipids, proteoglycans, collagen filaments and bundles to cells [Healy et al., 1992a]. Such gradient functional structure was also fabricated in CpTi and microtextured polyethylene terephthalate system [Jain et al., 2004].

In addition, a gradient structural system of Ti and TiN was developed [Clem et al., 2006]. During HA coating, a gradient functional layer was successfully fabricated [Yamada et al., 2001]. To promote these gradient functional (GF) and gradient structural (GS) transitions, there are many *in vivo*, as well as *in vitro*, evidences indicating that the surface titanium oxide is incorporated with mineral ions, water and other constituents of biofluids [McQueen et al., 1982; Liedberg et al., 1984; Sundgren et al., 1986; Hanawa, 1991]. Since a surface layer of TiO_2 is negatively charged, the calcium ion attachment can be easily achieved [Parsegian, 1983; Albrektsson et al., 1986]. Retrieved Ti implants showed that surface TiO_2 was incorporated with Ca and P ions [Uo et al., 2001], while *in vitro* treatment of TiO_2 in extra cellular fluids or simulated body fluid (SBF) for prolonged periods of incubation time resulted in the incorporation of Ca, P, and S ions into TiO_2 [McQueen et al., 1982; Liedberg et al., 1984; Sundgren et al., 1986; Wisbey et al., 1991; Hanawa, 1991; Healy et al., 1992b; Lu et al., 2004; Ng et al., 2005].

Without prolonged treatment, there are several methods proposed to relatively short-time incubation for incorporation of Ca and P ions. For example, TiO_2 can be electrochemically treated in an electrolyte of a mixture of calcium acetate monohydrate and calcium glycerophosphate [Li et al., 2004]. As a result of incorporation of Ca and P ions, bone-like hydroxyapatite can be formed in macro-scale [Spriano et al., 2005] or nano-dimension [Sato et al., 2006]. Again for reducing the incubation time, bone-like hydroxyapatite crystals can be formed by treating the TiO_2 surface with water and hydrogen plasma immersion ion implantation, followed by immersion in SBF [Xie et al., 2005], or by treating in hydrogen peroxide followed by SBF immersion [Rohanizadeh et al., 2004], or immersion in SBF while treating the TiO_2 surface with micro-arc oxidation and irradiation with UV light [Kim et al., 2005]. It is also known that P ions can be incorporated into TiO_2 while it is immersed in the human serum [Healy et al., 1992a].

Bony growth super-surface zones should have a same roughness as the roughness of receiving hard tissue through micro-porous texturing techniques. This area can be structured using nanotube concepts [Frosch et al., 2004; Macak et al., 2005; Oh et al., 2005]. Because this zone responds strongly to osseointegration, the structure, as well as the chemistry, should accommodate favorable osteoinductive reactions. Bone morphogenetic protein [Jetro, 1992; McAlarney et al., 1994; Klinger et al., 1996], and nano-apatite can be coated [Pham et al., 2003]. The zone may be treated by femtosecond laser machining [Hollander et al., 2006] to build a micro-scale three-dimensional scaffold which is structured inside the macro-porosities. Such scaffolding can be made of biodegradable material (such as, chitosan), which is incorporated with protein, Ca, P, apatite particles or other species possessing bone growth factors.

5.6 CONCLUSIONS

To meet cruicial requirements for successful implant developments and biofunctionality, mechanical and morphological gaps between foreign Ti implant surface and host receiving hard tissue should be gradually filled, so that retention of osseointegrated implant/bone interfacial zone should be strong and stress field at the interfacial zone can be minimized. Based on what has been done and researched in various implantology sectors, a new implant system was proposed.

REFERENCES

Adell R, Lekholm U, Rockler B, Brånemark PI. 1981. A 15-year study of osseointegrated implant in the treatment of the edentulous jaw. J Oral Surg 10:387–416.

Agarwal A, Dahotre NB. 2000. Laser surface engineering of titanium diboride coatings. Adv Mater Processes 158:43–45.

Albrektsson T, Brånemark PI, Hansson HA, Kasemo B, Larsson K, Lundstroem I, McQueen DH, Skalak R. 1983. The interface zone of inorganic implants *in vivo*: Titanium implants in bone. Ann Biomed Eng 11:1–27.

Albrektsson T. 1983. Direct bone anchorage of dental implants. J Prosth Dent 50:255–261.

Albreksson T, Hansson HA. 1986. An ultrastructural characterization of the interface between bone and sputtered titanium or stainless steel surfaces. Biomaterials 7:201–205.

Albrektsson T, Jacobsson M. 1987. Bone-metal interface in osseointegration. J Prosthet Dent 57:5–10.

Albrektsson T, Wennerberg A. 2004. Oral implant surfaces: Part 1—review focusing on topographic and chemical properties of different surfaces and *in vitro* responses to them. Intl J Prosthodont 17:536–543.

American Society for Metals. 1991. *Oxidation of Metals and Alloys.* Ohio ASM p.46.

Anselme K. 2000. Osteoblast adhesion on biomaterials. Biomaterials 21:667–681.

Ashby MF, Jones DRH. 1980. Engineering materials. An introduction to their properties and Applications. New York: Pergamon Press p.194–200.

Aziz-Kerrzo M, Conroy KG, Fenelon AM, Farrell AT, Breslin CB. 2001. Electrochemical studies on the stability and corrosion resistance of titanium-based implant materials. Biomaterials 22:1531–1539.

Baier RE. 1986. Modification of surfaces to meet bioadhesive design goals: a review. J Adhesion 20:171–186.

Banks BA. 1997. Improved texturing of surgical implants for soft tissues. LEW-15805. NASA Tech Briefs 21:70.

Bannon BP, Mild EE. 1983. Titanium alloys for biomaterial application: An overview, In: Titanium Alloys in Surgical Implants. Luckey HA, Kubli F, editors. ASTM STP 796, p.7–15.

Baro AM, Garcia N, Miranda R, Vázquez L, Aparicio C, Olivé J, Lausmaa J. 1986. Characterization of surface roughness in titanium dental implants measured with scanning tunneling microscopy at atmospheric pressure. Biomaterilas 7:463–466.

Bigerele M, Anselme K, Noël B, Ruderman I, Hardouin P, Iost A. 2002. Improvement in the morphology of Ti-based surfaces: a new process to increase *in vitro* human osteoblast response. Biomaterials 23:1563–1577.

Binon PP. 2000. Implants and components: entering the new millennium. Int J Oral Maxillofac Implants 15:76–94.

Bogdanski D, Köller M, Müller D, Muhr G, Bram M, Buchkremer HP, Stöver D, Choi J, Epple M. 2002. Easy assessment of the biocompatibility of Ni-Ti alloy by *in vitro* cell culture experiments on a functionally graded Ni-NiTi-Ti material. Biomaterials 23:4549–4555.

Brånemark PI. 1985. Introduction to osseointegration. In: Tissue-integrated protheses. Brånemark PI, editor. Chicago: Quintessence Pub. p.63–70.

Brockhurst PJ. 1980. Dental Materials: New Territories for Materials Science. In: Metals Forum. Australian Inst Metals 3:200–210.

Bruck SD. 1991. Biostability of materials and implants. Long-Term Effects of Med Imp 1:89–106.

Brunette DM. 1988. The effects of implant surface topography on the behavior of cells. Int J Oral Maxillofac Implants 3:231–246.

Brunski JB, Puleo DA, Nanci A. 2000. Biomaterials and biomechanics of oral and maxillofacial implants: current status and future developments. Intl J Oral Maxillofac Implants 15:15–46.

Burgess DS. 2005. InkJet Technique precludes microvessels and mirolenses. Technology World May:213.

Buser D, Schenk RK, Steinemann S, Fiorellinni JP, Fox CH, Stich H. 1991. Influence of surface characteristics on bone integration of titanium implants. A histomorphometric study in miniature pigs. J Biomed Mater Res 25:889–902.

Buser D, Nydegger T, Oxland T, Cochran DL, Schenk RK, Hirt HP, Sneitivy D, Nolte LP. 1999. Interface shear strength of titanium implants with a sandblasted and acid-etched surface: a biomechanical study in the maxilla of miniature pigs. J Biomed Mater Res 45:75–83.

Buttafoco L, Kolkman NG, Engbers-Buijtenhuijs P, Poot AA, Dijkstra PJ, Vermes I, Feijen J. 2006. Electrospinning of collagen and elastin for tissue engineering applications. Biomaterials 27:724–734.

Chang Y-S, Oka M, Kobayashi M, Gu H-O, Li Z-L, Nakamura T, Ikada Y. 1996. Significance of interstitial bone ingrowth under load-bearing conditions: a comparison between solid and porous implant materials. Biomaterials 17:1141–1148.

Cherhoudi B, Gould TR, Brunette DM. 1988. Effects of a grooved epoxy substratum on epithelial behavior *in vivo* and *in vitro*. J Biomed Mater Res 22:459–477.

Clem WC, Konovalov VK, Chowdhury S, Vohra YK, Catledge SA, Bellis SL. 2006. Mesenchymal stem cell adhesion and spreading on microwave plasma-nitrided titanium alloy. J Biomed Mater Res 76A:279–287.

Coddet C, Chaze AM, Beranger G. 1987. Measurements of the adhesion of thermal oxide films: application to the oxidation of titanium. J Mater Sci 22:2969–2974.

Cook SD, Thongpreda N, Anderson RC, Haddad RJ. 1988. The effect of post-sintering heat treatments on the fatigue properties of porous coated Ti-6Al-4V alloy. J Biomed Mater Res 22:287–302.

CRC Handbook of Chemistry and Physics. 1966. The 47th edition. Cleveland: The Chemical Rubber Co. p.D-54.

Deligianni DD, Katsala N, Ladas S, Sotiropoulou D, Amedee J, Missirlis YF. 2001. Effect of surface roughness of the titanium alloy Ti-6Al-4V on human bone marrow cell response and on protein adsorption. Biomaterials 22:1241–1251.

Denissen HW, Veldhuis AAH, van den Hooff A. 1986. Hydroxyapatite titanium implants. Proc. Int'l congress on Tissue Integration in Oral and Maxillofacial Reconstruction. May 1985, Brussels. Current Practice Series #29, Amsterdam: Excerta Media p.395–399.

Deporter D, Watson P, Pharoah M, Levy D, Todescan R. 1999. Five- to six-year results of a prospective clinical trial using the ENDOPORE dental implant and a mandibular overdenture. Clin Oral Implants Res 10:95–102.

De Putter, de Lange GL, de Groot K. 1986. Permucosla dental implants of dense hydroxy-apatite: Fixation in alveolar bone. Proc. Int'l congress on Tissue Integration in Oral and Maxillofacial Reconstruction. May 1985, Brussels. Current Practice Series #29, Amsterdam: Excerta Media p.389–394.

Douglass DL. 1995. A critique of internal oxidation in alloys during the post-Wagner era. Oxidation of Metals 44:81–111.

Draper CW, Poate JM. 1985. Laser surface alloying. Int Metal Reviews 30:85–108.

Drath DB, Karnovsky ML. 1975. Superoxide production by phagocytic leukocytes. J Exp Med 144:257–261.

Ducheyne P, Williams G, Martens M, Helsen J. 1984. *In vivo* metal-ion release from porous titanium-silver material. J Biomed Mater Res 18:293–308.

Ducheyne P, Healy KE. Surface spectroscopy of calcium phosphate ceramic and titanium implant materials. 1988. In: Surface characterization of biomaterials. Ratner BD, editor. Amsterdam: Elsevier Science. p.175–192.

Eliades T. 1997. Passive film growth on titanium alloys: physiochemical and biologic considerations. Int J Oral Maxillofac Implant 12:621–627.

Ellingsen JE. 1991. A study on the mechanism of protein adsorption to TiO_2. Biomaterials 12:593–596.

Eriksson C, Lausmaa J, Nygren H. 2001. Interactions between human whole blood and modified TiO_2-surfaces: Influence of surface topography and oxide thickness on leukocyte adhesion and activation. Biomaterials 22:1987–1996.

Ferguson AB, Akahoshi Y, Laing PG, Hodge ES. 1962. Characteristics of trace ions released from embedded metal implants in the rabbit. J Bone Joint Surg 44-A:323–336.

Fini M, Cigada A, Rondelli G, Chiesa R, Giardino R, Giavaresi G, Aldini N, Torricelli P, Vicentini B. 1999. *In vitro* and *in vivo* behaviour of Ca and P-enriched anodized titanium. Biomaterials 20:1587–1594.

Finke S, Feenstra K. 2002. Solid freedom fabrication by extrusion and deposition of semi-solid alloys. J Mater Sci 37:3101–3106.

Fraker AC, Ruff AW. 1973. Corrosion of titanium alloys in physiological solutions. In: Titanium Science and Technology, Vol. 4. New York: Plenum Press p.2447–2457.

Frosch K-H, Barvencik F, Viereck V, Lohmann CH, Dresing K, Breme J, Brunner E, Stürmer KM. 2004. Growth behavior, matrix production, and gene expression of human osteoblasts in defined cylindrical titanium channels. J Biomed Mater Res 68A:325–334.

Fujibayashi S, Neo M, Kim H-M, Kokubo K, Nakamura T. 2004. Osteoinduction of porous bioactive titanium metal. Biomaterials 25:443–450.

Galerie A, Fasasi A, Pons M, Caillet M. 1992. Improved high temperature oxidation resistance of Ti-6Al-4V by superficial laser alloying. In: Surface Modification Technologies V. Sudarshan TS, Braza JF, editors. The Institute of Materials pp.401–411.

Gaydos JM, Moore MA, Garetto LP, Oshida Y, Kowolik MJ. 2000. Bisphosphonate effect on neutrophil activation by titanium and hydroxyapatite implants. Jour Dent Res 79:225 (Abstract No. 890).

Gilbert JL, Berkery CA. 1995. Electrochemical reaction to mechanical disruption of titanium oxide films. J Dent Res 74:92–96.

Glantz P-O, Baier RE. 1986. Recent studies on nonspecific aspects of intraoral adhesion. J Adhesion 20:227–244.

Greene ND. 1983. Corrosion of surgical implant alloys: a few basic ideas. ASTM STP 859; In: Corrosion and degradation of implant materials: second symposium. Fraker AC, Griffin CD, editors. ASTM p.5–10.

Hanawa T. 1991. Titanium and its oxide film: A substrate for formation of apatite. In: The bone-biomaterial interface. Davies JE, editor. Toronto: Univ. of Toronto Press p.49–61.

Healy KE, Ducheyne P. 1992a. Hydration and preferential molecular adsorption on titanium *in vitro*. Biomaterials 13:553–561.

Healy KE, Ducheyne P. 1992b. The mechanisms of passive dissolution of titanium in a model physiological environment. J Biomed Mater Res 26:319–338.

Hekimoglu C, Anil N, Cehreli MC. 2004. Analysis of strain around endosseous implants opposing natural teeth or implants. J Prosthet Dent 92:441–446.

Henry P, Tan AE, Allan BP. 2000. Removal torque comparison of TiUnite and turned impants in the Greyhound dog mandible. Appl Osseointegration Res 1: 15–17.

Hohman MM, Shin M, Rutledge G, Brenner MP. 2001. Electrospinning and electrorically formed jets. Physics of Fluids 13:2201–2220.

Hollander DA, von Walter M, Wirtz T, Sellei R, Schmidt-Rohlfing B, Paar O, Erli H-J. 2006. Structural, mechanical and *in vitro* characterization of individually structured Ti-6Al-4V produced by direct laser forming. Biomaterials 27:955–963.

Ishizawa H, Fujiino M, Ogino M. 1995. Mechanical and histological investigation of hydrothermally treated and untreated anodic titanium oxide films containing Ca and P. J Biomed Mater Res 29:1459–1468.

Jain R, von Recum AF. 2004. Fibroblast attachment to smooth and microtextured PET and thin cp-Ti films. J Biomed Mater Res 68A:296–304.

Jasty M, Bragdon CR, Haire T, Mulroy RO, Harris WH. 1993. Comparison of bone ingrowth into cobalt chrome sphere and titanium fiber mesh porous coated cementless canine acetabular components. J Biomed Mater Res 27:639–644.

JETRO. 1992. Titanium surface reforming technology. New Technology Japan No. 92-02-100-08. 19:18.

JETRO. 1994. Ti-O coating on Ti-6Al-4V alloy by DC reactive sputtering method. New Technology Japan. No. 94-06-001-01. 22:18.

Kasemo B. 1983. Biocompatibility of titanium implants: surface science aspects. J Pros Dent 49:832–837.

Kasemo B, Lausmaa J. 1985. Metal selection and surface characteristics. In: Tissue-integrated protheses. Brånemark OI, editor. Chicago: Quintessence Pub. p.108–115.

Kasemo B, Lausmaa J. 1986. Surfaces science aspects on inorganic biomaterials. CRC Crit Rev Biocomp 2:335–380.

Keller JC, Young FA, Natiella JR. 1987. Quantitative bone remolding resulting from the use of porous dental implants. J Biomed Mater Res 21:305–319.

Keller JC, Dougherty WJ, Grotendorst GR, Wrightman JP. 1989a. *In vitro* cell attachment to characterized cpTi surfaces. A Adhesion 28:115–133.

Keller JC, Wrightman JP, Dougherty WJ. 1989b. Characterization of acid passivated cpTi surfaces. J Dent Res 68:872.

Keller JC, Draughn RA, Wrightman JP, Dougherty WJ. 1990. Characterization of sterilized CP titanium implant surfaces. Int J Oral Maxillofac Implants 5:360–369.

Kim H-W, Kim H-E, Knowles LC. 2004. Fluor-hydroxyapatite sol-gel coating on titanium substrate for hard tissue implants. Biomaterials 25:3351–3358.

Kim H-W, Kim H-E, Salih V, Knowles JC. 2005. Sol-gel-modified titanium with hydroxyapatite thin films and effect on osteoblast-like cell responses. J Biomed Mater Res 74A:294–305.

Klinger A, Steinberg D, Kohavi D, Sela MN. 1996. Adsorption of human salivary albumin to titanium-oxide. J Dent Res 75:273 (Abstract No. 2043).

Klokkevold PR, Nishimura RD, Adachi M, Caputo A. 1997. Osseointegration enhanced by chemical etching of the titanium surface. A torque removal study in the rabbit. Clin Oral Implants Res 8:442–447.

Klug KL, Ucok I, Gungor MN, Gulu M, Kramer LS, Tack WT, Nastac L, Martin NR, Dong H. 2004. The near-net-shape manufacturing of affordable titanium components for the M777 lightweight howitzer. J Metals 56:35–42.

Knabe C, Klar F, Fitzner R, Radlanski RJ, Gross U. 2002. In vitro investigation of titanium and hydroxyapatite dental implant surfaces using a rat bone marrow stromal cell culture system. Biomaterials 23:3235–3235.

Kohn DH, Ducheyne P. 1990. A parametric study of the factors affecting the fatigue strength of porous coated Ti-6Al-4V implant alloy. J Biomed Mater Res 24:1483–1501.

Kruger J. 1979. Fundamental aspects of the corrosion of metallic implants. ASTM STP 684. B.C. Syrett, A. Acharya ed. American Society for Testing and Materials. In: Corrosion and degradation of implant materials. p.107–127.

Ku C-H, Browne M, Gregson PI, Corbeil J, Pioletti DP. 2002. Effect of modification of oxide layer on NiTi stent corrosion resistance. J Biomed Mater Res (Appl Biomter) 43:433–440.

Kubaschewski O, Hopkins BE. 1962. Oxidation of metals and alloys. London: Butterworths. p.24.

Larsson C, Emanuelsson L, Thomsen P, Ericson L, Aronsson B, Rodahl M, Kasemo B, Lausmaa J. 1997. Bone response to surface-modified titanium implants: studies on the tisuue response after one year to machined and electropolished implants with different oxide thicknesses. J Mater Sci: Mater Med 8:721–729.

Larsson C, Esposito M, Liao H, Thomsen P. 2001. The titanim-bone interface *in vivo*. In: Brunette DM, Tengvall P, Textor M, Thomsen ed. Titanium in medicine: materials science, surface science, engineering, biological responsese, and medical applications. New York: Springer p.587–648.

Lausmaa GJ. 1986. Chemical composition and morphology of titanium surface oxides. Mat Res Soc Symp Proc 55:351–359.

Lausmaa GJ, Kasemo B. 1990. Surface spectroscopic characterization of titanium implant materials. Appl Surf Sci 44:133–146.

Lautenschlager EP, Monaghan P. 1993. Titanium and titanium alloys as dental materials. Intl Dent J 43:245–253.

Lee M, Dunn JCY, Wu BM. 2005. Scaffold fabrication by indirect three-dimensional printing. Biomaterials 26:4281–4289.

Leven RM, Virdi AS, Sumner DR. 2004. Patterns of gene expression in rat bone marrow stromal cells cultured on titanium alloy discs of different roughness. J Biomed Mater Res 70A:391–401.

Li H, Chang J. 2004. Fabrication and characterization of bioactive wollastonite/PHBV composite scaffolds. Biomaterials 25:5473–5480.

Li L-H, Kong Y-M, Kim H-W, Kim Y-W, Kim H-E, Heo S-J, Koak J-Y. 2004. Improved biological performance of Ti implants due to surface modification by micro-arc oxidation. Biomaterials 15:1867–1875.

Li J, Liao H, Fartash B, Hermansson L. 1997. Surface-dimpled commercially pure titanium implant and bone ingrowth. Biomaterials 18:691–695.

Li M, Mondrinos MJ, Gandhi MR, Ko FK, Weiss AS, Lelkes PI. 2005. Electropun protein fibers as matrices for tissue engineering. Biomaterials 26:5999–6008.

Liedberg B, Ivarsson B, Lundstrom I. 1984. Fourier transform infrared reflection absorption spectroscopy (FTIR-RAS) of fibrinogen adsorbed on metal and metal oxide surfaces. J Biochem Biophys Method 9:233–243.

Lim YJ, Oshida Y, Andres CJ, Barco MT. 2001. Surface characterizations of variously treated titanium materials. Int J Oral Maxillofac Imaplants 16:333–342.

Long M, Rack HJ. 1998. Review: Titanium alloys in total joint replacement—a materials science perspective. Biomaterials 19:1621–1639.

Lu Y-P, Li M-S, Li S-T, Wang Z-G, Zhu R-F. 2004. Plasma-sprayed hydroxyapatite + titania composite bond coat for hydroxyapatite coating on titanium substrate. Biomaterials 25:4393–4403.

Macak JM, Tsuchiya H, Taveira L, Ghicov A, Schmuki P. 2005. Self-organized nanotubular oxide layers on Ti-6Al-7Nb and Ti-6Al-4V formed by anodization in NH_4F solutions. J Biomed Mater Res 75A:928–933.

Maitz MF, Poon RWY, Liu XY, Pham M-T, Chu PK. 2005. Bioactivity of titanium following sodium plasma immersion ion implantation and deposition. Biomaterials 26:5465–5473.

Marchant RE. 1986. Cell attachment and interactions with biomaterials. J Adhesion 20:211–255.

Masuda T, Yliheikkaila PK, Fleton DA, Cooper LF. 1998. Generalizations regarding the process and phenomenon of osseointegration. Part I. *In vivo* studies. Int I Oral Maxillofac Implant 13:17–29.

McAlarney ME, Oshiro MA. 1994. Possible role of C3 in competitive protein adsorption onto TiO_2. J Dent Res 73:401 (Abstract No. 2397).

McQueen D, Sundgren JE, Ivarsson B, Lundstrom I, Af Ekenstam CB, Svensson A, Brånemark PI, Albrektsson T. 1982. Auger electron spectroscopic studies of titanium implants. In: Lee AJC, editor. Clinical applications of biomaterials. New York: Wiley p.179–185.

Meachim G, Williams DF. 1973. Changes in nonosseous tissue adjacent to titanium implants. J Biomed Mater Res 7:555–572.

Montero-Ocampo C, Loprez H, Salinas Rodriguez A. 1996. Effect of compressive straining on corrosion resistance of a shape memory Ni-Ti alloy in ringer's solution. J Biomed Mater Res 32:583–591.

Moroni A, Caja VL, Egger EL, Trinchese L, Chao EY. 1994. Histomorphometry of hydroxyapatite coated and uncoated porous titanium bone implants. Biomaterials 15:926–930.

Murray DW, Rae T, Rushton N. 1989. The influence of the surface energy and roughness of implants on bone resorption. J Bone Joint Surg 71B:632–637.

NASA Lewis Research Center. 1997. Sputter texturing to produce surfaces for bonding. NASA Tech Briefs. May:p.81.

Ng BS, Annergren I, Soutar AM, Khor KA, Jarfors AEW. 2005. Characterization of a duplex TiO_2/CaP coatings on Ti6Al4V for hard tissue replacement. Biomaterials 26:1087–1095.

Ni S, Chang J, Chou L. 2006. A novel bioactive porous $CaSiO_3$ scaffold for bone tissue engineering. J Biomed Mater Res 76A:196–205.

Nishiguchi S, Nakamura T, Kobayashi M, Kim H-M, Miyaji F, Kokubo T. 1999. The effect of heat treatment on bone-bonding ability of alkali-treated titanium. Biomaterials 20:491–500.

Oh S-H, Finōnes RR, Daraio C, Chen L-H, Jin S. 2005. Growth of nano-scale hydroxyapatite using chemically treated titanium oxide nanotubes. Biomaterials 26:4938–4943.

Oshida Y, Sachdeva R, Miyazaki S. 1992. Microanalytical characterization and surface modification of NiTi orthodontic archwires. J Biomed Mater Eng 2:51–69.

Oshida Y, Hashem A, Nishihara T, Yapchulay MV. 1994. Fractal dimension analysis of mandibular bones: toward a morphological compatibility of implants. J Biomed Mater Eng 4:397–407.

Oshida Y. 2000. Requirements for successful biofunctional implants. *Int'l Sym Advanced Biomaterials*. P.5.

Oshida Y. 2007a. Bioscience and Bioengineering of Titanium Materials. 1st ed. London: Elsevier.

Oshida Y. 2007b. Surface science and technology—Titanium dental implant systems. J Soc Titanium Alloys in Dentistry, Proc. 6th Int'l Sym. On Titanium in Dentistry 5:52–53.

Oshida Y. 2007c. unpublished data.

Oshida Y. 2007d. unpublished data.

Palmer RM, Plamer PJ, Smith BJ, 2000. A 5-year prospective study of astra single tooth implants. Clin Oral Implants Res 11:179–182.

Pan J, Leygraf C, Thierry D, Ektessabi AM. 1997. Corrosion resistance for biomaterial applications of TiO_2 films deposited on titanium and stainless steel by ion-beam-assisted sputtering. J Biomed Mater Res 35:309–318.

Parsegian VA. 1983. Molecular forces governing tight contact between cellular surfaces and subtrates. J Prosthet Dent 49:838–842.

Pham MT, Reuther H, Maitz MF. 2003. Native extracellular matrix coating on Ti surfaces. J Biomed Mater Res 66A:310–316.

Pilliar RM, Deporter DA, Watson PA, Valiquette N. 1991. Dental implant design-effect on bone remodeling. J Biomed Mater Res 25:467–483.

Rahal MD, Delorme D, Brånemark P-I, Osmond DG. 2000. Myelointegration of titanium implants: B lymphopoiesis and hemopoietic cell proliferation in mouse bone marrow exposed to titanium implants. Intl J Oral Maxillofac Implants 15:175–184.

Ratner BD. 1983. Surface characterization of biomaterials by electron spectroscopy for chemical analysis. Ann Biomed Eng 11:313–336.

Ratner BD, Johnston AB, Lenk TJ. 1987. Biomaterial surfaces. J Biomed Mater Res: Applied Biomater 21:59–90.

Rich A, Harris AK. 1981. Anomalous preferences of cultured macrophages for hydrophobic and roughened substrata. J Cell Sci 50:1–7.

Ringeisen BR, Chrisey DB, Piqué A, Krizman D, Bronks M, Spargo B. 2001. Direct write technology and a tool to rapidly prototype patterns of biological and electronic systems. Nanotech 1:414–417.

Rohanizadeh R, Al-Sadeq M, LeGeros RZ. 2004. Preparation of different forms of titanium oxide on titanium surface: Effects on apatite deposition. J Biomed Mater Res 71A:343–352.

Root BK, Metcalf JA. 1977. H_2O_2 release from human granulocytes during phagocytosis: Relationship to superoxide anion formation and cellular catabolism of

H_2O_2. Studies with normal and cytochalasin B-treated cells. J Clin Invest 60:1266–1279.

Sato M, Sambito MA, Aslani A, Kalkhoran NM, Slamovich EB, Webster TJ. 2006. Increased osteoblast functions on undoped and yttrium-doped nanocrystalline hydroxyapatite coatings on titanium. Biomaterials 27:2358–2369.

Schenk RK, Buser D. 1998. Osseointegration: a reality. Periodontology 17:22–35.

Schroeder A, Van Der Zypen E, Stich H, Sutter F. 1981. The reactions of bone, connective tissue and epithelium to endosteal implants with titanium sprayed surfaces. J Maxillofac Surg 9:15–25.

Simske SJ, Sachdeva R. 1995. Cranial bone apposition and ingrowth in a porous nickel-titanium implant. J Biomed Mater Res 29:527–533.

Skalak R. 1983. Biomechanical considerations in osseointegrated prostheses. J Prosthet Dent 49:843–848.

Skripitz R, Aspenberg P. 1998. Tesnile bond between bone and titanium. Acta Orthop Scand 69:2–6.

Stanford CM. 1994. Bone cell expression on titanium surfaces is altered by sterilization treatments. J Dent Res 73(5):1061–1071.

Steinmann SG. 1980. Corrosion of surgical implants—*in vivo* and *in vitro* tests. In: Evaluation of Biomaterials. Winter GD, Leray JL, de Groot K, editors. New York: John Wiley & Sons, p.1–34.

Solar RJ. 1979. Corrosion resistance of titanium surgical implant alloys: a review. In: Corrosion and degradation of implant materials, ASTM STP 684. Syrett BD, editor. Philadelphia: American Society for Testing and Materials p.259–273.

Spriano S, Bosetti M, Bronzoni M, Vernè E, Maina G, Bergo V, Cannas M. 2005. Surface properties and cell response of low metal ion release Ti-6Al-7Nb alloy after multi-step chemical and thermal treatments. Biomaterials 26:1219–1229.

Sukenik CN, Balachander N, Culp LA, Lewandowska K, Merritt K. 1990. Modulation of cell adhesion by modification of titanium surfaces with covalently attached self-assembled monolayers. J Biomed Mater Res 24:1307–1323.

Sul Y-T, Johansson CB, Jeong Y, Röser K, Wennerberg A, Albreksson T. 2001. Oxidized implants and their influence on the bone response. J Mater Sci: Mater Med 12:1025–1031.

Sul Y-T, Johansson CB, Jeong Y, Wennerberg A, Albrektson T. 2002a. Resonance frequency and removal torque analysis of implants with turned and anodized surface oxide. Clin Oral Implants Res 13:252–259.

Sul Y-T, Johansson CB, Albreksson T. 2002b. Oxidized titanium screws coated with calcium ions and their performance in rabbit bone. Int J Oral Maxillofac Implants 17:625–634.

Sul Y-T. 2003. The significance of the surface properties of oxidized titanium to the bone response: special emphasis on potential biochemical bonding of oxidized titanium implant. Biomaterials 24:3893–3907.

Sundgren J-E, Bodö P, Lundström I. 1986. Auger electron spectroscopic studies of the interface between human tissue and implants of titanium and stainless steel. J Colloid Interf Sci 110:9–20.

Sunny MC, Sharma CP. 1991. Titanium-protein interaction: change with oxide layer thickness. J Biomater Appl 5:89–98.

Sutherland DS, Forshaw PD, Allen GC, Brown IT, Williams KR. 1993. Surface analsyis of titanium implants. Biomaterials 14:893–899.

Taira M, Araki Y. 2005. Scaffolds for tissue engineering—Kinds and clinical application. J Dental Eng 52:27–30.

Testori T, Wiseman L, Woolfe S, Porter SS. 2001. A prospective multicenter clinical study of the osseitite implant: four-years interim report. Int J Oral Maxillofac Implants 16:193–200.

Tomashov ND. 1966. Theory of Corrosion and Protection of Metals: The Science of Corrosion. New York: The MacMillan Co., p.144.

Trépanier C, Tabrizian M, Yahia L'H, Bilodeu L, Piron DL. 1998. Effect of modification of oxide layer on NiTi stent corrosion resistance. J Biomed Mater Res (Apply Biomater) 43:433–440.

Tummler H, Thull R. 1986. Model of the metal/tissue connection of implants made of titanium or tantalum. Biological and Biochemical Performance of Biomaterials. Netherlands: Elsevier p.403–408.

Uo M, Watari F, Yokoyama A, Matsuno H, Kawasaki T. 2001. Tissue reaction around metal implant observed by X-ray scanning analytical microscopy. Biomaterials 22: 677–685.

van Rossen IP, Braak LH, de Putter C, De Groot K. 1990. Stress-absorbing elements in dental implants. J Prosthet Dent 64:198–205.

Villermaux F, Tabrizian M, Yahia L-H, Meunier M, Piron DL. 1997. Excimer laser treatment of NiTi shape memory alloy biomaterials. Apply Surf Sci 109/110: 62–66.

von Recum AF. 1990. New aspects of biocompatibility: motion at the interface. In: Clinical implant materials. Heimke G, Soltesz U, Lee AJC, editors. Amstrdam: Elseveier Science Pub. p.297–302.

Walboomers XF, Jansen JA. 2005. Bone tissue induction, using a COLLOSS®-filled titanium fibre mesh-scaffolding material. Biomaterials 26:4779–4785.

Wen X, Wang X, Zhang N. 1996. Microsurface of metallic biomaterials: a literature review. J Biomed Mater Eng 6:173–189.

West JM. 1986. Basic corrosion and oxidation, 2nd ed. London: John Wiley and Sons p.27–30.

Wisbey A, Gregson PJ, Peter LM, Tuke M. 1991. Effect of surface treatment on the dissolution of titanium-based implant materials. Biomaterials 12:470–473.

Wu L, Jing D, Ding J. 2006. A "room-temperature" injection molding/particulate leaching approach for fabrication of biodegradable three-dimensional porous scaffolds. Biomaterials 27:185–191.

Xie Y, Liu X, Huang A, Ding C, Chu PK. 2005. Improvement of surface bioactivity on titanium by water and hydrogen plasma immersion ion implantation. Biomaterials 26:6129–6135.

Yamada K, Imamura K, Itoh H, Iwata H, Maruno S. 2001. Bone bonding behavior of the hydroxyapatite containing glass-titanium composite prepared by the Cullet method. Biomaterials 22:2207–2214.

Yang Y, Cavin R, Ong LJ. 2003. Protein adsorption on titanium surfaces and their effect on osteoblast attachment. J Biomed Mater Res 67A:344–349.

Zhu X, Chen J, Scheideler L, Reichl R, Geis-Gerstorfer J. 2004. Effects of topography and composition of titanium surface oxides on osteoblast responses. Biomaterials 25:4087–4103.

Zinger O, Anselme K, Denzer A, Habersetzer P, Wieland M, Jeanfils J, Hardouin P, Landolt D. 2004. Time-dependent morphology and adhesion of osteoblastic cells on titanium model surfaces featuring scale-resolved topography. Biomaterials 25:2695–2711.

6

INJECTABLE HYDROGELS AS BIOMATERIALS

Lakshmi S. Nair[1,2], Cato T. Laurencin[1,2], and Mayank Tandon[3]

[1]Department of Orthopedic Surgery, University of Connecticut,
Connecticut
[2]Chemical, Materials and Biomolecular Engineering, University of
Connecticut, Connecticut
[3]Department of Biomedical Engineering, University of Virginia,
Virginia

Contents

6.1	Overview	180
6.2	Introduction	180
6.3	Injectable *In Situ* Forming Gels	182
	6.3.1 Photo-Gelling Polymers	183
	6.3.1.1 Hydrogels from Polymers with Photoactive Side Groups	184
	6.3.1.2 Hydrogels by Photopolymerization	185
	6.3.2 Hydrogels Formed by Fast Chemical Reaction/Physical Transitions	191
	6.3.3 Thermogelling Polymers	193
6.4	Conclusions	197
	References	197

Advanced Biomaterials: Fundamentals, Processing, and Applications, Edited by Bikramjit Basu,
Dhirendra S. Katti, and Ashok Kumar
Copyright © 2009 The American Ceramic Society

6.1 OVERVIEW

Injectable *in situ* cross-linkable gels are clinically highly desirable as they can be introduced into the body via a minimally invasive manner using endoscopic or percutaneous procedures. The development of ideal *in situ* gelling injectable system for biomedical applications that satisfy various requirements such as biocompatibility, and fast appropriate physical and mechanical properties as well as water content, and tunable degradation gelation kinetics is challenging. Several polymeric systems that respond to stimuli such as light, pH, ionic concentration, chemical/physical reaction as well as temperature are currently under development as injectable drug/protein/DNA delivery vehicles as well as cell carriers for tissue engineering. This chapter focuses on some of the recently developed injectable hydrogel systems that can undergo solid to gel transformation in response to light irradiation, chemical or physical reaction and temperature. Both synthetic and natural polymeric systems are discussed.

6.2 INTRODUCTION

Hydrogels are three-dimensional cross-linked hydrophilic polymer networks that have the ability to swell but do not dissolve in water. The unique swelling behavior and three-dimensional structure of hydrogels are derived from specific covalent chemical cross-links or a variety of physical cross-links (secondary forces, chain entanglement, crystalline formation) and therefore can be appropriately controlled. The interest in hydrogels for biomedical applications started during the later half of the twentieth centaury when Wichterle and Lim predicted the potential of hydrogels as unique biomaterials since they are highly compatible with living tissue [Wichterle and Lim, 1960]. Using 2-hydroxyethyl methacrylate and glycol dimethacrylate as model polymers, they demonstrated the ability to rationally design hydrogels for biomedical applications. The study also demonstrated the excellent tolerance of the body towards hydrogels; the non-degradable hydrogels got encapsulated in a fibrous capsule without eliciting any irritation to the surrounding tissue upon subcutaneous implantation. These hydrogels were subsequently used for developing soft contact lenses and the biocompatibility was clinically proven. The excellent biocompatibility of hydrogels can be attributed to some of its unique properties as summarized by Ulijin et al., [Ulijin et al., 2007]. These include their ability to:

  • Retain a large quantity of water within the matrix, enabling them to behave quite similar to natural living tissues [Hoffman, 2002].
  • provide a semi-wet, three-dimensional environment for molecular-level biological interactions [Zhang, 2004].
  • provide inert surfaces that prevent non-specific adsorption of proteins.

- provide a non-adhesive surface towards cells and allow for programmable cell adhesion upon attaching biological molecules to the hydrogel [Ratner et al., 2004].
- control the mechanical and physical properties by varying the cross-linking density as well as the type of cross-links.
- maintain a certain extent of structural integrity and elasticity.
- allow for increased diffusion of nutrients into the gel and cellular waste out of the gel due to the high equilibrium swelling when used as a cell delivery vehicle.

The commercial success of soft contact lenses raised significant interest in hydrogels as biomaterials. Subsequently, a wide range of hydrogels were developed using synthetic and natural hydrophilic polymers for various biomedical applications such as drug, gene, and protein delivery vehicles, as unique wound dressing materials, as well as scaffolds for tissue engineering [Peppas and Sahlin, 1996]. Hydrogels are highly suitable as wound dressings due to their ability to maintain a moist wound environment, to absorb exudate drainage, to allow oxygen transport, high permeability to provide appropriate medication (analgesia, anti-inflammatory/antibiotics) and to be easily removed without patient discomfort due to their low adherence to tissue. Hydrogels, due to their highly swollen three-dimensional environment with large pore size, porosity and high water content, closely resemble the environment of native tissue extracellular matrix (ECM). Hydrogels are therefore considered as potential materials for developing scaffolds for tissue engineering. Hydrogels are also suitable as protein delivery vehicles due to their ECM mimicking hydrated matrix, mild gelation process and high permeability.

Several synthetic non-degradable hydrogels based on methacrylate and polyethylene glycols were developed following the studies of Dr. Wichterle. Poly(ethylene glycol) (PEG) is one of the most extensively investigated synthetic hydrophilic polymers for biomedical applications due to its hydrophilicity, good tissue compatibility, non-toxicity and availability of reactive end groups for chemical functionalization. Among the natural hydrophilic macromolecules investigated for hydrogel formation, polysaccharides form the most prominent members [Coviello et al., 2007]. This is due to various advantages of polysaccharides such as non-toxicity, biocompatibility, availability in large variety of composition and properties, wide presence in living organisms, as well as due to the fact that they can be produced using recombinant DNA techniques [Coviello et al., 2007].

In addition to the wide range of hydrogels developed so far, these studies also led to the development of a major class of hydrogel system with unique stimuli sensitive properties for therapeutic and diagnostic applications. Stimuli sensitive polymers exhibit property changes in response to an external stimulus such as temperature, light, pH, salts, solvents, electric field, chemical as well as internal stimulus such as biochemical agents [Hoffman, 1991]. Among these, polymers sensitive to temperature, light, chemical and biological cues are highly preferred for biomedical applications. Stimuli sensitive hydrogels have been broadly classified into two systems: stimuli-responsive systems and stimuli-sensitive gelling systems.

Stimuli-responsive systems show marked swelling and de-swelling changes or degradation in response to various stimuli. The property has been used for controlling the release of entrapped molecules as well as pulsatile release of drugs or macromolecules from hydrogel depot systems. Bio-responsive hydrogels change properties (swelling/de-swelling, degradation) in response to selective biological recognition events such as nutrient, growth factor, receptor, antibody, enzyme or whole cell [Ulijin et al., 2007]. The release of insulin from bio-responsive hydrogels in response to raised blood sugar is one of the interesting systems developed [Fischel-Ghodsian et al., 1988]. Bio-responsive hydrogels are also used for bio-sensing applications. Kim et al., developed a whole cell sensing system based on the interaction of immobilized lymphocytes with target peptides [Kim et al., 2006]. Similarly, Hubbell et al., have developed a PEG-based ECM mimicking hydrogel scaffold that permits cell migration via the enzymatic cleavage of oligopeptides used as cross-linkers. These oligopeptides are cleavable by matrix metalloproteinases (MMPs), which belong to a family of enzymes that play a significant role during tissue remodeling. The presence of oligopeptides in the gel allows the invading cells to degrade the hydrogels by secreting MMPs, facilitating complete tissue regeneration [Lutolf and Hubbell, 2005]. Stimuli-responsive hydrogels, therefore, find applications in diagnostics, drug delivery and tissue regeneration.

In the case of stimuli-sensitive gelling systems, the aqueous polymer solution change into a gel in response to a particular stimulus, thus enabling the formation of gel *in situ*. The practical biomedical applications of these materials arise from their injectability that allows for non-invasive treatment strategies. An injectable *in situ*-gelling system can be injected into a complex defect site and gelled to form a solid structure of exactly the same dimension. The *in situ* formed gels generally show increased adhesion to surrounding tissue due to the intimate contact of the gel with the tissue during formation and by the mechanical interlocking resulting from surface micro-roughness [Elisseeff et al., 1999]. Biocompatible injectable stimuli-sensitive gelling polymers are potential biomaterials for drug delivery and tissue engineering applications.

This chapter reviews various types of injectable *in situ* gelling hydrogels currently being investigated as biomaterials, mainly for tissue regeneration with an emphasis on photo, chemical and thermo-gelling polymers.

6.3 INJECTABLE *IN SITU* FORMING GELS

Recent years saw an exponential increase in research towards developing *in situ* gelling materials due to their considerable applicability interest in such areas as protein and cell carriers, implants as well as other medical devices. Their advantages as protein delivery vehicle include ease of formulation, high-loading efficiency, ability to deliver protein in a non-invasive manner, suitable for sensitive proteins due to the mild gelling process, possibility of sustained or controlled protein delivery and the absence of any organic solvents.

Even though most of the earlier works using hydrogels were focused at using them as drug/protein delivery vehicles, the application of hydrogels as scaffolding materials for tissue engineering has attracted much attention recently. The concept of *in situ* generated implant strategy is highly unique and attractive since the implants (either cell or factor loaded) can be processed in the operating room, administered using a minimally invasive surgical procedure, and can be used to fill irregularly shaped defects as the implant is formed at the defect site [Cheung et al., 2007].

Hydrophilic polymers that can undergo gelation in response to different types of stimuli have been developed either by modifying existing polymers or by specifically designing polymers with stimuli sensitive units along the polymer chain. The various stimuli of interest include light (photo-polymerizing/photo-gelling systems), chemical agents (chemical and ionic cross-linking systems) as well as environmental stimuli present under the physiological condition (temperature, pH and ionic strength).

Visible or near ultra violet light induced photo-polymerization is one of the most extensively investigated *in situ* gelation process for developing injectable hydrogels. The photo-polymerizable systems are currently investigated for developing depot formulations [An and Hubbell, 2000], as biological adhesives [Ono et al., 2000] as well as for orthopaedic tissue engineering [Elisseeff et al., 2001].

Various chemical as well as physical processes are being investigated that enable the formation of hydrogels from hydrophilic polymers. These include using chemical polymerization reagents [Holland et al., 2007] or cross-linking agents as well as physical interactions between molecules.

Among the stimuli sensitive gelling systems, those responding to environmental stimuli are considered more biocompatible as they are able to change from liquid aqueous solutions to gel under physiological conditions without the addition of any chemicals or external stimulus. Temperature sensitive gelling systems, particularly those undergoing thermal transition at or near physiological temperature (37 °C), are the most extensively investigated and are the most preferred systems in this class [Ruel-Gariepy and Leroux, 2004].

6.3.1 Photo-Gelling Polymers

Photo-gelling biocompatible polymers form a versatile class of injectable biomaterials as the aqueous polymer solution can be introduced to the desired site via injection followed by photo-curing *in situ* using fiber optic cables and enabling a controllable as well as rapid gelation at physiological temperature and pH [Baroli, 2006]. Injectable photo-gelling systems have been extensively investigated as protein/cell delivery vehicles and as scaffolds for tissue engineering.

Different processes have been investigated to develop hydrogels from photo-labile polymers [Fisher et al., 2001]. The most extensively investigated processes include developing water soluble polymers with photoactive groups that can undergo cross-linking when irradiated with light of appropriate wave length and water soluble polymers with acrylic/methacrylic side groups that can undergo photo-polymerization via a radical chain polymerization mechanism initiated by appropriate photo-initiators.

6.3.1.1 Hydrogels from Polymers with Photoactive Side Groups.

These are mainly developed from hydrophilic polymers modified with photo-labile groups. Due to the mild gelation conditions and absence of non-toxic by-products or reagents during photo-gelation, this is an attractive strategy for developing injectable biomaterials. Most of the earlier studies using photo-gelling systems were focused to develop occlusive dressings that conform to the contour of the wound. Critical design criteria for these materials include fast gelation time, biocompatibility and ability to gel in the presence of low intensity radiation as well as at a narrow range of physiologically acceptable temperatures [Lu and Anseth, 1999].

Andreopoulos et al., have investigated unique chemical approaches to modify the hydrophilic, biocompatible, as well as non-degradable polymer "poly(ethylene glycol)"(PEG) to undergo photo-assisted cross-linking to form hydrogels. These injectable hydrogels were investigated as enzyme immobilization matrices, controlled drug delivery vehicles and antithrombogenic surfaces [Andreopoulos et al., 1996, 1998, 1999]. Photo cross-linked gels were prepared by the intermolecular photo-dimerization of various photo-labile groups attached to polymers including cinnamylidene, nitrocinnamate and anthracene. The PEG-nitro cinnamate system was found to be much more versatile than the cinnamylidine system due to its better thermal as well as storage stability and high photo-reactivity (~350 times) [Zheng et al., 2001]. The efficacy of PEG-nitrocinnamate system as a basic fibroblast growth factor delivery system was recently demonstrated. Long wave ultra violet radiation (365 nm) was used for photo-gelation and the resulting gels were found to be non-toxic to human neonatal fibroblast cells. The released growth factor maintained its activity as well as induced fibroblast proliferation and collagen production *in vitro* [Andreopoulos and Persaud, 2006].

In addition to synthetic polymers, natural polymers have also been modified to form photo-gelling systems. Ono et al., developed photo cross-linkable water soluble chitosan with a photoactive azide group as a biological adhesive [Ono et al., 2000]. Chitosan, a polyglycosamine derived from crustacean exoskeleton, is a highly versatile polymer for chemical modification due to the reactive amine side groups. Azide groups are unique for photo cross-linking, since upon photo-irradiation they will be converted into highly reactive nitrene groups which can under go rapid insertion reactions to form covalent cross-links. The efficacy of the chitosan photo-gels was compared to fibrin glue, a clinically used bio-adhesive. Compared to fibrin glue, the chitosan photo-gels were more effective in sealing air leakage from pinholes on isolated small intestine and aorta as well as from incisions on isolated trachea. Moreover, the gels were found to be non-toxic towards human skin fibroblasts, coronary endothelial cells and smooth muscle cells. The accelerating effect of chitosan-azide on wound healing was evaluated using a full thickness skin incision on the back of mice and subsequently covered with the polymer solution followed by photo-irradiation for 90 s. Significant wound contraction, accelerated closure, and healing was observed. Histological examination demonstrated the formation of advanced granulation tissue and epithelialization on chitosan hydrogel treated wounds [Ishihara et al., 2001]. The ability of the hydrogel to perform as a fibroblast growth factor delivery system while functioning as a wound dressing has also been demonstrated using healing-impaired diabetic mice [Obara et al., 2003].

Another interesting photo-gelling system developed by Haines et al., employs a uniquely designed peptide that can self-assemble into a hydrogel by forming intramolecular folded conformational state [Haines et al., 2005]. The peptide (2% w/v) when dissolved in aqueous medium remains unfolded and is stable to ambient light. Irradiation of solution with light <360 nm opens the photo-cage to trigger peptide folding to produce amphiphilic beta-hairpins that assemble to form a viscoelastic hydrogel. The hydrogel was also found to be cytocompatible as evidenced from *in vitro* studies [Haines et al., 2005].

These studies demonstrate the efficacy of photo-gelling injectable systems as protein delivery vehicles and wound dressings due to their mild gelation behavior and controllable swelling properties.

6.3.1.2 Hydrogels by Photopolymerization.

The most common strategy for developing an injectable photo-polymerizable system is by using a water soluble macromer having pendant acrylate groups along the polymer chain or as end groups. These photo-sensitive macromers are then polymerized in the presence of photo initiators (with or without photo sensitizers) upon exposure to long wavelength ultraviolet or visible radiation. Photo-polymerization further provides the benefit of spatial and temporal control of polymerization through controlling when and where the sample is exposed to the initiating light source.

One of the major concerns in developing photo-polymerizable systems as injectable biomaterials is the toxicity of the photo initiators. Bryant et al., investigated the cytocompatibility of several photoinitiators using cultured fibroblast cell lines [Bryant et al., 2000]. Photo initiators investigated include UV initiators such as 2,2-dimethoxy-2-phenylacetophenone (Irgacure 651), 1-hydroxycyclohexyl phenyl ketone (Irgacure 184), 2-methyl-1-[4-(methylthio)phenyl]-2-(4-morpholinyl)-1-propanone (Irgacure 907), and 2-hydroxy-1-[4-(hydroxyethoxy)phenyl]-2-methyl-1-propanone (Darocur 2959). The visible light initiators included camphorquinone (CQ), ethyl 4-N,N-dimethylaminobenzoate (4EDMAB) and triethanolamine (TEA) and the photo sensitizer isopropyl thioxanthone. At low photo initiator concentrations (<0.01% w/w), all the initiators were found to be cytocompatable except CQ, Irgacure 651 and 4EDMAB. When the photo initiators were coupled with low intensity initiating light (approximately 6 mWcm^{-2}) of 365 nm UV light and visible light of 470–490 nm (approximately 60 mWcm^{-2}), Darocur 2959 at concentrations <0.05% (w/w) and CQ at concentrations <0.01% (w/w) were found to be the most cytocompatible

UV and visible initiating systems, respectively. The cytocompatibility of Darocur 2959 was further confirmed by encapsulating chondrocytes in photo cross-linked PEG based gel prepared using 0.05% (w/w) Darocur 2959. When photo-polymerized for ten minutes with approximately $8\,mWcm^{-2}$ of 365 nm light, nearly all the chondrocytes survived in Darocur 2959 initiated gels. The good cytocompatibility of Darocur 2959 (also known as Irgacure 2959) was further confirmed using six different cell populations that are commonly used for tissue engineering applications [Williams et al., 2005]. The study confirmed that Irgacure 2959 cause minimal toxicity over a broad range of mammalian cell types and species. However, it has to be noted that different cell types showed variable responses to identical concentrations of Irgacure 2959 with fast dividing cells being more sensitive towards the initiator.

Due to the availability of less-toxic photo initiators, extensive research has undergone to develop photo-polymerizable injectable systems. Most of the studies were focused on synthetic hydrophilic polymer "PEG." The PEG-based polymers are highly preferred due to their availability in wide range of molecular weights as well as functionality, and consistent composition that allows the development of predictable gel properties [Cushing and Anseth, 2007]. The feasibility of transdermal photo-polymerization of polyethylene oxide (PEO) has been demonstrated [Elisseeff et al., 1999]. The study demonstrated that transdermal photo-polymerization through human skin is possible and is most efficient using visible light in the presence of visible light photo initiators. Mathematical modeling predicted that only two minutes of light exposure are required to photo-polymerize an implant underneath human skin. The efficacy of the system as a minimally-invasive injectable construct for plastic surgery, tissue engineering scaffolds, as well as drug delivery depots, was demonstrated using various animal models [Elisseeff et al., 1999].

One of the most extensively investigated applications for injectable photo cross-linkable systems is as cell delivery vehicles due to their ability to control gel formation, undergo gelation at milder conditions, allow localized delivery, protect the cells from the immediate external environment, and allow nutrient diffusion. Since materials that are capable of degrading *in vivo* are preferred for drug delivery and tissue engineering applications, most of the studies were focused on developing degradable, injectable photo cross-linking systems. Degradable, injectable and photo cross-linkable gel systems are usually prepared by incorporating ester groups [Davis et al., 2003; Sawhney et al., 1993] or enzymatically cleavable peptide linkages in the cross-link segments [West and Hubbell, 1999; Lutolf et al., 2003; Kurisawa et al., 1995].

Anseth, et al., demonstrated the greater efficiency of a degradable synthetic photopolymerizable hydrogel compared to a non-degradable hydrogel as a construct for cartilage-tissue engineering. Degradable injectable hydrogels were developed by photo polymerizing poly(ethylene glycol dimethacrylate) with a hydrolytically sensitive triblock copolymer, poly(lactic acid)-*b*-ethylene glycol)-*b*-poly(lactic acid) with acrylate end groups. Darocur 2959 was used as the photoinitiator. *In vitro* cell encapsulation studies using chondrocytes demonstrated

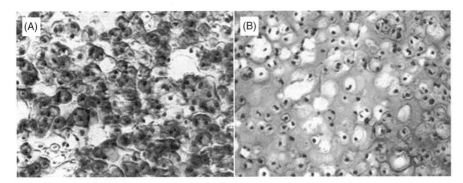

Figure 6.1. Histological analysis of chondrocytes photoencapsulated in PEG hydrogels with 15% macromer after 8 weeks *in vitro*. A. Stained with Safranin-O which stains proteoglycans red and B. Stained with Masson trichrome which stains collagen blue (×200). (See color insert.)

the highest production of collagen II by the encapsulated cells and homogeneous distribution of glycosamino glycans within the gels using degradable PEG-based injectable hydrogels compared to non-degradable PEG hydrogels [Bryant and Anseth, 2002, Bryant et al., 2003]. The feasibility of modulating the macroscopic properties and degradation behavior of degradable poly(ethylene glycol) hydrogels in order to optimize the properties of scaffolds for cartilage tissue engineering was demonstrated [Bryant et al., 2004; Rice and Anseth, 2004]. By increasing the macromer concentration, gels with initial compressive moduli of 60–55 kPa were obtained and incorporation of degradable cross-links into the network facilitated the diffusion of proteoglycans into the extracellular regions of the hydrogel. Figure 6.1 is the histological sections of chondrocyte encapsulated PEG hydrogels with 15% macromer after eight weeks in culture showing the formation of proteoglycans and collagen by the encapsulated cells [Bryant et al., 2004]. The study thus demonstrates the feasibility of tailoring the composition of the gels to control the degradation as well as temporal changes in the gel network structure.

PEG-based injectable photo cross-linkable hydrogels have also been found to be a potential cell carrier system for neural transplantation. Neural cells cultured within the three-dimensional polymer network created their own cellular microenvironment to survive, proliferate and differentiate to form neurons and glia that are electrophysologically responsive to neurotransmitters [Mahoney and Anseth, 2006]. Also, it has been demonstrated that by changing the degradation time of the hydrogels, the time-scale over which neural cells extend processes can be tuned from one to three weeks, since upon degradation gels provide space for cellular processes to extend through the three dimensional matrix. Figure 6.2 shows the spatial integration of the microtissue fluorescently labeled with calcein-AM (green-live) or ethidium bromide (red-dead) in the gel after 16 days in culture [Mahoney and Anseth, 2006].

A recent study demonstrated the minimally-invasive implantation of PEG hydrogel and subsequent chondrogenic differentiation of encapsulated

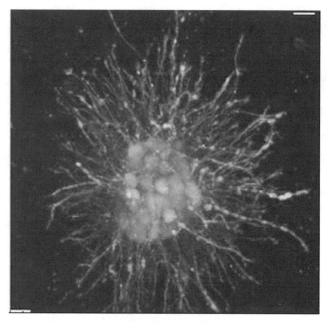

<u>Figure 6.2.</u> A dense plexus of processes emerged radially from aggregates to penetrate and grow through the hydrogel environment. Scale bar represents 20 mm.

mesenchymal stem cells in the subcutaneous tissue via transdermal photo polymerization [Sharma et al., 2007a]. High molecular-weight hyaluronic acid (HA) was used as a visco-supplement to increase the efficiency of injections and to hold the solution at the injection site during photopolymerization. Injectable PEG hydrogel was also used to deliver transforming growth factor-β3 (TGF-β3) to induce chondrogenesis of the mesenchymal stem cells. The study demonstrated the feasibility of forming cartilage tissue *in situ* using stem cells and appropriate injectable biomaterial. Figure 6.3 shows photo-polymerized hydrogel in subcutaneous tissue after three weeks of injection and the construct with a gross appearance similar to cartilage [Sharma et al., 2007a].

Apart from serving as a minimally-invasive injectable system, the versatility of a photo polymerization system allows for the development of multilayer constructs for tissue engineering. A co-culture system using bi-layered photo polymerized gels to organize zone specific chondrocytes in a stratified frame work has been studied [Sharma et al., 2007b]. The bi-layered constructs were first made by partially polymerizing the bottom layer followed by quickly adding the second layer and polymerizing them both. The bi-layered construct showed higher shear and compressive strength compared to homogeneous constructs and allowed separation of different cell layers to mimic the natural tissue structure [Sharma et al., 2007b].

One of the disadvantages of synthetic polymeric materials such as PEG as scaffolds for tissue engineering is the absence of any bioactive ECM molecules on

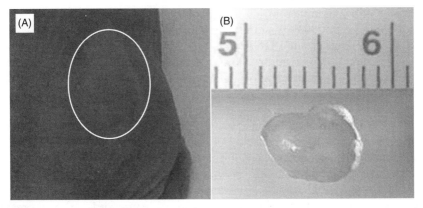

Figure 6.3. A. Hydrogel implant after photopolymerizing in the subcutaneous tissue for 3 weeks. B. Construct containing stem cells encapusulated in PEG hydrogel containing HA and TGF-B3.

PEG to provide cell-matrix interactions. A study investigated the feasibility of incorporating cell-adhesive peptide sequences to PEG-based hydrogels to biologically modulate cell adhesion. PEG macromers containing peptide sequence Arg-Gly- Asp (RGD) as well as macromers containing RGD and its synergy site Pro-His-Ser-Arg-Asn linked via a polyglycine sequence were used in the study to recapitulate the native spacing of the cell adhesive protein, fibronectin. The biologically-modified gels showed significant increase in osteoblast cell adhesion, proliferation and phenotype expression, compared to cells encapsulated in unmodified PEG gel [Benoit and Anseth, 2005]. Similarly, several other biologically active injectable gels based on degradable PEG have also been developed for tissue engineering applications [Nuttleman et al., 2005; Salinas et al., 2007; Hwang et al., 2006; Lee et al., 2006].

Anseth et al., have demonstrated the efficacy of injectable photogelling PEG-based degradable hydrogels as protein delivery vehicles. The ability to modulate drug release kinetics by engineering appropriate macromers and cross-linking densities has been demonstrated [Anseth et al., 2002].

Since delivery of plasmid DNA that encodes therapeutic proteins offer several advantages over protein delivery, studies were performed to evaluate the feasibility of delivering DNA using injectable photo cross-linkable gels [Quick and Anseth, 2003]. The advantages of plasmid DNA over proteins include the greater stability of DNA in a wide range of environments, better processability as the same procedure can be applied for administrating a wide range of plasmids that encodes for different proteins, more control over protein release *in vivo*, and considerable ease of production and purification of plasmid DNA. An injectable DNA delivery system would allow the local administration of plasmid DNA, thereby avoiding systemic interactions which significantly reduce the efficiency of the process. Apart from these advantages, the localized, sustained delivery of DNA enables continuous transfections leading to prolonged foreign gene expression allowing longer lasting therapeutic effect without repeated treatment [Quick and Anseth, 2003]. Photopolymerization has shown to increase the stability of encapsulated plasmid DNA when administrated *in vivo*. Moreover, since photointiatiated polymerization allows spatial and temporal control of gelation, the process could permit creation of patterned matrices *in vivo* with different concentrations of the transfecting agents as well as plasmids that encode several different tissue inducing proteins.

Even though photo gelation is a mild process, the encapsulated DNA was found to denature within the photo polymerized gel. It has been found that the denaturation of plasmid DNA is not due to the light used (~365 nm) but due to the free radicals that induce photo polymerization. Later studies by Anseth et al., revealed that addition of radical scavengers such as vitamin C and complexing plasmid DNA with transfection agents (such as protamine sulfate) could preserve the integrity of the plasmid DNA during photo polymerization. The feasibility of photo cross-linkable injectable gel to encapsulate and release plasmid DNA in an active, supercoiled form in a sustained manner has been demonstrated. Photo cross-linked PEG hydrogels released DNA for periods of six to one hundred days, with nearly linear or delayed burst release profiles and the released DNA exhibited high biological activity as evidenced from cell culture studies [Quick and Anseth, 2004].

Apart from synthetic polymers, several degradable natural polymers modified with acrylic groups have been investigated as injectable photo cross-linkable systems for biomedical applications [Leach et al., 2003]. Since natural polymers are present in many tissues, they provide a better biomimetic environment for tissue engineering application compared to synthetic polymers. The efficacy of hyaluronic acid based photo cross-linked gels as a potential matrix for creating a tissue engineered heart valve has been demonstrated by encapsulating valvular interstitial cells with high viability in photo cross-linked gels. High matrix and significant elastin production by the encapsulated cells were observed after six weeks in culture [Masters et al., 2005]. The efficacy of hyaluornic acid injectable gels for cartilage tissue engineering has also been demonstrated [Nettles et al., 2004]. A recent study demonstrated the efficacy of functionalized chondroitin sulfate as an efficient photo cross-linkable tissue adhesive system [Wang et al., 2007]. Chondroitin sulfate was functionalized with methacrylate groups for photo cross-linking and aldehyde groups for chemically bridging the hydrogel to the tissue proteins. *In vitro* and *in vivo* studies (in goat models) demonstrated the mechanical stability of the construct during tissue repair in cartilage defects [Wang et al., 2007].

Even though degradable injectable photo cross-linkable systems present unique advantages for a wide range of biomedical applications, some of the limitations of the system include residual high molecular weight compounds upon gel degradation, mild toxicity associated with the photoinitiators, limited control over the network evolution mechanism during chain-growth, and also light attenuation by the initiators restricting the maximum attainable cure depth of only a few millimeters [Rydholm et al., 2005; Baroli, 2006].

A new class of thiol-based system has been proposed to circumvent some of these limitations. The thiolated polymers can form degradable networks through Michael-addition-type reaction through acrylate, acrylamide or vinyl sulfone groups as well as by direct polymerization of thiol acrylates [Lutolf and Hubbell, 2003; Vernon et al., 2003]. The thiol-based systems enable the formation of a cross-linked network with better control over the cross-link density, eliminate high molecular weight degradation products as the degradable segments get incorporated throughout the network, could even eliminate the need for a photoinitiator, allow samples to be cured to depths exceeding ten cm, and therefore have significant potential as an *in situ* gelling system for cell encapsulation [Rydholm et al., 2005].

Another unique strategy to overcome the concerns of cell or tissue damage due to direct UV exposure is by forming an *in situ* gellable photo polymerizable system with a long induction period. Di-acrylated Pluoronic F127 has shown to have a long induction period after UV irradiation before macrosocpic gelation can occur. The polymer solution can therefore be injected after UV irradiation and will attain the gel state following injection [Lee and Tae, 2007]. Further studies on these unique injectable systems will demonstrate their potential for various biomedical applications.

6.3.2 Hydrogels Formed by Fast Chemical Reaction/Physical Transitions

The versatility of thiolated polymers allows for the development of *in situ* gelling polymers without using initiators. Michael type reaction has therefore been investigated to form *in situ* gels. A hyaluronic acid based hydrogel was formed *in situ* using thiolated hyaluronic acid [Shu et al., 2006]. However, the rate of gelation of thiolated polymers is very slow, making them less than optimal candidates as injectable systems. The addition of acrylated polymers to thiolated polymers significantly increased the rate of gelation, thereby making them suitable for use as injectable systems. Recently, Michael-addition has also been used to develop injectable *in situ* forming chitosan-based hydrogels. Chitosan was functionalized with acrylate groups and then reacted with thiolated poly(ethylene oxide) to form the *in situ* forming gels [Kim et al., 2007].

Polymerization of acrylated polymers can also be performed without photo irradiation in the presence of redox reagents, such as ammonium persulfate, as free radical generators. Biodegradable injectable hydrogel material based on the oligomer "oligo(poly(ethylene glycol) fumarate)" polymerized using redox reagents is another class of PEG-based biomaterial developed for treating cartilage lesions [Holland et al., 2005]. The efficacy of the injectable hydrogel system as an excellent protein delivery vehicle has also been demonstrated [Park et al., 2005]. Rabbit marrow mesenchymal stem cells encapsulated in the fumarate gels showed the ability to differentiate into chondrocytes in the presence of slowly released transforming growth factor-$\beta 1$ (TGF-$\beta 1$). The studies demonstrate the potential of the system for cartilage tissue engineering [Park et al., 2007].

Polymeric aldehydes derived from polysaccharides can be used for developing injectable fast gelling systems due to their chemical reactivity. Polymeric aldehydes are mainly developed using periodate chemistry from polysaccharides having vic-diols. An *in situ* gelling system formed by self cross-linking oxidized alginate and gelatin in the presence of small concentrations of borax without using any extraneous cross-linking agent has been reported [Balakrishnan and Jayakrishnan, 2005]. The fast gelling composition was found to be non-toxic as evidenced from *in vitro* cell culture studies. The ability of the gels to function as a heptocyte encapsulation matrix and as a wound dressing has been demonstrated [Balakrishnan et al., 2005]. The evaporative water loss through the gel has been found to be closer to the range appropriate to maintain proper fluid balance on the wound bed, indicating its potential as an injectable wound dressing. Moreover, the presence of borax has been shown to have some antibacterial properties promoting accelerated wound healing.

One of the potent applications of injectable systems is to act as barriers to prevent tissue adhesion following surgery or other injuries. An *in situ* gelling injectable hyaluronic acid-based system with marked *in vivo* anti-adhesion property was developed. The injectable system is based on hyaluornic acid-aldehyde and hyaluronic adipic dihydrazide. A fast gelation reaction occurs by mixing these two solutions due to the formation of a hydrazone compound. The system has also shown efficacy to be used as an effective drug delivery vehicle to enhance biological activity *in vitro* and *in vivo* [Yeo et al., 2007a,b]. Apart from HA, several other polysaccharides have also been investigated to develop injectable gels using similar chemistries [Ito et al., 2007].

Another versatile *in situ* gelling system developed is known as "click gels" based on "click chemistry." Room temperature gelation happens when hyaluronic acid (HA) bearing azido groups is reacted with an alkyne derivative of HA in the presence of catalytic amounts of cuprous chloride. The gelation is due to dipolar cycloaddition or Huisgen reaction, a type of click chemistry process. The study demonstrated the feasibility of varying the cross-linking density of the gel, as well as the efficacy of the gel as a drug and cell delivery vehicle [Crescenzi et al., 2007].

Another emerging technique for developing an *in situ* gelling system is based on enzyme-catalyzed cross-linking reaction. Several cross-linking systems using polymers containing glutaminamide and amines in the presence of transglutaminase (TG) and calcium ions as co-factors have been developed [Sperinde and Griffith, 1997; Sanborn et al., 2002; McHale et al., 2005]. A glutaminamide-functionalized poly(ethylene glycol) and poly(lysine-co-phenylalanine) was used by Sperinde and Griffith to form injectable gels in the presence of TG. TG mediated covalent cross-linking occurs via the formation of an amide linkage between the carboxy amide groups of peptidyl glutamine residues and primary amine of lysine residues. Several synthetic and natural polymers functionalized with tyramine, tyrosine or aminophenol side groups are currently under development that can form *in situ* gels by phenol or aniline derivative coupling using hydrogen peroxide as an oxidant catalyzed by horseradish perodidase (HRP) [Sofia et al., 2002; Kurisawa et al., 2005; Kobayashi et al., 2001; Jin et al., 2007].

Several protein-based self-assembling hydrogels are currently being investigated as unique, injectable biomaterials for wide range of applications. Most of these proteins/peptides self assemble in the presence of appropriate stimuli to form nanostructured matrices highly suitable for tissue engineering applications. A self-assembling peptide composed of typically 8–16 amino acids has been developed as an injectable system [Zhang, 2003]. The peptide will be in solution at low pH and osmolarity but rapidly assemble to form fibers of ~5–10 nm in diameter at physiological pH and osmolarity. The gels formed were found to be highly cytocompatible towards many types of mammalian cells [Holmes et al., 2000; Semino et al., 2003; Davis et al., 2005]. The potential of these injectable self-assembling gels as drug delivery vehicles has also been demonstrated [Nagai et al., 2006]. The studies demonstrate the versatility of chemical cross-linking systems as injectable biomaterials for biomedical applications.

6.3.3   Thermogelling Polymers

Thermogelation is one of the most favored and extensively investigated strategies for developing *in situ* gelling polymers. Pluoronics and various PEG-based polymers form the most widely investigated thermogelling polymers. Pluoronics present several advantages such as mild processing and gelling process, ability to increase the stability of encapsulated proteins, and good biocompatibility. The biomedical applications of Pluoronics based polymers as a drug or macromolecular delivery vehicle have been reviewed [Ruel-Gariepy and Leroux, 2004]. However, the low mechanical integrity of the gel, non-degradability, limited stability with quick dissolutions and high permeability limits its biomedical application [Liu et al., 2007].

Several degradable block co-polymers with hydrolytically sensitive blocks such as poly(lactic acid/glycolic acid) or poly(caprolactone) as the hydrophobic units and poly(ethylene glycol) as the hydrophilic units were therefore developed [Cohn et al., 2006; Jeong et al., 2000; Chen et al., 2005]. The thermogelling properties, combined with their biocompatibility and biodegradability, make these polymers potential candidates for various applications. Furthermore, these polymers have significant potential as injectable drug delivery vehicles due to the ability of these polymers to solubilize highly hydrophobic drugs.

Another unique approach to incorporate thermogelling properties to macromolecules is by grafting PEG to various polymers. Bhattarai et al. were able to develop thermo-reversible hydrogels from chitosan functionalized with PEG. PEG grafting significantly increased the solubility of chitosan at neutral pH and enabled gelation at physiological pH [Bhattarai et al., 2005a,b]. However, further cross-linking using genipin has been suggested for developing protein delivery vehicles due to the high permeability of the PEG-grafted gels. Mikos et al. have developed a thermosensitve triblock copolymeric system by combining methoxy poly(ethylene glycol) with poly(propylene fumarate). The system provides the additional advantage of further chemical cross-linking using fumarate double bonds. The thermogels are being evaluated as chondrocyte delivery vehicles

[Behravesh et al., 2002; Fisher et al., 2004]. PEG-grafted polyphosphazenes form another class of injectable biodegradable hydrogels developed for biomedical applications. The unique feature of these hydrogels is that the versatility of polyphosphazenes would enable the development of systems with controllable degradation and release profiles for drug/cell delivery applications [Sohn et al., 2004; Park and Song., 2006; Kang et al., 2006a,b].

Another non-degradable polymer extensively investigated as a thermogelling system is based on Poly(N-isopropylacryamide) (pNiPAAm) or its copolymers [Schild, 1992]. The low biocompatibility and non-degradability of the homo-polymer limits the *in vivo* applications of pNiPAAm; however, several copolymeric systems are currently under evaluation as potential injectable thermosensitve polymers. A promising system recently developed is a copolymer of NiPAAm with water-soluble chitosan. The polymer has shown to undergo gelation at 37 °C and the efficacy of the system as a cell delivery vehicle has also been demonstrated. The feasibility of using the system for the minimally invasive treatment of vesicouretral reflux with an endoscopic procedure through a single injection has been suggested [Cho et al., 2004]. Copolymer of NiPAAm with gelatin has also been investigated as a thermogelling injectable biodegradable system for cell encapsulation. Encapsulated smooth muscle cells showed high proliferation and matrix synthesis in the case of gels with high pNiPAAm to gelatin ratio presumably due to the hydrophobicity of NiPAAm units leading to larger aggregates within the matrix and thereby providing high porosity and pore size structure to the matrix [Ohya et al., 2005].

Many natural polymers exhibit innate thermosensitve gelation process and therefore have been investigated as *in situ* gelling systems. Methyl cellulose is a biocompatible polysaccharide that exhibits thermo gelling properties. The thermogelation of methyl cellulose has been attributed to the hydrophobic interaction between polymeric molecules containing methoxy groups. As the temperature of the aqueous solution of the polymer increases to 37 °C, hydrogen bonds between the polymer and surrounding solvent break, and hydrophobic interaction between the polymer chains led to gel formation. This simple sol–gel transition in methyl cellulose has been used for developing injectable biomaterials. A fast gelling, injectable system was developed by blending methyl cellulose with HA (to take advantage of the unique visocoelastic properties of HA) for intrathecal delivery of bioactive molecules [Gupta et al., 2006; Shoichet et al., 2007]. Bioactive methyl cellulose derivatives were also prepared by chemically grafting protein to methyl cellulose backbone after periodate oxidation. The oxidized and functionalized methyl cellulose promoted neuronal adhesion, proliferation and viability and hence has potential for neuronal tissue engineering [Stabenfeldt et al., 2006].

Hydroxy butyl chitosan (HBC) is another class of temperature-sensitive water soluble polysaccharide that is attracting significant attention. Dang et al. evaluated the feasibility of encapsulating mesenchymal stem cells and intervertebral disk cells in rapidly gelling HBC composition as an injectable matrix/cell therapeutic for treating degenerative disk disease. The gels maintained a certain extent of mechanical integrity and the encapsulated cells proliferated and produced a matrix within the gel during a period of up to two weeks [Dang et al., 2006].

Another chitosan-based thermogelling system that is attracting significant attention is chitosan-glycerophosphate mixture [Chenite et al., 2000; 2001]. The uniqueness of the system lies in the transformation of pH-gelling cationic chitosan solution into a thermally sensitive, pH-dependent gel forming solution capable of gelling at physiological temperature without any chemical modification or cross-linking. To produce thermo-gelling solution, polyols bearing single anionic groups such as glycerol-, sorbitol, fructose or glucose-phosphate salts are slowly added to a chitosan solution at a low temperature. The mechanism of gelation has been attributed to a combination of favorable hydrogen bonding, electrostatic interactions and hydrophobic interactions between polymer chains and with the polyols. The thermogelling chitosan-glycerophosphate solution can be easily administered endoscopically within the body or through injections to form *in situ* gelling systems. The injectable system has been found to form homogeneous gel implants after injection in many body compartments—subcutaneously, intrarticularly, intra-muscularly, as well as in bone and cartilage defects. The good cytocompatibility of the gel was established using *in vitro* cell culture studies. The mild gelling process of chitosan–glycerophosphate makes it a potential delivery vehicle for bioactive proteins. A study investigated the efficacy of chitosan-glycerophosphate to deliver BMP-2 ectopically in a subcutaneous pouch in rats. Figure 6.4 shows the feasibility of chitosan-glycerophosphate to subcutaneously deliver active BMP-2, leading to de novo cartilage and bone formation in an ectopic site [Chenite et al., 2000].

Chitosan-glycerophosphate solution, when mixed with whole blood, has shown to coagulate *in situ* within 15 minutes when applied to cartilage defects *in vivo* [Hoemann et al., 2007]. Furthermore, the chitosan-glycerophosphate-blood mixture was found to have tissue adhesivity with minimal gel shrinkage, showing its potential as an injectable scaffold for cartilage tissue engineering. The chitosan-glycerophosphate-blood mixture has also been investigated to treat marrow-stimulated chondral defects in rabbit and sheep cartilage repair models. The application of chitosan-glycerophosphate-blood has been found to significantly increase more cellular and hyaline repair leading to cartilage repair well integrated with a porous subchondral bone structure compared to marrow stimulation alone [Hoemann et al., 2005]. The increased healing of chondral defects using chitosan-glycerophosphate-blood has been attributed to greater levels of provisional tissue vascularization and bone remodeling activity due to the presence of *in situ* gels [Chevrier et al., 2007].

This author's laboratory has developed a similar injectable thermo-gelling system based on chitosan using inorganic phosphate salts as the neutralizing and thermo-gelling agent [Nair and Laurencin, 2007]. The *in situ* gelling system was developed by adding ammonium hydrogen phosphate (AHP) to a chitosan solution at a low temperature. The system has been found to be highly versatile, with gelling time varying from five minutes to several hours at 37 °C, by varying the concentration of the phosphate salt. Compared to the chitosan-glycerophosphate

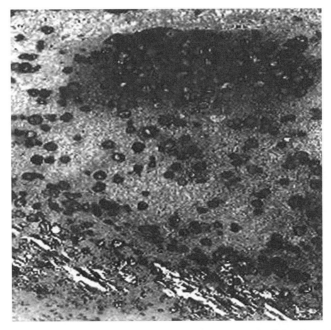

Figure 6.4. Toluidine blue stain of C/GP gel with 30 lg BP demonstrated an abundance of chondrocytes encompassed by a territorial cartilagenous matrix. (10×) (See color insert.)

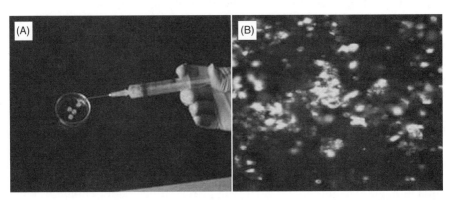

Figure 6.5. A. Demonstrates the injectability of the hdyrogel using a 21 guage needle. B. Human foreskin fibroblast cells encapsulatedin chitosan-ammonium hydrogen phosphate thermogels after 3 days in culture. Cells stained green (live cells) and cells stained red (dead cells). (See color insert.)

system, the concentration of the inorganic phosphate salt required to achieve thermogelation has been found to be significantly lower. The injectability of the system as well as the feasibility of using chitosan—AHP thermogels as a cell delivery vehicle has been demonstrated [Nair et al., 2007]. Figure 6.5a shows the feasibility of injecting chitosan-phosphate solution using a 21-guage needle and

6.5b shows human foreskin fibroblast cells encapsulated in the gel after three days in culture stained using Live Dead staining. The ability of the chitosan-AHP system to undergo fast gelation at physiological temperature without chemically modifying the polymer and at very low concentrations of AHP makes this system highly suitable as a protein and cell delivery vehicle.

6.4 CONCLUSIONS

The last decade saw a tremendous growth in developing unique biocompatible injectable hydrogels for biomedical applications due to the several advantages of *in situ* forming gels compared to implantable systems. Injectable systems responding to various stimuli such as light, chemical/physical reactions, as well as temperature, have been investigated. The feasibility of tuning the degradation and gelation time as well as the water content of the gels, coupled with the mild gelation process and ability to deliver them in a minimally invasive manner, make them potential protein and cell carrier vehicles. The most important parameters that determine the suitabilit of the injectable gel for tissue engineering and drug delivery applications include rate of gelation, degradability, rate of degradation, extent of water content, non-toxicity of the process, as well as physical and mechanical properties of the gel. Each of the developed systems has its own disadvantages and advantages depending on the end application. Even though many of the gels show good biocompatibility, the ability of the gels to mimic the viscoelastic properties of various tissues will be a crucial parameter that will determine their applicability as tissue engineering scaffolds.

REFERENCES

An Y, Hubbell JA. 2000. Intraarterial protein delivery via intimally adherent bilayer hydrogels. J Control Release 64: 205–215.

Andreopoulos FM, Beckman EJ, Russell AJ. 1998. Light induced tailoring of PEG hydrogel properties. Biomaterials 19: 1343–1352.

Andreopoulos FM, Deible CR, Stauffer MT, Weber SG, Wagner WR, Beckman EJ. 1996. Photoscissable hydrogel synthesis via rapid photopolymerization of novel PEG-based polymers in the absence of photoinitiators. J Am Chem Soc 118: 6235–6240.

Andreopoulos FM, Persaud I. 2006. Delivery of basic fibroblast growth factor from photoresponsive hydrogel scaffolds. Biomaterials 27:2468–2476.

Andreopoulos FM, Roberts MJ, Bentley MD, Harris JM, Beckman EJ, Russell AJ. 1999. Photoimmobilization of Organophosphorous Hydrolase within a PEG-based hydrogel. Biotechnol Bioeng 65: 579–588.

Anseth KS, Metters AT, Bryant SJ, Martens PJ, Elisseeff JH, Bowman CN. 2002. *In situ* forming degradable networks and their application in tissue engineering and drug delivery. J Control Release 78: 199–209.

Balakrishnan B, Jayakrishnan A. 2005. Self-cross-linking biopolymers as injectable *in situ* forming biodegradable scaffolds. Biomaterials 26: 3941–3951.

Balakrishnan B, Mohanty M, Umashankar PR, Jayakrishnan A. 2005. Evaluation of an *in situ* forming hydrogel wound dressing based on oxidized alginate and gelatin. Biomaterials 26: 6335–6342.

Baroli, B. 2006. Photopolymerization of biomaterials: issues and potentialities in drug delivery, tissue engineering, and cell encapsulation applications. J Chem Technol Biot 81: 491–499.

Behravesh E, Shung AK, Jo S, Mikos AG. 2002. Synthesis and characterization of triblock copolymers of methoxy poly(ethylene glycol) and poly(propylene fumarate). Biomacromolecules 3: 153–158.

Benoit DS, Anseth KS. 2005. The effect on osteoblast function of colocalized RGD and PHSRN epitopes on PEG surfaces. Biomaterials 26: 5209–5220.

Bhattarai N, Matsen FA, Zhang M. 2005a. PEG-grafted chitosan as an injectable thermoreversible hydrogel. Macromol Biosci 5: 107–111.

Bhattarai N, Ramay HR, Gunn J, Matsen FA, Zhang M. 2005b. PEG-grafted chitosan as an injectable thermosensitive hydrogel for sustained protein release. J Control Release 103: 609–624.

Bryant SJ, Nuttelman CR, Anseth KS. 2000. Cytocompatibility of UV and visible light photoinitiating systems on cultured NIH/3T3 fibroblasts *in vitro*. J Biomater Sci Polym Ed. 11: 439–457.

Bryant SJ, Anseth KS. 2002. Hydrogel properties influence ECM production by chondrocytes photoencapsulated in poly(ethylene glycol) hydrogels. J Biomed Mater Res 59: 63–72.

Bryant SJ, Durand KL, Anseth KS. 2003. Manipulations in hydrogel chemistry control photoencapsulated chondrocyte behavior and their extracellular matrix production. J Biomed Mater Res 67: 1430–1436.

Bryant SJ, Bender RJ, Durand KL, Anseth KS. 2004. Encapsulating chondrocytes in degrading PEG hydrogels with high modulus: engineering gel structural changes to facilitate cartilaginous tissue production. Biotechnol Bioeng 86: 747–755.

Chen S, Singh J. 2005. Controlled delivery of testosterone from smart polymer solution based systems: *In vitro* evaluation. Int J Pharm 295: 183–190.

Chenite A, Buschmann M, Wang D, Chaput N, Kandani N. 2001. Rheological characterization of thermogelling chitosan/glycerolphosphate solution. Carbohydr Polym 46: 39–47.

Chenite A, Chaput C, Wang C, Combes C, Buschmann MD, Hoemann CD, Leroux JC, Atkinson BL, Binette F, Selmani A. 2000. Novel injectable neural solutions of chitosan form biodegradable gels *in situ*. Biomaterials 21: 2155–2161.

Cheung H, Lau K, Lu T, Hui D. 2007. A critical review on polymer-based bio-engineered materials for scaffold development. Composites 38: 291–300.

Chevrier A, Hoemann CD, Sun J, Buschmann MD. 2007. Chitosaneglycerol phosphate/blood implants increase cell recruitment, transient vascularization and subchondral bone remodeling in drilled cartilage defects. OsteoArthr and Cartilage 15: 316–327.

Cho JH, Kim SH, Park KD, Jung MC, Yang WI, Han SW, Noh JY, Lee JW. 2004. Chondrogenic differentiation of human mesenchymal stem cells using athermosensitive poly(N-isopropylacrylamide) and water-soluble chitosan copolymer. Biomaterials 25: 5743–5751.

Cohn D, Lando G, Sosnik A, Garty S, Levi A. 2006. PEO-PPO-PEO-based poly (ether ester urethane)s as degradable reverse thermo-responsive multiblock copolymers. Biomaterials 27: 1718–1727.

Coviello T, Matricardi P, Marianecci C, Alhaique F. 2007. Polysaccharide hydrogels for modified release formulations. J of Control Release 119: 5–24.

Crescenzi V, Cornelio L, Di Meo C, Nardecchia S, Lamanna R. 2007. Novel hydrogels via click chemistry: synthesis and potential biomedical applications. Biomacromolecules 8: 1844–1850.

Cushing MC, Anseth KS, Melinda C. 2007. Hydrogel Cell Cultures. Science 316: 1133–1134.

Dang JM, Sun DD, Shin-Ya Y, Sieber AN, Kostuik JP, Leong KW. 2006. Temperature-responsive hydroxybutyl chitosan for the culture of mesenchymal stem cells and inter-vertebral disk cells. Biomaterials 27:406–418.

Davis KA, Burdick JA, Anseth KS. 2003. Photoinitiated crosslinked degradable copoly-mer networks for tissue engineering applications. Biomaterials 24: 2485–2495.

Davis ME, Motion JP, Narmoneva DA, Takahashi T, Hakuno D, Kamm RD, Zhang S, Lee RT. 2005. Injectable self-assembling peptide nanofibers create intramyocardial microenvironments for endothelial cells. Circulation 1:442–450.

Elisseeff J, Anseth K, Sims D, McIntosh W, Randolph M, Langer R. Transdermal photo-polymerization for minimally invasive implantation. 1999. In: Proceedings of the Na-tional Academy of Sciences of the United States of America: p 3104–3107.

Elisseeff J, McIntosh W, Fu K, Blunk BT, Langer R. 2001. Controlled-release of IGF-I and TGF-beta1 in a photopolymerizing hydrogel for cartilage tissue engineering. J Orthop Res 19: 1098–1104.

Fischel-Ghodsian F, Brown L, Mathiowitz E, Brandenburg D, Langer R. 1988. Enzymati-cally Controlled Drug Delivery. In: Proceedings of the National Academy of Sciences of the United States of America: 2403–2406.

Fisher JP, Dean D, Engel PS, Mikos AG. 2001. Photoinitiated polymerization of bio-materials, Annu Rev Mater Res 31: 171–181.

Fisher JP, Jo S, Mikos AG, Reddi AH. 2004. Thermoreversible hydrogel scaffolds for articu-lar cartilage engineering. J Biomed Mater Res A 71: 268–274.

Gupta D, Tator CH, Shoichet MS. 2006. Fast-gelling injectable blend of hyaluronan and methylcellulose for intrathecal, localized delivery to the injured spinal cord. Biomaterials 27: 2370–2379.

Haines LA, Rajagopal K, Ozbas B, Salick DA, Pochan DJ, Schneider JP. 2005. Light activated hydrogel formation via the triggered folding and self-assembly of a designed peptide. J Am Chem Soc 127: 17025–17029.

Hoemann CD, Hurtig M, Rossomacha E, Sun J, Chevrier A, Shive MS, Buschmann MD. 2005. Chitosaneglycerol phosphate/blood implants improve hyaline cartilage repair cartilage in ovine microfracture defects. J Bone Joint Surg Am 87: 2671–2686.

Hoemann CD, Sun J, McKee MD, Chevrier A, Rossomacha E, Rivard GE, Hurtig M, Buschmann MD. 2007. Chitosaneglycerol phosphate/blood implants elicit hyaline cartilage repair integrated with porous subchondral bone in microdrilled rabbit defects. Osteoarthr Cartilage 15: 78–89.

Hoffman AS. 1991. Environmentally sensitive polymers and hydrogels. MSR Bulletin 16:42–46.

Hoffman AS. 2002. Hydrogels for biomedical applications. Adv Drug Deliver Rev 54: 3–12.

Holland TA, Bodde EW, Baggett LS, Tabata Y, Mikos AG, Jansen JA. 2005. Osteochondral repair in the rabbit model utilizing bilayered, degradable oligo(poly(ethylene glycol) fumarate) hydrogel scaffolds. J Biomed Mater Res 75: 156–167.

Holland TA, Bodde EW, Cuijpers VM, Baggett LS, Tabata Y, Mikos AG, Jansen JA. 2007. Degradable hydrogel scaffolds for in vivo delivery of single and dual growth factors in cartilage repair. Osteoarthr Cartilage 15: 187–197.

Holmes TC, De Lacalle S, Su X, Liu G, Rich A, Zhang S. 2000. Extensive neurite outgrowth and active synapse formation on self-assembling peptide scaffolds. Proc Natl Acad Sci USA 6:6728–6733.

Hwang NS, Varghese S, Zhang Z, Elisseeff J. 2006. Chondrogenic differentiation of human embryonic stem cell-derived cells in arginine-glycine-aspartate-modified hydrogels. Tissue Eng 12: 2695–2706.

Ishihara M, Nakanishi K, Ono K, Sato M, Kikuchi M, Saito Y, Yura H, Matsui T, Hattori H, Uenoyama M, Kurita A. 2002. Photocrosslinkable chitosan as a dressing for wound occlusion and accelerator in healing process. Biomaterials 23: 833–840.

Ito T, Yeo Y, Highley CB, Bellas E, Kohane DS. 2007. Dextran-based in situ cross-linked injectable hydrogels to prevent peritoneal adhesions. Biomaterials 28: 3418–3426.

Jeong BM, Lee DS, Bae YH, Kim SW. 2000. In situ gelation of PEG-PLGA-PEG triblock copolymer aqueous solutions and degradation thereof. J Biomed Mater Res 50: 171–177.

Jin R, Hiemstra C, Zhong Z, Feijen J. 2007. Enzyme-mediated fast in situ formation of hydrogels from dextran-tyramine conjugates. Biomaterials 28: 2791–2800.

Kang GD, Cheon SH, Khang G, Song SC. 2006a. Thermosensitive poly(organophosphazene) hydrogels for a controlled drug delivery. Eur J Pharm Biopharm 63: 340–346.

Kang GD, Cheon SH, Song SC. 2006b. Controlled release of doxorubicin from thermosensitive poly(organophosphazene) hydrogels. Int J Pharm 319: 29–36.

Kim H, Cohen RE, Hammond PE, Irvine DJ. 2006. Live Lymphocyte Arrays for Biosensing. Adv Func Mater 16: 1313–1323.

Kim MS, Choi YJ, Noh I, Tae G. 2007. Synthesis and characterization of in situ chitosan based hydrogel via grafting of carboxyethyl acrylate. J Biomed Mater Res A. 2007 May 25;

Kobayashi S, Uyama H, Kimura S. 2001. Enzymatic polymerization. Chem Rev 101: 3793–3818.

Kopecek J. 2002. Swell gels. Nature 417: 388–391.

Kurisawa M, Terano M, Yui N. 1995. Doublestimuli-responsive degradable hydrogels for drug-delivery—interpenetrating polymer networks composed of oligopeptide-terminated poly(ethylene glycol) and dextran. Macromol Rapid Commun 6: 663–666.

Kurisawa M, Chung JE, Yang YY, Gao SJ, Uyama H. 2005. Injectable biodegradable hydrogels composed of hyaluronicnacid-tyramine conjugates for drug delivery and tissue engineering. Chem Commun 34: 4312–4314.

Leach JB, Bivens KA, Patrick CW, Schmidt CE. 2003. Photocrosslinked hyaluronic acid hydrogels: natural, biodegradable tissue engineering scaffolds. Biotechnol Bioeng 82: 578–89.

Lee HJ, Lee JS, Chansakul T, Yu C, Elisseeff JH, Yu SM. 2006. Collagen mimetic peptide conjugated photopolymerizable PEG hydrogel. Biomaterials 27: 5268–5276.

Lee S, Tae G. 2007. Formulation and in vitro characterization of an *in situ* gelable, photo polymerizable Pluoronic hydrogel suitable for injection. J Controlled Release 119: 313–319.

Liu Y, Lu W, Wang JC, Zhang X, Zhang H, Wang X, Zhou T, Zhang Q. 2007. Controlled delivery of recombinant hirudin based on thermo-sensitive Pluoronic F127 hydrogel for subcutaneous administration: in vitro and in vivo characterization. J Control Rel 117: 387–395.

Lu S, Anseth KS. 1999. Photopolymerization of multilaminated poly(HEMA) hydrogels for controlled release. J Control Release 57: 291–300.

Lutolf MP, Hubbell JA. 2003. Synthesis and physicochemical characterization of end linked poly(ethylene glycol)-co-peptide hydrogels formed by Michael-type addition. Biomacromolecules 4: 713–22.

Lutolf MP, Hubbell JA. 2005. Synthetic biomaterials as instructive extracellular microenvironments for morphogenesis in tissue engineering. Nat Biotechnol 23: 47.

Lutolf MP, Raeber GP, Zisch AH, Tirelli N, Hubbell JA. 2003. Cellresponsive synthetic hydrogels. Adv Mater 5: 888–892.

Mahoney MJ, Anseth KS. 2006. Three-dimensional growth and function of neural tissue in degradable polyethylene glycol hydrogels. Biomaterials 27: 2265–2274.

Masters KS, Shah DN, Leinwand LA, Anseth KS. 2005. Crosslinked hyaluronan scaffolds as a biologically active carrier for valvular interstitial cells. Biomaterials 26: 2517–2525.

McHale MK, Setton LA, Chilkoti A. 2005. Synthesis and in vitro evaluation of enzymatically cross-linked elastin-like polypeptide gels for cartilaginous tissue repair. Tissue Eng 11: 1768–1779.

Nair LS, Laurencin CT. Methods for regulating gelation of polysaccharide solutions and uses thereof. International patent applied January, 2007.

Nair LS, Sterns T, Ko J, Laurencin CT. 2007. Development of Injectable thermogelling chitosaninorganic phosphate solutions for biomedical applications Biomacromolecules 8(12):3779–3785, 2007.

Nagai Y, Unsworth LD, Koutsopoulos S, Zhang S. 2006. Slow release of molecules in selfassembling peptide nanofiber scaffold. J Control Release. 115:18–25.

Nettles DL, Vail TP, Morgan MT, Grinstaff MW, Sefton LA. 2004. Photocrosslinkable hyaluronan as a scaffold for articular cartilage repair. Ann Biomed Eng 32:391–397.

Nuttelman CR, Tripodi MC, Anseth KS. 2005. Synthetic hydrogel niches that promote hMSC viability. Matrix Biol 24: 208–218.

Obara K, Ishihara M, Ishizuka T, Fujita M, Ozeki Y, Maehara T, Saito Y, Yura H, Matsui T, Hattori H, Kikuchi M, Kurita A. 2003. Photocrosslinkable chitosan hydrogel containing fibroblast growth factor-2 stimulates wound healing in healing-impaired db/db mice. Biomaterials 24: 3437–3444.

Ohya S, Matsuda T. 2005. Poly (N-isopropylacrylamide) (PNIPAM)-grafted gelatin as thermoresponsive three-dimensional artificial extracellular matrix: molecular and formulation parameters vs. cell proliferation potential. J Biomater Sci Polym Ed 16: 809–827.

Ono K, Saito Y, Yura H, Ishikawa K, Akaike T, Kurita A, Ishihara M. 2000. Photocrosslinkable chitosan as a biological adhesive. J Biomed Mater Res 49: 289–295.

Park H, Temenoff JS, Holland TA, Tabata Y, Mikos AG. 2005. Delivery of TGF-beta1 and chondrocytes via injectable, biodegradable hydrogels for cartilage tissue engineering applications. Biomaterials 26: 7095–7103.

Park H, Temenoff JS, Tabata Y, Caplan AI, Mikos AG. 2007. Injectable biodegradable hydrogel composites for rabbit marrow mesenchymal stem cell and growth factor delivery for cartilage tissue engineering. Biomaterials 28: 3217–3222.

Park KH, Song SC. 2006. Morphology of spheroidal hepatocytes within injectable, biodegradable and thermosensitive poly(organophosphazene) hydrogel as cell delivery vehicle. J Biosci Bioeng 101: 238–242.

Peppas NA, Sahlin JJ. 1996. Hydrogels as mucoadhesive and bioadhesive materials: a review. Biomaterials 17: 1553–1561.

Quick DJ, Anseth KS. 2003. Gene delivery in tissue engineering: a photopolymer platform to coencapsulate cells and plasmid DNA. Pharm Res 20: 1730–1737.

Quick DJ, Anseth KS. 2004. DNA delivery from photocrosslinked PEG hydrogels: Encapsulation efficiency, Release profiles and DNA quality. J Control Release 96:341–351.

Ratner BD. 2004. Biomaterials Science: An Introduction to Materials in Medicine, 2nd ed., London: Elsevier/Academic Press.

Rice MA, Anseth KS. 2004. Encapsulating chondrocytes in copolymer gels: bimodal degradation kinetics influence cell phenotype and extracellular matrix development. J Biomed Mater Res 70: 560–568.

Ruel-Gariepy E, Leroux JC. 2004. *In situ* forming hydrogels—review of temperature sensitive systems. Eur J Pharm Biopharm 58: 409–426.

Rydholm AE, Bowman CN, Anseth KS. 2005. Degradable thiol-acrylate photopolymers: polymerization and degradation behavior of an *in situ* forming biomaterial. Biomaterials 26: 4495–4506.

Salinas CN, Cole BB, Kasko AM, Anseth KS. 2007. Chondrogenic differentiation potential of human mesenchymal stem cells photoencapsulated within poly(ethylene glycol)-arginine-glycine-aspartic acid-serine thiol-methacrylate mixed-mode networks. Tissue Eng 13: 1025–1034.

Sanborn TJ, Messersmith PB, Barron AE. 2002. *In situ* crosslinking of a biomimetic peptide-PEG hydrogel via thermally triggered activation of factor XIII. Biomaterials 23: 2703–2710.

Sawhney AS, Pathak CP, Hubbell JA. 1993. Bioerodible hydrogels based on photopolymerized poly(ethylene glycol)-co-poly (alpha-hydroxy acid) diacrylate macromers. Macromolecules 6: 581–587.

Semino CE, Merok JR, Crane GG, Panagiotakos G, Zhang S. 2003. Functional differentiation of hepatocyte-like spheroid structures from putative liver progenitor cells in thres-dimensional peptide scaffolds. Differentiation. 71:262–270.

Schild HG. 1992. Poly(N-isopropylacrylamide): experiment, theory and application. Prog Polym Sci 17: 163–249.

Sharma B, Williams CG, Khan M, Manson P, Elisseeff JH. 2007a. *In vivo* chondrogenesis of mesenchymal stem cells in a photopolymerized hydrogel. Plast Reconstr Surg 119: 112–120.

Sharma B, Williams CG, Kim TK, Sun D, Malik A, Khan M, Leong K, Elisseeff JH. 2007b. Designing zonal organization into tissue-engineered cartilage. Tissue Eng 13: 405–414.

Shoichet MS, Tator CH, Poon P, Kang C, Douglas Baumann M. 2007. Intrathecal drug delivery strategy is safe and efficacious for localized delivery to the spinal cord. Prog Brain Res 161: 385–392.

Shu XZ, Ahmad S, Liu Y, Prestwich GD. 2006. Synthesis and evaluation of injectable, *in situ* crosslinkable synthetic extracellular matrices for tissue engineering. J Biomed Mater Res 79: 902–912.

Sofia SJ, Singh A, Kaplan DL. 2002. Peroxidase-catalyzed cross-linking of functionalized polyaspartic acid and polymers. J Macromol Sci-Pure Appl Chem A 39: 1151–1181.

Sperinde JJ, Griffith LG. 1997. Synthesis and characterization of enzymaticaly corss-linked poly(ethylene glycol) hydrogels. Macromolecules 30: 5255–5264.

Stabenfeldt SE, Garcia AJ, LaPlaca MC. 2006. Thermoreversible lamininfunctionalized hydrogel for neural tissue engineering. J Biomed Mater Res 77A: 718–725.

Ulijin RV, Bibi N, Jayawarna V, Thornton PD, Todd SJ, Mart RJ, Smith AM, Gough JE. 2007. Bioresponsive hydrogels. Materials Today 10: 40–48.

Vernon B, Tirelli N, Bachi T, Haldimann D, Hubbell JA. 2003. Waterborne, *in situ* crosslinked biomaterials from phase-segregated precursors. J Biomed Mater Res 64: 447–456.

Wang DA, Varghese S, Sharma B, Strehin I, Fermanian S, Gorham J, Fairbrother DH, Cascio B, Elisseeff JH. 2007. Multifunctional chondroitin sulphate for cartilage tissue-biomaterial integration. Nat Mater 6:327–328.

West JL, Hubbell JA. 1999. Polymeric biomaterials with degradation sites for proteases involved in cell migration. Macromolecules 32: 241–244.

Wichterle O, Lim D. 1960. Hydrophilic gels for Biological use. Nature 185:117–118.

Williams CG, Malik AN, Kim TK, Manson PN, Elisseeff JH. 2005. Variable cytocompatibility of six cell lines with photoinitiators used for polymerizing hydrogels and cell encapsulation. Biomaterials 26: 1211–1218.

Sohn YS, Kim JK, Song R, Jeong B. 2004. The relationship of thermosensitive properties with structure of organophosphazenes. Polymer 45: 3081–3084.

Yeo Y, Adil M, Bellas E, Astashkina A, Chaudhary N, Kohane DS. 2007a. Prevention of peritoneal adhesions with an *in situ* cross-linkable hyaluronan hydrogel delivering budesonide. J Control Release 120: 178–185.

Yeo Y, Bellas E, Highley CB, Langer R, Kohane DS. 2007b. Peritoneal adhesion prevention with an *in situ* cross-linkable hyaluronan gel containing tissue-type plasminogen activator in a rabbit repeated-injury model. Biomaterials. 28: 3704–3713.

Zhang S. 2003. Fabrication of novel biomaterials through molecular self-assembly. Nat Biotechnol 21:1171–1178.

Zhang S. 2004. Hydrogels: Wet or let die. Nat Mater 3: 7–8.

Zheng Y, Andreopoulos FM, Micic M, Huo Q, Pham SM, Leblanc RM. 2001. A Novel Photoscissile Poly(ethylene glycol)-Based Hydrogel. Adv Funct Mater 11: 37–40.

7

NANOMATERIALS FOR IMPROVED ORTHOPEDIC AND BONE TISSUE ENGINEERING APPLICATIONS

Lijie Zhang, Sirinrath Sirivisoot,
Ganesh Balasundaram, and Thomas J. Webster

*Divisions of Engineering and Orthopedics, Brown University,
Providence, Rhode Island*

Contents

7.1 Overview	206
7.2 Introduction	206
7.2.1 Problems With the Current Orthopedic Implants	207
7.2.2 Reasons for Implant Failures	207
7.2.2.1 Loosening of the Implant	208
7.2.2.2 Osteolysis	210
7.2.2.3 Other Complications (Wear of Articulating Surfaces, Fractures, etc.)	212
7.3 Nanomaterials for Improved Orthopedic and Bone Tissue Engineering Applications	212
7.3.1 Nanostructured Ceramics	213
7.3.1.1 Special Surface Properties of Nanophase Ceramics for Improved Orthopedic Implants	213
7.3.1.2 Enhanced Mechanical Properties of Nanophase Ceramics	217
7.3.2 Nanostructured Metals	220
7.3.3 Nanostructured Polymers	223
7.3.3.1 Nanostructured Biodegradable Polymers as Bone Tissue Engineering Scaffolds	223

Advanced Biomaterials: Fundamentals, Processing, and Applications, Edited by Bikramjit Basu,
Dhirendra S. Katti, and Ashok Kumar
Copyright © 2009 The American Ceramic Society

7.3.3.2 Nanostructured and Injectable Hydrogels as Bone Tissue
Engineering Scaffolds   225
7.3.4 Nanostructured Composites   226
7.3.5 Role of Chemistry   228
7.4 Future Challenges   231
References   233

7.1 OVERVIEW

With the strikingly increasing number of elderly patients and the relatively high percentage of orthopedic revision procedures performed around the world, conventional materials which have many shortcomings cannot satisfy the high requirements necessary for current orthopedic implants. Novel nanomaterials with basic structures below 100 nm exhibit superior mechanical, cytocompatibility and electrical properties over conventional micron-materials, thus potentially serving as improved orthopedic implants. To date, a wide range of nanostructured ceramics, metals, polymers, organic materials and composites have been investigated and have shown promise towards lowering the rate of implant failures by promoting early, quick osseointegration. Thus, due to the potentially numerous applications of nanomaterials as orthopedic implants and other tissue engineering applications, they have been proposed as the next generation of improved tissue growing materials. This chapter will give an overview of contemporary developments of various nanomaterials for improved orthopedic and bone tissue engineering applications.

7.2 INTRODUCTION

As an emerging interdisciplinary field, bone tissue engineering has evoked increasing interest from scientists wishing to develop biological substitutes that restore, maintain, or improve bone cell functions. It is widely known that natural bone is a well-organized matrix that consists of a protein-based soft hydrogel template (i.e., collagen) and hard inorganic components—specifically, hydroxyapatite. The special structure of natural bone supplies unique physical properties (such as Young's modulus, elasticity, and strength) in order to support various mechanical loading [1]. Novel biomaterials that biomimic the nano-structure of natural bone have, thus, been investigated and have shown promise as improved orthopedic implants.

In the following sections, the problems with current orthopedic implants will be introduced. Then, the main part of this chapter will focus on a variety of nanomaterials (nanostructured ceramics, metals, polymers, composites, and so on) that have been tested for better orthopedic implant efficacy. Important future research directions concerning nanomaterials will be presented in the last section.

7.2.1   Problems With the Current Orthopedic Implants

With the rapid development of orthopedic implant technology, various bone implant surgeries and procedures (such as for healing bone fractures, repairing defects, and inserting hip and knee replacements) are routinely performed. The first hip replacement was conducted in 1923. However, the most significant breakthrough happened in the 1960s with the introduction of the ultra-low friction cemented arthroplasty by John Charnley [2,3]. Since then, as one of the most important surgery advances of last century, this orthopedic implant technology has rescued a myriad of people suffering intense pain and limited mobility from arthritis. The American Academy of Orthopedic Surgeons reported that in the United States alone, in just a four-year period, there was a 19.7% increase in hip replacements performed from nearly 274,000 procedures in 1999 (including 168,000 total hip replacements and 106,000 partial hip replacements) to 328,000 procedures in 2003 (including 220,000 total hip replacements and 108,000 partial hip replacements) [4]. The total number of hip replacements is projected to almost double by 2030 to 272,000 procedures [4], a staggering number as well as a trend unavoidably accompanied by increasing hospitalization costs.

Although orthopedic implants have become more successful over the recent decades, it is important to note that current orthopedic implant technology has not been perfected. While 90% of hip and knee replacements can last ten to fifteen years on average, and implant joints for some patients have endured for more than 20 years with no problems, occasionally hip or knee replacement implants may fail immediately after surgery [5]. Considering the endurance of current orthopedic implants, younger and more active patients (men under 60-years-old and women under 55-years-old) will inevitably need more than one revision surgery in their lives. For example, in the United States, nearly 11% of hip replacements (36,000 revisions for 328,000 replacements) and 8% of knee replacements (33,000 revisions for 418,000 replacements) were revision procedures of previously failed hip and knee replacements in 2003 [5]. A similar trend occurs in other industrialized countries as well. Due to the strikingly increasing number of patients who need various medical implants and the relatively high percentage of revision procedures performed around the world, it is urgent to develop a new generation of orthopedic implant technology and a set of materials that can significantly lengthen the service lifetime of orthopedic implants and, thus, dramatically reduce patient pain and health insurance costs.

7.2.2   Reasons for Implant Failures

Many reasons can lead to implant failures. For example, in the early stage of implant surgery, many acute complications, severe host responses (such as infection and inflammation), prosthesis dislocations, and surgery failures (such as improper placement and cement extrusion) may lead to implant failure [6]. After several years, various additional reasons including implant loosening, osteolysis (softening of the bone tissue), wear of articulating surfaces and biomaterial fracture become the main reasons necessitating revision surgery [6]. In other words, based on clinical data collected by the Canadian Joint Replacement Registry (CJRR) in 2004, the most common reasons for revision of a total hip replacement were loosening of the implant (55%), followed by osteolysis (33%), implant wear and tear (30%), instability/dislocation (17%), bone and implant fracture (12%), and infection (10%) [7]. Since some patients have more than one reason necessitating orthopedic implant revision surgery, the aforementioned percentages do not add up to 100%.

7.2.2.1 Loosening of the Implant.
Generally, one crucial criterion for the long-term success of orthopedic implants is the forming of sufficient bonding of the implant to juxtaposed bone—a process known as osseointegration which was initially described as a direct structural and functional bone-to-implant contact under load by Per-Ingvar Branemark [8]. Osseointegration plays an important role in minimizing the motion-induced damage to surrounding tissues. Insufficient bonding to juxtaposed bone may lead to a mismatch of mechanical properties between implant materials and surrounding bone tissues [9].

As a result, a variety of implant-loosening conditions originating from stress and strain imbalances may frequently take place. Several factors such as surface roughness of the fixture, overloading and infection [10,11] can be related to loss of acquired osseointegration and even failure of osseointegration. Most commonly, surface properties of implant materials have been intimately related to the success of osseointegration between an endosseous implant and bone. There are numerous studies elucidating that surface roughness of implant materials affects the rate of osseointegration and biomechanical fixation [12–17]. Since traditional orthopedic implant materials have been chosen based on their mechanical properties and biological inertness, there has not been enough concern about their chemical structure and surface properties. Thus, loosening of implants (such as for the socket or femoral component) has been frequently observed when conventional micron-structured materials are used in total hip replacements.

On the other hand, the formation of a fibrous soft tissue capsule which originates from excessive secretion of fibrous tissue from inflammatory cells is another vital factor that leads to insufficient osseointegration and eventually causes loosening of implants (Figure 7.1) [9,19].

After implanting biomaterials into a surgical site, it is inevitable to damage the surrounding tissue and cause injury. Then, various host responses such as infection and inflammation are triggered (Figure 7.1). Initially, neutrophils and macrophages arrive at the injury site and begin to attempt to phagocytose the implant material; when they fail to engulf this large mass, they fuse together to form giant cells and interrogate again the implant to wall it off from the surrounding tissue. At the same time, giant cells send out chemical messengers (cytokines) to recruit other cells to "help" them. In response to cytokines, fibroblasts (which are in charge of secreting and synthesizing collagen into the extracellular matrix comprising the soft tissue capsule [18]) arrive and generate a collagen capsule, the first sign of a new tissue. The final stage of the process is

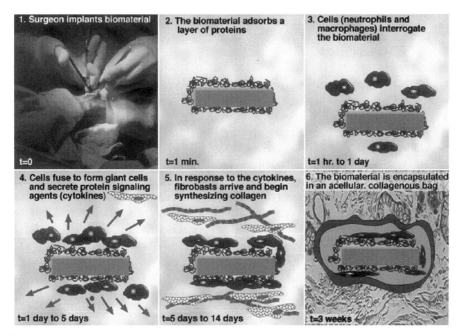

Figure 7.1. The foreign body reaction towards implanted biomaterials. 1) A biomaterial is implanted and damage to surrounding tissue occurs. 2) In seconds to minutes, non-specific proteins from body fluids are adsorbed on the implant surface. 3) Neutrophils and macrophages try to interrogate the material. 4) Failing to interrogate the material, cells fuse to form giant cells and concurrently secrete cytokines to signal other kinds of cells. 5) and 6) Fibroblasts arrive and fabricate a collagenous bag to insulate the material from the surrounding tissue. Fig. adapted from [19].

that the implant is completely encapsulated in an acellular, avascular collagen bag about 50–200 micrometers thick [19]. The fibrous capsule prevents sufficient bonding between an implant surface and juxtaposed bone and frequently leads to clinical failure of orthopedic implants. Consequently, repelling fibroblasts that can cause an inflammatory reaction is necessary at the surface of a newly implanted orthopedic device [9]. Controlling protein adsorption by surface modification is an effective method for attracting desirable cells onto the implant surface and minimizing the functions of fibroblasts, such as their adhesion and secretion of fibrous tissue [9,20].

Therefore, numerous research efforts in bone tissue engineering have focused on surface modification (or altering the implant surface topography and chemistry of implant materials, including the development of novel nanophase materials "that is, materials with basic structural units, grains, particles, fibers or other constituent components in the range of 1–100 nm [42]" such as nanophase metals, ceramics, and polymers, and so on. These materials have been critical in the overall design and synthesis of bone-like composites which possess not only mechanical properties similar to those of physiological bone but also cytocompatible surface properties in order to more successfully promote cell adhesion and tissue integration [21–23],

7.2.2.2 Osteolysis. As a late-appearing complication, osteolysis induced by wear particles of implant materials has been regarded as one of the most common complications and the leading reasons for revision surgery after primary replacement [26–29]. It can cause severe bone loss which eventually results in implant instability and failure. Metals, ceramics and polymers (such as polyethylene, a material used for acetabular components in hip replacements) are widely accepted as a source of prosthetic particles and serve as a major contributor to bone resorption. These wear particles appear most commonly at the bearing surface, but are also at host-implant or implant-implant interfaces. Figure 7.2 shows the osteolysis process caused by biomaterial wear debris.

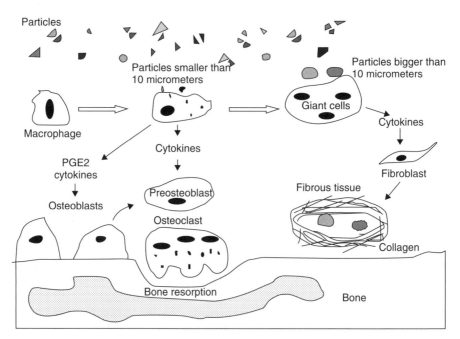

Figure 7.2. Schematic of biomaterial wear debris activating macrophages and inducing osteolysis. Particulate debris is generated from wear of arthroplasty components, metal corrosion or polymer degradation. Particles <10μm are engulfed directly by macrophages but can not be digested easily. Consequently, macrophages begin to release interleukins (IL-1, IL-6), prostaglandin E_2 (PGE$_2$), and tumor necrosis factors (TNF) which then mediates bone resorption via osteoclasts [29]. On the other hand, macrophages form giant cells to phagocytose large particles (>10μm) and then secrete cytokines to signal fibroblasts to synthesize collagen to result in a fibrous tissue capsule around the implant. Redrawn from [24,25]. It remains to be seen what happens when particles are less than 100nm (in non agglomerated form).

Macrophages are believed to play a key role during osteolysis (shown in Figure 7.1). But there exists a critical number of active macrophages necessary for osteolysis since only one disturbed macrophage and its neighboring osteoclast would not cause osteolysis. For instance, clinical experience indicates that osteolysis cannot happen if the wear rate of the polyethylene cup is below 0.05 mm per year. In contrast, osteolysis frequently occurs if the wear rate exceeds 0.2 mm per year [30]. Moreover, studies have also illustrated that there exists a critical size for bioactive particles that can trigger cellular responses and finally result in osteolysis. Macrophages have evolved to detect and phagocytose bioactive particles in the size range of 0.5–10 μm. Particles larger than 10 μm or less than 0.5 μm are relatively less active for macrophages. Particles larger than 10 μm will cause giant cell responses which lead to the formation of fibrous tissue (see details in 7.2.2.1) without osteolysis. In addition, particles with sharp edges are more active than spherical particles [20,29].

It is apparent that minimizing the generation of wear particles in the interfacial tissues is a basic approach to preventing osteolysis. Therefore, there has been much effort to design alternative wear-resistant bearing materials in order to reduce the production of wear particles from the bearing area. The metal-on-metal, ceramic-on-ceramic or ceramic-on-polyethylene implants have been developed to prevent osteolysis and have been shown to produce less wear particles in vitro or in vivo than the conventional metal-on-polyethylene materials [138–139]. For example, a five-year prospective randomized study in the U.S. revealed that osteolysis greatly decreased from 14.0% of patients with metal-on-polyethylene bearings to 1.4% patients with alumina-on-alumina ceramic bearings [139]. In addition, a variety of nanocomposites (such as zirconia-toughened alumina nanocomposites [140], ceria-stabilized tetragonal zirconia–alumina nanocomposites [141] or hydroxyapatite coated ceria-stabilized tetragonal zirconia–alumina nanocomposites [142]) have shown promise as bearing materials with excellent cytocompatibility and low wear rates. Furthermore, metal-on-metal bearings also exhibit low wear rates (such as 0.004 mm per year compared with 0.1 mm per year for polyethylene [138]).

But there still exists many concerns about the generation of metal implant ions or corrosion for metal combinations, which may lead to implant failure in the long term. Recent studies reported that special surface coatings (i.e., TiN, CrN or diamond-like carbon coatings) on titanium alloys may improve the performance of metal-on-metal bearings [143–144]. Moreover, except designing novel artificial joint materials with more wear-resistant features, there are other possible strategies that may address the problem of osteolysis, including preventing debris from accessing the bone-implant interface through extensive bone growth and, thus, decreasing cellular reaction to such wear debris [26].

Some preliminary results of the effects of nanoparticle wear debris on osteoblasts and on other cells have been reported [31–33]; such studies showed a less adverse effect on osteoblast viability for nano compared to micro particle wear debris. Although the effects of nanoparticulate wear debris at the bone-implant interface are not totally understood, to date, the biologically-inspired features of nanomaterials has motivated wide investigation for their applications in orthopedic implants. Further investigation of the influence of nanoparticulate wear debris on bone cell health is necessary to effectively minimize osteolysis as well as fully realize the benefits of nanotechnology in orthopedic implant/applications [34,35].

7.2.2.3   Other Complications (Wear of Articulating Surfaces, Fractures, etc.).

The relative motion of some orthopedic implants is impossible to avoid and the resulting mechanical load is extremely large (especially at the articulating surface of hip or knee implants). The more active and young the patients receiving orthopedic implants, the higher the risk of articulating bearing surface wear and periprosthetic fractures [36]. In fact, wear of articulating bearing surfaces has commonly evoked our attention. From the basic mechanical viewpoint, adhesive wear, abrasive wear, third body wear, wear fatigue and corrosion are five major mechanisms causing wear of articulating bearing surfaces [37]. Modification of polyethylene and substitution of metal-metal or ceramic-ceramic bearings for polyethylene may both help to improve the wear-resistant property of implant materials.

Several investigations have revealed that periprosthetic femoral fractures accompanied with total hip replacements are more common after revision surgeries than after primary replacements [40,41]. So with the increasing number of revision surgeries, it is expected that periprosthetic femoral fractures will become more common than before. Since mechanical properties (including strength, toughness, and ductility) of implant materials are closely related to the above complications and have influences on the long-term success of an orthopedic implant, synthesizing various orthopedic implant materials which biomimic the mechanical properties of natural bone is rather desirable.

It should be realized that each previously mentioned complication for orthopedic implants are widely related to each other. That is, the high rate of implant fractures is usually accompanied by a loose implant [38,39]; loosening of implants can also be caused by osteolysis or inflammation; wear particle generation (see section 7.2.2.2) and inflection [5] often coexist with wear of articulating surfaces. Therefore, reducing the influence of one complication may have positive effects on preventing other complications and finally improving the long-term success of orthopedic implants.

7.3   NANOMATERIALS FOR IMPROVED ORTHOPEDIC AND BONE TISSUE ENGINEERING APPLICATIONS

Nanomaterials are materials with basic structural units, grains, particles, fibers or other constituent components in the range of 1–100 nm [42]. Compared to respective conventional micron-scale materials, they can exhibit enhanced mechanical properties, cytocompatibility, and electrical properties which make them suitable for orthopedic implants. Next, the research investigating the use of nanomaterials in the orthopedic tissue engineering fields is extensively reviewed.

7.3.1   Nanostructured Ceramics

Ceramics are non-metallic inorganic materials which have excellent cytocompatibility and possibly biodegradability properties in the physiological environment that makes them attractive for orthopedic applications. For these reasons, they have been widely adopted as orthopedic implants (known as bioceramics for several decades). According to the tissue response in an osseous environment, bioceramics can be classified in three groups: bioactive ceramics (such as hydroxyapatite (HA), tricalcium phosphate (TCP), bioglasses, HA/TCP bi-phase ceramics, and glass-ceramics); biopassive ceramics (such as alumina, titania and zirconia); and biodegradable ceramics (such as TCP).

Although traditional bioceramics have long served as bone substitutes and filler materials, structural forms, and surface coatings in orthopedic applications [43], there often exists a variety of implant failures due to insufficient osseointegration, osteolysis, as well as implant wear (see section 7.2.2). There are many reasons to use nanophase ceramics to overcome these traditional implant failures. As we know, 70% of the human bone matrix is composed of inorganic crystalline hydroxyapatite which is typically 20–80 nm long and 2–5 nm thick [18]. Additionally, other components in the bone matrix (such as collagen and noncollagenous proteins (laminin, fibronectin, vitronectin)) are nanometer-scale in dimension [9]. Therefore, novel nanophase ceramics (grain sizes less than 100 nm in diameter) which biomimic the nanostructure of natural bone have become quite popular in orthopedics. Present researchers have shown that nanostructured alumina, titania, ZnO and HA can greatly enhance osteoblast adhesion and promote calcium/phosphate mineral deposition [14–16,44–48]. It is believed that the special surface topography, increased wettability and better mechanical properties of nanoceramics may contribute to enhanced osteoblast functions. Obviously nanostructured ceramics may become a new generation of more promising and efficient orthopedic material. In the following section, the advantages of various nanostructured ceramics compared to conventional ceramics will be discussed.

7.3.1.1   Special Surface Properties of Nanophase Ceramics for Improved Orthopedic Implants.   With decreased grain size as well as decreased pore diameter, nanophase ceramics have increased surface area, surface roughness (shown in Figure 7.3) and number of grain boundaries at the surface.

For example, from the results of extensive characterization studies (Table 7.1), increased surface roughness and improved surface wettability (decreased contact angles) are evident in nanophase compared to conventional alumina, HA and titania [16]. In the case of ZnO, atomic force microscopy (AFM) root-mean-square roughness values of nanophase and microphase ZnO were 32 and 10 nm, respectively [57]. Additionally, a 23 nm grain size alumina had approximately 50% more surface area for cell adhesion than that of a 177 nm grain size alumina; similarly, a 32 nm grain size titania had nearly 35% more surface area than that of a 2.12 μm grain size titania [14] while nanophase ZnO had 25% more surface area than that of microphase ZnO [57].

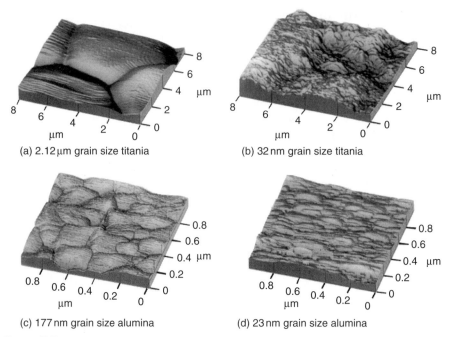

Figure 7.3. Atomic force microscopy images of titania and alumina. (a) and (c) represent conventional titania and alumina, respectively, and (b) and (d) represent nanophase titania and alumina, respectively. Adapted from [14].

TABLE 7.1. Nanophase and Conventional Ceramic Structure and Surface Wettability, Data is From [16]

Material	Porosity (%)	Pore diameter (nm)	Surface roughness (nm)	Contact angle (degrees)
24 nm alumina	4.5	0.69	20	6.4 ± 0.7
45 nm alumina	3.4	1.11	19	10.8 ± 1.3
167 nm alumina	2.4	2.94	17	18.6 ± 0.9
39 nm titania	4.1	0.98	32	2.2 ± 0.1
97 nm titania	3.8	1.91	24	18.1 ± 3.2
4520 nm titania	3.2	23.3	16	26.8 ± 2.8
67 nm HA	1.1	0.66	17	6.1 ± 0.5
132 nm HA	1.1	1.98	11	9.2 ± 0.4
179 nm HA	1.1	3.10	10	11.5 ± 1.1

In order to illustrate the advantages of nanophase ceramics in terms of surface properties for orthopedic applications, calcium phosphate derivatives are perfect examples—such as HA, tricalcium phosphate, calcium carbonate and bioglass which have extensive applications in orthopedic implants [49]. Since they share a similar crystal structure and chemical composition to natural bone, calcium phosphate ceramics have been considered the most popular coating materials on traditional implant metals as well as in pure form for bone graft substitutes. For example, HA and TCP (α- or β-crystalline) can serve as bone tissue engineering scaffolds to facilitate new bone formation and as a coating on femoral (metal) or socket (polymer) prostheses to inhibit complications related to osteolysis [50]. HA and TCP have a relatively high rate of degradation *in vivo* as well, making them promising in drug eluting biodegradable bone graft therapies.

Furthermore, HA has been shown to have good osteoconductive properties since their surfaces can undergo selective chemical reactivity with surrounding tissues, resulting in a tight bond between bone and the implant [51]. Thus, new bone formation will be promoted by such a bonded interface [52–53]. Moreover, it has been demonstrated that osseoinductivity of calcium phosphate ceramics is strongly related to their surface properties. Higher amounts of surface porosity, increased surface roughness and improved wettability of nanophase ceramics have positive effects on the osseointegration of calcium phosphate ceramics with juxtaposed bone. The nanometer-sized grains and high volume fraction of grain boundaries in nanostructured HA can increase osteoblast adhesion, proliferation, and mineralization [54]. For example, Webster et al. showed that there was significantly enhanced osteoblast adhesion and strikingly inhibited fibroblast adhesion on nanophase HA (67 nm) compared to conventional HA (179 nm HA) after four-hour cell culture studies [16].

Some *in vivo* studies also demonstrated that nanocrystalline HA can serve as an osteoconductive coating on tantalum scaffolds to accelerate new bone formation compared to uncoated or conventional micron size HA coated tantalum [131]. As shown in Figure 7.4, nanocrystalline HA coatings promote more new bone growth in the rat calvaria than that on uncoated and conventional HA coated tantalum after a six-week implantation time [131]. Apparently, the special surface properties of nanophase ceramics contribute to efficiently enhancing new bone growth regardless of whether the studies were conducted *in vitro* or *in vivo*.

In addition, enhanced osteoclast-like cell functions (such as synthesizing tartrate-resistant acid phosphatase (TRAP) and formation of resorption pits) on naophase HA have also been observed compared to conventional HA [46]. In contrast, decreased functions of fibroblasts have been observed on nanophase compared to conventional HA [46]. Since excessive secretion of fibrous tissue from fibroblasts causes the formation of a detrimental fibrous tissue capsule which can contribute to loosening of implants, decreased fibroblast functions on nanophase HA may contribute to a better bone-implant interface. Recently, a bioresorbable nano-crystalline HA paste was used as a valuable addition to TCP-HA ceramic granules for acetabular bone grafting in animal models. That study showed that the nano-crystalline HA paste resulted in better acetabular cup stability than the pure allografts and at the same time didn't cause adverse biological reactivity [55]. Histology slides of human cancellous bone revealed that the nano-crystalline HA paste appeared to be a suitable bone substitute for bone defects

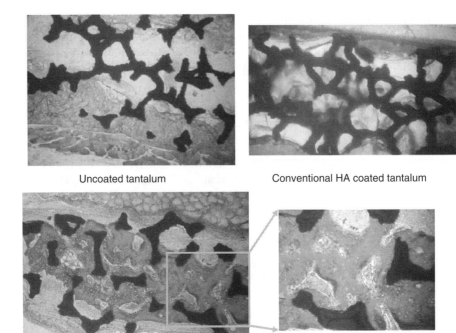

| Uncoated tantalum | Conventional HA coated tantalum |

| Nanocrystalline HA coated tantalum | Nanocrystalline HA coated tantalum |

Figure 7.4. Histology of rat calvaria after 6 weeks of implantation of uncoated tantalum, conventional HA coated tantalum and nanocrystalline HA coated tantalum. Greater amounts of new bone formation occurred in the rat calvaria with implanting nanocrystalline HA coated tantalum compared to uncoated and conventional HA coated tantalum. Red represents new mineralized bone and blue represents unmineralized tissue. Adapted and redrawn from [131]. (See color insert.)

or cavities since it showed good tissue incorporation, high biocompatibility and rapid osseointegration [56].

To demonstrate the versatility of nano ceramics, similar tendencies also appeared for nanophase alumina, zirconia and titania. A 51% increase in osteoblast adhesion and a 235% decrease in fibroblast adhesion in a four-hour period were observed on alumina as grain size decreased from 167 to 24 nm [16]. Moreover, osteoblast adhesion increased by 146% and 200% on nanophase zirconia (23 nm) and titania (32 nm) compared to microphase zirconia (4.9 µm) and titania (4.1 µm), respectively, when normalized to projected surface area [57]. Furthermore, increased collagen synthesis, alkaline phosphatase activity and calcium mineral deposition by osteoblasts were observed on nanophase zirconia, titania and alumina (theta + delta crystalline phase) compared to conventional equivalents [48,57].

To determine the role of nano ceramics in fighting implant infection, various bacteria functions were recently investigated on nanophase ceramics. For instance, *Staphylococcus epidermidis* (a common bacterium in human skin) forms a thick extracellular matrix and eventually a biofilm around bone implants [58], which leads to implant failure. Thus, decreased *Staphylococcus epidermidis* functions on implants are desirable. Nanophase zinc oxide and titania have indeed been observed to significantly inhibit *Staphylococcus epidermidis* functions [57].

It was elucidated that the special surface topography as well as wettability of nanophase ceramics may be the main reason for the promoted bone cell and inhibited bacteria functions on nanoceramics. At the tissue-implant interface, the first and necessary step for success is the adsorption of specific proteins. Many researchers have demonstrated that the protein adsorption process depends on surface properties (such as hydrophilicity, charge density, roughness, and surface energy) [60,61]. For instance, on hydrophilic and high nanorough surfaces, studies have shown maximum vitronectin, fibronectin and laminin adsorption [16,60,61]. Specifically, the highest concentration of vitronectin (a protein known to mediate anchorage-dependent cell adhesion) adsorption on nanophase ceramics may explain the subsequent enhanced osteoblast adhesion on nanophase ceramics [16]. Secondly, proteins will interact with specific cell membrane receptors (integrins) to aid in cell adhesion on the substrate and at the same time inhibit other nonspecific cell adhesion. It is apparent that surface properties are closely related to anchorage-dependent cell (such as osteoblasts and osteoclasts) adhesion to a biomaterial surface. After that, cell proliferation, differentiation, and extracellular matrix deposition can happen and will lead to a successful integration with surrounding tissue. Many current attempts, therefore, have focused on nanosurface modifications of conventional orthopedic materials in order to promote anchorage-dependent osteoblast adhesion on implant surfaces. Importantly, promising results have been observed on nano ceramics without any modification; it is their raw surface that works.

7.3.1.2 Enhanced Mechanical Properties of Nanophase Ceramics.

Mechanical properties (such as hardness, ductility, stiffness, bending, compressive and tensile strengths) of biomaterials play a crucial role in the long-term success of orthopedic implants. Many attempts and efforts have ensued to improve mechanical properties of current metals, ceramics and polymers in order to biomimic those of physiological bone. Unlike metals, ceramics (such as alumina and HA) have little ductility and have low fracture toughness ($0.8–1.2\,\text{MPa·m}^{-1/2}$ for HA). They cannot tolerate damage and are vulnerable to crack initiation and propagation. They, therefore, cannot be applied in some loading-bearing applications. Table 7.2 shows the mechanical properties of traditional ceramics compared to natural bone as well as to other implant materials.

To date, it is well known that decreasing grain sizes into the nanoscale (diameter >12–20 nm) increases strength, hardness and plasticity for both metals and ceramics. Theoretically, the well-known empirical Hall-Petch equation which relates yield stress (σ_y) to average grain size (d) can exhibit remarkably increased strength when reducing grain size from the micronmeter to the nanometer regime [63]:

TABLE 7.2. Comparison of Mechanical Properties of Ceramics and Bone and Other Orthopedic Materials

Material	Modulus of elasticity/stiffness (GPa)	Bending strength (MPa)	Ductility (%)	Hardness (knoop hardness number)
Cortical bone	10–16	140	0–2	
Ceramics				
Alumina	380	550	0	2100
Zirconia	170	350	0	1160
Hydroxyapatite	34.5	200	0	
Metals				
Implant alloy (Co-Cr-Mo)	240	825	10	430
Stainless steel annealed (316L)	190	485	40	235
Ti-6Al-4V (ELI)	110	900	12	325
Polymers				
Polymethyl methacrylate (PMMA)	3	55	0–2	
Polyethylene (UHMW)	12	44	400	

Adapted from [62].

$$\sigma_y = \sigma_0 + \frac{k}{\sqrt{d}} \qquad (7.1)$$

Here σ_0 is a friction stress and k is a constant. Hardness and grain size also have the above similar relationships. Many experimental results partly confirmed the above theoretical predictions. For example, as grain size is reduced to nanoscale dimensions, the hardness of nanocrystalline metals (such as copper, palladium and silver) typically increases and can be a factor of two to five higher than conventional metals [59,75–76]. Karch and Birringer reported that an increased value of hardness and remarkably high values of fracture toughness (~14 MPa·m$^{-1/2}$) were observed for nanocrystalline titania [63]. Reducing the grain size of tetragonal zirconia polycrystals (Y-TZP) from commercially used 0.3 μm to 10 nm enhanced deformation rates by a factor of two and provided a material with superplasticity properties [63]. Webster et al. also reported the modulus of elasticity of 23 nm grain size alumina decreased by 70% compared to that of 177 nm grain size alumina [15]. However, since flaws such as pores, dislocations, and other defects of nanocrystalline ceramics frequently occur, sometimes strength or hardness values of nanocrystalline ceramics deviate from Hall-Petch predictions. This phenomena is called the inverse Hall-Petch effect, namely, a decrease in strength or hardness as grain size is decreased below ~10 nm [54]. Controlling manufacturing parameters may avoid the inverse Hall-Petch effect.

TABLE 7.3. Coefficient of Friction for Different Bearing Couples Used in Total Hip Replacements

Bearing couples	Coefficient of friction
Cartilage-cartilage	0.002
CoCr-UHMWPE*	0.094
Zirconia-UHMWPE	0.09–0.11
Alumina-UHMWPE	0.08–0.12
CoCr-CoCr	0.12
Alumina-alumina	0.05–0.1

Data obtained from Park and Lakes, 1992 [132] and Streicher et al., 1992 [133], [74].
*UHMWPE, ultra-high molecular weight polyethylene.

Currently, the most widely used bearing couples in hip replacements are metal-on-polyethylene components. However, as we know, wear debris originating from polyethylene causes foreign body reactions around the implant that frequently influence the longevity of orthopedic implants. Consequently, many researchers have focused on evaluating alternative materials for articulating surfaces and lowering the wear rate of articulating components in order to reduce wear-related complications to improve the life expectancy of bone implants [64]. Generally, low wear rates can be achieved by using materials with high hardness. Clearly, ceramics have rather high hardness compared to other implant materials (see previously shown Table 7.2). For this reason, ceramics such as alumina are widely evaluated as wear-resistant articulating materials considering their high hardness, chemical inertness, respectable strength, and fracture toughness [65]. For instance, metal-on-metal implants with ceramic coatings (such as nanostructured diamond), ceramic-on-ceramic, and ceramic-on-polyethylene couples have been studied (Table 7.3). It has been shown that the wear rates of ceramic-on-polyethylene and further ceramic-on-ceramic systems [66] are noticeably lower than for metal-on-polyethylene systems of total hip prostheses.

Moreover, since grain size and porosity can be closely related to wear behavior of ceramics, many investigations on the wear resistance of alumina ceramics have focused on the role of nanophase ceramics. By reducing the grain size as well as decreasing porosity, the wear characteristics can be significantly improved [67–71]. For example, Al_2O_3-SiC nanocomposites have been shown to have much greater resistance to surface fracture than conventional ceramics [65]. Polycrystalline phased-stabilized zirconia from nanoparticles has improved ductility, fracture toughness and wear-resistance compared to current-generation zirconia [72].

In this light, nanostructured diamond and diamond-like carbon coatings on cobalt-chrome and titanium alloys can be considered for potential orthopedic applications [54] due to their excellent mechanical properties compared to conventional microscale implant materials. They are one of the hardest, strongest, and most wear-resistant materials, and also have suitable biocompatibility and corrosion resistance. Through using chemical vapor deposition (CVD) technology, a nanostructured diamond film with high hardness, enhanced toughness and good adhesion to alloys can be obtained. Catledge et al. have demonstrated that nanostructured diamond films can be tailored on metallic surfaces with hardness values ranging from 10 GPa to 100 GPa by changing the feed gas (N_2/CH_4) ratio [73]. The above excellent properties of nanostructured diamond make it promising as a coating for load-bearing articulating surfaces [54] in orthopedic implants.

In summary, nanoceramics can offer significantly improved mechanical properties, good wear properties, as well as excellent biocompatibility compared to conventional ceramics. Although further investigations of nanoceramics are needed to justify and apply them into real orthopedic applications, nanoceramics are clearly promising future orthopedic materials.

7.3.2 Nanostructured Metals

Artificial joints or prostheses have employed a variety of metallic components because of their durability, physical strength and physiological inertness. For example, titanium, Ti alloys (such as Ti6Al4V), metal alloys (such as CoCrMo) and stainless steel are commonly used in orthopedics. Most metallic components such as hip ball and sockets are made of stainless steels or titanium, which allows bone ingrowth. Commercially pure titanium and Ti6Al4V alloys are the two of the most common titanium-based implant biomaterials [77].

Because of the fact that titanium is not ferromagnetic, titanium implants can be safely examined with magnetic resonance imaging, which makes them especially useful for long-term implants. Moreover, titanium develops an oxide layer in contact with water or air, resulting in high biocompatibility. Thus, titanium and titanium alloys are considered the best choice for manufacturing permanent non-biodegradable implants [77,78]. Importantly, the modulus of elasticity of titanium can be exploited to closely match the modulus of the bone [79]. However, the stiffness of titanium alloys is still more than twice that of bone.

The micro or nanoscale surface properties of metals, just like ceramics, such as surface composition and topography, can affect bone formation. Coatings and/or surface modifications are interrelated with topography and surface energy. For this reason, it is very difficult to determine how these affect—as an independent factor—the final bone formation result [77]. The topographical features obtained on the metal implant surface can range from nanometers to millimeters, which are far below the size of osteoblasts but have been shown to promote bone formation [80].

Numerous treatment processes, including machining or micromachining, particle blasting, Ti plasma spraying, HA plasma spraying, chemical or electrochemical etching, and anodization are available to modify Ti surface topography. In addition, anodizing titanium under different conditions can change the nature of the oxide layer (thickness, porosity and crystallinity) on the nanoscale to strongly affect *in vivo* bone formation [77].

The topography of an implant surface can be defined in terms of form, waviness and roughness (Figure 7.5), with the waviness and roughness often presented

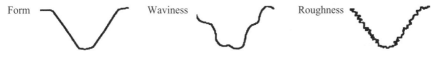

Figure 7.5. From Wennerberg & Albrektsson (2000). Adapted from [82].

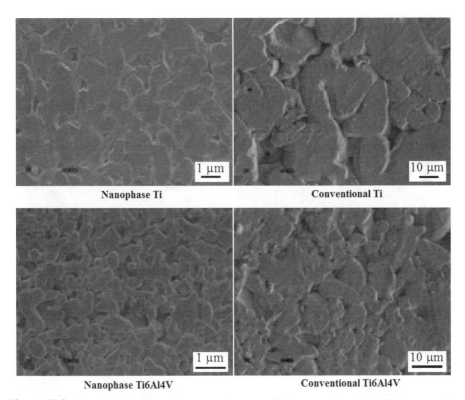

Figure 7.6. Scanning electron microscopy images of Ti compacts and Ti6Al4V compacts. Increased nanostructured surface roughness was observed on nanophase compared to conventional Ti and Ti6Al4V, Adapted from [17].

together under the term texture [81]. Affected by the surface roughness, the composition of the initially adsorbed protein layers and the orientation of the molecules adsorbed on the implant surfaces, have been shown to be an important factor for osseointegration.

For example, compared with conventional metals, nanophase Ti, Ti6Al4V (Figure 7.6) and CoCrMo have greatly increased surface roughness (Table 7.4) and have been shown to significantly promote osteoblast function [17]. The dimensions of nanometer surface features gave rise to larger amounts of interparticulate voids (with fairly homogeneous distribution) on nanophase Ti and Ti6Al4V, unlike the corresponding conventional Ti and Ti6Al4V compacts;

TABLE 7.4. Surface Roughness of Metal Compacts [17]

Substrate	Surface roughness (rms; nm)
Ti (nano)	11.9
Ti (conv.)	4.9
Ti6Al4V (nano)	15.2
Ti6Al4V (conv.)	4.9
CoCrMo (nano)	356.7
CoCrMo (conv.)	186.7

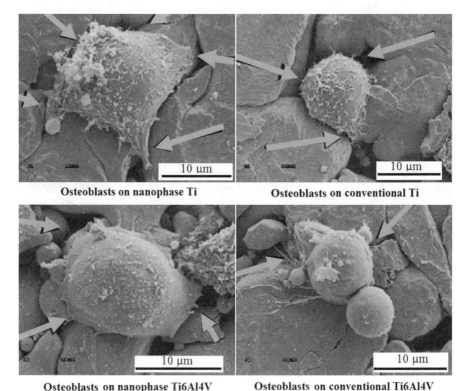

Osteoblasts on nanophase Ti   Osteoblasts on conventional Ti

Osteoblasts on nanophase Ti6Al4V   Osteoblasts on conventional Ti6Al4V

Figure 7.7. Scanning electron microscopy images of osteoblasts on nanophase and conventional metals (Ti and Ti6Al4V) after 1 hour culture. More spread osteoblasts can be observed on nanophase metals than conventional metals. Arrows point to particle boundaries where cell protrusions are seen. Adapted and redrawn from [17].

rather these latter compacts revealed fewer interparticulate voids with a non-homogeneous distribution [17].

Figure 7.7 shows the osteoblast morphology on nanophase and conventional metals. Obviously, osteoblasts spread well on nanophase Ti and Ti6Al4V, which have increased roughness and surface particles boundaries. Therefore, similar to ceramics, these nano properties are promising for bone formation.

However, despite these promises there may be some problems with certain titanium alloys. For example, Hong et al. reported that Ti surfaces are excessively highly thrombogenic [83], leading to more rapid collagenous encapsulation and faster remineralization. Some researchers have discussed the potential cytotoxicity associated with the vanadium element in Ti6Al4V [77]. When Ti6Al4V was compared with commercially pure Ti [84], gingival fibroblasts demonstrated a rounded cell shape and a reduced area of spreading on the alloy, presumably because of a minor toxicity to vanadium or aluminum. In this light, it is important to mention that fibroblast adhesion has been shown to be lower on nano compared to conventional metals.

7.3.3 Nanostructured Polymers

Polymers are a class of synthetic materials characterized by their high versatility [85] and, thus, have been widely applied in orthopedics. They can mechanically secure components of hip replacements into bone—as in bone cements such as injectable polymethylmethacrylate (PMMA)—and can line acetabular cups for smooth articulation with metallic femoral head components (such as in UHMWPE). However, there also exists many disadvantages related to traditional polymers used in orthopedic implants. For example, PMMA suffers from fatigue-related cracking and impact-induced breakage due to its poor setting and fixation [86]. Furthermore, PMMA can also elicit a host response due to release of toxic monomers and necrosis of the surrounding tissue caused by exothermic polymerization *in vivo* [87]. Increased articulation-induced wear of UHMWPE frequently leads to osteolysis (see section 7.2.2.2) [88].

Therefore, further development of various polymer alternatives that could improve osseointegration is necessary, not only for fracture fixation but also as bone tissue engineering scaffolds. For this reason, polymers—such as polylactic acid (PLA), polyglycolic acid (PGA), poly(lactic-co-glycolic acid) (PLGA) and various hydrogels—currently generate more interest from scientists to investigate their potentials as bone tissue engineering scaffolds to repair bone defects due to their excellent biocompatibility, suitable mechanical properties, biodegradability and ease of modification for different applications.

An ideal bone repair scaffold should be biocompatible to minimize local tissue response but maximize osseointegration, and be biodegradable after new bone formation. As will be described, an important consideration in scaffold design is providing a polymer nanoscale framework for cellular interactions.

7.3.3.1 Nanostructured Biodegradable Polymers as Bone Tissue Engineering Scaffolds. One of the most common polymers used as a biodegradable biomaterial has been PLGA [85]. It has high biocompatibility, the ability to degrade into harmless monomer units, and a useful range of mechanical properties,

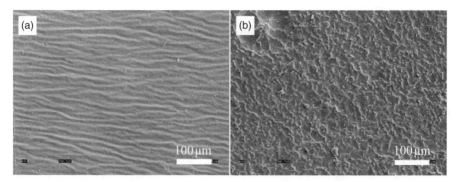

Figure 7.8. Scanning electron microscopy images of chemically treated and conventional untreated PLGA surfaces. (A) Conventional PLGA (feature dimensions ~10–15 μm) and (B) chemically treated nanostructured PLGA (feature dimensions ~50–100 nm). Scale bar is 100 μm. Adapted from [95].

depending on the copolymer ratio. Recently, this copolymer and its homopolymer derivatives, PLA and PGA, have received substantial attention for skeletal repair and regeneration. Various techniques—such as particulate leaching, textile technologies or three-dimensional (3D) printing techniques—have successfully created 3D porous matrices from PLGA and its derivatives [89–92]. For instance, with the simplicity of the polymer casting and phase separation processes, a robust nanofibrous poly(l-lactic acid) (PLLA) scaffold can be prepared [93]. These nanofibrous scaffolds have a collagen-like 3D structure, high porosity and a suitable surface structure for osteoblast attachment, proliferation, and differentiation.

In addition, several studies have shown that nanostructured PLGA (Figure 7.8) which is prepared by chemical etching procedures can promote vascular endothelial and smooth muscle cell adhesion compared to the conventional PLGA [94–95].

Further investigation demonstrated that nanostructured PLGA can adsorb significantly more vitronectin and fibronectin from serum compared to conventional PLGA, just as the aforementioned nano ceramics and metals do [93]. This increase in protein adsorption may help explain enhanced osteoblast adhesion observed on PLGA with nano-surface roughness. In addition, significantly increased chondrocyte functions—adhesion, proliferation and matrix synthesis—have been observed on NaOH-treated nanostructured PLGA [97]. Furthermore, improved osteoblast functions have also been observed on nanophase titania/PLGA composites which make them promising as bone tissue engineering scaffold materials [98]. At the same time, it was found that fibroblast density decreased on nanophase PLGA, polyurethane and polycaprolactone which may inhibit the formation of a fibrous tissue capsule [99]. Obviously, because nanostructured PLGA has excellent biocompatibility properties (above that of traditional PLGA) and ease of degradability, it has been considered as a new generation of tissue engineering scaffold for numerous tissue engineering composite applications especially for bone and articular cartilage.

7.3.3.2 Nanostructured and Injectable Hydrogels as Bone Tissue Engineering Scaffolds.
Polymeric hydrogels have excellent biocompatibility which makes them useful in orthopedic applications (such as for injectable bone repair and cartilage reconstruction) [100]. Natural hydrogels (such as collagen and gelatin) are the main components of extra cellular matrices (ECM) of mammalian tissues including bone, cartilage, and so on [101]. Through a technique called electrospinning, nanofibrous scaffolds [104] can be successfully created from various synthetic and natural polymers such as gelatin and collagen (Figure 7.9).

Several studies have shown that protein and cell interactions are promoted by nanofibrous scaffolds that biomimic the ECM [102–103]. On the other hand, studies have demonstrated that using self-assembling peptide KLD-12 hydrogels for encapsulating chondrocytes can support chondrocyte differentiation and promote the synthesis of a cartilage-like extracellular matrix for cartilage repair [105].

In addition, various synthetic hydrogels such as poly(2-hydroxyethyl methacrylate) (pHEMA) were modified to have nanofeatures for orthopedic applications. For example, some studies have created an injectable nanostructured pHEMA-hydrogel scaffold which incorporates novel self-assembled helical rosette nanotubes (HRNs) into hydrogels to fill bone fractures and repair bone defects [106]. The nanoscale, tubular architecture of HRNs on and in hydrogels can provide a topography that improves protein adsorption and an environment

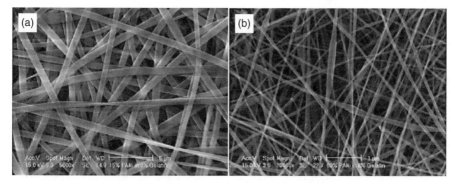

Figure 7.9. Scanning electron microscopy images of electrospun polyaniline-contained gelatin nanofibers. (A) polyaniline-gelatin blend fibers with ratios of 15:85 and (B) polyaniline-gelatin blend fibers with ratios of 60:40. This Fig. shows that the electrospun fibers are homogeneous while 60:40 fibers were electrospun with beads [104]. Scale bars = 5 μm for (A) and 1 μm for (B).

that resembles an extracellular matrix surrounding cells *in vivo*. Results revealed that HRNs coated on and embedded in hydrogels significantly improved osteoblast adhesion even at a low concentration of 0.001 mg/ml [106]. These HRN incorporate hydrogels can also solidify at body temperatures, thus, allowing for aqueous injection and *in situ* bone healing. Thus, it has been anticipated that such nanostructured hydrogels are promising for bone tissue engineering applications.

7.3.4   Nanostructured Composites

Bone is a natural nanostructured matrix composite made from calcium-phosphate apatite mineral which is reinforced with collagen fibers. Cells in the body are accustomed to interacting with composite materials that have nanostructured features, thus, one way to closely mimic the properties of natural bone tissues is by using nanocomposite biomaterials. Such composite biomaterials are engineered materials consisting of two or more distinct materials with significantly different physical or chemical properties that provide desirable overall mechanical, chemical, biological, and physical properties. Such composites may contain reinforcing phases embedded within a matrix phase. The reinforcing material can be either fibers or particles, for example, carbon nanofibers, carbon nanotubes, helical rosette nanotubes (HRN), or ceramic nanoparticles (such as hydroxyapatite or calcium phosphates). The matrix can be metal, ceramic, or polymer, but most biomedical composites have polymeric matrices. The majority of composites used in biomaterial applications are intended for the purposes of bone repair.

Polymer composite materials offer a desired high strength and bone-like elastic properties, potentially leading to a more favorable bone remodeling response. For example, polyethylene (PE) is a polymeric material which, in different grades—namely, HDPE (high-density polyethylene), UHMWPE (ultra-high-molecular-weight polyethylene), and LDPE (low-density polyethylene)—can be used as an implant [107]. Unfortunately, osseointegration of this polymer is low. Thus, normally its attachment to bone should be mechanical in nature. However, in many studies bioactivated PE has been obtained by adding bioactive materials to PE, such as, hydroxyapatite-reinforced high-density polyethylene (HAPEX). In addition, some studies investigated nanostructured titanium as a bioactive coating on UHMWPE and polytetrafluoroethylene (PTFE) [134]. For instance, Reising et al. demonstrated that a nanostructured Ti coating created by a new ionic plasma deposition (IPD) method can significantly improve osteoblast functions compared to conventional Ti or the uncoated polymer (Figure 7.10) [134].

Minerals of calcium phosphates are frequently used as an additive to polymeric matrices. Calcium phosphates (CaP) are a major constituent of natural bone. Therefore, they show great potential as a supplement in orthopedic applications, including bone replacements, bone cements, and scaffolds for tissue engineering [108–109]. Thus, they are very popular as bioactive ceramic materials. For example, the chemical composition of hydroxyapatite (HA) makes it more stable against resorption. On the other hand, tricalcium phosphate (TCP) is partially

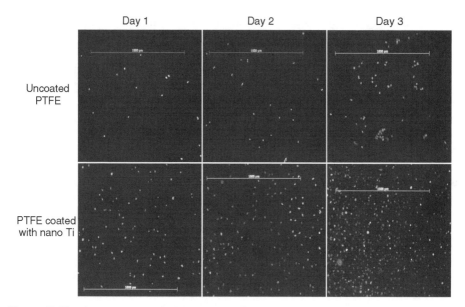

<u>Figure 7.10.</u> Fluorescent microscope images of improved osteoblast proliferation on PTFE coated with nano Ti using ionic plasma deposition (IPD) compared to conventional uncoated PTFE. Scale bars = 1000 μm. Adapted from [134].

resorbable and frequently used as bone substitutes [110]; in particular, β-TCP is known to be biocompatible, osteoconductive, and osteoinductive [111].

β-tricalcium phosphate-reinforced high-density polyethylene (β-TCP/ HDPE) is one of the new biomaterials that can replace bone tissues. Homaeigohar et al. concluded that inserting TCP particles into the structure of PE is beneficial for both structural compatibility and biological performance. Also, the results from this study provided a basis for further studies in the *in vivo* field towards using this composite as a bone graft substitute in orthopedic surgery [112]. Murugan et al. demonstrated the possibilities of bone paste production incorporating a composite of HA nanocrystals and chitosan, which is an organic polymer, using a wet chemical synthesis method at low temperature. The rate of bioresorption of HA was improved by the addition of chitosan. It was anticipated that this kind of composite can act as a bioresorbable bone substitute with superior bioactivity and osteoconductivity *in vivo* [113]. Moreover, Jabbari et al. grafted HA nanoparticles with hydrophilic unsaturated poly(ethylene glycol) oligomers to improve their suspension stability and interfacial bonding in an aqueous hydrogel solution. They hypothesized that hydrogel/apatite nanocomposites are the ideal biomaterial to mimic the physio-chemical and biological properties of the bone matrix for bone regeneration [114]. It is possible to dope even nanostructured hydroxyapatite with ions such as carbonate, sodium, and magnesium to create a material closely resembling the composition of the surrounding hard tissue.

Another highly studied ceramic material in composites is zirconium dioxide or zirconia (ZrO_2). It enhances fracture toughness in polymers or other ceramics. A novel orthopedic bioceramic is the zirconia (ZrO_2)-hydroxyapatite (HA) composite which has good biocompatibility properties [115]. CaP and phosphate-based glass composite coatings have been shown to strengthen ZrO_2 and to improve biocompatibility. The proliferation and alkaline phosphatase activities of osteoblasts on such composite coatings were improved by approximately 30–40% when compared to ZrO_2 substrates alone, and were comparable to the pure HA coating. These findings suggest that the CaP and P-glass composites are potentially useful for coating traditional biomaterials used as a hard tissue implant, due to their morphological and mechanical integrity, enhanced bioactivity, and favorable responses of osteoblast-like cells [116]. Kong et al. studied HA-added zirconia-alumina (ZrO_2-Al_2O_3) nanocomposites in load-bearing orthopedic applications. The HA-added zirconia-alumina nanocomposites contained biphasic calcium phosphates (BCP) of HA/TCP and had higher flexural strength than conventionally mixed HA-added zirconia-alumina composites. *In vitro* tests showed that the proliferation and differentiation of osteoblasts on this nanocomposite gradually increased as the amount of HA added increased [117].

Synthetic biodegradable polymers are widely utilized in the fabrication of scaffolds for bone tissue engineering [118]. Because carbon nanotubes (CNTs) have a very high strength to weight ratio for greater mechanical properties, they can be used as a reinforcing material for polymer composites. For example, Webster et al. developed a carbon nanofiber reinforced polycarbonate urethane (PU) composite in an attempt to determine the possibility of using either carbon nanofibers or strips of CNTs, as either neural or orthopedic prosthetic devices. The results have shown that such composite biomaterials have the potential to promote osteoblast functions [119]. Also, Shi et al. used single-walled carbon nanotubes (SWNTs) as reinforcing materials for poly(propylene fumarate) (PPF). Such composites are used as an injectable highly porous scaffold for load-bearing bone repair [120]. Moreover, it is believed that electrical stimulation enhances osteoblast function on such CNT composites. Conductivity of polylactic acid (PLA), which is an insulator, can be enhanced by adding CNTs. Studies have shown that osteoblast proliferation increased significantly on such composites after exposing them to electrical stimulation [121]. Thus, great promise exists for many nanocomposites for orthopedic applications.

7.3.5 Role of Chemistry

In bone tissue engineering, nanotechnology is also being used in conjunction with changes in implant surface chemistries. For example, for titanium, the surface oxide layer has many qualities regarded as important for optimal reactions with bone. The excellent biocompatibility of Ti-based materials can be attributed to the high corrosion resistance (low metal ion release) and, moreover, to the good bone-binding ability of TiO_2 which covers the implant surface. An electrochemical method known as anodization or anodic oxidation (Figure 7.11) is a

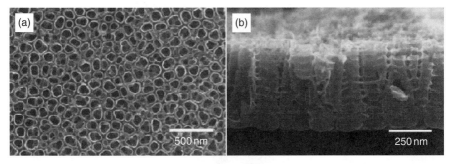

<u>Figure 7.11.</u> Scanning electron microscopy images of the short-nanotube layer formed by anodization of titanium in 1 M H_2SO_4 + 0.15 wt % HF at 20 V. (a) Top-view and (b) cross-section. Adapted from [122].

well-established surface nano-modification technique for metals like titanium to produce protective layers that possibly enhance bone growth [122].

Essentially, electrochemical approaches have been reported to form highly-defined porous TiO_2 layers. Under specific electrochemical conditions, self-organized TiO_2 nanotube layers can be grown on Ti simply by the anodization of Ti in dilute HF electrolytes. With this approach, TiO_2 layers could be grown consisting of tubes with a diameter of ~100 nm and a length of ~500 nm. This oxide layer that forms on titanium implants can be manipulated chemically and there has been speculation about whether the biological properties of the oxide surface may then be changed, and even improved, as a result. The significance of surface chemistry can be illustrated by the varied cellular responses reported on different titanium alloys, different grades of c.p. titanium, and different bulk metals. Chemical modification of titanium surfaces by their treatment in simulated body fluid, covalent attachment of biological molecules, changes in the surface ion content, and alkali treatment have all been reported to affect cellular responses to the implant [123–125]. It is noteworthy that this approach is successful not only for Ti, but also for other metals and for the formation of nanotube layers on biomedical Ti alloys such as Ti-6Al-4V and Ti-6Al-7Nb [126]. In this light, it is important to note that to date many studies highlighting the ability of nanomaterials to increase tissue growth have been performed on nano, compared to conventional materials of the same chemistry.

Another emerging area, still at the experimental stage, is the use of photolithography to produce micro and nano-fabricated surfaces [127]. Such surfaces, made of silicon and titanium, incorporate intentional surface chemical and topographical features in the nano- and micrometer scales and provide greater opportunities to control cell behavior.

The biological performance of biomedical implants strongly depends on the first interaction occurring when implant surfaces come into contact with a biological environment. Extra-cellular matrix proteins that contain the cell-binding domain RGD have a critical role in mediating cell behavior because they regulate gene expression by signal transduction set in motion by cell adhesion to proteins

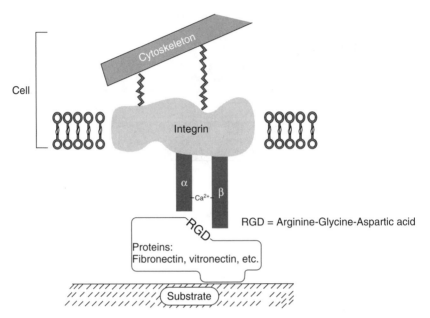

Figure 7.12. Surface properties affecting protein conformation and bioactivity. Adapted from [128].

adsorbed on biomaterial [128]. Interactions between cell-membrane integrins and extracellular proteins are often facilitated by the RGD sequence. These interactions are important for the adhesion of many cells types. Integrin-mediated cell attachment influences and regulates cell migration, growth, differentiation, and apoptosis [128]. Various proteins—such as all types of collagen, fibronectin, and vitronectin—are known to be particularly important in mediating osteoblast adhesion; importantly, RGD is contained in all of these proteins and is recognized by cell membrane integrin receptors. Capitalizing on the use of such sequences may enhance cell targeting and adhesion to specific receptors, and also cell behavior via activation of specific signaling cascades, as shown in Figure 7.12.

The central hypothesis of biomimetic surface engineering is that peptides that mimic part of the extra-cellular matrix affect cell attachment to the material, and that surfaces or 3D matrices modified with these peptides can induce tissue formation according to the cell type seeded on the material. Therefore, extensive research over the last decade has been performed on the incorporation of adhesion promoting oligopeptides onto the biomaterial surfaces. Further, the major advantage of using small peptides (such as RGD) with respect to larger peptides or proteins is their resistance to proteolysis and their ability to bind with high affinities to integrin receptors. Combining this approach (covalently linking peptides) with the use of nanomaterials has maximized cell responses.

In conclusion, as shown in Figure 7.13, nanomaterials have favorable surface chemistry, nano structure and bioactive surfaces as well as improved various

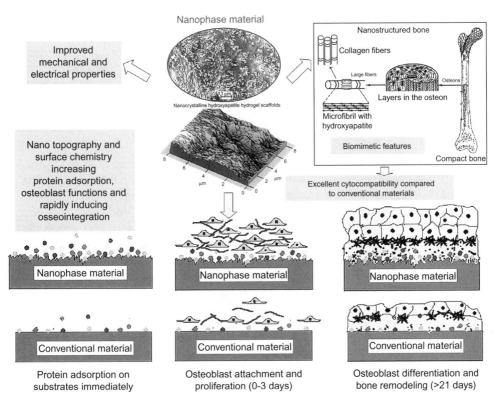

Figure 7.13. Schematic illustration of the proposed mechanism of the superior properties of nanomaterials over conventional materials to improve orthopedic applications. Compared to conventional micron-scale materials, nanomaterials have enhanced mechanical, cytocompatibility and electrical properties, which make them suitable for orthopedic and bone tissue engineering applications. The nano and bioactive surfaces of nanomaterials mimicking bones can promote greater amounts of protein adsorption and efficiently stimulate more new bone formation than conventional materials. Redrawn from [135–137]. (See color insert.)

other properties (such as electrical and mechanical) compared to respective conventional materials. These superior properties of nanomaterials provide great promise to use them as the next generation of biomaterials for a wide range of tissue engineering applications.

7.4   FUTURE CHALLENGES

Nanotechnology applications are entering industrial production, mainly for diagnostics, drugs, and other medical therapies. Particularly for orthopedic applications, nano-meter scale modifications of implant surfaces would improve durability and biocompatibility.

Although nanostructured implant materials may have many potential advantages in the context of bone tissue engineering, it is important to remember that studies on nanophase materials have only just begun; there are still many other issues regarding health that must be answered. Most importantly, influences of nanoparticulates on human health are not well understood, whether exposure occurs through the manufacturing of nanophase materials or through the implantation of nanophase materials. Clearly, detailed studies in this context are required if nanoparticles are to be used in these systems [129].

Interactions of nanoparticles with biomolecules—such as DNA, RNA or proteins—are also more likely with decreasing particle size. A number of reports on cellular uptake of micro- and nano- sized particles have been published. Reports on particle uptake by endothelial cells, pulmonary epithelium, intestinal epithelium, alveolar macrophages, other macrophages, nerve cells and other cells are available [129]. Further, it is expected that transport of nanoparticles across the blood-brain barrier (BBB) is possible by either passive diffusion or by carrier-mediated endocytosis.

Nanoparticles may also become loose through the degradation of implanted polymeric materials through oxidation and / or hydrolysis which accelerates exposure of materials [35]. Corrosion of metals once implanted can also cause the release of nanoparticulates and, thus, contribute to toxicity in biological environments. Oxidation accelerates the degradation of metals and the release of metal ions such as Al^{3+}, Ni^{2+}, Cr^{6+}, and Co^{2+}.

In addition, nanoparticles can be generated at artificial joints where friction between two surfaces is high. The outcome of micron-sized wear debris on bone health has been well-studied for several decades. For instance, ultra high-molecular-weight polyethylene often used as acetabular cups become brittle through oxidation and, thus, become susceptible to wear. Conventional size wear debris (i.e., micron) triggers osteolysis as well as further wearing (third-body wear).

In contrast, the influence of nanoparticulate wear debris—or particles in general—on bone cell health is only just beginning to be understood. It has been speculated that the effects of nanotubes on lungs are more toxic than quartz dust. One study also showed that nanometer titania particles (50 nm) and carbon nanotubes (20 × 100 nm) induced morphological changes in neutrophils and decreased the overall cell survival rate [130].

On the contrary, other studies have also demonstrated increased cell viability in the presence nanometer, compared with conventional particles [35]. Specifically, nanophase materials did not stimulate cytotoxicity but even redeemed the toxic effects observed on osteoblast viability in the presence of conventionally sized particles. In this study, osteoblast proliferation was not negatively influenced by alumina and titania nanoparticles, whereas conventional particles of the same chemistry and crystalline phase increased cell death and slowed cell proliferation. The potential lack of nanoparticle toxicity was also demonstrated on coatings of pigment-grade titania particles as nanorods and nanodots of titania (<50 nm) which did not result in as much lung inflammation when compared with larger particle sizes (>300 nm) [35].

Obviously, further tests and studies concerning the toxicity of nanophase materials need to be conducted and expanded before the benefits of nanotechnology in orthopedic applications can be realized. However, it is important to emphasize that such studies need accurate comparisons when determining health influences of nanometer compared with conventionally-sized particles of the same size and crystallinity.

In summary, despite the challenges that lie ahead, significant evidence now exists elucidating that nanomaterials represent an important growing area of research that may improve bonding between an implant and surrounding bone. Even if nanophase materials do not provide the ultimate answer for increasing bone cell responses, research has provided a tremendous amount of information concerning bone cell recognition with nanostructured surfaces that will most certainly aid in improving orthopedic implant efficacy.

REFERENCES

1. Joos, U., Wiesmann, H. P., Szuwart, T. and Meyer, U., Mineralization at the interface of implants, *Int. J. Oral Maxillofac. Surg.*, volume: 35, 2006, pp. 783–790.

2. Charnley, J., Anchorage of the fermoral head prosthesis to the shaft of the femur, *Journal of bone joint surgery*, volume: 42B, 1960, pp. 28–30.

3. Charnley, J., Surgery of the hip-joint: present and future developments, *Br. Me. J.*, volume: 5176, 1960, pp. 821–826.

4. Frankowski, J. J. and Watkins-Castillo, S., Primary total knee and hip arthroplasty projections for the U.S. population to the year 2030, American Academy of Orthopaedic Surgeons, Rosemont, IL, reviewed by T. P. Sculco and S. M. Sporer, August 23, 2002.

5. AAOS online, http://www.aaos.org/research/research.asp

6. Bozic, K. J., Rubash, H. E., Berry, J., Saleh, K. J. and Durbhakula, S. M., Modes of failure in revision hip and knee replacement.

7. Revisions of Hip and Knee Replacements in Canada, Canadian Joint Replacement Registry Analytic Bulletin: Canadian Institute for Health Information, June 2004, pp. 1–20.

8. Branemark, P. I., Adell, R., Albrektsson, T., Lekholm, U., Lundkvist, S. and Rockler, B., Osseointegrated titanium fixtures in the treatment of edentulousness, *Biomaterials*, volume: 4, 1983, pp. 25–28.

9. Webster, T. J., Nanophase ceramics: the future orthopedic and dental implant material. Advances in Chemical Engineering, pp. 125–166, J. Y. Ying (eds.), *Academic Press: A Harcourt Science and Technology company*, 2001.

10. Esposito, M., Hirsh, J. M., Lekholm, U. and Thomsen, P., Biological factors contributing to failures of osseointegrated oral implants (I): Success criteria and epidemiology, *European Journal of Oral Sciences*, volume: 106, 1998, pp. 527–551.

11. Esposito, M., Hirsh, J. M., Lekholm, U. and Thomsen, P., Biological factors contributing to failures of osseointegrated oral implants (II): Etiopathogenesis, *European Journal of Oral Sciences*, volume: 106, 1998, pp. 721–764.

12. Cochran, D. L., Schenk, R. K., Lussi, A., Higginbottom, F. L. and Buser, D., Bone response to unloaded and loaded titanium implants with a sandblasted and acid-etched surface: a histometric study in the canine mandible, *J. Biomed. Mater. Res.*, volume: 40, 1998, pp. 1–11.

13. Wennerberg, A., Hallgren, C., Johansson, C. and Danelli, S., A histomorphometric evaluation of screw-shaped implants each prepared with two surface roughnesses, *Clin. Oral Implants Res.*, volume: 9, 1998, pp. 11–19.

14. Webster, T. J., Siegel, R. W. and Bizios, R., Osteoblast adhesion on nanophase ceramics, *Biomaterials*, volume: 20, 1999, pp. 1221–1227.

15. Webster, T. J., Siegel, R. W. and Bizios, R., Design and evaluation of nanophase alumina for orthopaedic/dental applications, *Nanostructured Materials*, volume: 12, 1999, pp. 983–986.

16. Webster, T. J., Siegel, R. W. and Bizios, R., Specific proteins mediate osteoblast adhesion on nanophase ceramics, *J. Biomed. Mater. Res.*, volume: 51, 2000, pp. 475–483.

17. Webster, T. J. and Ejiofor, J. U., Increased osteoblast adhesion on nanophase metals: Ti, Ti6Al4V, and CoCrMo, *Biomaterials*, volume: 25, 2004, pp. 4731–4739.

18. Kaplan, F. S., Hayes, W. C., Keaveny, T. M., Boskey, A., Einhorn, T. A. and Iannotti, J. P., Form and function of bone. Orthopedic basic science, pp. 127–185, S. P. Sinmon, (eds.). *American Academy of Orthopaedic Surgeons*, 1994.

19. Castner, D. G. and Ratner, B. D., Biomedical surface science: Foundations to frontiers, *Surface Science*, volume: 500, 2002, pp. 28–60.

20. Chun, A. L., Helical Rosette Nanotubes: An investigation towards its application in orthopaedics, Purdue university (thesis), May 2006.

21. Hayakawa, T., Yoshinari, M., Kiba, H., Yamamoto, H., Nemoto, K. and Jansen, J. A., Trabecular bone response to surface roughened and calcium phosphate (Ca-P) coated titanium implants, *Biomaterials*, volume: 23, 2002, pp. 1025–1031.

22. Meyer, U., Wiesmann, H. P., Fillies, T. and Joos, U., Early tissue reaction at the interface of immediately loaded dental implants, *Int. J. Oral Maxillofac Implants*, volume: 18, 2003, pp. 489–499.

23. Gu'ehennec, L. L., Soueidan, A., Layrolle, P. and Amouriq, Y., Surface treatments of titanium dental implants for rapid osseointegration, Dental Materials, 2006, doi:10.1016/j.dental

24. Loosening & Osteolysis: Osteolysis (Aseptic Loosening), AAOS online.

25. Hanson, S. R., Lalor, P. A., Niemi, S. M., Northup, S. J., Ratner, B. D. and Spector, M., et al., Testing biomaterials. pp. 221. Biomaterials science: An introduction to materials and medicine, B. D. Ratner, A. S. Hoffman, F. J. Schoen, J. E. Lemons, (eds.). New York: *Academic Press*.

26. Zhu, Y. H., Chiu, K. Y. and Tang, W. M., Review article: polyethylene wear and osteolysis in total hip arthroplasty, *Journal of Orthopaedic Surgery*, volume: 9, number: 1, 2001, pp. 91–99.

27. Harris, W. H., The problem is osteolysis, *Clin. Orthop.*, volume: 311, 1995, pp. 46–53.

28. David, V., Jarka, N. and Olga, K., Periprosthetic osteolysis and its association with the molecule RANKL expression. Physiological research pre-press article.

29. Bronson, J. G., Breakthrough technology: searching for artificial articular cartilage, *Orthopedic Technology Review*, volume: 1, number: 1, 1999.

30. Anaheim and Calif. Rosemont, Polyethylene: the past, present and future. In: orthopaedic proceedings, 66th Annual Meeting, American Academy of Orthopaedic Surgeons. Academy of Orthopaedic Surgeons, 2001, 445–468.

31. Gutwein, L. G. and Webster, T. J., Increased viable osteoblast density in the presence of nanophase compared to conventional alumina and titania particles, *Biomaterials*, volume: 25, number: 18, 2004, pp. 4175–4183.

32. Gutwein, L. G. and Webster, T. J., Osteoblast and chrondrocyte proliferation in the presence of alumina and titania nanoparticles, *Journal of Nanoparticle Research*, volume: 4, 2002, pp. 231–238.

33. Tamura, K., Takashi, N. and Akasaka, T., et al., Effects of micro/nano particle size on cell function and morphology, *Key Engr. Mat.*, 2004, 254–256, 919–922.

34. Warheit, D. B., Nanoparticles: health impacts? *Materials Today*, 2004, pp. 32–35.

35. Sato, M. and Webster, T. J., Nanobiotechnology: implications for the future of nanotechnology in orthopedic applications, *Expert Rev. Medical Devices*, volume: 1, number: 1, 2004, pp. 105–114.

36. Lindahl, H., Garellick, G., Regnér, H., Herberts, P. and Malchau, H., Three hundred and twenty-one periprosthetic femoral fractures, *J. Bone Joint Surg. Am.*, volume: 88, 2006, pp. 1215–1222.

37. Implant wear in total joint replacement: clinical and biologic issues, material and design considerations, edited by T. M. Wright and S. B. Goodman. Chapter 22: what are the wear mechanisms and What control them? (2001) ISBN number 0-89203-261-8. Available online: http://www4.aaos.org/product/details_page.cfm?code=02522 &dlink=ImpWear.cfm

38. Bethea, J. S., Deandrade, J. R., Fleming, L. L., Lindenbaum, S. D. and Welch, R. B., Proximal femoral fractures following total hip arthroplasty, *Clin. Orthop. Relat. Res.*, volume: 170, 1982, pp. 95–106.

39. Beals, R. K. and Tower, S. S., Periprosthetic fractures of the femur. An analysis of 93 fractures. *Clin. Orthop. Relat. Res.*, volume: 327, 1996, pp. 238–246.

40. Learmonth, I. D., The management of periprosthetic fractures around the femoral stem, *J. Bone Joint Surg. Br.*, volume: 86, 2004, pp. 13–19.

41. Herberts, P. and Malchau, H., Long-term registration has improved the quality of hip replacement: a review of the Swedish THR Register comparing 160,000 cases, *Acta Orthop Scand.*, volume: 71, 2000, pp. 111–121.

42. Siegel, R. W. and Fougere, G. E., Mechanical properties of nanophase metals, *Nanostruct. Mater.*, volume: 6, 1995, pp. 205–216.

43. Lemons, J. E., Bioceramics: is there a difference? *Clinical Orthopedics and Related Research*, volume: 261, 1990, pp: 153–158.

44. Webster, T. J., Ergun, C., Doremus, R. H., Seigel, R.W. and Bizios, R., Enhanced functions of osteoblasts on nanophase ceramics, *Biomaterials*, volume: 21, 2000, pp. 1803–1810.

45. Webster, T. J., Siegel, R. W. and Bizios, R., Nanoceramic surface roughness enhances osteoblast and osteoclast functions for improved orthopedic/dental implant efficacy, *Scripta Mater.*, volume: 44, 2001, pp. 1639–1642.

46. Webster, T. J., Ergun, C., Doremus, R. H., Seigel, R. W. and Bizios, R., Enhanced osteoclast-like functions on nanophase ceramics, *Biomaterials*, volume: 22, 2001, pp. 1327–1333.

47. Gutwein, L. G., Webster, T. J., Increased viable osteoblast density in the presence of nanophase compared to conventional alumina and titania particles, *Biomaterials*, volume: 25, 2004, pp. 4175–4183.

48. Webster, T. J., Hellenmeyer, E. L., Price, R. L., Increased osteoblast functions on theta+delta nanofiber alumina, *Biomaterials*, volume: 26, 2005, pp. 953–960.

49. Hamadouche, M., Sedel, L., Ceramics in oethopaedics, *J. Bone Joint Surg. Br.*, volume: 82-B, 2000, pp. 1095–1099.

50. Willert, H. G., Bertram, H., Buchhorn, G. H., Osteolysis in alloarthroplasty of the hip: the role of bone cement fragmentation, *Clin Orthop*, volume: 258, 1990, pp. 108–121.

51. Hulbert, S. F., Hench, L. L., Forbers, D. and Bowman, L. S., History of bioceramics, *Ceramics international*, volume: 8, number: 4, 1982, pp. 131–140.

52. Chang, C. K., Wu, J. S., Mao, D. L. and Ding, C. X., Mechanical and histological evaluations of hydroxyapatite-coated and noncoated Ti-6Al-4V implants in tibia bone, *J. Biomed. Mater. Res.*, volume: 56, number: 1, 2001, pp. 17–23.

53. Cook, S. D., Thomas, K. A., Kay, J. F. and Jarcho, M., Hydroxyapatite-coated porous titanium for use as an orthopedic biologic attachment system, *Clin. Orthop. Relat. Res.*, volume: 230, 1988, pp. 303–312.

54. Catledge, S. A., Fries, M. D., Vohra, Y. K., Lacefield, W. R., Lemons, J. E., Woodard, S. and Venugopalan, R., Nanostructured Ceramics for Biomedical Implants, *Journal of Nanoscience and Nanotechnology*, volume: 2, 2002, pp. 293–312.

55. Chris Arts, J. J., Verdonschot, N., Schreurs, B. W., Buma, P., The use of a bioresorbable nano-crystalline hydroxyapatite paste in acetabular bone impaction grafting, *Biomaterials*, volume: 27, 2006, pp: 1110–1118.

56. Huber, F.-X., Belyaev, O., Hillmeier, J., Kock, H.-J., Huber, C., Meeder, P.-J. and Berger, I., First histological observations on the incorporation of a novel nanocrystalline hydroxyapatite paste OSTIM® in human cancellous bone, *BMC Musculoskeletal Disorders*, 2006, 7:50 doi:10.1186/1471-2474-7-50

57. Colon, G., Ward, B. C., Webster, T. J., Increased osteoblast and decreased Staphylococcus epidermidis functions on nanophase ZnO and TiO2, *J. Biomed. Mater. Res. A.*, volume: 78, number: 3, 2006, pp. 595–604.

58. Donlan, R. M. and Costerton, J. W., Biofilms: Survival mechanisms to clinically relevant microorganisms, *Clinical Microbiol Rev.*, volume: 15, 2002, pp. 167–193.

59. Nieman, G. W., Processing and mechanical behavior of nanocrystalline Cu, Pd and Ag. (Ph. D thesis), Northwestern University, 1991.

60. Luck, M., Paulke, B. R., Schröder, W., Blunk, T., Müller, R. H., Analysis of plasma protein adsorption on polymeric nanoparticles with the different surface characteristics, *J. Biomed. Mater. Res.*, volume: 39, 1998, pp. 478–485.

61. Lopes, M. A., *J. Biomed. Mater. Res.*, volume: 45, number: 4, 1999, pp. 370–375.

62. Cooke, F. W., Ceramics in orthopedic surgery, *Clinical orthopaedics and related research*, volume: 276, 1992, pp. 135–146.

63. Weertman, J. R. and Averback, R. S., Mechanical properties, pp. 323. Nanomaterials: sythesis, properties and applications, A. S. Edelstein and R. C. Cammarata (eds.), London: *Institue of Physics Publishing*, 1998.

64. Wallbridge, N., Dowson, D., The walking activity of patients with artificial hip joints, *Eng. Med.*, volume: 11, 1982, pp. 95–96.

65. Dogan, C. P., Hawk, J. A., Role of composition and microstructure in the abrasive wear of high-alumina ceramics, *Wear*, volume: 225–229, 1999, pp. 1050–1058.

66. Sedel, L., Kerboul, L., Christel, P., Meunier, A. and Witvoet, J., Alumina-on-alumina hip replacement, *J. Bone Joint Surg. Br.*, volume: 72B, 1990, pp. 658–663.

67. Xu, H. H. K., Wei, L. and Jahanmir, S., Influence of grain size on the grinding response of alumina, *J. Am. Ceram. Soc.*, volume: 79, 1996, pp. 1307–1313.

68. Xu, H. H. K., Jahanmir, S. and Wang, Y., Effect of grain size on scratch interactions and material removal in alumina, *J. Am. Ceram. Soc.*, volume: 78, 1995, pp. 881–891.

69. Xiong, F., Manory, R. R., Ward, L., Terheci, M. and Lathabai, S., Effect of grain size and test configuration on the wear behavior of alumina. *J. Am. Ceram. Soc.*, volume: 80, 1997, pp. 1310–1312.

70. Mukhopadhyay, A. K. and Mai, Y-W., Grain size effect on abrasive wear mechanisms in alumina ceramics, *Wear*, volume: 162–164, 1993, pp. 258–268.

71. He, Y., Winnubst, L., Burggraaf, A. J. and Verweij, H., Influence of porosity on friction and wear of tetragonal zirconia polycrystal, *J. Am. Ceram. Soc.*, volume: 80, number: 2, 1997, pp. 377–380.

72. Park, J. B. and Lakes, R. S., Biomaterials: An Introduction, New York: *Plenum Press*, 1992.

73. Streicher, R. M., Senlitsch, M. and Schon, R., Articulation of ceramic surfaces against polyethylene, pp. 118–123. Bioceramics and the Human Body. A. Ravaglioli and A. Krajewsk (eds.), New York: *Elsevier Applied Science*, 1992.

74. Grim, M. J., Orthopedic biomaterials, in: Standard handbook of biomedical engineering and design. 15.1–15.22.

75. Nieman, G. W., Weertman, J. R. and Siegel, R. W., Microhardness of Nanocrystalline Palladium and Copper Produced by Inert-Gas Condensation, *Scr. Metall.*, volume: 23, 1989, pp. 2013–2018.

76. Nieman, G. W., Weertman, J. R. and Siegel, R. W., Mechanical behavior of nanocrystalline Cu and Pd, *J. Mater. Res.*, volume: 6, 1991, pp. 1012–1027.

77. Vanzillotta, P. S., Soares, G. A., Bastos, I. N., Simão, R. A. and Kuromoto, N. K., Potentialities of some surface characterization techniques for the development of titanium biomedical alloys, *Materials Research*, volume: 7, number: 3, 2004, pp. 437–444.

78. Tengvall, P., Textor, M. and Brunette, D. M., Titanium in medicine, *Springer*, 2001.

79. Steinemann, S. G., Titanium: the material of choice? *Periodontol*, volume: 7, 2000, pp. 7–21.

80. Rompen, E., Domken, O., Degidi, M., Farias Pontes, A. E. and Piattelli, A., The effect of material characteristics, of surface topography and of implant components and connections on soft tissue integration: a literature review, *Clinical oral implants research*, volume: 17, number: 2, 2006, pp. 55–67.

81. Thomas, T., Rough Surfaces, *Imperial College Press*, 2nd edition London, 1999.

82. Wennerberg, A. and Albrektsson, T., Suggested guidelines for the topographic evaluation of implants surfaces, *The International Journal of Oral & Maxillofacial Implants*, volume: 15, number: 3, 2000, pp. 331–344.

83. Hong, J., andersson, J., Ekdahl, K. N., Elgue, G., Axen, N., Larsson, R. and Nilsson, B., Titanium is a highly thrombogenic biomaterial: Possible implications for osteogenesis, *Thrombosis Haemostasis*, volume: 82, number: 1, 1999, pp. 58–64.

84. Eisenbarth. E., Meyle. J., Nachtigall, W. and Breme, J., Influence of the surface structure of titanium materials on the adhesion of fibroblasts, *Biomaterials*, volume: 17, 1996, pp. 1399–1403.

85. Laurencin, C. T., Ambrosio, A. M. A., Borden, M. D. and Cooper, J. A. Jr., Tissue Engineering: Orthopedic Applications. *Annu. Rev. Biomed. Eng.*, volume: 1, 1999, pp. 19–46.

86. Unwin, P. S., The recent advantages in bone and joint implant technology. Cost-effective titanium component technology for leading-edge performance, M. Ward-Close (ed.), Bury St. Edmunds & London: *Professional engineers publishing limited for the institution of mechanical engineers*, 2000.

87. Dunn, M. G. and Maxian, S. H., Biomaterials used in orthopedic surgery, pp. 229–252. Implantation biology. The host response and biomedical devices, Greco, R. S. (ed.), Boca Paton: *CRC Press, Inc.*, 1994.

88. Davidson, J. A., Poggie, R. A., Mishra, A. K., Abrasive wear of ceramic, metal and UHMPE bearing surfaces from third-body bone, PMMA bone cement and titanium debris. *Biomed. Mater. Eng.*, volume: 4, 1994, pp. 213–229.

89. Coombes, A. D. and Heckman, J. D., Gel casting of resorbable polymers, *Biomaterials*, volume: 13, 1992, pp. 217–224.

90. Devin, J. E., Attawia, M. A. and Laurencin, C. T., Three-dimensional degradable porous polymer-ceramic matrices for use in bone repair, *J. Biomater. Sci. Polymer Ed.*, volume: 7, 1996, pp. 661–669.

91. Mikos, A. G., Thorsen, A. J., Czerwonka, L. A., Bao, Y. and Langer, R., Preparation and characterization of poly (l-lactic acid) foams, *Polymer*, volume: 35, 1994, pp. 1068–1077.

92. Thompson, R. C., Yaszemski, M. J., Powers, J. M. and Mikos, A. G., Fabrication of biodegradable polymer scaffolds to engineer trabecular bone, *J. Biomater. Sci. Polymer Ed.*, volume: 7, 1995, pp. 23–38.

93. Chen, V. J. and Ma, P. X., Nano-fibrous poly(l-lactic acid) scaffolds with interconnected spherical macropores, *Biomaterials*, volume: 25, 2004, pp. 2065–2073.

94. Miller, D. C., Thapa, A., Haberstroh, K. M. and Webster, T. J., Enhanced functions of vascular and bladder cells on poly-lactic-co-glycolic acid polymers with nanostructured surfaces, *IEEE Trans Nanobioscience*, volume: 1, number: 2, 2002, pp. 61–66.

95. Thapa, A., Miller, D. C., Webster, T. J. and Haberstroh, K. M., Nano-structured polymers enhance bladder smooth muscle cell function, *Biomaterials*, volume: 24, 2003, pp. 2915–2926.

96. Miller, D. C., Haberstroh, K. M. and Webster, T. J., Mechanism(s) of increased vascular cell adhesion on nanostructured poly(lactic-*co*-glycolic acid) films, *J. Biomed. Mater. Res. A.*, volume: 73, number: 4, 2005, pp. 476–484.

97. Park, G. E., Pattison, M. A., Park, K. and Webster, T. J., Accelerated chondrocyte functions on NaOH-treated PLGA scaffolds, *Biomaterials*, volume: 26, number: 16, 2005, pp. 3075–3082.

98. Liu, H., Slamovich, E. B. and Webster, T. J., Increased osteoblast functions among nanophase titania/poly(lactide-*co*-glycolide) composites of the highest nanometer surface roughness, *J. Biomed. Mater. Res. A.*, volume: 78, number: 4, 2006, pp. 798–807.

99. Vance, R. J., Miller, D. C., Thapa. A., Haberstroh, K. M. and Webster, T. J., Decreased fibroblast cell density on chemically degraded poly(lactic-*co*-glycolic acid), polyurethane, and polycaprolactone, *Biomaterials*, volume: 25, 2004, pp. 2095–2103.

100. Li, J., Polymeric hydrogels. In Engineering materials for biomedical applications, pp. 7.1–7.18, T. S. Hin (ed.), *World Scientific*, 2004.

101. Lee, K. Y. and Mooney, D. J., Hydrogels for tissue engineering, *Chemical Reviews*, volume: 101, number: 7, 2001, pp. 1869–1879.

102. Stevens, M. M. and George, J. H., Exploring and engineering the cell surface interface, *Science*, volume: 310, 2005, pp. 1135–1138.

103. Bonzani, I. C., George, J. H. and Stevens, M. M., Novel materials for bone and cartilage regeneration, *Current Opinion in Chemical Biology*, volume: 10, 2006, pp. 1–8.

104. Lia, M., Guob, Y., Weib, Y., MacDiarmidc, A. G. and Lelkes, P. I., Electrospinning polyaniline-contained gelatin nanofibers for tissue engineering applications, *Biomaterials*, volume: 27, 2006, pp. 2705–2715.

105. Kisiday, J., Jin, M., Kurz, B., Hung, H., Semino, C. and Zhang, S., et al., Self-assembling peptide hydrogel fosters chondrocyte extracellular matrix production and cell division: implications for cartilage tissue repair. *Proc. Natl. Acad. Sci.*, volume: 99, 2002, pp. 9996–10001.

106. Zhang, L., Ramsaywack, S., Fenniri, H. and Webster, T. J., Enhanced osteoblast adhesion on self-assembled nanostructured hydrogel scaffolds, *Tissue engineering*, in press, 2007.

107. Yamada, S., Heymann, D., Bouler, J. N. and Daculsi, G.D., Osteoclastic resorption of calcium phosphate ceramics with different hydroxyapatite/tricalcium phosphate ratios, *Biomaterials*, volume: 18, pp. 1037–1041.

108. Ramachandra, R. R., Roopa, H. N. and Kannan, T. S., Solid state synthesis and thermal stability of HAP and HAP-β-TCP composite ceramic powders, *Journal of materials science Materials in medicine*, volume: 8, 1997, pp. 511–518.

109. Tampieri, A., Celloti, G., Szontagh, F. and Landi, E., Sintering and characterization of HA and TCP bioceramics with control of their strength and phase purity, *Journal of materials science, Materials in Medicine*, volume: 8, 1997, pp. 29–37.

110. Cuneyt, A. T., Korkusuz, F., Timucin, M. and Akkas, N., An investigation of the chemical synthesis and high-temperature sintering behavior of calcium hydroxyapatite (HA) and Tricalcium phosphate (TCP) bioceramic, *Journal of materials science, Materials in medicine*, volume: 8, 1997, pp. 91–96.

111. Hench, L. L., Bioceramics, *Journal of the American Ceramic Society*, volume: 81, 1998, pp. 705–1728.

112. Homaeigohar, S. SH., Shokrgozar, M. A., Sadi, A. Y., Khavandi, A., Javadpour, J. and Hosseinalipour, M., *In vitro* evaluation of biocompatibility of beta-tricalcium phosphate-reinforced high-density polyethylene; an orthopedic composite, *Wiley Periodicals Inc.*, 2005.

113. Murugan, R. and Ramakrishna, S., Bioresorbable composite bone paste using polysaccharide based nano hydroxyapatite, *Biomaterials*, volume: 25, number: 17, 2004, pp. 3829–3835.

114. Esmaiel, J., Aqueous Based Hydrogel/Apatite Nanocomposite Scaffolds for Guided Bone Regeneration, Topical H #256d (TH014)—Biomedical Applications of Nanotechnology (Bionanotechnology), *AIChE Annual Meeting, Cincinnati, OH, Oct.* 30–Nov 4, 2005.

115. Quan, R., Yang, D. and Miao, X., Biocompatibility of graded zirconia-hydroxyapatite composite, *Chinese journal of reparative and reconstructive surgery*, volume: 20, number: 5, 2006, pp. 569–573.

116. Kim, H. W., Georgiou, G., Knowles, J. C., Koh, Y. H. and Kim, H. E., Calcium phosphates and glass composite coatings on zirconia for enhanced biocompatibility, *Biomaterials*, volume: 25, number: 18, 2004, pp. 4203–4213.

117. Kong, Y. M., Bae, C. J., Lee, S. H., Kim, H. W. and Kim, H. E., Improvement in biocompatibility of ZrO_2-Al_2O_3 nano-composite by addition of HA, *Biomaterials*, volume: 26, number: 5, 2005, pp. 509–517.

118. Mistry, A. S. and Mikos, A. G., Tissue engineering strategies for bone regeneration, advances in biochemical engineering/biotechnology 2005, pp. 94, 1–22.

119. Webster, T. J., Waid, M. C., McKenzie, J. L., Price, R. L. and Ejiofor, J. U., Nanobiotechnology: carbon nanofibres as improved neural and orthopaedic implants, *Nanotechnology*, volume: 15, 2004, pp. 48–54.

120. Shi, X., Hudson, J. L., Spicer, P. P., Tour, J. M., Krishnamoorti, R. and Mikos, A.G., Injectable nanocomposites of single-walled carbon nanotubes and biodegradable polymers for bone tissue engineering, *Biomacromolecules*, volume: 7, number: 7, 2006, pp. 2237–4.

121. Supronowicz, P. R., Ajayan, P. M., Ullmann, K. R., Arulanandam, B. P., Metzger, D. W. and Bizios, R., Novel current-conducting composite substrates for exposing osteoblasts to alternating current stimulation, *Journal of biomedical materials research*, volume: 59, volume: 3, 2002, pp. 499–506.

122. Tsuchiya, H., Macak, J. M., Muller, L., Kunze, J., Muller, F., Greil, P., Virtanen, S. and Schmuki, P., Hydroxyapatite growth on anodic TiO2 nanotubes, *Journal of biomedical materials research A.*, volume: 77, 2006, pp. 534–541.

123. Serro, A. P. and Saramago, B., Influence of sterilization on the mineralization of titanium implants induced by incubation in various biological model fluids, *Biomaterials*, volume: 24, 2003, pp. 4749–4760.

124. Barber, T. A., Golledge, S. L., Castner, D. G. and Healy, K. E., Peptide modified p (AAm-co-EG/AAc) IPNs grafted to bulk titanium modulate osteoblast behavior in vitro, *J. Biomed. Mater. Res.*, volume: 64, 2003, pp. 38–47.

125. Lu, X., Leng, Y., Zhang, X., Xu, J., Qin, L. and Chan, C. W., Comparative study of osteoconduction on micromachined and alkalitreated titanium alloy surfaces *in vitro* and in vivo, *Biomaterials*, volume: 26, 2005, pp. 1793–1801.

126. Macak, J. M., Tsuchiya, H., Taveira, L., Ghicov, A. and Schmuki, P., Self-organized nanotubular oxide layers on Ti-6Al-7Nb and Ti-6Al-4V formed by anodization in NH4F solutions, *J. Biomed. Mater. Res.*, 2005, volume: 75, pp. 928–933.

127. Winkelmann, M., Gold, J. and Hauert, R., Chemically patterned, metal oxide based surfaces produced by photolithographic techniques for studying protein- and cell-surface interactions I: Microfabrication and surface characterization, *Biomaterials*, volume: 24, 2003, pp. 1133–1145.

128. Balasundaram, G. and Webster, T. J., A perspective on nanophase materials for orthopedic implant applications, *J. Mater. Chem.*, volume: 16, 2006, pp. 3737–3745.

129. Hoet, P. H., Bruske-Hohlfeld, I. and Salata, O.V., Nanoparticles—known and unknown health risks, *J. Nanobiotechnology.*, volume: 2, 2004, pp. 2–12.

130. Tamura, K., Takashi, N. and Akasaka, T., Effects of micro/nano particle size on cell. function and morphology, *Key Engr. Mat.*, volume: 254, 2004, pp. 919–922.

131. Sato, M., Nanophase hydroxyapatite coatings for dental and orthopedic applications [Ph.D. thesis]. School of Materials Engineering, Purdue University, West Lafayette, IN, 2006.

132. Park, J. B. and Lakes, R. S., Biomaterials: An Introduction, New York: *Plenum Press*, 1992.

133. Streicher, R. M., Senlitsch, M. and Schon, R., Articulation of ceramic surfaces against polyethylene, pp. 118–123. Bioceramics and the human body. Ravaglioli, A. and Krajewsk, A. (eds.), New York: *Elsevier Applied Science*, 1992.

134. Reising, A., Yao, C., Storey, D. and Webster, T. J., Greater osteoblast long-term functions on ionic plasma deposited nanostructured orthopedic implant coatings, *J. Biomed. Mater. Res. A.*, volume: 87A, number 1, 2008, pp. 78–83. Epub ahead of print.

135. Spencer, N. D. and Textor, M., Surface modification, surface analysis, and biomaterials. http://www.textorgroup.ch/pdf/publications/journals/22/Spencer_MatDay_1998.pdf

136. Bronzino, J. D., Biomedical Engineering Handbook. *CRC Press*, 1995, pp. 274.706.

137. Vincent, J., Materials technology from nature. Metals and Materials, *Institute of Materials*, 1990.

138. Learmonth, I. D., Young, C. and Rorabeck, C., The operation of the century: total hip replacement, *Lancet*, volume: 370, 2007, pp. 1508–1519.

139. D'Antonio, J., Capello, W., Manley, M., Naughton, M. and Sutton, K., Alumina ceramic bearings for total hip arthroplasty, *Clinical orthopaedics and related research*, number: 436, 2005, pp. 164–171.

140. Affatato, S., Torrecillas, R., Taddei, P., Rocchi, M., Fagnano, C., Ciapetti, G. and Toni, A., Advanced nanocomposite materials for orthopaedic applications, a long-term *in vitro* wear study of zirconia-toughened alumina, *J. Biomed. Mater. Res. Part B (Appl. Biomater.)*, volume: 78B, 2006, pp. 76–82.

141. Tanaka, K., Tamura, J., Kawanabe, K., Nawa, M., Oka, M., Uchida, M., Kokubo, T. and Nakamura, T., Ce-TZP/Al$_2$O$_3$ nanocomposite as a bearing material in total joint replacement, *J. Biomed. Mater. Res. (Appl. Biomater.)*, volume: 63, 2002, pp. 262–270.

142. Takemoto, M., Fujibayashi, S., Neo, M., Suzuki, J., Kokubo, T. and Nakamura, T., Bone-bonding ability of a hydroxyapatite coated zirconia–alumina nanocomposite with a microporous surface. *J. Biomed. Mater. Res.*, volume: 78A, 2006, pp. 693–701.

143. Österle, W., Klaffke, D., Griepentrog, M., Gross, U., Kranz, I. and Knabe, CH., Potential of wear resistant coatings on Ti6Al4V for artificial hip joint bearing surfaces, *Wear*, volume: 264, 2008, pp. 505–517.

144. Sokolowska, A., Rudnicki, J., Niedzielski, P., Boczkowska, A., Boguslawski, G., Wierzchon, T. and Mitura, S., TiN-NCD composite coating produced on the Ti6Al4V alloy for medical applications, *Surf. Coat. Technol.*, volume: 200, 2005, pp. 87–89.

Section II

8

INTRODUCTION TO PROCESSING OF BIOMATERIALS

Dhirendra S. Katti, Shaunak Pandya, Meghali Bora, and Rakesh Mahida

Department of Biological Sciences and Bioengineering, Indian Institute of Technology, Kanpur, Kanpur, India

Contents

Abbreviations	246
8.1 Overview	247
8.2 Introduction	247
8.3 Processing of Biomaterials	248
8.3.1 Metals	248
8.3.1.1 Introduction	248
8.3.1.2 Metal Processing	249
8.3.1.2.1 Processing of Ores to Get Raw Metals	249
8.3.1.2.2 Processing of Raw Materials	250
8.3.1.2.3 Surface Finishing	250
8.3.2 Ceramics	251
8.3.2.1 Introduction	251
8.3.2.2 Processing	251
8.3.2.2.1 Preparation of Powders	251
8.3.2.2.2 Forming (Shaping) and Sintering of Powders	252
8.3.2.2.3 Surface Treatment	252
8.3.2.2.4 Other Processing Techniques	253

Advanced Biomaterials: Fundamentals, Processing, and Applications, Edited by Bikramjit Basu, Dhirendra S. Katti, and Ashok Kumar
Copyright © 2009 The American Ceramic Society

8.3.3 Polymers   254
    8.3.3.1 Introduction   254
    8.3.3.2 Processing   254
        8.3.3.2.1 Basic Steps of Processing   254
        8.3.3.2.2 Surface Treatment   255
8.3.4 Biocomposites   256
    8.3.4.1 Introduction   256
    8.3.4.2 Classification   256
    8.3.4.3 Manufacturing   256
        8.3.4.3.1 Fiber/Particle Reinforced Composites   256
        8.3.4.3.2 Metal Matrix Composites   256
    8.3.4.4 Processing/Surface Treatments   260
8.3.5 Sterilization   260
8.4 Processing for Scale   260
    8.4.1 Micro/Nano Surface Modification   260
        8.4.1.1 Introduction   260
        8.4.1.2 Types of Surface Modification   262
            8.4.1.2.1 Surface Chemistry   262
            8.4.1.2.2 Surface Topography   265
    8.4.2 Micro/Nano Fabrication   268
8.5 Conclusion and Future Directions   269
8.6 Brief Overview of Chapters in the Section on Processing   270
    Further Reading   271
    Acknowledgment   271
    References   271

Abbreviations

CAD	Computer aided design	MMC	Metal matrix composite
CAM	Computer aided machining	NIPAM	N-Isopropylacrylamide
Cermet	Ceramic + Metal	nm	Nanometer
CMC	Ceramic matrix composite	PAN	Polyacrylonitrile
CNT	Carbon nanotubes	PDLLA	Poly (D,L-lactic acid)
ECM	Extracellular matrix	PDMS	Poly (dimethylsiloxane)
ELD	Electrolytic deposition	PEEK	Poly (etheretherketone)
EPD	Electrophoretic deposition	PET	Poly (ethylene terephthalate)
FDM	Fused deposition modeling	PLGA	Poly (lactic-co-glycolic acid)
FGM	Functionally graded material	PLLA	Poly (L-lactic acid)
FN	Fibronectin	PMMA	Poly (methylmethacrylate)
GFOGER	Glycine–Phenylalanine–Hydroxyproline-Glycine-Glutamate–Arginine	PVC	Poly (vinyl chloride)
		RFGD	Radio frequency glow discharge
HAp	Hydroxyapatite	SFF	Solid freeform fabrication
LENS	LASER engineered net shaping	SLA	Stereolithography
		SLS	Selective laser sintering
MEMS	Micro-electro-mechanical systems		

8.1 OVERVIEW

In recent years, improved understanding of structure function relationship in tissues, tissue organization as well as biomaterial-host tissue interactions have had a large influence on the selection, design and processing of biomaterials. Most biomaterials need to undergo treatments that can enable them to possess properties and form/shape that is appropriate for the desired biomedical application. Therefore, transformation of biomaterials to the final device often requires a series of processing steps such as purification, fabrication, finishing, and sterilization. These processing methods normally vary with the type of biomaterial used. Biomaterials are generally classified into four types—metals, ceramics, polymers, and composites—with each type being conventionally processed by discrete methods. However, the choice of a processing technique for a specific biomaterial-based device depends on the physicochemical properties of the material as well as on the end application. This chapter provides an introduction to the section on processing of biomaterials and briefly discusses the conventional methods for processing metals, ceramics, polymers and composites. In addition, the chapter discusses processing/fabrication techniques that are used to manufacture devices at the micro/nanometer scale that are gaining increasing importance in the biomaterial-based device industry.

8.2 INTRODUCTION

The field of biomaterials has seen three generations of biomaterials ranging from glass eye and wooden teeth in the nineteenth century to advanced biomaterials like cell-seeded scaffolds in the twenty-first century [1]. Until the dawn of the twenty-first century, the materials used as biomaterials were non-viable metals, ceramics, polymers or their combinations in different physical forms. The evolution of biomaterials with time has resulted in the development of improved fabrication techniques. Conventional fabrication techniques of common biomaterials—metal-forging, casting, molding; ceramics-casting [2]; polymers-spinning, phase separation and composites-molding—have been modified or replaced by newer techniques which can process a wide variety of materials and fabricate biomaterials that are more amicable for biomedical applications—rapid prototyping, electrophoretic deposition [3] and laser assisted techniques [4]. The function of biomaterials has also gradually evolved from conventional replacement to more challenging repair and regeneration with the scale of biomaterial application moving down from whole organ to tissue level. The challenging applications often demand post-fabrication processing of biomaterials to improve surface finish, inertness, biocompatibility, and strength [5, 6], thereby leading to the development of surface processing techniques [1].

The cellular scale response that implanted biomaterials receive is mainly governed by their surface properties (chemistry and physical characteristics) [7–9]. Improved understanding of the effect of biomaterial surface on cellular fate processes has demonstrated that cells interact with implanted biomaterial via surface integrin receptors and show changes in cellular fate processes depending on the type and scale (macro/micro/nano) of the interaction [9, 10]. Therefore, via modifications in surface chemistry/topography of biomaterials, it is possible to alter cellular fate processes such as adhesion, migration and proliferation [11–20]. These cues were substantially implemented in designing biomaterials to improve biointegration and biocompatibility which in turn led to the development of advanced processing techniques. Initially, strategies for modification of surface topography involved different types of lithography and other surface etching techniques, whereas modification of surface chemistry involved various grafting techniques.

The last few decades have witnessed a rapid growth in the area of micro/ nanotechnology that has significantly influenced the field of bioengineering. This has, in turn, initiated the utilization of sophisticated tools (such as novel lithographic techniques, direct writing to create surface nanotopography) that can enable improved contact guidance [21, 22] of cells on biomaterials when compared to conventional surface modification techniques. Improved properties demonstrated by these micro/nano surface modified implants [23] has also opened up new methods to fabricate biomaterial-based devices having dimensions in the cellular and sub-cellular scale (or more precisely micrometer and nanometer scale) applications.

This chapter is meant to provide the reader with an introduction to the area of biomaterial processing and to enable a better understanding of other chapters in this section. In the first part, various conventional as well as advanced processing techniques (manufacturing, finishing, and sterilization) for four major classes of materials (metals, ceramics, polymers, and composites) used as biomaterials has been explained in brief. The second part of this chapter discusses advanced techniques used for micro/nanometer scale modification and fabrication.

8.3 PROCESSING OF BIOMATERIALS

8.3.1 Metals

8.3.1.1 Introduction. Metals, as biomaterials, have been used for a wide variety of biomedical applications. For example, in orthopedics, metals are used for bone and joint replacement in the form of fracture fixation plates, simple metallic wires, and screws. Besides orthopedic applications, metals are also used in other biomedical applications such as dental implants, electrodes in neural implants, in heart valves, and in pacemakers [24].

Most biomedical applications of metals demand some basic properties like, non-toxicity/biocompatibility, corrosion resistance and good mechanical properties that include static and cyclic load-bearing capabilities, tensile yield and ultimate strength, modulus of elasticity, fatigue endurance limit and toughness [28]. Since the aforementioned properties are largely influenced by the processing that the metal undergoes, it is essential to understand the processing of metals that are to be used for biomedical applications.

8.3.1.2 Metal Processing [24–26]. Metal processing in the context of biomedical implant includes conversion of metal ores, present in earth's crust, into final implant device through various steps such as extraction of raw metal, forming and casting operation, heat treatment and precipitation hardening, and finally surface finishing with or without inert coatings (Figure 8.1).

8.3.1.2.1 PROCESSING OF ORES TO GET RAW METALS. Metals are available in the earth's crust in an impure form called metal ores. These ores are commonly present as metal oxides and are often associated with impurities. Water flow and gravity-based separation are used to remove sand and further processing methods, such as electrostatic separator, extraction, vacuum processing and remelting, are used to convert the ore into raw metal [24].

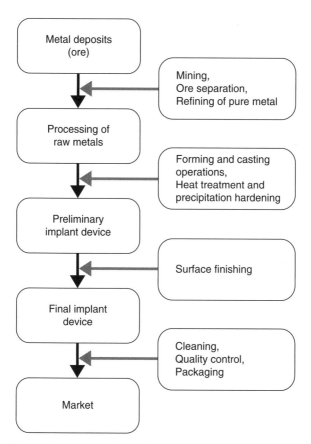

Figure 8.1. Schematic representation of conventional processing pathway of metals.

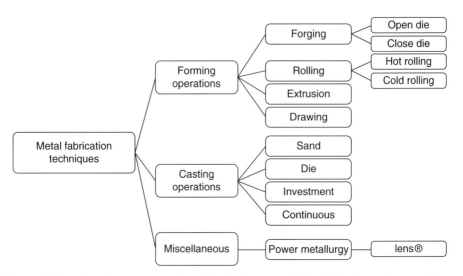

Figure 8.2. Schematic representation of techniques used for fabricating primary devices (bars, wires, sheets, rods, plates and tubes) from raw metal.

8.3.1.2.2 PROCESSING OF RAW MATERIALS [1, 25, 26]. Various forming and castings steps (Figure 8.2) are used to produce stock shapes from raw metal that are subsequently converted into primary devices such as bars, wires, sheet, rods, plates and tubes.

The strength of these stock shapes is improved by heat treatment and pre-cipitation hardening. Conventional metal fabrication techniques that involved the use of dyes for the production of stock shapes are being gradually replaced with modern techniques such as computer-aided machining (CAM/CAD) and automated processing for fabrication of preliminary implants [27, 29–32]. These modern techniques reduce production cost, processing time and shop-floor area, while providing greater manufacturing flexibility and precision on the shapes of the primary devices. The primary devices, once formed, then undergo surface finishing to incorporate desired changes in surface properties and aesthetics of the device.

8.3.1.2.3 SURFACE FINISHING. Surface finishing is the method of processing of stock shapes/preliminary devices to improve physicochemical properties [33] such as corrosion resistance, friction control, wettability, adhesion, and appear-ance. The two main types of surface modification techniques are adding/altering the surface and removing/reshaping the surface. However, there are other surface finishing techniques that are specifically used at lower scales (micro/nano-meter scale) and have been included under the section on 'processing by scale' in this chapter.

Metal processing techniques are gradually changing from the conventional techniques to more sophisticated techniques such as CAD/CAM and rapid prototyping that have enabled the fabrication of metallic implants with desired properties at high precision. Moreover, the recent fabrication techniques allow for synthesis of metal alloys which combines the desirable properties of constituent metals, thereby fostering potential for new horizons in the field. Along with these developments, novel surface modification techniques have also been developed to improve the surface property and functionality of an implant to improve biointegration. Hence, the modern techniques for metal fabrication hold promise for the future and will hopefully continue to improve the development of metal-based devices for biomedical applications.

8.3.2 Ceramics

8.3.2.1 *Introduction.* Basic composition of hard tissue includes natural polymers—such as collagen—and ceramics—such as hydroxyapatite—which impart strength to the tissue. Ceramics are inorganic, non-metallic biomaterials with a wide range of properties such as inertness, bioactivity, high strength, wear resistance and durability. These properties have led to their use in a wide range of biomedical applications such as orthopedic implants, neurostimulaters, pacemakers, artificial heart valves and cochlear implants. The most commonly used ceramic biomaterials are alumina, zirconia, pyrolytic carbon, bioglass, hydroxyapatite, and triclacium phosphate.

There are a number of techniques available for the processing of ceramics and the choice of an appropriate technique is largely driven by the properties desired from the ceramic. Although the basic steps of fabrication of ceramics can be similar, post-fabrication modifications can differ depending on the ultimate use of the biomaterial device [34].

8.3.2.2 *Processing.* Ceramics are currently used as biomaterials in a number of forms and compositions. Processing of ceramics is critical because this generally controls the final properties and functions of the finished ceramic product. Hence, it is important to understand the basic mechanism occurring in each step of processing to obtain the final product with desirable properties (microstructure and architecture) in a reproducible manner.

Broadly, ceramic processing techniques involve, preparation of powders, shaping and sintering of ceramic components and surface treatment of product.

8.3.2.2.1 PREPARATION OF POWDERS. This first step involves processing of raw ceramic materials to obtain uniform size of power, which can be further processed for shaping and sintering. The conventional methods of powder preparation include crushing, grinding, milling and screening, spray drying, freeze drying, and solution-precipitation (Figure 8.3) [35]. These processing techniques appropriately control purity, particle size and particle size distribution, which in turn enable homogeneous microstructure and high-sintered density. The method of preparation of powders can also influence the structure over many length scales, ranging from particle size to macroscopic dimensions of the material, which in turn can influence biomaterial host tissue interactions. Hence, powder

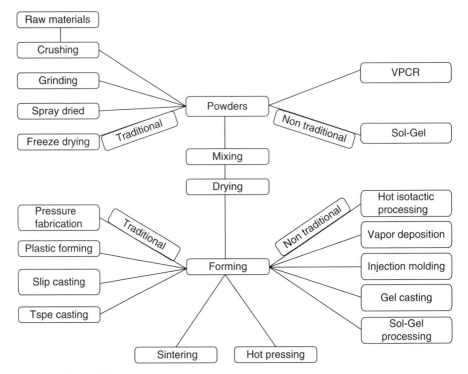

Figure 8.3. Schematic representation of ceramic processing techniques.

preparation can have a significant influence on the performance of the ultimate ceramic device/implant.

8.3.2.2.2 FORMING (SHAPING) AND SINTERING OF POWDERS. The preparation of powders culminates in the formation of a solid ceramic product. Solvent/binder is then added to the solid ceramic product to provide a specific shape. These forming processes can be broadly categorized into two types: traditional and non-traditional (Figure 8.3). The product formed after the forming process is known as "green ware [1]." Subsequently, this product then undergoes a heat treatment (called firing or sintering) for the removal of water and binders from the rigid finished product.

8.3.2.2.3 SURFACE TREATMENT. Various techniques have been developed to alter the surface characteristics (chemistry and topography) of ceramics to improve the functionality of the final device. Some of the major surface modification techniques include laser treatment [36], metal ion treatment [37], and acid treatment [41]. Laser treatment can be used to alter the surface of final products obtained from ceramics for controlling thermal gradients and cooling rates, for example, alumina-based ceramics [36]. Metal ions and their complexes can be used for the modification of ceramic surfaces, for example, Al^{3+} complexes are used for surface modification of SiC or Si_3N_4 particles [37]. Similarly, acid treatment can be used for the surface modification of ceramics such as zirconium [41].

8.3.2.2.4 OTHER PROCESSING TECHNIQUES. In addition to the aforementioned conventional processing techniques for ceramics, there are several other approaches that have been developed for the fabrication of ceramic products. Some of these techniques have been briefly explained in this section.

One such non-conventional technique is microwave processing, wherein pressureless sintering is done at low temperatures. This type of processing saves energy and reduces process cycle time. Other advantages include volumetric heating, a wide range of controlled heating rates, tailored microstructures, atmosphere control, and the ability to reach very high temperatures [38].

In addition to microwave processing, other ceramic processing techniques that have been reported include solid freeform fabrication (SFF) techniques—such as stereolithography (SLA), selective laser sintering (SLS), three-dimensional printing (3DP), direct ink-jet printing, robocasting, fused deposition modeling (FDM) and micro-pen writing [39]—ultra pressing, ultra rapid densification in inductively coupled plasma, direct casting, dynamic compaction of powders using high pressure shock waves, and electrodeposition [35].

One of the more recent ceramic processing techniques that is gaining increasing importance is electrodeposition, wherein thin ceramic films can be deposited on material surfaces. These techniques are gaining increasing importance as they are rapid and cost-effective processes that provide an easy scale-up option along with flexibility in the shapes of finished products. The two electrodeposition techniques that have been used for ceramics processing are electrophoretic deposition (EPD) and electrolytic deposition (ELD) [40]. In EPD, charged particles in a liquid move towards an electrode under the influence of electric field and deposition takes place due to particle coagulation. In ELD, solutions of metal salts produce colloidal particles from electrode reactions and deposition occurs on the substrate as a thin ceramic film. EPD allows shaping of free-standing objects as well as deposition of films, layers, and coatings on substrates. An interesting feature of EPD is the ability to engineer step-graded and functionally-graded materials/components. Due to the advantages offered by these electrodeposition techniques, they are being used for a number of other non-biomedical applications including electronic, optical, and electrochemical applications [40].

Conventional methods for powder synthesis like crushing and grinding do not produce materials with desirable microstructure. Hence, newer methods such as vapor phase chemical reactions (VPCR) and sol-gel methods have been developed that can produce fine powders with controlled microstructure in the finished ceramic product. In addition, these fabrication methods produce products with high purity, smaller defects, controlled microstructure, homogeneous particle size distribution and reproducibility, while requiring fewer fabrication steps. It is projected that the colloidal processing of powders and automation of the existing techniques for processing ceramics will contribute significantly to the development of advanced ceramics. Future research in ceramic processing would include designing of models for quantitative studies, development of novel forming processes for providing improved properties, newer formulations for power synthesis, and optimization at different scale-levels, including nanometer scale and lower.

8.3.3 Polymers

8.3.3.1 Introduction. Among all available biomaterials, polymeric materials present the greatest diversity in properties and processing techniques. The diversity in properties enables the use of polymers in a variety of applications, including long term implantable devices in neurological, cardiovascular, ophthalmic and reconstructive pathologies, as well as for devices to be used in short term applications such as hemodialysis, coronary angiogenesis, blood oxygenation, electrosurgery, wound treatment and dental implants. For any given application, polymers need to be processed into a form that is appropriate for that particular application. This manipulation of the material can be physical, chemical, thermal or mechanical, depending on the end application of the polymer.

There are several reported methods for the processing of polymers; for example, fibers can be processed by spinning; films and sheets by extrusion and calendering; and fabrication of specific shapes by molding methods. The basic steps involved in the processing of polymers have been briefly explained in the following section. In addition to the processing of polymers to generate specific forms, it is also important to understanding the surface characteristics (composition and structure) of a polymer as the processed polymer (biomaterial) primarily interacts with the neighboring microenvironment through its surface. Some of the important surface modification methods have been briefly explained later in this section.

8.3.3.2 Processing

8.3.3.2.1 BASIC STEPS OF PROCESSING [42–44]. The basic steps involved in polymer processing can be can be categorized as follows:

1. Pre-shaping—A form of polymeric material is produced by application of heat and/or pressure that can be shaped in the further steps.
2. Shaping—The pre-shaped polymeric material can be shaped by the techniques such as die forming, molding and casting, and surface treatments.
3. Post-shaping—The shaped polymeric material is further modified by processes such as welding, bonding, fastening, decorating, cutting, milling, drilling, dying and gluing to obtain the desired finished product.

To improve the properties of polymers, additional materials are often added to the polymer during its processing. These additives (i.e., plasticizers, stabilizers, fillers, lubricants, and foaming agents) can enhance the physical, chemical and mechanical properties of the final polymer [45].

Although the aforementioned steps of processing are commonly applicable to most polymeric biomaterials, there can be special applications wherein the processing of polymers can be relatively unique. One such example is that of processing polymers for the fabrication of scaffolds to be used in tissue engineering applications. Scaffolds are usually made from biodegradable polymers and act as a transient ECM that provides support and guidance for the growth of seeded cells that eventually leads to the formation of new tissue. Hence the polymers used for the fabrication of scaffolds are necessarily biocompatible and biodegradable while providing mechanical strength (especially important in the case of hard tissue regeneration) and being intrinsically transient in nature. In addition to these properties, more recent scaffolding systems are associated with proteins such as growth factors that govern tissue growth. The association of proteins with scaffolds limits the processing conditions in terms of temperature and usage of solvents, thereby making the processing more challenging. Various techniques that have been previously reported for the fabrication of scaffold are: fiber bonding, solvent casting and salt leaching, phase separation, freeze drying, membrane lamination, melt molding, and *in situ* polymerization [46, 47].

8.3.3.2.2 SURFACE TREATMENT [48]. Polymeric materials also undergo various surface finishing processes (Figure 8.4) with the aim of improvement of appearance, biocompatibility and biointegration.

Polymers, being chemically and physically versatile, have been used in a variety of biomedical applications. Due to the versatility of polymers and the growth in the biomedical device industry, the processing of polymeric biomaterials has experienced an exponential growth in the past few decades. Future development should involve machinery design, process analysis and optimization to enable the fabrication of polymeric products with improved properties.

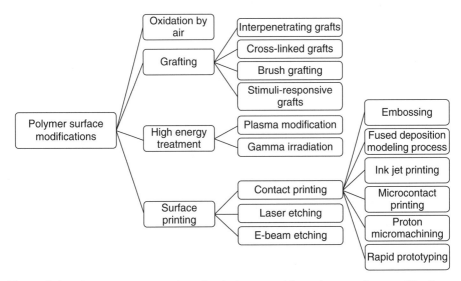

Figure 8.4. Schematic representation of techniques used for polymer surface modifications.

8.3.4   Biocomposites

8.3.4.1   Introduction. Metals, ceramics and polymers when used independently as biomaterials can have certain limitations. Hence, the search for an ideal biomaterial led to the development of biocomposites that are materials made up of physical combinations of conventional materials. Biocomposites generally consist of two phases, a matrix (base) phase in which there is an embedded reinforcing phase that is normally made up of particles or fibers [49] and hence in the final composite material both phases remain separate at the macro scale. Tailoring of composition and structure of both phases can be done to obtain specific physicomechanical properties and hence desired biological response. Thus the composition, synthesis and processing of biocomposites are aspects that must be carefully considered while designing a composite for biomedical applications.

8.3.4.2   Classification. Though composites can be classified in various ways, depending on the type of reinforcing phase they can be classified as follows: [1, 44, 50–53]

- Fiber Reinforced
  - Continuous fiber reinforced (long fibers extending throughout matrix phase) Alignment of long fibers gives anisotropy to the properties of final composite.
  - Discontinuous fiber reinforced (short fibers dispersed in matrix phase) Random orientation of short fibers gives isotropy to the properties of final composite.
- Particle Reinforced [54]
  - Small particles or whiskers dispersed throughout the matrix phase.

8.3.4.3   Manufacturing

8.3.4.3.1   FIBER/PARTICLE REINFORCED COMPOSITES [1, 44]. In general, the procedure for fabrication of composites involves reinforcing and matrix phase mixing, compaction and consolidation. However, the manufacturing technique can vary with final biocomposite composition. For example, composites that use thermoplastic materials as the continuous phase or need to be resistant to water intrusion are not fabricated by open mold processes [1]. Figure 8.5 provides a schematic of the processing techniques used for fiber/particle reinforced composites.

Curing (cross linking of matrix phase material) may be used *in situ* or post fabrication to reduce degradation and increase strength. Depending on the type of composite material, curing may be induced by light, heat, electron beam or x-ray.

8.3.4.3.2   METAL MATRIX COMPOSITES [52, 55–57]. Though Metal Matrix Composites (MMCs) are classified under fiber or particle reinforced composites,

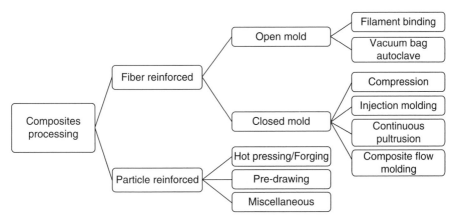

Figure 8.5. Schematic representation of composite processing techniques.

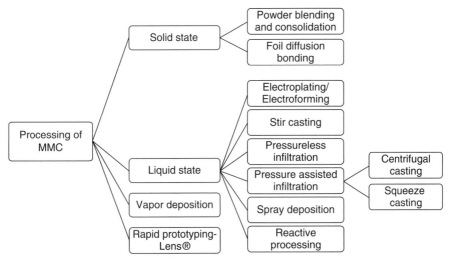

Figure 8.6. Schematic representation of processing techniques used for manufacturing MMCs.

they possess unique manufacturing techniques (Figure 8.6) by virtue of metals being their continuous phase. Depending on the properties desired in the final composite, processing can vary from conventional metal processing to advanced rapid prototyping.

Discontinuous MMC's can be produced with standard metalworking techniques, such as extrusion, forging or rolling as stated in the section 8.3.1.2 on metals in this chapter. However, functionally graded MMC's [58] (in which the composition and microstructure change gradually from one side to the other) and cermets can be manufactured using techniques such as LENS® [59]. In addition to the aforementioned techniques, there are other processing techniques that have been used for the fabrication of specific biocomposites as shown in Table 8.1.

TABLE 8.1. Novel Processing Techniques for Fabrication of Biocomposites

Sr. No	Fabrication method	Matrix phase	Reinforcement phase	Application	Comments	Reference
1.	**Textile preforming (braiding) and Pultrusion**	Epoxy	Carbon fiber/ Kevlar fibers	Orthopedic implants	Functionally graded composite rods can be produced	[60]
2.	**Hot pressing/ forging**	PLLA	HAp	Orthopedic implants	Possible to change the porosity, PLLA molecular weight and amorphous/ crystal-line ratio	[61]
3.	**Flow molding**	PEEK	Carbon fiber	Medical screws	—	[49]
4.	**Mixing and incubation**	Calcium phosphate and fibrin glue(Tissucol^tm) mixture	—	Bone tissue engineering	—	[62]
5.	**Insitu polymerizetion** of resin matrix monomers by light/heat application	Bisphenol A-glycidyl methacrylate	64% barium Aluminum fluoride glass	Dental restorative material	—	[63]
6.	**Sol-gel processing** followed by **electrospinning** technique	TiO_2	MWNT-COOH	Improves the catalytic property of titania	Mechanism of crystallization not clear	[64]

	Technique	Material		Advantage	Remarks	Ref.
7.	**Pre drawing** technique	Polypropylene	SiO_2	High tensile strength, improved particle dispersion	—	[65]
8.	**Supercritical CO$_2$ injection** system	Poly(DL-lactic acid) (PDLLA)	Live murine C2C12 cells	Incorporation of mammalian cells into the scaffold fabrication step at any stage of polymer processing	Time-dependent survival of the cells in supercritical CO_2	[66]
9.	**Electrophoretic deposition** (EPD)	TiO_2,CNT mixture	—	Laminate coating of various metal	This method is an additive process and can be used to deposit nanostructures on metals	[3]
10.	**Novel combustion synthesis**	Mullite (TiB_2)	Zircona	Endothermic reaction can be carried out	Unlike normal combustion technique, this method can be used for reactions other than exothermic	[67]

259

8.3.4.4 Processing/Surface Treatments. The surface of biocomposites can be modified by methods that are applicable both pre- and post-fabrication. The goal of these surface treatments is mainly for improving biocompatibility and integration as well as bond strength between the two phases. The methods used for surface finishing of composites vary with the type of composite, such as CMC or MMC. Examples of such methods are provided under individual material sections of this chapter.

The following methods are examples of surface treatment techniques that have been used to improve adhesion between filler resin and implanted composite for repairing of the latter in dentistry [6]: air-borne particle abrasion (50 μm Al_2O_3) and silica coating (30 μm SiO_2, CoJet®-Sand).

In the recent past, composites have gained increased importance as biomaterials because they possess a combination of desirable properties of both the individual components. Hence their processing techniques primarily depend on their composition and end use. General processing involves manufacturing of matrix phase, manufacturing of reinforcement phase, embedding of reinforcement phase in matrix phase, and, finally, curing of composite to improve strength and decrease degradation rate. Unlike conventional molding techniques, newer techniques like pultrusion and resin injection molding are capable of producing a composite with highly aligned reinforcement phase, uniform cross sectional area, as well as functionally graded composites. Just as in conventional biomaterials, biocomposites also can undergo various types of surface treatments post fabrication to improve tissue biomaterial interactions [9]. It is projected that more advanced methods such as micro/nanofabrication techniques hold promise for the production of next generation biocomposites.

8.3.5 Sterilization

Biomaterials that are intended for applications that involve direct contact with human tissue or body fluids demand proper sterilization techniques to prevent chances of infection and undesirable immune response. The selection of an appropriate sterilization method usually depends on the chemical composition and end use of the material. In the case of biocomposites that are made up of a mixture of two or more chemically distinct materials, this selection becomes even more challenging. The method of choice is normally the one that provides good sterilization while minimally compromising on the desirable properties of the biocomposites. Table 8.2 enlists some of the commonly used sterilization methods for biomaterials.

8.4 PROCESSING FOR SCALE

8.4.1 Micro/Nano Surface Modification

8.4.1.1 Introduction. After the implantation of a device, biomaterial-tissue interaction events occur at different time and length scales as shown in Figure 8.7. Some of these events occur within a fraction of a second while others

TABLE 8.2. Commonly Used Sterilization Methods Along with Their Advantages and Limitations

Method	Advantage	Limitation	Comments	References
Ethanol 70%	No adverse effect on polymer, metal or ceramic	Does not adequately eliminate hydrophilic viruses and bacterial spores	Limited to surface disinfection	[68]
Dry Heat	No adverse effect on strength of ceramic/composite	Adversely affects most biomaterials' composition	—	[69]
Autoclave	No adverse effect on composition of ceramic/composite	Adversely affects compressive strength of ceramic/composite	—	[69]
Ethylene oxide	No adverse effect on composition of most biomaterials	Residual deposition is hazardous and can lead to shrinkage of polymer macrostructures	Relatively better when compared to ethanol, dry heat and autoclaving	[68]
Gamma irradiation	—	Causes surface roughening in ceramics and metals. Causes decrease in molecular weight, and increase in cross-linking, density and melting point of polymers	Widely used for implant materials	[61, 68, 70]
Electron beam irradiation	—	Same as above	Less used	[70]
Radio frequency glow discharge (RFGD) plasma sterilization	Does not alter 3-D morphology of composite macro-structures	Effective only on surfaces due to poor penetration power	Very effective in etching prions and endotoxins from surfaces	[68, 70]

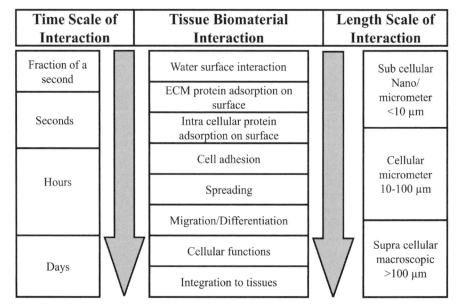

Time Scale of Interaction	Tissue Biomaterial Interaction	Length Scale of Interaction
Fraction of a second	Water surface interaction	Sub cellular Nano/ micrometer <10 μm
	ECM protein adsorption on surface	
Seconds	Intra cellular protein adsorption on surface	
Hours	Cell adhesion	Cellular micrometer 10-100 μm
	Spreading	
	Migration/Differentiation	
Days	Cellular functions	Supra cellular macroscopic >100 μm
	Integration to tissues	

Figure 8.7. Tissue biomaterial interactions: events occurring at the tissue biomaterial interface at varying time and length scales.

can take as long as few days [10]. The fast initial response is generally governed by the surface chemistry of the implanted biomaterial/device. Surface chemistry modulates adhesion and signaling of cells which in turn controls phenotype and cell function while degree of adhesion modulates proliferation and differentiation [9]. Therefore, alterations on the surface of a biomaterial can modulate cell behavior/function, which in turn governs the tissue response to the implant/device. Hence, it is important to understand cell-biomaterial surface interaction to enable better integration of the implant/device.

Cell behavior/function such as adhesion, cell morphology, migration, orientation, and differentiation are influenced by biomaterial surface topography and surface chemistry [71]. This has been evidenced in the native environment wherein fibrous proteins present in the ECM of tissue have diameters in the micrometer range, while mineral particles present in the ECM of bone tissue have diameters in the nanometer range and both of these scales (fiber-micrometer and mineral particle-nanometer) have a different effect on cell behavior, though the exact mechanism is still not well understood. Therefore, surface chemistry and surface topography [72, 73] are important design considerations during the development of a biomaterial-based implant to improve integration and compatibility.

8.4.1.2 Types of Surface Modification [1, 7, 10, 74]

8.4.1.2.1 SURFACE CHEMISTRY. To date several ways of modifying surface chemistry have been explored [1, 7, 9, 15]. Changes in surface chemistry can pro-

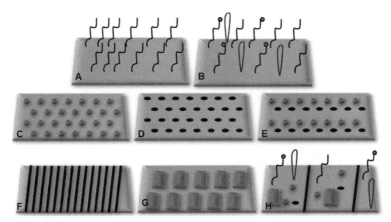

Figure 8.8. Surface modifications of biomaterials: surface chemistry (A-B) and topography (C-H). (A) Single molecule grafting, (B) Multi-molecule grafting (e.g., RGD and PHSRN), (C) Patterned nano-islands, (D) Patterned pits, (E) Patterned pits and nano-islands, (F) Patterned channels, (G) Patterned pillars and (H) Combinatorial approach.

mote or deter protein/cell adhesion onto the implant depending on the bioactive moieties present on the surface, that is, functionalities such as NH_2, COOH, CH_3 and OH or amino acids such as RGD, RADS, RGDS and PHSRN. The surface chemistry of biomaterials can be modulated using surface grafting techniques as shown in Figure 8.8 (A–B).

Following is the list of different techniques that are used to tailor surface chemistry of the biomaterials.

- Noncovalent coatings
  - Solvent deposition
  - Langmuir-Blodgett film deposition
  - Vapor deposition of metals and carbon
- Covalently attached coatings
- Radiation, plasma and photo-grafting
- Thin film deposition
- Application of a surface chemical gradient
- Self-assembled films: They give highly ordered structures on specific substrates, for example alkanethiols array arranged on gold
- Surface chemical reaction
- Soft lithography-micro contact printing of alkanesthiols on gold
- Chemical grafting (ozonization)
- Surface modification via aminolysis

Table 8.3 lists some of the surface chemistry modifications [16, 20, 22, 84] that have been reported for biomaterials.

TABLE 8.3. Different Types of Surface Chemistry Modifications on Biomaterials.

Surface chemistry	Fabrication methods used	Material used	Dimensions	References
Peptides	Covalent linking on PLGA scaffold by aminolysis	RGD	—	[11]
	Covalent linking on titatium surface via Poly(OEGMA) as linker	$\alpha_5\beta_1$-integrin-specific FN fragment $FNIII_{7-10}$	~135 A° thick	[79]
	Coating on titanium surfaces using silicone based adhesive	GFOGER collagen-mimetic peptide	Surface density $123.2 \pm 6.2\, ng/cm^2$	[80]
Protein/ polysaccharide tracks	Photolithography followed by silanization and coating on quartz or glass	Laminin or fibronectin	2–25 µm width	—
	Plasma etching and Photo-immobilization	Hyaluronan	25 or 5 mm wide and 35 nm thick	[19]
Grooves and chemical pattern	Photolithography and reactive ion etching, silanization	Amino-silane and methyl-silane coated quartz	Square grooves 2.5–50 µm width 0.1–6.0 µm depth	[18]
	Photolithography anisotropic etching, polymer micro- molding, treatment with alkanethiols	Ti, Au-coated polyurethane treated with ibronectin, alkane thiols	V-shaped grooves 5, 50 µm width	
Micro patterning of cells	Laser-guided particle deposition Ink jet printing	Chinese Hamster ovary and embryonic motoneuron cells	Deposition in patterns	[81] [82]

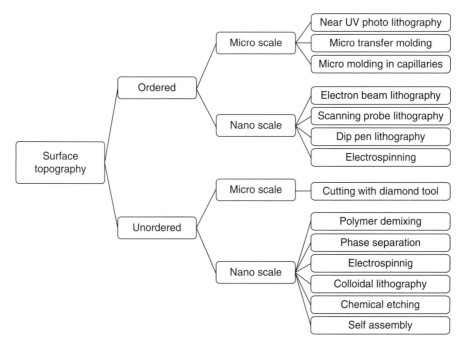

Figure 8.9. Schematic representation of types of topographical modification and techniques used for their fabrication.

8.4.1.2.2 SURFACE TOPOGRAPHY [48, 75–78]. Addition or subtraction of material at the surface leads to surface roughness. Although photolithography has been widely used for generating surface topographies, new methods that allow for more precise control of topography at the micro/nano scale [Figure 8.8 (C-H), Figure 8.9] have also been developed.

As previously stated, surface topography can significantly influence cell behavior and as a consequence biomaterial-tissue interaction and eventual device integration with tissue. Hence, a variety of methods have been developed for the modulation of surface topography including plasma methods. Among the plasma methods, a wide choice is available for use, such as plasma sputtering and etching, plasma implantation, plasma deposition, plasma polymerization, laser plasma deposition and plasma spraying. The main advantage of surface modification using plasma-based techniques is that they do not affect the bulk properties or composition of the biomaterial [85]. Table 8.4 lists some of the surface topography modifications [16, 20, 22, 84] that have been reported for biomaterials.

Contrary to the belief that surface modifications can significantly influence cell response, there have been reports that surface modification may not influence biointegration or biomaterial host tissue response. Parker et al. studied implants that were surface treated with RFGD plasma or fibronectin coating and demonstrated that none of the surface treatment methods significantly influenced tissue reaction around the implant [14]. In a similar study with surface modified silicon

TABLE 8.4. Different Types of Surface Topography Modifications on Biomaterials

Surface topography	Fabrication methods used	Material used	Dimensions	References
General roughness	**Metal**-acid etching, nitriding, plasma-etching, electro- polishing, ion beam etching	—	—	[8, 83]
	Polymer-sand blasting, polymer casting, scratching, plasma treatment			[8, 84]
Grooves	Photolithography and reactive ion etching	PDMS cast of silicon original	Square grooves 2, 5, 10 µm width 0.5 µm depth	—
	Photolithography and anisotropic etching	Ti-coated silicon	Square and V-shaped grooves, 7 and 39 µm repeat spacing with 3 or 10 µm depth	
	Photolithography and anisotropic etching	Poly-lysine-coated quartz	Square grooves 1 µm width 1 µm depth	
	Electron-beam lithography and wet etching	PDMS cast of silicon original	Square grooves 2, 5, 10 µm width 0.5 µm depth	
	UV and glow discharge treatment	Serum-coated glass	2 µm width 2 µm depth	
	Cutting with diamond or tungsten	Poly-D-lysine coated chrome plated quartz	0.13–4.01 µm width 0.1–1.17 µm depth	
	Laser holographic technique used to define masks for X-ray lithography and reactive ion etching	Quartz and poly-L-lysine coated quartz	130 nm width 100–400 nm depth	

Feature	Method	Material	Dimensions	Ref.
Grooves and Pits	Photolithography and anisotropic etching	Titanium-coated epoxy replicas of silicon original	V-shaped grooves 35–165 μm width 30–120 μm depth V-shaped pits 35–270 μm width and 30–120 μm depth	—
Ridges	Photolithography and reactive ion etching Evaporative coating	Polystyrene cast of silicon original Silicon oxide on Polystyrene PMMA	0.5–100.0 μm width 0.03–5.0 μm height 4 μm width 50 nm height 1–18 μm steps	—
Steps	Photolithography and reactive ion etching			—
Waves	Solution polymerization	PDMS gels of varying softness	Softer gels had smaller waves while hard gel had larger waves	—
Wells and Nodes	Photolithography and etching	PDMS replicas of silicon original	2, 5 μm diameter round nodes, 0.38 and 0.46 μm high respectively 8 μm round well, 0.57 μm deep Square nodes 7, 25, or 50 μm width 0.5, 1.5, 2.5 μm height	—
Pillars and Pores	Laser modification	Polycarbonate, polyetherimide	Circular pillars and pores 1–50 μm diameter	—
	Laser ablation used in conjunction with masks made by electron-beam lithography, reactive ion etching	PMMA, PET, polystyrene		
Pores	Micro porous filter: Nylon dip-coated with PVC/PAN copolymer	Uncoated and silicon coated filters	0.2–10 μm diameter	—
Spheres	Particle settling	Poly(NIPAM) particles on polystyrene surface	0.86–0.63 μm diameter when temperature raised from 25 to 37°C	—
Cylinders	Fiber-optic light conduit–fused quartz cylindrical fibers placed on agarose-covered cover slips	Fused quartz	12–13 or 25 μm radii	—

and poly (lactic acid), Parker et al. demonstrated that application of periodic or random micro grooves to polymer implants had no beneficial effect on peri-implant tissue healing [87]. Although there are some reports on the limited influence of surface modification on cell behavior, a large majority of reports support the fact that surfaces of biomaterial-based implants can significantly influence cell and tissue response. Hence, there have been efforts to understand and develop improved methods for surface modification. Also, since most of the cell–biomaterial interactions occur at the micrometer and nanometer length scale, there has been a strong motivation to understand and develop methods for processing as well as for fabrication at these length scales.

8.4.2 Micro/Nano Fabrication [88]

Although fabrication of micro/nanometer scale devices for electronics/electromechanical applications have been extensively reported, their use in biomedical applications is more recent and is projected to grow exponentially in the near future. The fabrication techniques at the micro/nanometer scale use either the top-down or the bottom-up approach to fabricate micro/nano structures. The top-down approach involves starting with a bulk material/biomaterial and arriving at the desired length scale by reduction in material content (subtractive process), whereas the bottom-up approach involves starting at a molecular scale and building on that to arrive at the desired length scale (additive process). The fabrication techniques for biomedical devices were initially limited to manufacturing of polymeric drug delivery devices but have now been expanded to multiple applications including fabrication of smart devices such as BIOMEMS and BIONEMS [90]. Micro/nanometer scale fabrication techniques like LENS(r) have found use in production of implantable devices with controlled surface architecture. These techniques hold promise in the production of micro/nanometer scale scaffolds [12, 86], micro-fluidics for artificial vascularization and, implantable microchips as self-regulated drug devices.

Broadly, microfabrication techniques can be divided into two types:

- Surface micromachining—is an additive process in which fabrication of structures is done via deposited thin films.
- Bulk micromachining—is a subtractive process in which fabrication of structures is done by selective removal of material from the bulk material.

Table 8.5 enlists some of the various micro/nano-meter scale biomedical structures along with their respective fabrication techniques [23, 89].

After establishing that surface chemistry and topography of biomaterials can be tailored to provoke a favorable cellular response, this concept has gained significant importance in the design of advanced biomaterials. As a consequence, numerous methods have emerged that can precisely tailor biomaterial surface chemistry and topography. However, it is expected that as our understanding of cellular responses to surface chemistry and topography improves, the designing

TABLE 8.5. Fabrication Techniques of Various Micro/Nano Devices

Device	Fabrication techniques
Microneedles, Micropumps/Microvalves, Implantable microchip	Micromachining techniques adopted from microelectronics industry
Liposomes	High pressure homogenization, microemulsion method and high speed stirring
Nanofibers	Electrospinning, drawing, self assembly, phase separation and template synthesis
Dendrimes	Convergent synthesis and divergent synthesis
Nanotubes and fullerenes	Chemical vapor deposition, electric arc discharge and laser ablation
Nanogels	Emulsion polymerization and crosslinking reaction of preformed polymer fragments
Nanocrystals	Wet comminution, precipitation, disintegration and milling

of biomaterial surfaces (chemistry and topography) will develop simultaneously, thereby leading to improved biomedical devices.

8.5   CONCLUSION AND FUTURE DIRECTIONS

Newly developed biomaterials have revolutionized the field of biomedical devices in the past few years. Hence, the selection, manufacturing and processing of biomaterials has gained increased importance in the recent past. After the selection of an appropriate biomaterial, their processing and fabrication techniques are the parameters that can significantly influence the performance/function in the intended final application. These processing techniques can be fairly diverse for biomaterials due to the diversity in type of biomaterials—metals, ceramics, polymers, composites. However, for all of these classes of biomaterials, conventional methods of processing can have limitations for use in biomedical applications. Hence, newer techniques that offer advantages such as desired mechanical and chemical properties, precise control on device dimensions, and improved reproducibility have been developed.

On a parallel front, the modification of implant surfaces for improved integration with neighboring tissue has witnessed significant progress. A variety of methods have been developed to modify surface chemistry and topography at both the macro as well as the micro/nanometer scale. Newer fabrication techniques at the micro/nanometer scale have also led to improved devices such as advanced drug delivery systems, scaffolds for tissue engineering applications, and biosensors. Nanotechnology borrowed from the electronics industry has been used extensively for fabrication of micro/nanometer scale structures like micro pumps, valves, implantable chips (Bio-MEMS/NEMS), self-regulated drug delivery devices, and micro needles. In the future, it is expected that the processing techniques (especially micro/nanometer scale processing) may play an important role in the development of next-generation biomaterials with the potential to interact with cells at cellular, as well as sub-cellular, scales.

8.6 BRIEF OVERVIEW OF CHAPTERS IN THE SECTION ON PROCESSING

Following this introductory chapter, this section on processing consists of chapters that describe some emerging manufacturing techniques such as Laser Assisted Net Shaping (LENS) as well as processing involved in designing biomaterials for applications such as bioactive scaffolds and polymeric drug delivery systems.

The chapter written by R. Banerjee (University of North Texas, U.S.) demonstrates how novel near-net shape processing technologies, such as laser-engineered net shaping (LENS™) can be utilized to rapidly manufacture custom-designed functionally-graded unitized implants with site-specific properties. The chapter also discusses the mechanical properties, the electrochemical response, wear resistance and biocompatibility of laser-deposited beta Ti alloys and metal-matrix composites for orthopedic applications.

After reviewing the present status of the development of bioinert ceramics for Total HIP joint Replacement (THR), the chapter by Omer Van Der Biest (Katholieke Universiteit Leuven, Belgium) and his co-workers, largely focuses on the design principles of Electrophoretic deposition as a novel processing route to develop functionally gradient materials (FGM) based on biocompatible ceramics. The processing issues to select optimal parameters to obtain gradient in composition and properties for small-to-large scale ZrO_2/Al_2O_3 based implant materials are discussed.

In the chapter written by Pio González (Universidade de Vigo, Lagoas-Marcosende, Vigo, Spain) and co-workers, bioinspired ceramics for bone tissue replacement are discussed. The chapter focuses on biomorphic silicon carbide ceramics fabricated from bio-derived cellulose templates that can be applied as scaffolds for bone substitution because of their lightweight, high-strength and interesting biocompatibility with natural tissues. The chapter discusses the microstructure, chemical composition, and mechanical properties of different types of biomorphic silicon carbide ceramics along with the *in vitro* biocompatibility test data.

The chapter by Artemis Stamboulis (University of Birmingham, Birmingham, UK) and co-workers discusses the design and characterization of ionomeric glasses with a focus on the crystallization aspects of the glasses.

The chapter by Dhirendra Katti (Indian Institute of Technology, Kanpur, India) and co-workers describes the processing of polymeric systems for the synthesis of nanofibers that are to be used as scaffolding systems for tissue engineering applications. The chapter emphasizes electrospinning techniques and discusses the various polymeric systems that have been used to generate nanofibers which in combination with cells have been applied for the regeneration of musculoskeletal tissue.

The chapter by Ashok Kumar (Indian Institute of Technology, Kanpur, India) and co-workers describes a novel processing technique applicable to polymeric systems for the generation of supramacroporous biomaterials. The chapter discusses the processing technique—known as "cryogelation"—and discusses various polymeric systems that have been used for the synthesis of cryogels, along with their applications.

FURTHER READING

1. Ratner BD, Schoen FJ, Hoffman AS, and Lemons JE, eds., Biomaterials Science: An Introduction to Materials in Medicine, Elsevier Academic Press, 2004.
2. Callister WD Jr, ed., Materials Science and Engineering, An Introduction, John Wiley and Sons, Inc., 1997.
3. Gonsalves KE, Halberstadt CR, Laurencin CT, and Nair LS, eds., Biomaedical Nanostructures, Wiley-Interscience, 2007.
4. Vadgama P, ed., Surface and Interface for Biomaterials, CRC Press, 2005.

ACKNOWLEDGMENT

Corresponding author DSK would like to acknowledge Indian Institute of Technology Kanpur, Department of Science and Technology, India and Department of Biotechnology (DBT), India for the research grants received. Authors SP and MB would like to acknowledge All India Council for Technical Education (AICTE) and RM would like to acknowledge DBT, India for providing Research Assistantship.

REFERENCES

1. Ratner BD, Schoen FJ, Hoffman AS, Lemons JE. Biomaterials Science: An Introduction to Materials in Medicine. Elsevier Academic Press; 2004. p 67–83; 181–195; 201–215.
2. Geiger G. Powder Synthesis and Shape Forming of Advanced Ceramics. American Ceramic Society Bulletin; 2004;62–65.
3. Johann C. Nanostructured carbon nanotube/TiO_2 composite coatings using electrophoretic deposition (EPD). J Nanopart Res 2008;10:99–105.
4. Laoui T, Santos E, Osakada K, Shiomi M, Morita M, Shaik SK, Tolochko NK, Abe F. Properties of Titanium implant models made by LASER processing. Rapid Manufacturing 2004;475–484.
5. Singh R, Dahotre NB. Corrosion degradation and prevention by surface modification of biometallic materials. J Mater Sci: Mater Med 2007;18:725–751.

6. Ozcan M, Alander P, Vallittu PK, Huysmans MC, Kalk W. Effect of three surface conditioning methods to improve bond strength of particulate filler resin composites. J Mater Sci: Mater Med 2005;16:21–27.

7. Vasita R, Katti DS. Improved biomaterials for tissue engineering applications: Surface modification of polymers. Curr Topics Med Chem 2008;8:341–353.

8. Pesakova V, Kubies D, Hulejova H, Himmlova L. The influence of implant surface properties on cell adhesion and proliferation. J Mater Sci: Mater Med 2007;18: 465–473.

9. Roach P, Eglin D, Rohde K, Perry CC. Modern biomaterials: a review—bulk properties and implications of surface modifications. J Mater Sci: Mater Med 2007;18:1263–1277.

10. Palsson BQ, Bhatia SN. Tissue Engineering. Pearson Education; 2003. p 270–289.

11. Yoon JJ, Song SH, Lee DS, Park TG. Immobilization of cell adhesive RGD peptide onto the surface of highly porous biodegradable polymer scaffolds fabricated by a gas foaming/salt leaching method. Biomaterials 2004;25:5613–5620.

12. Sarkar S, Lee GY, Wong JY, Desai TA. Development and characterization of a porous micro-patterned scaffold for vascular tissue engineering applications. Biomaterials 2006;27:4775–4782.

13. Kulkarni SS, Orth R, Ferrari M, Moldovan NI. Micropatterning of endothelial cells by guided stimulation with angiogenic factors. Biosens Bioelectron 2004;19:1401–1407.

14. Parker JATC, Walboomers XF, Von den Hoff JW, Maltha JC, Jansen JA. Soft tissue response to microtextured silicone and poly-l-lactic acid implants: fibronectin pre-coating vs. radio-frequency glow discharge treatment. Biomaterials 2002;23:3545–3553.

15. Bin L, Ma Y, Wang S, Moran PM. A technique for preparing protein gradients on polymeric surfaces: effects on PC12 pheochromocytoma cells. Biomaterials 2005;26: 1487–1495.

16. Yoshihiro I. Surface micropatterning to regulate cell functions. Biomaterials 1999;20: 2333–2342.

17. Jager M, Zilkens C, Zanger K, Krauspe R. Significance of nano- and microtopography for cell-surface interactions in orthopaedic implants. J Biomed Biotechnol 2007;2007: 1–19.

18. Charest JL, Eliason MT, Garc AJ, King WP. Combined microscale mechanical topography and chemical patterns on polymer cell culture substrates. Biomaterials 2006; 27:2487–2494.

19. Barbucci R, Torricellib P, Finib M, Pasquia D, Faviac P, Sardellac E, d'Agostinoc R, Giardino R. Proliferative and re-defferentiative effects of photo-immobilized micro-patterned hyaluronan surfaces on chondrocyte cells. Biomaterials 2005;26:7596–7605.

20. Giordano C, Sandrini E, Busini V, Chiesa R, Fumagalli G, Giavaresi G, Fini M, Giardino R, Cigada A. A new chemical etching process to improve endosseous implant osseointegration: in vitro evaluation on human osteoblast-like cells. Int J Artif Organs 2006;29:772–780.

21. Uttayarat P, Toworfe GK, Dietrich F, Lelkes PI, Composto RJ. Topographic guidance of endothelial cells on silicone surfaces with micro- to nanogrooves: orientation of actin filaments and focal adhesions. J Biomed Mater Res A 2005;75A:668–680.

22. Flemming RG, Murphy CJ, Abrams GA, Goodman SL, Nealey PF. Effects of synthetic micro- and nano-structured surfaces on cell behaviour. Biomaterials 1999;20:573–588.

23. Gonsalves KE, Halberstadt CR, Laurencin CT, Nair LS. Biomedical Nanostructures. Wiley-Interscience; 2007. p 139–183.

24. Ratner BD, Schoen FJ, Hoffman AS, Lemons JE. Biomaterials Science An Introduction To Materials In Medicine. Elsevier Academic Press; 1996. p 139–141.

25. Kalpakjian S. Manufacturing Engineering and Technology. Addison-Wesley Publishing Company; 1995. p 265–317; 357–359; 381–389; 417–430; 499–512.

26. Beddoes J, Bibby M J. Principles of Metal Manufacturing Processes. Viva Books Private Ltd; 2000. p 99–100; 103–107; 115–117; 121–127; 173–181.

27. Groover MP, Zimmers EW. CAD/CAM: Computer-Aided Design and Manufacturing. Prentice-Hall of India Private Ltd; 1991. p 1–3; 53–56.

28. Pilliar RM. Modern metal processing for improved load bearing surgical implants. Biomaterials 1991;12:95–100.

29. Giannatsis J, Dedoussis V. Additive fabrication technologies applied to medicine and health care: a review. Int J Adv Manuf Technol 2007;1–12.

30. Roy R, Agrawal D, Cheng J, Gedevanishvili S. Full sintering of powdered-metal bodies in a microwave field. Nature 1999;399:668–670.

31. Yang S. Metering and dispensing of powder; the quest for new solid freeforming techniques. Powder Tech 2007;178:56–72.

32. Takahashi R. State of the art in hot rolling process control. Contr Eng Prac 2001;9: 987–993.

33. Nie X. Thickness effects on the mechanical properties of micro-arc discharge oxide coatings on aluminium alloys. Surf Coating Tech 1999;116–119:1055–1060.

34. Bartolo P, Bidanda B. Bio-Materials and Prototyping Applications. Springer; 2008. p 1–14.

35. Biswas D. Development of novel ceramic processing. J Mater Sci Lett 1989;24: 3791–3798.

36. Triantafyllidis D, Li L, Stott HF. Surface treatment of alumina based ceramics using combined laser sources. Appl Surf Sci 2002;186:140–144.

37. Zhang Y. Surface modification of ceramic powders by complexes of metal ions in aqueous media. J Mater Sci Lett 2002;21:1723–1725.

38. Isabel KL, Yuval C, Otto CW, Gengfu X. Microwave processing of ceramics. Adv Sci Tech 2006;45:857–862.

39. Peng YHX, Yang L, Su B. Fabrication of three dimensional inter-connective porous ceramics via ceramic green machining and bonding. J Eur Ceram Soc 2008;28: 531–537.

40. Boccaccinia IZ. Application of electroproretic and electrolytic deposition techniques in ceramics processing. Curr Opin Solid State Mater Sci 2002;6:251–260.

41. Randon J, Blanc P, Paterson R. Modification of ceramic membrane surfaces using phosphoric acid and alkyl phosphonic acids and its effects on ultrafiltration of BSA protein. J Membr Sci 1995;98:119–129.

42. Griskey RG. Polymer Processes: Extrusion in Polymer Process Engineering. Chapman and Hall 1995;278–447.

43. Carraher CE. Introduction to Polymer Chemistry. CRC press; 2007. p 429–469.

44. Callister WD. Jr. Materials Science and Engineering, An Introduction. John Wiley and Sons; 1997. p 488–498; 510–544.

45. Grulke EA. Polymer Process Engineering. PTR Prentice Hall; 1994. p 7–17.

46. Atala A. Methods of Tissue Engineering. Academic Press; 2002. p 681–738.

47. Robert PL, Robert L. Princliples of Tissue Engineering. Academic Press; 2000. p 251–260.

48. Vadgama P. Surface and Interface for Biomaterials. CRC Press; 2005. p 29–57; 40–49; 150–182; 389–411; 447–461; 719–740.

49. Ramakrishna S, Huang ZM, Kumar GV, Batchelor AW, Meyer J. An Introduction to Biocomposites. Imperial College Press; 2004.

50. Jones DW. Dental Composite Biomaterials. J Can Dent Assoc 1998;64:732–734.

51. Opdam NJM, Roeters JJM, de Boer T, Pesschier D, Bronkhorst E. Voids and porosities in class I micropreparations filled with various resin composites. Operative Dentistry 2003;28.

52. Witte F, Feyerabend F, Maier P, Fischer J, Stormer M, Blawert C, Dietzel W, Hort N. Biodegradable magnesium–hydroxyapatite metal matrix composites. Biomaterials 2007;28:2163–2174.

53. Evans SL, Gregson PJ. Composite technology in load-bearing orthopaedic implants. Biomaterials 1998;19:1329–1342.

54. Wang M, Joseph R, Bonfield W. Hydroxyapatite-polyethylene composites for bone substitution effects of ceramic particle size and morphology. Biomaterials 1998;19: 2357–2366.

55. Taha MA, El-Mahallawy NA. Metal-matrix composites fabricated by pressure-assisted infiltration of loose ceramic powder. J Mater Process Tech 1998;73:139–146.

56. Aghajanian MK, Rocazella MA, Burke JT, Keck SD. The fabrication of metal matrix composites by a pressureless infiltration technique. J Mater Sci 2004;26:447–454.

57. Hashim J. The production of cast metal matrix composite by a modified stir casting method. Jurnal Teknologi A 2007;35A:9–20.

58. Liu W, DuPont JN. Fabrication of functionally graded TiC/Ti composites by laser engineered net shaping. Scripta Materialia 2003;48:1337–1342.

59. Xiong Y, Smugeresky JE, Ajdelsztajn L, Schoenung JM. Fabrication of WC–Co cermets by laser engineered net shaping. Mater Sci Eng A 2008;493:261–266.

60. Boss JN, Ganesh VK. Fabrication and properties of graded composite rods for biomedical applications. Compos Struct 2006;74:289–293.

61. Ignjatovic N, Uskokovik D. Synthesis and application of hydroxyapatite/polylactide composite biomaterials. Appl Surf Sci 2004;238:314–319.

62. Nihouannen DL. Micro-architecture of calcium phosphate granules and fibrin glue composites for bone tissue engineering. Biomaterials 2006;27:2716–2722.

63. Casselli DS, Worschech CC, Paulillo LA, Dias CT. Diametral tensile strength of composite resins submitted to different activation techniques. Braz Oral Res 2006;20: 214–218.

64. Aryal S, Kim CK, Kim KW, Khil MS, Kim HY. Multi-walled carbon nanotubes/TiO_2 composite nanofiber by electrospinning. Mater Sci Eng 2007;28:75–79.

65. Ruan WH, Mai YL, Wang XH, Rong MZ, Zhang MQ. Effects of processing conditions on properties of nano-SiO_2/polypropylene composites fabricated by pre-drawing technique. Composites Science and Technology 2007;67:2747–2756.

66. Ginty PJ, Howard D, Upton CE, Barry JJA, Rose FRAJ, Shakesheff KM, Howdle SM. A supercritical CO_2 injection system for the production of polymer/mammalian cell composites. J Supercri Fluids 2008;43:535–541.

67. Zaki ZI. Novel route for combustion synthesis of zirconia–mullite/TiB_2 composites. J Alloy Comp 2009;467:288–292.

68. Holy CE, Cheng C, Davies JE, Shoichet MS. Optimizing the sterilization of PLGA scaffolds for use in tissue engineering. Biomaterials 2001;22:25–31.

69. Alonso LM, Carrodeguas RG, Menocal JADG, Perez JAA, Manent SM. Effect of sterilization on the properties of CDHA-OCP-β-TCP biomaterial. Mater Res 2007;10: 15–20.

70. Goldman M, Gronsky R, Pruitt L. The influence of sterilization technique and ageing on the structure and morphology of medical-grade ultrahigh molecular weight polyethylene. J Mater Sci: Mater Med 1998;9:207–212.

71. Evelyn KFY, Leong KW. Significance of synthetic nanostructures in dictating cellular response. Nanomedicine: Nanotechnology, Biology, and Medicine 2005;1:10–21.

72. Hirao M, Sugamoto K, Tamai N, Oka K, Yoshikawa H, Mori Y, Sasaki T. Macrostructural effect of metal surfaces treated using computer-assisted yttrium-aluminumgarnet laser scanning on bone-implant fixation. J Biomed Mater Res A 2005;73A:213–22.

73. Hamilton DW, Chehroudi B, Brunette DM. Comparative response of epithelial cells and osteoblasts to microfabricated tapered pit topographies *in vitro* and *in vivo*. Biomaterials 2007;28:2281–2293.

74. Barbucci R, Pasqui D, Wirsen A, Affrossman S, Curtis A, Tetta C. Micro and nano structured surfaces. J of Mat Sci: Mat in Med 2003;14:721–725.

75. Bae B, Chun BH, Kim D. Surface characterization of microporous polypropylene membranes modified by plasma treatment. Polymer 2001;42:7879–7885.

76. Norman JJ, Desai TA. Methods for fabrication of nanoscale topography for tissue engineering scaffolds. Ann Biomed Eng 2006;34:89–101.

77. Dalby MJ, Gadegaard N, Tare R, Andar A, Riehle MO, Herzyk P, Wilkinson CDW, Oreffo ROC. The control of human mesenchymal cell differentiation using nanoscale symmetry and disorder. Nat Mater 2007;6:997–1003.

78. Takashi I, Okasaki S. Pushing the limits of lithography. Nature 2000;406:1027–1031.

79. Petrie TA, Raynor JE, Reyes CD, Burns KL, Collard DM, Garcı AJ. The effect of integrin-specific bioactive coatings on tissue healing and implant osseointegration. Biomaterials 2008;2849–2857.

80. Reyes CD, Petriea TA, Burnsa KL, Schwartzb Z, Garcı AJ. Biomolecular surface coating to enhance orthopaedic tissue healing and integration. Biomaterials 2007; 28:3228–3235.

81. Chrisey DB. Materials Processing: The power of direct writing. Science 2000;289: 879–881.

82. Xu T, Jin J, Gregory C, Hickman JJ, Boland T. Inkjet printing of viable mammalian cells. Biomaterials 2005;26:93–99.

83. Cui FZ, Luo ZS. Biomaterials modification by ion-beam processing. Surf Coating Tech 1999;112:278–285.

84. Schroder K, Meyer-Plath A, Keller D, Ohl A. On the applicability of plasma assisted chemical micropatterning to different polymeric biomaterials. Plasmas and Polymers 2002;7:103–125.

85. Chu PK, Chen JY, Wang LP, Huang N. Plasma-surface modification of biomaterials. Mater Sci Eng 2002;36:143–206.

86. Ma PX. Biomimetic materials for tissue engineering. Adv Drug Deliv Rev 2008; 60:184–198.

87. Parker JATC, Walboomers XF, Von den Hoff JW, Maltha JC, Jansen JA. Soft-tissue response to silicone and poly-L-lactic acid implants with a periodic or random surface micropattern. J Biomed Mater Res 2002;61:91–98.

88. Zachary HJ, Nicholas A, Peppas A. Microfabricated drug delivery devices. Int J Pharm 2005;306;15–23.

89. Lu Y, Chen SC. Micro and nano-fabrication of biodegradable polymers for drug delivery. Adv Drug Deliv Rev 2004;56:1621–1633.

90. Wang GJ, Chen CL, Hsu SH, Chiang YL. Bio-MEMS fabricated artificial capillaries for tissue engineering. Microsyst Technol 2005;12:120–127.

9

LASER PROCESSING OF ORTHOPEDIC BIOMATERIALS

Rajarshi Banerjee[1] and Soumya Nag[2]

[1]*Department of Materials Science and Engineering, University of North Texas, Denton, Texas, USA*
[2]*Department of Materials Science and Engineering, Ohio State University, Columbus, Ohio, USA*

Contents

9.1	Overview	278
9.2	Introduction	279
9.3	Laser Processing of Orthopedic Biomaterials	282
	9.3.1 Novel Processing Technology—Laser Engineered Net Shaping (LENS™)	282
	9.3.2 Proposed Design of Functionally-Graded Hip Implant	285
	9.3.3 Laser Processed Ti-Nb-Zr-Ta Alloys	286
	9.3.3.1 Details of Processing and Characterization Methods Used	286
	9.3.3.2 Microstructure and Mechanical Properties	287
	9.3.3.3 Deformation Mechanisms	290
	9.3.3.4 Corrosion Resistance of LENS™ Deposited Ti-Nb-Zr-Ta Alloys	296
	9.3.3.5 XPS Studies of the Passive Oxide Film on LENS™ Deposited TNZT	298
	9.3.3.6 Preliminary *In Vitro* Studies on LENS™ Deposited TNZT	302

Advanced Biomaterials: Fundamentals, Processing, and Applications, Edited by Bikramjit Basu, Dhirendra S. Katti, and Ashok Kumar
Copyright © 2009 The American Ceramic Society

9.3.4 Laser Processed Titanium Boride Reinforced Ti-Nb-Zr-Ta
       Metal-matrix Composites   304
      9.3.4.1 Wear Resistance of Titanium Alloys and Titanium
            Matrix Composites   304
      9.3.4.2 Titanium Boride Reinforced Ti-Nb-Zr-Ta Composites   305
      9.3.4.3 Tribological Behavior of Ti-Nb-Zr-Ta + TiB Composites   309
      9.3.4.4 Summary of Ti-Nb-Zr-Ta + TiB Composites   317
9.4 Conclusions   318
9.5 Future Perspectives   319
    Acknowledgments   319
    References   320

9.1 OVERVIEW

In the area of load-bearing orthopedic implant applications, both novel metallic and non-metallic biomaterials as well as novel processing technologies can have a substantial impact. While there has been a significantly large volume of research in recent years on the development of novel titanium alloys, especially based on the beta phase of titanium, for implant applications there has been rather limited research on the development and application of newer processing technologies for fabricating such implants. The newer generation beta titanium alloys that are being actively researched for biomedical applications typically contain completely biocompatible (non-toxic) alloying elements such as niobium, zirconium, tantalum, molybdenum, iron, and tin. These alloys also exhibit a substantially lower elastic modulus that is much closer to that of bone (10–40 GPa) as compared with the previous generation alloys, such as Ti-6Al-4V.

On the processing side, while orthopedic implants are conventionally fabricated using traditional metal-working processing technologies such as casting and forging, the advent of novel processing technologies such as direct deposition of metallic powders using a laser-based deposition process (for example, the laser engineered net shaping or LENS™ process) can substantially impact implant fabrication. Thus, while traditional processes are typically subtractive in nature with material being removed (machined) from a big block of metal into the final shape of the implant, processes such as LENS™ based on additive manufacturing permit the fabrication of a three-dimensional near-net shape component directly from a computer-aided design file in a single step. Furthermore, the use of laser-deposition based additive manufacturing also allows for the fabrication of custom-designed compositionally and *functionally graded* implants with *site-specific* properties, a concept that can revolutionize the processing of orthopedic implants.

In this chapter, some of the salient features of laser-deposition of orthopedic biomaterials will be discussed. In addition to the processing aspects, the core of this chapter is devoted to the properties of laser-deposited beta titanium alloys and metal-matrix composites, in the context of their suitability for use in orthopedic implants.

9.2 INTRODUCTION

Due to demographic changes, there is a worldwide increase in the average age of the population, leading to a rapidly increasing number of surgical procedures involving prosthesis implantation. Human joints are prone to degenerative and inflammatory diseases that result in pain and stiffness of joints [1]. Approximately 90% of the population over the age of 40 suffers from some degree of degenerative joint disease [2]. Typically such premature degenerative diseases result in degradation in the mechanical properties of the joint that has been subjected to excessive loading conditions or from failure of normal biological repair processes. Since the natural joints cannot function optimally, the joint surfaces are replaced by artificial biomaterials through arthoplastic surgery [1]. This has resulted in an urgent need for improved biomaterials and manufacturing technologies for orthopedic implants such as hip, knee, and shoulder implants.

Furthermore, since such geometrically-complex implants have different property requirements at different locations, their manufacturing becomes particularly challenging. The design and manufacture of these medical devices is complicated by a host of inter-related factors, including regulatory requirements, patient quality of life considerations, durability, weight of the device, cost, and constraints of manufacturing. In order to achieve the best balance of all these factors, compromises often have to be made in the design and development of orthopedic implants. However, the advent of novel additive near-net shape manufacturing processes, such as the laser engineered net shaping (LENS™) process [3,4] is expected to have a substantial impact on the design and development of a new generation of orthopedic implants and other medical devices. Furthermore, by employing such near-net shape processing technologies, it is possible to manufacture custom-designed implants with site-specific properties. Such a novel processing approach is expected to have a substantial impact on the development of next-generation orthopedic implants and is the primary motivation for this chapter.

Typically the manufacturing of a hip implant is a multi-stepped process that may take weeks [5–8]. The starting raw material is typically a casting or forging in the rough shape of the femoral stem part of the hip implant. This casting or forging is polished to remove scales and rough edges leftover from the casting or forging process [9]. Usually, a skilled craftsman is required for carrying out the polishing job. Subsequently, the stem of the implant is passed through a fluorescent penetrate inspection (FPI) for surface defects such as cracks, porosity, and other imperfections. Following the FPI test, the stem is exposed to sand-blasting in order to give the implant an uneven surface finish for better bonding with the porous coating that is subsequently sprayed on the surface of the implant. The stem is initially sprayed with a binder followed by a layer of metal beads made of either cobalt-chromium alloy or titanium. The stem is then sintered to allow for the porous coating to adhere to the implant surface.

Subsequently, the taper or top of the stem is machined to precise measurements using a lathe, followed by a final polishing step. The stem is then put through a bath of nitric acid to remove any undesirable materials left behind during the manufacturing process. The other components of the hip implant are also manufactured in a series of steps. The femoral head, which is the component that replaces the top of the natural thigh bone, can be manufactured in approximately one week. The acetabular cup, which replaces the hip socket of the pelvic bone, consists of a metallic shell (typically titanium base) with a medical grade ultra-high molecular weigh polyethylene (UHMWPE) liner. While the metallic shell takes three to four weeks to manufacture, the liner takes about two weeks. It should be emphasized that these various processes involve considerable time and therefore expensive. Additionally, most of the processes are subtractive in nature and involve significant waste of materials, consequently increasing the cost of manufacturing.

One of the key manufacturing challenges for hip implants is the strongly contrasting property requirements at different locations of the implant. The components of a typical hip (femoral) implant used for a total joint replacement (TJR) are the femoral stem, the femoral head, and the acetabular cup [10] as shown schematically in Figure 9.1. The property requirements for these individual components are listed below [11]:

1. Femoral stem: low elastic modulus (close to bone modulus), high strength, good ductility, good fatigue resistance, good fracture toughness, good corrosion resistance, no cyto-toxic reactions with the bone tissue, excellent osseo-integration (attachment to the bone).
2. Femoral head: excellent wear resistance, good fracture toughness, good corrosion resistance, no cyto-toxic reactions with the bone tissue.
3. Acetabular cup: good corrosion resistance, no cyto-toxic reactions with the bone tissue, excellent osseo-integration, and, excellent wear resistance to the counterface material of the femoral head.

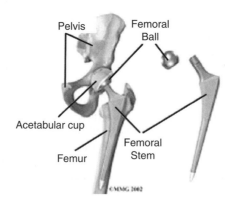

Figure 9.1. Schematic representation of typical hip implant showing the femoral head (or ball), femoral stem and acetabular cup.

Traditionally, the differences in the property requirements of these components have warranted the use of very different materials and processing routes for these components resulting in the unavoidable formation of abrupt interfaces between types of materials. Localized wear at these interfaces may cause debris formation which is a great concern from the health and safety point of view.

For example, while the femoral stem is often made of titanium alloys, such as Ti-6Al-4V, the poor wear resistance of this alloy prevents its use for femoral head applications. Therefore, more wear-resistant materials are used for the femoral head, such as ceramics (e.g., alumina or zirconia) or cobalt-chromium alloys. However, while alumina or zirconia ceramic femoral heads offer excellent wear-resistance, these ceramics do not have the same level of fracture toughness as their metallic counterparts leading to problems such as fracture of these heads in use. This has even lead to the recall of hip implants using zirconia femoral heads [12–14]. Furthermore, the use of a ceramic femoral head attached to a metallic femoral stem also leads to an undesirable abrupt ceramic/metal interface in the hip implant.

From the materials perspective, while the use of titanium-base alloys had been quite beneficial for such implants, most of the materials that are currently in use, such as Ti-6Al-4V, were originally developed for other applications such as for aircraft engines. Consequently, in general the biomaterials that have been used to date possess a less than optimum combination of biocompatibility and mechanical properties, representing a fairly unfavorable compromise regarding the necessary balance of properties for application in orthopedic implants. The ideal biomaterial for orthopedic implant applications, especially for load-bearing joint replacements, is expected to exhibit excellent biocompatibility with no adverse cytotoxicity, excellent corrosion resistance, and a good combination of mechanical properties such as high strength and fatigue resistance, low modulus, good ductility, and good wear resistance [1,15]. The two primary Ti base alloys used in implants today are commercially pure (C.P.) titanium and Ti-6Al-4V ELI (extra low interstitial impurity content). Recent studies show that the release of both V and Al ions from Ti-6Al-4V might cause long-term health problems, such as peripheral neuropathy, osteomalacia, and Alzheimer diseases [16,17].

Another issue with the existing Ti-base orthopedic alloys is that their modulus is significantly higher than that of bone tissue (~10–40 GPa), leading to *stress-shielding* that can potentially cause bone resorption and eventual failure of the implant [18]. Thus, there is currently a substantial thrust directed towards the development of completely biocompatible low modulus implant alloys. β-Ti alloys exhibit a substantially lower modulus as compared with stainless steels, cobalt-based alloys and also conventional $\alpha\beta$ alloys, such as Ti-6Al-4V. Recently developed biocompatible β-Ti alloys developed for this purpose include Ti-12Mo-6Zr-2Fe [19], Ti-15Mo-5Zr-3Al [20], Ti-15Mo-3Nb-3O [21], Ti-13Nb-13Zr [22], and Ti-35Nb-5Ta-7Zr [23]. Interestingly, while the role of microstructure in determining the properties has been well-recognized and critically addressed in the field of structural materials, in the case of implant alloys, the role of the microstructure and the influence of processing on the microstructure has been sparsely addressed in the literature. Therefore, there is an urgent need for the development of a better understanding of microstructural evolution and property-microstructure relationships in implant alloys as a function of processing.

As noted above, the need for prosthesis implants such as hip implants is increasing at an alarming rate. While currently existing hip implants function appropriately, they do not represent the best compromise of required properties. Furthermore, presently the manufacturing of implants is largely via subtractive technologies involving substantial material wastage leading to increased costs and time of production. Therefore, an imperative need exists for functionally-graded hip implants representing a better balance of properties and manufactured via novel additive manufacturing technologies based on near-net shape processing.

Some specific problems associated with currently employed implant manufacturing processes and the consequent compromise in properties are listed below:

1. The manufacturing is based on conventional casting and forging of components followed by material removal steps via subtractive technologies such as precision machining. These technologies not only involve substantial wastage of material but are also limited to monolithic components without any compositional/functional changes within the same component.

2. Diverse property requirements at different locations on an implant are satisfied by joining different components (for example, femoral stem and femoral head) made of different materials in a total hip replacement system. This always leads to the formation of chemically abrupt interfaces that are detrimental to the properties of the implant.

The current manufacturing route for hip implants does not allow for custom-designing for specific patients with rapid turnaround times. Consequently, instead of custom-designing the implant, the surgeon is often forced to adapt the pre-existing design to fit the patient's requirements. This can become particularly challenging if the required physical dimensions of the implant differ substantially from those of the standard manufactured ones, such as implants to be used for children.

9.3 LASER PROCESSING OF ORTHOPEDIC BIOMATERIALS

9.3.1 Novel Processing Technology—Laser Engineered Net Shaping (LENS™)

Similar to rapid prototyping technologies such as stereolithography, the LENS™ process [3,24] begins with a CAD design file of a three-dimensional component, which is electronically sliced into a series of layers. The information about each of these layers is transmitted to the manufacturing assembly. A metal or alloy substrate is used as a base for depositing the component. A high power laser (capable of delivering several hundred watts of power) is focused on the substrate to create a melt pool into which the powder feedstock is delivered through an inert gas flowing through a multi-nozzle assembly. The nozzle is designed such that the powder streams converge at the same point on the focused laser beam. Subsequently, the substrate is moved relative to the laser beam on a computer-controlled stage to deposit thin layers of controlled width and thickness [24].

There are four primary components of the LENS™ assembly: the laser system, the powder delivery system, the controlled environment glove box, and the motion control system. A 750W Nd:YAG laser, which produced near-infrared laser radiation at a wavelength of 1.064 µm, is typically used for the depositions. The energy density is in the range of 30,000 to 100,000 W/cm^2. The oxygen content in the glove box is maintained below 10 ppm during the depositions. The powder flow rates are typically 2.5 g/min while the argon volumetric flow rate is maintained at three litres/min. The LENS™ offers a unique combination of near-net shape manufacturing and rapid solidification processing that can be particularly useful for manufacturing orthopedic implants. A schematic representation of the LENS™ process is shown on the top of Figure 9.2.

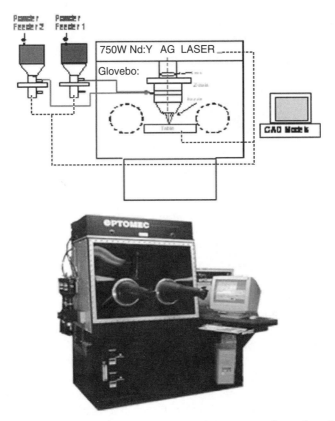

Figure 9.2. Schematic representation and image of the LENS™ laser deposition system. [Rajarshi Banerjee et al. *Laser Deposited Ti-Nb-Zr-Ta Orthopedic Alloys* (J. Bio. Mater. Res., 78A (2), 2006), 298.]

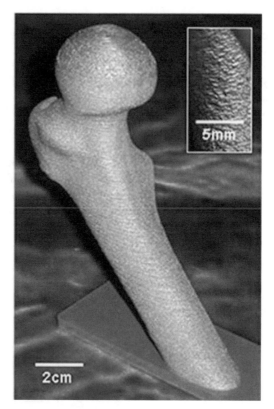

Figure 9.3. LENS™ deposited hip (femoral) implant with internal cavity. [Optomec Design Company, Albuquerque, New Mexico, U.S.]

There the two powder feeders along with the laser setup and the visual monitor is drawn. The actual picture of the LENS equipment is shown in the bottom part of the figure. The LENS™ process has been commercialized by the company Optomec Inc., based in the United States, and has been demonstrated to be a viable processing technology for fabrication of orthopedic implants, e.g., femoral hip implants. For example, a prototype hollow femoral implant made from Ti-6Al-4V using LENS™ is shown in Figure 9.3.

One of the key strength of LENS™ processing is that by using a powder-feeder system consisting of multiple hoppers, it is possible to process compositionally-graded and consequently functionally-graded materials. Thus, by controlling the deposition rates from individual hoppers, it is possible to design compositionally graded materials as demonstrated in a number of previous papers on laser-processed compositionally-graded titanium alloys [25–26]. From the viewpoint of orthopedic implants, compositionally-graded alloys can be particularly beneficial since they will enable the development of custom-designed orthopedic implants with site-specific properties. Furthermore, engineering functional gradation in these implants will allow for a single unitized component to be manufactured without any chemically or structurally abrupt interfaces leading to enhanced properties and performance.

9.3.2   Proposed Design of Functionally-Graded Hip Implant

Since there are distinct property requirements at different locations of the femoral (hip) implant, satisfying all these requirements in a monolithic implant is rather challenging. However, using the LENS™ process with multiple powder feeders, it might be possible to produce a functionally-graded implant in its near-net shape form with site-specific properties. Firstly, the idea is to fabricate the basic core structure of the femoral stem and head assembly using LENS™. This core-structure can also be hollow, similar to the prototype shown in Figure 9.3. However, instead of Ti-6Al-4V, the material of choice for the core of the femoral stem and head assembly will be based on the newer generation beta-Ti alloys, such as those based on the Ti-Nb-Zr-Ta system. This alloy system exhibits a low modulus and consists of completely biocompatible alloying elements. Both solid geometries as well as stems with internal cavities can be processed in order to achieve an optimum balance of mechanical properties. Since the surface of the femoral stem is required to exhibit excellent osseointegration properties, additional roughness can be introduced on the surface of the stem by laser depositing lines of the same alloy in the form of a grid. The pattern of these lines/grid can be optimized for achieving the best potential of osseointegration based on trial *in vitro* studies.

As discussed previously, one of the primary requirements of the femoral head (ball part of the ball-socket joint) is excellent wear resistance, especially against the internal surface of the acetabular cup. Titanium and its alloys typically exhibit rather poor wear resistance. Therefore, the femoral head is often made of ceramic or a Co-Cr-Mo based alloy which exhibit very good wear resistance. The acetabular cup is often made of titanium with the internal surface coated with a special polyethylene (UHMWPE). While the use of a ceramic femoral head improves the wear resistance, it typically exhibits poor fracture toughness and the joint between the head and the stem (made of Ti alloy) creates a weak interface between two dissimilar materials. A more appropriate approach might be to manufacture the core of the femoral stem and head assembly in the form of a single monolithic component and use surface engineering to improve the wear resistance of the base Ti alloy locally in the femoral head section. Thus, as discussed before, the LENS™ process will be used to initially deposit an integrated femoral stem-head assembly using the Ti-Nb-Zr-Ta based beta-Ti alloy and subsequently, a boride (or carbide) reinforced Ti-Nb-Zr-Ta alloy will be deposited in a graded fashion on the femoral head section of the implant. In this manner, the core of the femoral head will be made of the same tough β-Ti alloy as the structural core of the femoral stem while the surface of the femoral head will comprise of a hard and wear-resistant metal-matrix composite. An ideal candidate for the outer layers of the wear-resistant femoral head is the Ti-Nb-Zr-Ta-B system, which forms hard titanium boride precipitates within the soft beta titanium matrix and substantially enhances its wear resistance.

Based on the above discussion, it is evident that basically two types of materials will need to be processed using LENS™ for these functionally-graded implants. The individual materials that will eventually be integrated into the femoral hip implant are listed below:

1. Beta titanium based Ti-Nb-Zr-Ta alloys deposited using LENS™ from a blend of elemental powders.
2. Metal-matrix composites based on titanium boride reinforced Ti-Nb-Zr-Ta alloys deposited using LENS™ and compositionally graded composites with gradations from Ti-Nb-Zr-Ta to Ti-Nb-Zr-Ta + TiB (borides) deposited using LENS™.

9.3.3   Laser Processed Ti-Nb-Zr-Ta Alloys

9.3.3.1   Details of Processing and Characterization Methods Used. The specific alloy composition chosen was Ti-35Nb-7Zr-5Ta (wt%) (henceforth referred to as TNZT), based on the good balance of properties reported for the conventionally-processed material of this composition [27]. All the LENS™ depositions were carried out on a commercially procured Ti-6Al-4V alloy substrate. The LENS™ unit used for these depositions was manufactured by Optomec Inc., Albuquerque, New Mexico. The *in situ* alloys were deposited from a blend of pure elemental Ti, Nb, Zr, and, Ta powders mixed in the ratio of 53 wt% Ti + 35 wt% Nb + 7 wt% Zr + 5 wt% Ta. The elemental powder feedstock used for these depositions are as follows:

Ti: 99.9% pure, −150 mesh (from Alfa Aesar)
Nb: 99.9% pure, −200 × 325 mesh (from Reading alloys)
Zr: 99.8% pure, −140/+325 mesh (from CERAC)
Ta: 99.98% pure, −100 mesh (from Alfa Aesar)

The laser power used in these depositions was ~350 W. The hatch width (gap between two successive passes of the laser beam), layer spacing (the gap between two successive layers deposited), and travel speed (the speed at which the substrate is moved with respect to the laser beam), used for all depositions were 0.38 mm, 0.25 mm, and, 635 mm/min, respectively. The LENS™ deposited alloys had a cylindrical geometry with a diameter of 12 mm and a height of 30 mm. Tensile specimens were machined from the as-deposited cylinders and tested in tension to failure by fracture. The tensile specimens were machined as per ASTM standards, E-8(00) with the dimensions of the gage being 3.6 mm diameter × 20.6 mm length. These specimens were subsequently characterized in detail by scanning electron microscopy (SEM), orientation imaging microscopy (OIM), and transmission electron microscopy (TEM). The SEM/OM studies were carried out in a FEI/Philips XL-30 SEM equipped with a field emission gun (FEG) source, an electron backscatter EBSD detector, as well as an EDS detector. Sample preparation for TEM studies involved drilling of 3 mm diameter cylinders by Electro-discharge Machining (EDM), followed by sectioning of thin discs from these cylinders, which were subsequently mechanically thinned and ion-milled to electron transparency in a Gatan Duo Mill. The TEM specimens were characterized in a Philips CM200 TEM at an operating voltage of 200 keV.

9.3.3.2 Microstructure and Mechanical Properties.

The microstructure of the LENS™-deposited TNZT sample is shown in the backscatter SEM image in Figure 9.4a [28]. It is evident from this image that the as-deposited alloy is primarily single phase with no substantial compositional inhomogeneity. The same was confirmed by x-ray diffraction (XRD) studies on the same sample. A representative XRD pattern from this sample is shown in Figure 9.4(b). This XRD pattern indicates the presence of a single β phase in the as-deposited TNZT sample. The composition of the alloy, as determined from EDS studies in the SEM, was found to be Ti-34%Nb-7%Zr-7%Ta (all in wt%). (The error associated with the measurement of compositions using EDS in a SEM is typically ~1–2%.) As compared with the target composition, there is a marginal increase in the Zr and Ta contents in the LENS™ deposited alloy, presumably due to the differences in the flow rate of Zr and Ta powders as compared with Ti and Nb powders.

Nevertheless, considering that this chemically complex alloy was deposited *in situ* from a blend of elemental powders, the composition is within reasonable limits of the target composition. In addition, the oxygen contents of these samples, measured using were ~0.16 wt%. A bright-field TEM micrograph of the as-deposited sample is shown in Figure 9.5a. This image shows a grain boundary between two β grains. A selected area diffraction (SAD) pattern recorded along the [113] β zone axis is shown in Figure 9.5b. In this SAD pattern, in addition to the primary reflections arising from the β matrix, secondary precipitate reflections are also visible along the $g = (21\text{-}1)\beta$ vector. The intensity profile along the $g = (21\text{-}1)\beta$ vector is shown in Figure 9.5b below the SAD pattern. These secondary reflections are present at the 1/3 and 2/3 $(21\text{-}1)\beta$ as well as at the 1/2 $(21\text{-}1)\beta$ locations and other equivalent vectors. While the secondary reflections at the 1/3 and 2/3 $(21\text{-}1)\beta$ positions can be attributed to precipitates of the ω phase in the β matrix, the reflections at 1/2 $(21\text{-}1)\beta$ positions can be attributed to nanometer-scale precipitates of the α phase within the same β matrix [26,29]. Therefore, it can be concluded that in the as-deposited condition, these alloys consist predominantly of a β matrix with nanometer-scale ω and α precipitates.

The engineering stress-strain curve for the as-deposited tensile sample is shown in Figure 9.6. The corresponding mechanical properties of this sample have been tabulated as insets in the same figure. The alloy exhibits a relatively low modulus, ~55 GPa, but reasonably high yield (~814 MPa) and tensile (UTS ~834 MPa) strengths. These strength values are substantially higher than those reported for alloys of similar composition in the solution-treated condition while the modulus is comparable. The yield strength and UTS of Ti-35Nb-7Zr-5Ta in

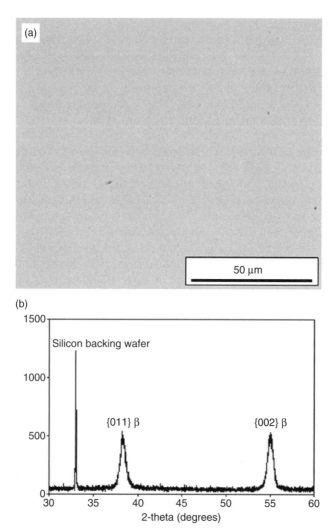

Figure 9.4. (a) Backscatter SEM image of LENS™ as-deposited TNZT alloy. (b) X-ray diffraction plot from the same as-deposited TNZT alloy indicating a single β phase. [Rajarshi Banerjee et al. *Laser Deposited Ti-Nb-Zr-Ta Orthopedic Alloys* (J. Bio. Mater. Res., 78A (2), 2006), 298.]

the solution-treated condition have been reported to be 530 MPa and 590 MPa respectively [1,27,30]. It has also been reported that the yield and tensile strength of these alloys increase with oxygen content. Thus, with 0.46 wt% oxygen in the alloy, the yield strength has been reported to be ~937 MPa and UTS ~1014 MPa in the solution-treated condition [27]. Since the oxygen content in the LENS™ deposited TNZT alloys is not as high as 0.46 wt%, the increased strength in these samples cannot be solely attributed to the oxygen content. Other possible reasons for increased strength are the presence of the fine scale ω and α phases. However,

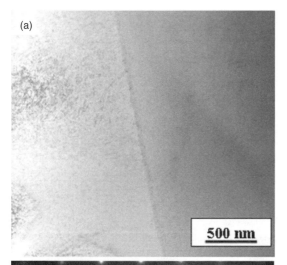

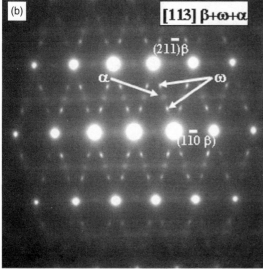

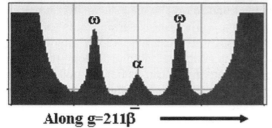

Figure 9.5. (a) Bright field TEM micrograph showing a grain boundary between two grains of β in the LENS™ as-deposited sample. (b) [113] zone axis SAD pattern from the β matrix showing secondary reflections from the nanoscale ω and α precipitates present in this sample. An intensity profile along the $g = (21\text{-}1)\beta$ axis is shown below the SAD pattern. [Rajarshi Banerjee et al. *Laser Deposited Ti-Nb-Zr-Ta Orthopedic Alloys* (J. Bio. Mater. Res., 78A (2), 2006), 298.]

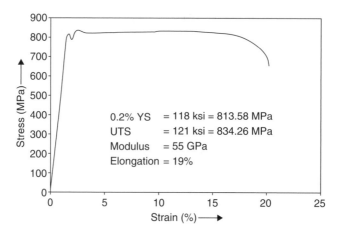

Figure 9.6. An engineering stress-strain curve for the LENS™ deposited TNZT tensile sample. [Rajarshi Banerjee et al. *Laser Deposited Ti-Nb-Zr-Ta Orthopedic Alloys* (J. Bio. Mater. Res., 78A (2), 2006), 298.]

it should be noted that these nanometer-scale precipitation products have been reported in other conventionally-processed TNZT alloys which exhibited a similar modulus but a substantially lower strength [30,31]. In the stress-strain plot shown in Figure 9.6, there is a dip in the plot just after yielding (initiation of plastic deformation). This dip in the stress can be attributed to the classic yield point phenomena, which is often observed in case of metals and alloys exhibiting a *bcc* crystal structure [32].

9.3.3.3 Deformation Mechanisms. In order to investigate the reason for the enhanced strength in greater detail, SEM-OM and TEM studies have been carried out on the LENS™ deposited samples post tensile testing. A cross-section OM map of a tensile specimen, recorded from the gauge section, is shown in Figure 9.7a. The viewing direction is parallel to the tensile axis. This OM map has been pseudo-colored based on the crystallographic orientations (Euler angles) of the different regions of the sample. Regions exhibiting the same crystallographic orientation are depicted in the same color. The map shown in Figure 9.7a is a direct image of the grains in this sample. The average grain size is ~50 μm as determined by the TSL OIM Analysis software based on ASTM standards for grain size measurement. In addition to the grain size and morphology, the actual crystallographic orientations of the different grains can be determined as shown in the pole figures for the β phase in Figure 9.7b. This pole figure corresponds to grains in a region of 1 mm × 1 mm of the gage section. The {001}β, {011}β, {111}β, and, {112}β pole figures are shown. These pole figures indicate that there is a preferential alignment of the {001} poles for a substantial number of the β grains nearly perpendicular to the substrate, or parallel to the tensile axis.

Thus, most of the β grains seen in Figure 9.7a have a <001> axis along the viewing direction that is parallel to the tensile axis. This preferential alignment of

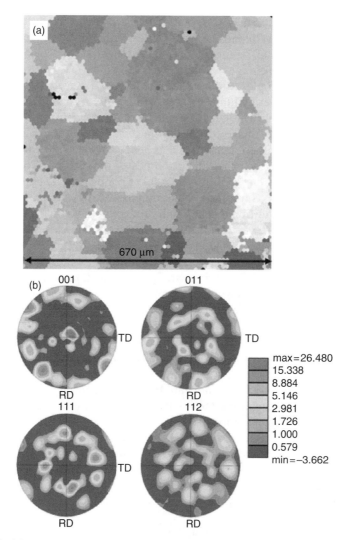

Figure 9.7. (a) Pseudo-colored OIM map from the cross-section of the tensile-tested LENS™ deposited TNZT sample viewed parallel to the tensile axis. The β grains are clearly visible in this map. (b) {001}, {011}, {111}, and, {112}β pole figures from the same sample exhibiting a strong <001> texture. [Rajarshi Banerjee et al. *Laser Deposited Ti-Nb-Zr-Ta Orthopedic Alloys* (J. Bio. Mater. Res., 78A (2), 2006), 298.] (See color insert.)

the β grains indicates the possible presence of a <001> texture in the as-deposited sample. OM maps were acquired at three different locations on the sample and in each map ~50–100 grains were analyzed. Furthermore, it should be noted that these maps covered areas ranging from 0.7 mm × 0.7 mm to 1 mm × 1 mm. Since the gage section of the tensile specimen has a diameter of ~3 mm, these maps represented substantial fractions of the gage section. In all cases, the pole figures indicated the preferential <001> orientation of the β grains. Such a <001> texture has been previously reported for LENS™ deposited Ti-Cr alloys [33] and is likely a result of the preferential texture resulting from the alloy solidification. Furthermore, this <001> texture might influence the deformation mechanisms in these LENS™ deposited samples and could lead to the enhanced yield and tensile strengths observed experimentally. However, more detailed studies are required in order to investigate these aspects of the deformation behavior.

A bright-field TEM image of the tensile tested TNZT sample is shown in Figure 9.8a. A large number of distinct shear bands are clearly visible in this TEM image. The presence of such shear bands indicates deformation dominated by a slip mechanism and also slip localization in shear bands. A SAD pattern recorded along the $[113]\beta$ zone axis from the same sample is shown in Figure 9.8b. In this diffraction pattern, in addition to the primary reflections arising from the β matrix, additional reflections are also visible along the $g = (21\text{-}1)\beta$ vector and vectors of the same type. A intensity profile along the $g = (21\text{-}1)\beta$ vector is also shown in Figure 9.8b. From this intensity profile, it is evident that while the secondary reflections at the $1/2 (21\text{-}1)\beta$ locations are quite distinct, those at the 1/3 and 2/3 $(21\text{-}1)\beta$ locations are much lower in intensity and not as distinct as in case of the as-deposited LENS™ sample prior to tensile testing (refer to the SAD pattern and the intensity profile in Figure 9.5b). Therefore, it appears that while well-defined α precipitates, giving rise to the secondary reflections at the $1/2 (21\text{-}1)\beta$ locations, are present after the tensile testing, the ω precipitates, giving rise to the secondary reflections at the 1/3 and 2/3 $(21\text{-}1)\beta$ locations, are not as well-defined. The intensity at these locations appears to be streaked along the $g = (21\text{-}1)\beta$ vector. Furthermore, comparing the relative intensity of the ω reflections before and after tensile testing, it appears that the ω precipitates are likely to be of smaller size in the tensile tested samples as compared to the LENS™ as-deposited sample. The reduction in the average size of the ω precipitates is likely to be a consequence of shearing of these precipitates by the dislocations during plastic flow. Such precipitate shearing at the nanoscale would consequently result in slip localization and the formation of shear bands that is experimentally observed in the tensile-tested samples.

The dislocations within the shear band have been imaged under two-beam imaging conditions in the TEM and these results have been shown in Figure 9.9. A two-beam bright-field TEM image recorded using $g = (011)\beta$ near the $[1\text{-}11]\beta$ zone axis is shown in Figure 9.9a. The shear bands and the dislocations within the shear bands are clearly visible in this diffraction contrast image. Another set of two images from the exact same location, recorded using two different two-beam imaging conditions are shown in Figures 9.9b and 9.9c. Thus, while Figure 9.9b shows the two-beam bright-field image recorded using $g = (011)\beta$ near the $[3\text{-}11]\beta$ zone axis, Figure 9.9c has been recorded using $g = (\text{-}1\text{-}21)\beta$ near the $[3\text{-}11]\beta$ zone axis. The dislocation contrast within the shear band, running almost parallel to the edge of the TEM foil, is visible in Figure 9.9b but is invisible in the same region in Figure 9.9c. The invisibility criterion for $g = (\text{-}1\text{-}21)\beta$ suggests that most of these dislocations possibly have a burgers vector of the type $1/2<111> \beta$ as would be

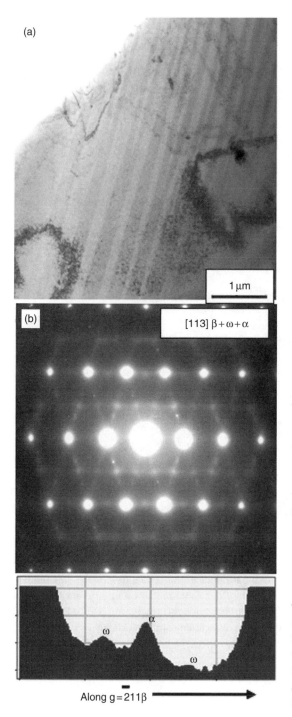

(a)

1 μm

(b)

[113] β+ω+α

α

ω

ω

Along g=211β‾

Figure 9.8. (a) Bright field TEM micrograph from the tensile-tested LENS™ deposited TNZT sample showing a large number of shear bands after the deformation. (b) [113] zone axis SAD pattern from the β matrix showing secondary reflections from the nanoscale ω and α precipitates present in this sample. An intensity profile along the g = (21-1)β axis is shown below the SAD pattern. Note the substantial reduction in the intensity of ω reflections in this pattern as compared with a similar SAD pattern prior to deformation (refer to Fig. 5(b)). [Rajarshi Banerjee et al. *Laser Deposited Ti-Nb-Zr-Ta Orthopedic Alloys* (J. Bio. Mater. Res., 78A (2), 2006), 298.]

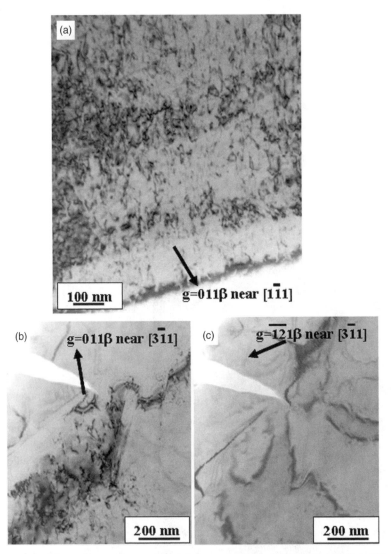

<u>Figure 9.9.</u> (a) Bright-field two-beam image recorded using $g = (011)\beta$ showing diffraction contrast from the dislocations within the shear bands in the tensile deformed TNZT sample. A set of bright-field images recorded from the exact same region using different two-beam imaging conditions are shown in (b) and (c). (b) has been recorded using $g = (011)\beta$ while (c) has been recorded using $g = (-1-21)\beta$. While the dislocation contrast is clearly visible in (b), it is invisible in (c). [Rajarshi Banerjee et al. *Laser Deposited Ti-Nb-Zr-Ta Orthopedic Alloys* (J. Bio. Mater. Res., 78A (2), 2006), 298.]

expected in such *bcc* alloys. Similar invisibility conditions have been observed at other locations in the same sample when imaging using $g = \{112\}\beta$ type two-beam conditions [28].

Finally, an additional feature observed in these LENS™ deposited samples was the presence of a modulated contrast as shown in Figures 9.10a and 9.10b. Figure 9.10a is a lower magnification bright-field TEM image showing the shear bands and the modulated contrast in the background. A higher magnification

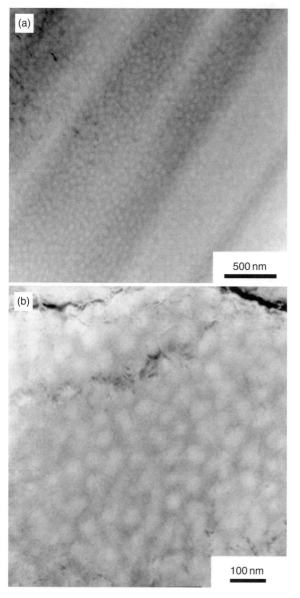

500 nm

100 nm

Figure 9.10. (a) Bright-field TEM image of a highly refined scale modulated contrast within the β matrix in addition to the contrast arising from the shear bands. (b) A higher magnification image of the same modulated contrast. This contrast could possibly be associated with fine scale dendrites in the β matrix of this LENS™ deposited alloy. [Rajarshi Banerjee et al. *Laser Deposited Ti-Nb-Zr-Ta Orthopedic Alloys* (J. Bio. Mater. Res., 78A (2), 2006), 298.]

image of the modulated contrast is shown in Figure 9.10b. This modulated contrast occurs at a highly refined scale in this material (<50 nm as seen in Figure 9.10b). While the origin of this modulated contrast is the subject of ongoing investigations, based on its appearance it can be speculated that this contrast is arising from a highly-refined dendritic solidification of this alloy. Such refined scale dendrites are likely in LENS™ deposited alloys due to the rapid solidification rates inherent to the process [3,24].

9.3.3.4 Corrosion Resistance of LENS™ Deposited Ti-Nb-Zr-Ta Alloys.

Anodic polarization tests were carried out on LENS™ deposited TNZT, CP Ti and Ti-6Al-4V ELI samples and also on the boride reinforced TNZT samples. The specimens used were in the form of discs with a diameter of 15 mm and were polished to a surface finish of 0.3 μm. The samples were then cleaned ultrasonically and were employed as the working electrode in the test cell. The tests were carried out in two different media, 0.1 N HCl and a simulated body solution known as the Ringers Solution. The Ringers solution has a composition of NaCl 9 g/l, KCl 0.43 g/l, $CaCl_2$ 0.24 g/l, $NaHCO_3$ 0.2 g/l [34]. The anodic polarization test was performed from an initial potential of −1.5 Volts to 5 V at room temperature at a scan rate of 0.166 mV/s and the current density was recorded continuously. A saturated calomel electrode was used as a reference electrode and a platinum wire as a counter electrode. The tests were repeated to ensure the reproducibility of the data obtained. A detailed spectroscopic analysis using X-Ray photoelectron spectroscopy was performed on the corrosion product (oxide layer) formed on the TNZT alloy.

Anodic polarization plots for the three materials in 0.1 N HCL, LENS™ deposited TNZT, CP Ti and Ti-6Al-4V are shown in Figure 9.11. All the three

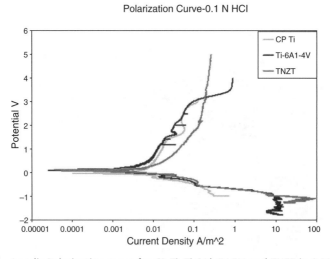

Polarization Curve-0.1 N HCl

Figure 9.11. Anodic Polarization curve for CP-Ti, Ti-6Al-4V ELI and TNZT in 0.1 N HCl. [Sonia Samuel, (M.S. Thesis, Dept of Mater. Sci. and Eng., University of North Texas, 2007)]

materials tested showed a clear active to passive transition at E_{Corr} values close to 0 V. There is not much significant difference in the free potential E_{corr} values for these materials. The active-to-passive transition corresponds to the formation of a passive protective oxide film on the surface of the material. In the case of the conventional alloys Ti-6Al-4V and CP-Ti, the film that forms breaks down at a potential close to 1.5 V, typically referred to as the breakdown potential, while in the case of LENS™ deposited TNZT alloys the passive film does not show any breakdown up to a voltage of 5 V and above. The critical current density values for CP Ti and Ti-6Al-4V are ~8.4 uA/m^2 and ~5.3 uA/m^2, respectively, whereas that of TNZT is marginally higher, ~10.4 uA/m^2. Though the critical current density of TNZT alloys are higher than CP-Ti and Ti-6Al-4V, the E_{tp} or the transpassive potential for this alloy is higher than 5 V, while E_{tp} for Ti-6Al-4V and CP Ti are ~1.3 and ~1.5 V respectively. Thus it can be concluded that LENS™ deposited TNZT forms a more adherent surface oxide layer, exhibiting better corrosion resistance in 0.1 N HCl as compared to CP-Ti and Ti-6Al-4V.

Anodic polarization tests were also performed in simulated body fluid (Ringer's solution). The materials compared were Ti-6Al-4V ELI, TNZT and boride reinforced TNZT composite. The processing and tribological properties of the boride reinforced TNZT composite have been discussed in the succeeding section. The testing Ringer's solution used comprised of NaCl 9 g/l, KCl 0.43 g/l, CaCl$_2$ 0.24 g/l, and, NaHCO$_3$ 0.2 g/l. Similar to the case of the testing in 0.1 N Hcl, described previously, the potential was measured with reference to a Saturated Calomel electrode and was varied from –2V to 5V with a scan rate as low as 0.166 mV/s. Current density was plotted simultaneously and the resulting anodic polarization curves for the three materials are shown in Figure 9.12. All three

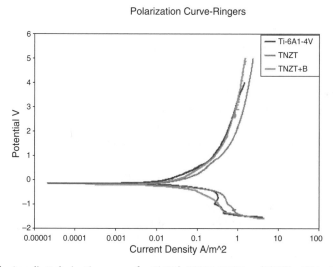

Figure 9.12. Anodic Polarization curve for Ti-6Al-4V ELI, TNZT and TNZT + 2B in Ringers Solution. [Sonia Samuel, (M.S. Thesis, Dept of Mater. Sci. and Eng., University of North Texas, 2007)]

materials show a clear active to passive transition at E_{Corr} values close to 0 V. There is no significant difference in the free potential values, E_{corr} for these materials. In contrast to testing in 0.1 N HCl, in Ringers Solution none of the three materials, Ti-6Al-4V, TNZT, or TNZT + 2B, exhibited any breakdown of the protective oxide film formed on the surface even at potentials as high as 5 V. The critical current density value for TNZT alloy (~17 uA/cm^2) is marginally higher than that observed for Ti-6Al-4V (~14 uA/cm^2). Ti-6Al-4V and TNZT + 2B (~15.36 uA/cm^2) exhibited similar critical current densities. The anodic polarization curve shows no breakdown suggesting the formation of a very stable passive oxide film on the surface. Thus, it can be inferred that all the three materials are highly corrosion resistant in Ringers solution. The typical values of E_{tp} or E_{br}, (breakdown potential) reported under similar conditions of testing in Ringer's solution, for Stainless Steels and Co-Cr-Mo alloys are ~300–500 mV, which can easily be reached in the body in the case of an inflammation [35]. The substantially higher values (>5 V) of E_{tp} for Ti-6Al-4V, TNZT and TNZT + 2B indicate that these materials have superior corrosion resistance in simulated body fluid conditions.

9.3.3.5 *XPS Studies of the Passive Oxide Film on LENS™ Deposited TNZT.* The superior biocompatibility and corrosion resistance of titanium alloys are attributed to the stable and dense passive oxide film that forms on the surface in the presence of an oxidizing media. The bio-adhesion of titanium is achieved by free OH$^-$ groups that are available in the pH region from 2.9 to 12.7 on the surface of the oxide layer. These groups react with the bio molecules and are influenced by the chemical and biological characteristics of the surface film. The interaction of the surface oxide film with the bio molecules from the body fluids generates a film called the bio film. The host body initiates a series of reactions in response to this bio film thereby enabling the development of the interface between the implant and the surrounding tissue.

Typical hostile bio-responses after implant surgery include the buildup of monocytes and macrophages (after one day), formation of granulation tissue containing fibroblasts and type III collagens (after five days) and finally attack of foreign body giant cells. Thus, from the perspective of biocompatibility, it is important to develop a better understanding of the properties of the oxide film forming on the surface of the implant alloy. These properties include composition, thickness and the structure of the oxide layer. Surface analytical techniques, such as x-ray photoelectron spectroscopy (XPS), can be effectively used to probe the thin surface oxide layers, created by anodic polarization tests on these LENS™ deposited TNZT alloys [36]. There have been several studies related to the oxide layer forming on electrochemically tested (or treated) Ti-6Al-4V alloys. In most cases, the results indicate that the surface oxide layer on Ti-6Al-4V comprises mainly of TiO_2 with small amounts of sub oxides TiO and Ti_2O_3. Hence, in the present case, a detailed XPS analysis of the surface oxide layer formed on LENS™ deposited TNZT has been carried out.

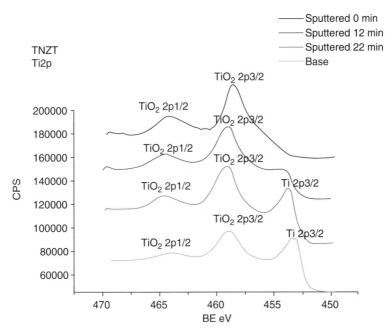

<u>Figure 9.13.</u> XPS Spectra of Ti2p on the oxide and base TNZT. [Sonia Samuel, (M.S. Thesis, Dept of Mater. Sci. and Eng., University of North Texas, 2007)]

The XPS runs were carried out on a Thermo VG Scientific ESCALAB MKII spectrometer system using a standard Al-Kα X-ray source at 280 W and electrostatic analysis in constant pass energy mode of 200 eV for survey scans and 20 eV for regional scans. Argon sputtering was carried out for different time intervals to assess the chemical compositions at different sputtered depths in a systematic manner. The elements scanned for were C1s, O1s, Ti2p, Nb3d, Ta4f and Zr4f. XPS scans were also performed on the surface of the base material without the oxide layer for comparison. Carbon was present as a contaminant, and as expected, the amount of carbon decreased with increasing sputter depth.

In Figure 9.13, XPS spectra corresponding to the energy window for the Ti2p peak are shown, for sputter time periods of zero, twelve and twenty-two minutes on the surface oxide of the TNZT alloy subjected to electrochemical testing. For comparison, in the same figure, the spectra corresponding to the base TNZT alloy without the oxide layer, sputtered for a time interval of 30 minutes is also shown. As observed from the spectra, the TiO_2 2p3/2 ($E_b = 458.4$ eV) [37] peak is observed on the surface (zero minutes sputtering) as well as after sputtering for 22 minutes into the oxide layer. The peak corresponding to metallic titanium is observed with a binding energy of $E_b = 453.7$ eV [37] after sputtering into the oxide layer for 22 minutes. The metallic titanium peak is also observed in case of the base material (without oxide layer). These results indicate that 22 minutes of sputtering presumably removes the oxide layer and the base metallic alloy begins. Also the presence of TiO_2 even after sputtering for 22 minutes suggests the presence of a

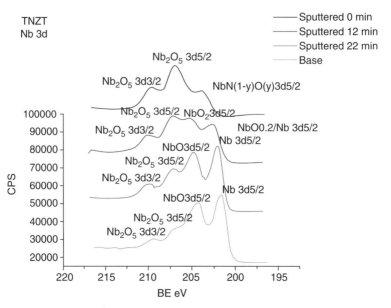

Figure 9.14. XPS Spectra of Nb3d on the oxide and base TNZT. [Sonia Samuel, (M.S. Thesis, Dept of Mater. Sci. and Eng., University of North Texas, 2007)]

mixed metal + oxide layer. Figure 9.14 shows the XPS spectra corresponding to the Nb3d peak after different sputtering time periods of zero, twelve and twenty-two minutes into the surface oxide layer of the LENS™ deposited TNZT alloy. The surface of the oxide layer showed the presence of Nb_2O_5 3d5/2 ($E_b = 207.01$ eV) oxide and an oxy-nitrile of the composition NbN(1-y)O(y) 3d5/2. ($E_b = 203.6$ eV). After sputtering for 12 minutes and beyond into the oxide layer, other types of niobium oxides are detected including, NbO_2, NbO0.2Nb and NbO. Metallic Nb peak appears after sputtering for 22 minutes into the oxide layer. As in the case of titanium, niobium oxide peaks are detected in the XPS spectra even after a sputtering of 30 minutes into the oxide layer suggesting the presence of a mixed metal + oxide layer. In the case of the elements Zr and Ta XPS spectra were collected for conditions similar to those used for Ti and Nb as shown in Figures 9.15 and 9.16. In the case of Zr the oxide present in the surface passive layer was found to be ZrO_2 and after sputtering for about 22 minutes into the oxide layer, the peaks corresponding to the metallic Zr was detected, as seen in Figure 9.15. Interestingly in case of Ta, as seen in Figure 9.16, while Ta_2O_5 was the oxide present in the surface passive layer, metallic tantalum was also detected even for 0 mins sputtering. This can be explained based on the fact that since Ta is a much more noble metal as compared to Ti, Nb, or Zr, there is a substantially reduced tendency for the oxidation of this alloying element in the surface passive layer forming on the LENS™ deposited TNZT alloy. A summary of the different oxides detected in the passive oxide layer on the surface, based on the XPS studies, is shown in Table 9.1.

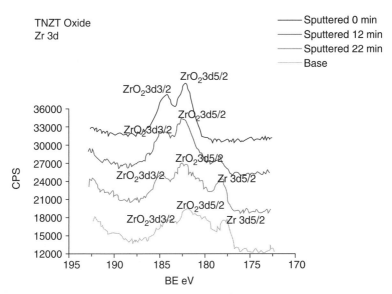

Figure 9.15. XPS Spectra of Zr3d on the oxide and base TNZT. [Sonia Samuel, (M.S. Thesis, Dept of Mater. Sci. and Eng., University of North Texas, 2007)]

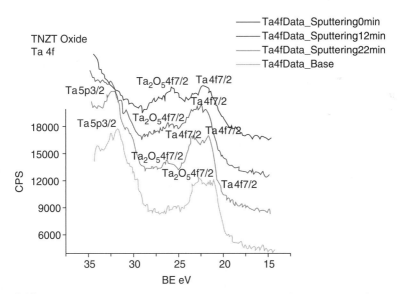

Figure 9.16. XPS Spectra of Ta4f on the oxide and base TNZT. [Sonia Samuel, (M.S. Thesis, Dept of Mater. Sci. and Eng., University of North Texas, 2007)]

TABLE 9.1. Analysis of the XPS Spectra: A Summary of the Different Oxides Detected in the Passive Oxide Layer on the Surface

Sputtering time (min)	Ti based	Nb based	Ta based	Zr based
0	TiO_2	Nb_2O_5, $NbN(1-y)O(y)$	Ta_2O_5, Ta	ZrO_2
12	TiO_2, Ti	Nb_2O_5, NbO_2, $NbO0.2/Nb$	Ta_2O_5, Ta	ZrO_2
22	TiO_2, Ti	Nb_2O_5, NbO, Nb	Ta_2O_5, Ta	ZrO_2, Zr
Base	TiO_2, Ti	Nb_2O_5, NbO, Nb	Ta_2O_5, Ta	ZrO_2, Zr

9.3.3.6 *Preliminary In Vitro Studies on LENS™ Deposited TNZT.* Bone formation is a complex process involving the migration of bone cells to the bone surfaces termed as bone proliferation of the osteoprogenitor cells and their subsequent differentiation into osteoblasts. Hence assessing the extent of bone proliferation and bone differentiation on the surface of a material of interest is a method to evaluate its biocompatibility. In this study, primary rat bone marrow cells isolated from the femurs of Sprague Dawley rats were seeded in T-75 flasks and subsequently incubated. Seeded cells were then detached and resuspended in media to achieve a seeding density of 10,000 cells /cm^2 and added on to the Ti-6Al-4V and TNZT disk samples. Following this the disks were incubated for 6 hours to allow for cell adhesion. The disks were then transferred to well plates used as positive controls. After the fourth and the seventh day or (third and the sixth day) the disks were treated with a lysing agent and cells grown on top of the disks were scraped and the lysate was pippetted out. A Pico green assay kit was used to quantitatively determine the amount of double stranded DNA present in the cultured cells. Alkaline phosphate, an enzyme found in the early stages of osteoblast formation, was used as an early marker of the differentiation of bone marrow stromal cells into osteoblast cells. This experiment was repeated twice to ensure the reproducibility in the test results.

In the first set of data obtained, shown in Figure 9.17a, it was observed that rate of bone proliferation measured as a function of the amount of DNA present in the cultured cells was higher in the case of LENS™ deposited TNZT alloys when compared to the control Ti-6Al-4V ELI after four days. However, after seven days, both the Ti-6Al-4V and TNZT exhibited almost the same rate of bone proliferation. The rate of bone differentiation studied using Alkaline Phosphate enzyme as a marker showed a significant amount of ALP enzyme in the TNZT sample when compared to the Ti-6Al-4V, indicating enhanced bone differentiation after a period of seven days. As seen from Figure 9.17b, the amount of ALP enzyme that was present in case of the Ti-6Al-4V sample was relatively lower than that present in the TNZT sample. These preliminary *in vitro* results are quite encouraging and suggest that laser deposited TNZT alloys are biocompatible since they aid both in bone cell proliferation and differentiation. The second sets of experiments were also done under conditions similar to those used for the first set of tests and the results from these experiments are shown in Figures 9.18a and 9.18b. The PicoGreen DNA assays (Invitrogen) have been used to measure total

(a)

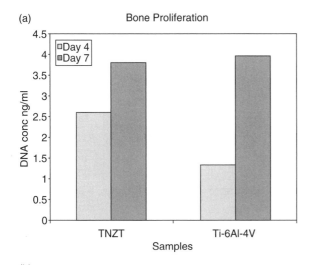

(b)

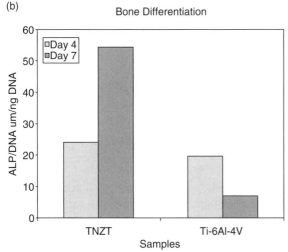

Figure 9.17. (a) Bone cell proliferation and (b) Bone cell differentiation results from the first test. [Sonia Samuel, (M.S. Thesis, Dept of Mater. Sci. and Eng., University of North Texas, 2007)]

DNA concentration, which is correlated to the cell number grown on the surfaces. Studies of DNA were performed after three and six days of bone cell seeding. The results are presented as shown in Figure 9.18. The ALP assays are used to measure the ALP production per ng DNA for each sample used to indicate the bone cell differentiation. It was observed that the TNZT samples allow for substantially enhanced bone cell differentiation of bone marrow stem cells as compared to the Ti-6Al-4V ELI control samples. In contrast, cell growth on TNZT samples is not as good as those grown on control samples in this second set of experiments. These results suggest that the laser deposited Ti-35Nb-7Zr-5Ta alloy promotes the osteogenic potential of bone marrow stem cells compared to the Ti-6Al-4V ELI alloy.

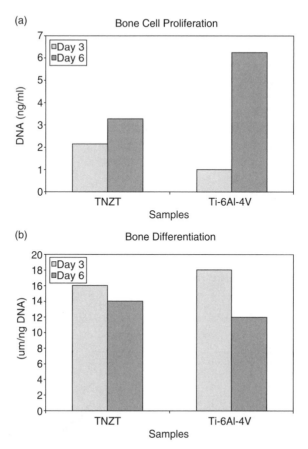

<u>Figure 9.18.</u> (a) Bone cell proliferation and (b) Bone cell differentiation results from the second test. [Sonia Samuel, (M.S. Thesis, Dept of Mater. Sci. and Eng., University of North Texas, 2007)]

9.3.4   Laser Processed Titanium Boride Reinforced Ti-Nb-Zr-Ta Metal-matrix Composites

9.3.4.1 Wear Resistance of Titanium Alloys and Titanium Matrix Composites. As discussed previously, titanium alloys, including beta alloys, typically exhibit rather poor wear resistance, consequently limiting their application in the femoral head. Frictional behavior of some selected orthopedic biomaterials has been studied by Rack and Long [38,39]. The four titanium alloys they studied were Ti-35Nb-8Zr-5Ta with slightly different compositions (TNZT and TNZTO), a metastable β-Ti alloy (21SRX) and Ti-6Al-4V ELI (Extra Low Interstitial). The steady state dynamic coefficient of friction values in sliding contacts for the metastable β-Ti alloys were always higher than that of the Ti-6Al-4V alloy under all conditions of contact stresses tested. Post-wear testing the surfaces exhibited

extensive plastic deformation accompanied with micro-plowing and micro-cracking perpendicular to the sliding direction.

In addition, shear delamination and smearing with transfer of material from the wear surface to the counterpart material was also observed. Surface topography analysis showed that the roughness of the metastable Ti alloys tested were higher than that for the Ti-6Al-4V alloy [39]. Also the TNTZ alloys were subjected to different heat treatments in order to study the effect of heat treatment/microstructure on wear resistance. The wear loss measurements indicate that heat treatment is not a practical way to improve the wear resistance of the Titanium alloys. The TNTZ and the Ti-6Al-4V alloys were then subjected to thermal oxidation to study the effect of an oxide layer on wear resistance. Results indicate that the presence of an oxide layer greatly improves the wear resistance of both TNZT alloys as well as that of Ti-6Al-4V [40].

In addition to base titanium alloys, previous research has been devoted to the study of hard boride reinforcements in the Ti matrix. Sliding wear properties of TiB/Ti-6Al-4V metal matrix layer fabricated using laser cladding and laser melt injection were evaluated in a previous study [41] and showed an improvement in the tribological properties of this MMC layer. The results of the wear studies reported highlighted the excellent wear resistance of the Laser engineered TiB/Ti-6Al-4V MMC layers [41]. Hence these composites combine the high strength and stiffness of the borides with the toughness and damage tolerance of the Ti-alloy matrix and offer attractive properties including increased stiffness and substantially enhanced *wear resistance*. Using the laser-engineered net shaping (LENS™) process, it has been successfully demonstrated that *in-situ* TiB reinforced Ti alloy composites can be fabricated in a single step [42,43]. These laser-deposited composites exhibit a substantially refined distribution of reinforcing TiB precipitates as compared to their conventionally processed (e.g., ingot processing) counterparts. Furthermore, by employing novel near-net shape processing technologies, such as LENS™, it becomes possible to not only rapidly and efficiently manufacture custom-designed implants, but also to functionally-grade those to exhibit required site-specific properties. Therefore, the current effort is directed towards the processing, characterization, and, measurement of the tribological properties of laser-deposited, boride reinforced, TNZT composites based on the nominal matrix composition Ti-35Nb-7Zr-5Ta (all in wt %). Sliding wear resistance and friction behavior were examined under a wide range of post-processing and testing conditions such as varying the concentrated interfacial load, the effect of ex-situ annealing on the tribological properties, and the role of counterpart material. The tribological properties have been correlated to the surface microstructure under these conditions.

9.3.4.2 *Titanium Boride Reinforced Ti-Nb-Zr-Ta Composites.* LENS™ deposition of the metal-matrix composites were carried out from a powder feedstock consisting of a blend of elemental pure Ti, Nb, Zr and Ta powders with Titanium Boride (TiB$_2$) mixed in the ratio of 51 wt% Ti + 35 wt% Nb + 7 wt%

TABLE 9.2. Hardness and Initial Mean Hertzian Contact Stresses (p_m) for Ti-6Al-4V ELI and TNZT 2B

Alloy	Hardness (VHN)	p_m (GPa) for Si_3N_4 balls	p_m (GPa) for SS 440 C balls
Ti-6Al-4V ELI	320	0.95	0.90
TNZT 2B	375	1.01	0.95

TABLE 9.3. Heat Treatment Conditions for Ti-6Al-4V ELI and TNZT 2B for Wear Testing

Alloy	Heat treatment
Ti-6Al-4V ELI	As deposited
Ti-6Al-4V ELI	600 °C/10 hours/FC/Oxide Layer
Ti-6Al-4V ELI	600 °C/10 hours/FC/Oxide Layer removed
TNZT 2B	As deposited
TNZT 2B	600 °C/10 hours/FC/Oxide Layer
TNZT 2B	600 °C/10 hours/FC/Oxide Layer removed

Zr + 5 wt% Ta + 2 wt% B. The total weight of pre-blended powders per deposit was ~300 gm. The processing conditions used were similar to those discussed previously for the Ti-Nb-Zr-Ta alloys. The as-deposited specimens were subsequently characterized using SEM, OIM, and, TEM. Post-wear testing, the SEM studies of the worn and unworn surfaces were carried out in a FEI Sirion SEM equipped with an EDS detector. Their indentation hardness (VHN) values for these samples are listed in Table 9.2. Friction and wear behavior of TNZT + 2B and Ti-6Al-4V ELI were determined using a Falex (Implant Sciences) ISC-200 Tribometer. This tribometer is a pin-on-disk type configuration which measures the sliding friction coefficients on planar surfaces. The details of the wear tests are discussed elsewhere [44]. Also, some of the polished samples were subjected to separate heat treatments in air before testing, shown in Table 9.3. The heat-treatments carried out on the TNZT + 2B and Ti-6Al-4V ELI samples had a two-fold objective, namely to study the influence of α precipitates and the surface oxide layer, formed as a result of the heat treatment on the resulting friction and wear behavior.

The microstructure of the LENS™-deposited TNZT + 2B alloy at different magnifications is shown in the backscatter SEM images in Figure 9.19 [44]. Figure 9.19a shows a low magnification backscattered image of the boride composite while Figure 9.19b shows a higher magnification view of the microstructure consisting of the coarser primary boride precipitates and the finer scale eutectic boride precipitates dispersed in a matrix. Furthermore, while the finer scale eutectic borides exhibit a uniform contrast in the backscatter SEM images, the coarser primary boride precipitates exhibit strong contrast variations within the same precipitate suggesting a possibility of compositional variation within the same

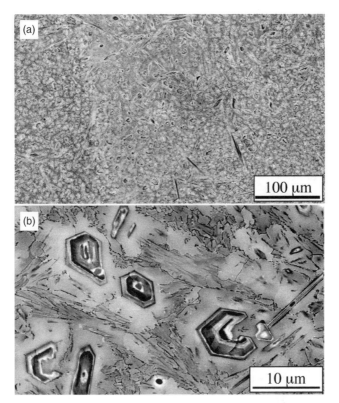

Figure 9.19. (a) Lower magnification and (b) higher magnification backscatter SEM images of LENS™ as-deposited TNZT + 2B alloy composites showing both coarser primary borides exhibiting contrast within the same boride precipitate as well as finer scale eutectic borides. [Sonia Samuel et al. *Wear Resistance of Laser Deposited Boride Reinforced Ti-Nb-Zr-Ta Alloy Composites for Orthopedic Implants* (to appear in Mater. Sci. Eng. C, 2007)]

boride. In addition, the matrix also exhibits variations in contrast. Thus, while the regions adjoining the primary boride precipitates exhibit a lighter contrast, the regions a further distance exhibit a relatively darker contrast. There is also a clustering of the eutectic boride precipitates within these regions of darker contrast, as clearly visible in Figure 9.19b. SEM-EDS studies revealed that the composition of the matrix to be Ti-34%Nb-7%Zr-7%Ta (all in wt%). Figure 9.20 shows the results of EDS studies carried out on one of the primary boride precipitates.

The SEM image of the specific boride precipitate analyzed is shown in Figure 9.20a together with the line across which the compositional variation was measured using SEM-EDS. The compositional profile across this line is shown in Figure 9.20b and has been divided into distinct zones within the boride precipitate, exhibiting the different contrasts in Figure 9.20a. On either sides of the boride, the composition of the matrix is Ti-33Nb-7Zr-9Ta which is marginally enriched in Ta as compared with the average alloy composition (~7 wt% Ta). The

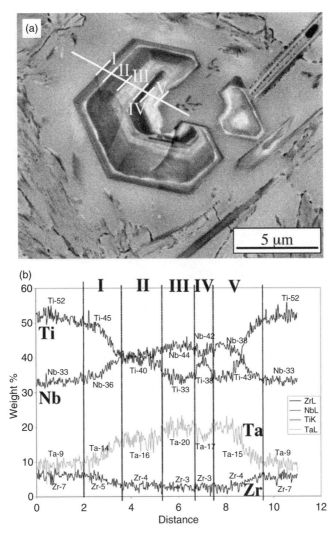

Figure 9.20. (a) High magnification backscatter SEM image of a single primary boride in the LENS™ as-deposited TNZT + 2B alloy exhibiting a strong contrast within the boride. (b) EDS compositional profile across the white line, shown in (a), distinguishing the contrast within the boride arising from a compositional modulation with regions richer in Nb and Ta exhibiting a brighter contrast while regions relatively richer in Ti and Zr exhibiting a darker contrast in the backscatter SEM image. [Sonia Samuel et al. *Wear Resistance of Laser Deposited Boride Reinforced Ti-Nb-Zr-Ta Alloy Composites for Orthopedic Implants* (to appear in Mater. Sci. Eng. C, 2007)]

relatively higher Ta content of the matrix in the vicinity of the primary boride precipitates is also indirectly indicated by the lighter contrast in these regions (adjacent to the primary borides) seen in the SEM backscatter image in Figure 9.19b. Within the boride precipitate, there are distinct alternating bands of dark and bright contrast. It should be noted that in the profile shown in Figure 9.20b, the composition of the boride does not include the boron content (since it cannot be quantified by EDS) and thus has been scaled to Ti + Nb + Zr + Ta = 100 wt%.

The boride precipitate can be divided into five distinct composition zones based on the bands of different contrast visible in Figure 9.20a. In Figure 9.20b, Zone I corresponds to the first band and exhibits a continually decreasing Ti and Zr content while the Nb and Ta contents increase. In Zone II, the composition appears to be nominally constant and approximately equal to Ti-40Nb-4Zr-16Ta. However, it should be noted that the composition of these bands might not be constant along the direction normal to surface. Therefore, it is not possible to accurately determine the composition of these bands using SEM-EDS but rather use these measurements as a qualitative indicator. In band III, the Nb and Ta contents increase while that of Ti and Zr decreases. The reverse trend is observed in case of band IV, wherein Ti and Zr increase while Nb and Ta decrease. Finally, band V exhibits the same trend as band III. Overall the compositional changes in these bands within the boride precipitate appear to follow an alternating trend of increasing and decreasing Ti and Zr (or decreasing and increasing Nb and Ta). The origin of these compositional modulations within the same boride precipitate is currently under investigation.

9.3.4.3 *Tribological Behavior of Ti-Nb-Zr-Ta + TiB Composites.* Typical friction curves are shown in Figure 9.21 for as-deposited Ti-6Al-4V ELI and TNZT + 2B sliding against Si_3N_4 [44].

The friction coefficients immediately increased to high values of ~0.4 and 0.5 for Ti-6Al-4V and TNZT + 2B, respectively. With continued sliding, their steady-state friction coefficients leveled off at ~0.5 and 0.6, respectively, for the remainder of the tests. These are relatively high friction coefficient values for Ti-based alloys, especially those with TiB precipitate reinforcements. This behavior would suggest an increased amount of abrasive wear due to precipitate pull-out causing accelerated third body debris generation trapped inside the sliding contact. To confirm this possible mechanism(s), SEM of the wear surfaces was conducted on both alloys.

Figures 9.22 and 9.23 show (a) low and (b) high magnification SEM images of the Ti-6Al-4V ELI and TNZT + 2B wear tracks, respectively.

In the case of Ti-6Al-4V ELI (Figure 9.22), the low and high magnification images of the wear track show evidence of surface deformation due to ductile layering and smearing, common in repeated sliding contacts for Ti-6Al-4V alloys [41]. In contrast, the TNZT + 2B wear track morphology shown in Figure 9.23 exhibits more severe wear, which, like the friction coefficient, is a surprising result

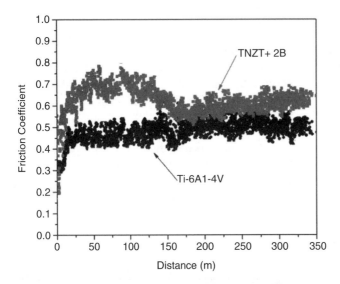

Figure 9.21. Wear plots showing the friction behavior as a function of distance of Ti-6Al-4V ELI and TNZT + 2B with Si_3N_4 counterface balls. [Sonia Samuel et al. *Wear Resistance of Laser Deposited Boride Reinforced Ti-Nb-Zr-Ta Alloy Composites for Orthopedic Implants* (to appear in Mater. Sci. Eng. C, 2007)]

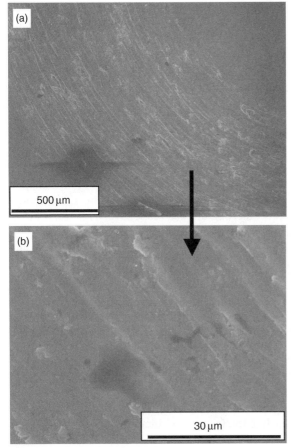

Figure 9.22. (a) Lower magnification and (b) higher magnification secondary SEM images of Ti-6Al-4V ELI wear tracks after friction studies using Si_3N_4 counterface balls. [Sonia Samuel et al. *Wear Resistance of Laser Deposited Boride Reinforced Ti-Nb-Zr-Ta Alloy Composites for Orthopedic Implants* (to appear in Mater. Sci. Eng. C, 2007)]

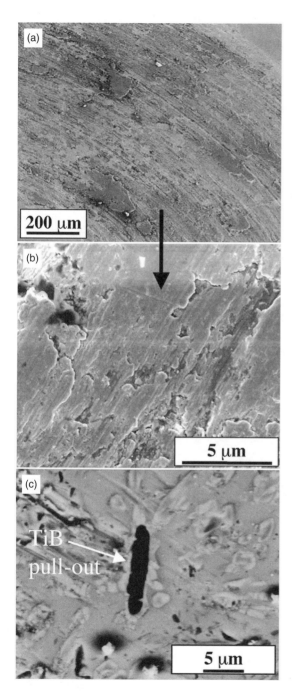

Figure 9.23. (a) Lower magnification and (b) higher magnification secondary SEM images of LENS™ as-deposited TNZT + 2B wear tracks after friction studies using Si₃N₄ counterface balls. (c) Region in the wear track clearly exhibiting evidence of boride pull-out from the softer β-Ti matrix. [Sonia Samuel et al. *Wear Resistance of Laser Deposited Boride Reinforced Ti-Nb-Zr-Ta Alloy Composites for Orthopedic Implants* (to appear in Mater. Sci. Eng. C, 2007)]

due to the harder and more resistant TiB precipitates. One possible explanation for this behavior is the pull-out of the harder TiB precipitates from the matrix resulting in third body wear, which would accelerate abrasive wear events by ploughing and deep grooving, as shown in Figure 9.23b. The SEM image in Figure 9.23c confirms that one of several TiB precipitates (~10 μm on edge) being pulled-out of the matrix inside the wear track, which is in agreement with previous observations of boride pull out from the matrix of Ti-6Al-4V reinforced with TiB$_2$ [41]. From these results, it was surmised that the Si$_3$N$_4$ ball, much harder than would be active in a hip prosthesis contact where a ultra-high molecular weight polyethylene (UHMWPE) coated surface is typically the wearing counterface, was responsible for precipitate pull-out from the Ti-6Al-4V matrix. Therefore, the use of a softer SS 440C counterface against the candidate alloys will be addressed below.

In order to lower the friction and wear of Ti-6Al-4V ELI and the TNZT + 2B, the samples were heat treated at 600 °C for ten hours in air to promote the formation of toughened oxide layers and finer α precipitates in TNZT + 2B. SEM images of the oxidized TNZT + 2B surface, not shown, could not resolve the very small α precipitates through the oxide layer. However, after removal of the oxide layer via mechanical polishing, the fine scale α precipitates could be resolved using high resolution SEM imaging. Typical friction coefficient curves of the alloys sliding against Si$_3$N$_4$, shown in Figure 9.24, are much lower than the non-oxidized alloys. After an initial run-in period, the steady-state friction coefficients are ~0.23

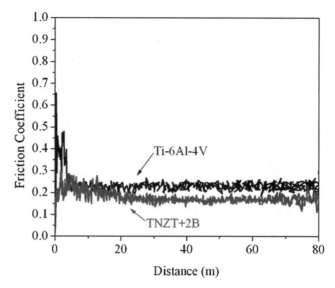

Figure 9.24. Wear plots showing the friction behavior as a function of distance of oxidized surfaces (600 °C/10 hrs) of Ti-6Al-4V ELI and TNZT + 2B with Si$_3$N$_4$ counterface balls. [Sonia Samuel et al. *Wear Resistance of Laser Deposited Boride Reinforced Ti-Nb-Zr-Ta Alloy Composites for Orthopedic Implants* (to appear in Mater. Sci. Eng. C, 2007)]

and 0.17 out to 80 m sliding distance for Ti-6Al-4V ELI and the TNZT + 2B, respectively. These are very low friction coefficients typically exhibited for oxidized titanium materials [45]. In addition, these friction coefficients show much less fluctuations compared to their as-synthesized state, suggesting a more stable sliding interface without debris in the contact. The values are also consistent with the corresponding wear track morphologies shown in Figures 9.25 and 9.26.

Based on these SEM images, both wear track morphologies exhibit a change in mechanism to mild oxidative wear, which suppresses the previous plastically dominated wear mechanisms shown for the as-synthesized alloys. The toughened

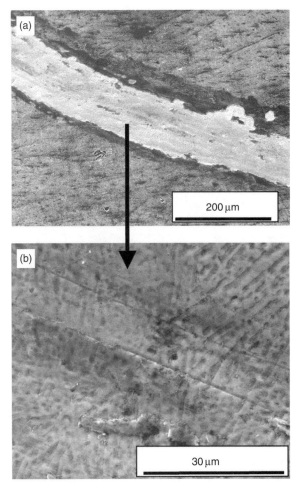

Figure 9.25. (a) Lower magnification and (b) higher magnification secondary SEM images of wear tracks on the surface of oxidized Ti-6Al-4V ELI after friction studies using Si_3N_4 counter-face balls. [Sonia Samuel et al. *Wear Resistance of Laser Deposited Boride Reinforced Ti-Nb-Zr-Ta Alloy Composites for Orthopedic Implants* (to appear in Mater. Sci. Eng. C, 2007)]

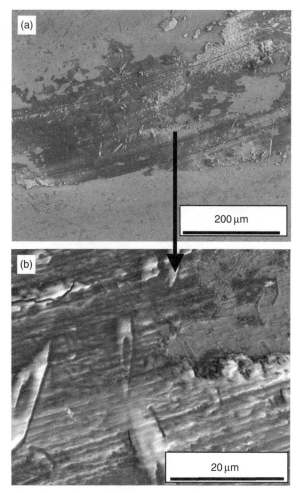

Figure 9.26. Lower magnification (a) and (b) higher magnification secondary SEM images of wear tracks on the surface of oxidized TNZT + 2B after friction studies using Si$_3$N$_4$ counterface balls. [Sonia Samuel et al. *Wear Resistance of Laser Deposited Boride Reinforced Ti-Nb-Zr-Ta Alloy Composites for Orthopedic Implants* (to appear in Mater. Sci. Eng. C, 2007)]

titanium oxide layers, like the rutile phase have been shown to be very effective in lowering the friction coefficients (~0.2) and wear rates [45]. This narrowed the wear tracks with no significant third body debris formation that might result in severe abrasive wear. Thus the titanium oxide layer acted as a lubricous oxide and prevented boride particles from being potentially pulled out of the matrix, and thereby improved the wear resistance considerably for both Ti-6Al-4V ELI and TNZT + 2B. Lastly, there were no significant differences in the wear track morphologies between the alloys outside of some patchy regions in TNZT + 2B that did not contribute to the overall friction behavior.

While the improvement in wear resistance of the TNZT + 2B material after oxidation against a substantially harder Si_3N_4 counterface material is promising, it is quite likely that in a real implant, such an oxide layer might spall during the sliding of the femoral head against the internal surface of the acetabular cup, a highly undesirable attribute. Therefore, the critical issue is to determine the wear resistance of the TNZT + 2B composite against a softer, more realistic, counterface materials, such as SS440C (H~10 GPa). Table 9.2 lists the hardness and Hertzian contact stresses for both TNZT + 2B and Ti-6Al-4V with respect to the two different counterfaces namely Si_3N_4 and SS440C. This contacting condition is expected to be more representative of an actual ball and socket joint. Figure 9.27 show typical friction coefficient curves for the alloys sliding against a SS 440C counterface ball after removal of the titanium oxide layers by a light mechanical polish.

The initial friction coefficients of both Ti-6Al-4V and TNZT + 2B are approximately 0.1, however the friction coefficient of Ti-6Al-4V began to deviate at ~15 m sliding distance. A continual steady increase in the friction coefficient occurs up to ~0.4 to 0.6, similar to the values shown in the as-synthesized condition in Figure 9.21. These higher and more fluctuating values suggest increased abrasive wear and debris generation. In contrast, the initial friction coefficient of TNZT + 2B alloy remained at a very low steady-state value of ~0.13 for the entire test, instead of the high values (~0.6) shown in Figure 9.21 for the as-deposited condition. Thus, the softer steel counterface eliminated the TiB precipitate

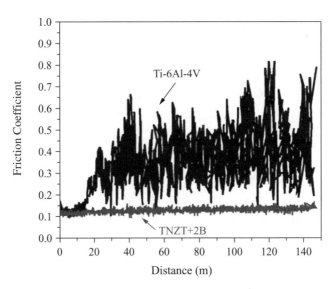

Figure 9.27. Wear plots showing the friction behavior as a function of distance of Ti-6Al-4V ELI and TNZT + 2B with SS440 stainless steel counterface balls. [Sonia Samuel et al. *Wear Resistance of Laser Deposited Boride Reinforced Ti-Nb-Zr-Ta Alloy Composites for Orthopedic Implants* (to appear in Mater. Sci. Eng. C, 2007)]

pull-out, third body abrasive wear observed with the harder Si_3N_4 counterface. The corresponding SEM images of the wear tracks shown in Figures 9.28 and 9.29 for Ti-6Al-4V ELI and TNZT + 2B, respectively, corroborate the friction behavior.

The wear track morphology of Ti-6Al-4V ELI in Figure 9.28 shows more extensive plastic deformation, microplowing and cutting, all typical processes associated with an abrasive wear mechanism. Conversely, the TNZT + 2B wear track shown in Figure 9.29 exhibits less severity in wear. It is apparent that the

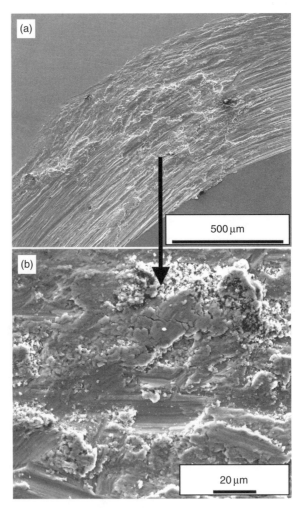

Figure 9.28. (a) Lower magnification and (b) higher magnification secondary SEM images of Ti-6Al-4V ELI wear tracks after friction studies using SS440 counterface balls. [Sonia Samuel et al. *Wear Resistance of Laser Deposited Boride Reinforced Ti-Nb-Zr-Ta Alloy Composites for Orthopedic Implants* (to appear in Mater. Sci. Eng. C, 2007)]

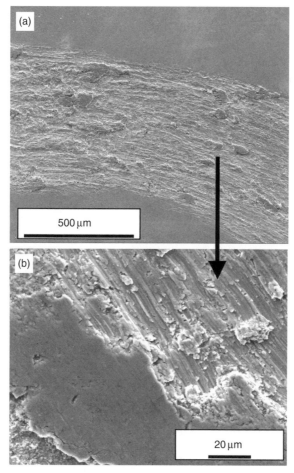

Figure 9.29. (a) Lower magnification and (b) higher magnification secondary SEM images of TNZT + 2B wear tracks after friction studies using SS440 counterface balls. [Sonia Samuel et al. *Wear Resistance of Laser Deposited Boride Reinforced Ti-Nb-Zr-Ta Alloy Composites for Orthopedic Implants* (to appear in Mater. Sci. Eng. C, 2007)]

surface morphology has undergone a plastic shear deformation mechanism usually associated with less wear volume removal. This is evident by examining some of the larger surface depressions with plastic flow process. These results show that much lower friction coefficient and improved wear resistance can be obtained by using a softer counterface material in case of TNZT + 2B as-synthesized state, when compared to Ti-6Al-4V ELI alloys.

9.3.4.4 Summary of Ti-Nb-Zr-Ta + TiB Composites. The summary of Ti-Nb-Zr-Ta + TiB Composites is as follows:

1. As deposited LENS™ TNZT + 2B has borides precipitates that contain compositionally segregated regions of higher Ti(Zr) or Ta(Nb) weight percent,

2. Using Si_3N_4 balls, there is TiB precipitate pullout resulting in accelerated third body abrasive wear with higher friction coefficients.

3. Using 440C stainless steel balls drastically improved the friction coefficients of as deposited TNZT + 2B, eliminating the effect of "three body abrasive wear" and resulting in superior wear resistance when compared to Ti-6Al-4V ELI.

4. Oxide film improves the wear resistance of both TNZT + 2B and Ti-6Al-4V ELI.

9.4 CONCLUSIONS

The present article demonstrates the feasibility and advantages of using laser engineered net shape processing (LENS™) for orthopedic biomaterials. This relatively new manufacturing technology allows for the deposition of metallic biomaterials with refined microstructures and in some cases preferential crystallographic texture, which in turn lead to enhanced mechanical properties. In this article, the specific focus has been on the laser deposition of newer generation beta titanium alloys, such as those based on the Ti-Nb-Zr-Ta system. These newer generation alloys not only exhibit a much lower elastic modulus (~50–60 GPa) as compared to conventionally used Ti-6Al-4V (~110 GPa), but also consist of completely biocompatible alloying additions with minimal toxicity. Along the growth direction during deposition, the LENS™ deposited Ti-35Nb-7Zr-5Ta alloys exhibit a higher strength as compared with alloys of similar composition processed via more conventional techniques, while still maintaining a low modulus. The corrosion resistance of these laser-deposited alloys is also comparable to, if not better than, conventionally processed Ti-6Al-4V ELI and commercially pure Ti (Grade 2). Preliminary *in vitro* biocompatibility studies also indicate that these laser-deposited alloys are comparable to conventionally used alloys and might actually lead to better cell differentiation. Furthermore, by introducing a homogeneous distribution of hard ceramic precipitates, such as borides, into the same metallic Ti-35Nb-7Zr-5Ta base matrix to form metal-matrix composites, the wear resistance of these alloys can be substantially enhanced. A higher wear resistance would allow the use of these materials in a number of applications including the femoral head part of the hip implant, or in other words, the ball part of the ball-socket joint. This in turn leads to the possibility of manufacturing a unitized, compositionally and functionally-graded, femoral (hip) implant with site specific properties. In such an implant the femoral stem would consist of a hollow Ti-35Nb-7Zr-5Ta based structure with a low elastic modulus, while the femoral head would be graded from a core consisting of the softer and tough base Ti-35Nb-7Zr-5Ta alloy while the outer surface of the head consisted of wear-resistant boride-reinforced metal matrix composite layers based on the same base alloy composition with boron additions to it.

9.5 FUTURE PERSPECTIVES

Laser-assisted direct metal deposition techniques such as LENS™ offer great potential as future manufacturing technologies for orthopedic implants and other biomaterials. The use of LENS™ would not only allow for the design and development of compositionally and functionally-graded implants with site-specific properties, as discussed in the previous section, but also lead to the availability of custom-designed implants for specific patient needs. Thus, since LENS™ is based on the concepts of three-dimensional stereolithography and is capable of reconstructing a 3D shape from a computer CAD file in a relatively short period of time, this processing technology can be quite easily adapted to manufacture custom-designed implants. It is possible to envision a scenario in the future where a detailed 3D tomographic description of the implant required for a specific patient can be generated in the doctor's hospital, electronically transmitted to a LENS™ based manufacturing setup at a different location, processed at the manufacturing facility directly from the CAD file, and then shipped back to the hospital in a rather short period of time for the surgical implantation. If successful, this has the potential of revolutionizing the orthopedic implants industry of the future. One of the drawbacks of LENS™ processing is the effective cost of production associated with orthopedic implants. However, with the rapidly increasing efficiency of lasers and the obvious advantages from an environmental and conservation point of view, LENS™ and related near-net shape processing technologies based on additive manufacturing are becoming increasingly popular and are very promising for the future.

ACKNOWLEDGMENTS

The authors take this opportunity to express their gratitude to a number of people without whose support this work would not have been possible. First and foremost, the authors gratefully acknowledge the support, encouragement, and, guidance from Professor Hamish Fraser at the Ohio State University for this work on laser deposition of orthopedic biomaterials. The authors would also like to acknowledge Dr. Thomas Scharf from the University of North Texas (UNT) for his guidance and support in the tribology work, Dr. Seifollah Nasrazadani (UNT) for support with the corrosion studies, Dr. Mohamed El Bouanani (UNT) for support with the XPS studies, and Dr. Kytai Ngyugen from the University of Texas at Arlington for support in carrying out the *in vitro* studies. The authors would also like to acknowledge the excellent work by graduate students, both past and present, working on this program over a period of time and at different institutions. These include Sonia Samuel and Anantha Puthucode at UNT and Davion Hill at the Ohio State University.

REFERENCES

1. M. J. Long and H. J. Rack, "Titanium alloys in total joint replacement—a materials science perspective," *Biomater.*, 19, 1621–1639 (1998).
2. E. W. Lowman, "Osteoarthiritis," *J. Amer. Med. Acad.*, 157, 487 (1955).
3. D. M. Keicher and J. E. Smugeresky, "The laser forming of metallic components using particulate materials," *JOM*, 49(5), 51 (1997).
4. M. Hedges, Orthopaedic Product News, www.opnews.com, art. 126, Sep. 2003.
5. www.jointreplacement.com.
6. R. H. Rothman, et al., "Total Hip Arthroplasty using Two Different Cementless Tapered Stems," *Clin orthop*, (393), 121–7 (Dec 2001).
7. Investigational Device Review, *Biomet Inc.* (Sept 25, 1986).
8. W. Head, et al., "Mechanical Properties and Clinical Evaluation of Isostatic Molded ArCom Polyethylene," *J. Bone Joint Surg.*, 74A, 849–863 (1992).
9. Modern Casting, A publication of *American Foundry Society*, 29–32 (Feb 2003)
10. H. C. Amstutz, "Trapezoidal-28 total hip replacement," *J. Bone Joint Surg*, 62A, 670–673 (1980).
11. D. W. Hoeppner and V. Chandrasekaran, "Fretting in orthopaedic implants: a review," *Wear*, 173, 189–197 (1994).
12. http://www.fda.gov/cdrh/recalls/zirconiahip.html
13. http://arthritis.about.com/od/news/a/hipimplants.htm
14. I. C. Clarke, M. Manaka, D. D. Green, P. Williams, G. Pezzotti, Y. H. Kim, M. Ries, N. Sugano, L. Sedel, C. Delauney, B. Ben Nissan, T. Donaldson, and G. A. Gustafson, "Current Status of Zirconia Used in Total Hip Implants," *Jour. Bone & Joint Surg. Am*, 85, 73–84 (2003).
15. K. Wang, "The Use and Properties of Titanium and Titanium Alloys for Medical Applications in the USA," *Mater. Sci. and Eng.*, A213, 134–137 (1996).
16. S. Rao, T. Ushida, T. Tateishi, Y. Okazaki, and S. Asao, "Effect of Ti, Al and V ions on the relative growth rate of fibroblasts (L 929) and osteoblasts (MC 3 T 3-E 1) cells," *Bio-med. Mater. Eng.*, 6, 79 (1996).
17. P. R. Walker, J. Leblanc, and M. Sikorska, "Effects of Aluminum and Other Cations on the structure of Brain and Liver Chromatin," *Biochemistry*, 28, 3911 (1989).
18. W. F. Ho, C. P. Ju, and J. H. Chern Lin, "Structure and properties of cast binary Ti-Mo alloys," *Biomater.*, 20, 2115–2122 (1999).
19. K. Wang, L. Gustavson, and J. Dumbleton, "The characterization of Ti-12Mo-6Zr-2Fe. A new biocompatible titanium alloy developed for surgical implants," *Beta Titanium in the 1990's*, The Mineral, Metals and Materials Society, Warrendale, Pennsylvania, 2697–2704 (1993).
20. S. G. Steinemann, P-A. Mäusli, S. Szmukler-Moncler, M. Semlitsch, O. Pohler, H-E Hintermann, and S-M Perren, "Beta-titanium alloy for surgical implants," *Beta*

Titanium in the 1990's, The Mineral, Metals and Materials Society, Warrendale, Pennsylvania, 2689–2696 (1993).

21. J. C. Fanning, "Properties and processing of a new metastable beta titanium alloy for surgical implant applications: TIMETAL™ 21SRx," *Titanium 95': Science and Technology*, 1800–1807 (1996).

22. A. K. Mishra, J. A. Davidson, P. Kovacs, and R. A. Poggie, "Ti-13Nb-13Zr: a new low modulus, high strength, corrosion resistant near-beta alloy for orthopaedic implants," *Beta Titanium in the 1990's*, The Mineral, Metals and Materials Society, Warrendale, Pennsylvania, 61–72 (1993).

23. T. A. Ahmed, M. Long, J. Silverstri, C. Ruiz, and H. J. Rack, "A new low modulus biocompatible titanium alloy," *Titanium 95': Science and Technology*, 1760–1767 (1996).

24. M. Griffith, M. E. Schlienger, L. D. Harwell, M. S. Oliver, M. D. Baldwin, M. T. Ensz, M. Esien, J. Brooks, C. E. Robino, J. E. Smugeresky, W. Hofmeister, M. J. Wert, and D. V. Nelson, *Materials And Design*, 20(2–3), 107 (1999).

25. R. Banerjee, P. C. Collins, D. Bhattacharyya, S. Banerjee, and H. L. Fraser, "Microstructural evolution in laser deposited compositionally graded α/β titanium-vanadium alloys," *Acta. Mater.*, 51, 3277–3292 (2003).

26. R. Banerjee, D. Bhattacharyya, P. C. Collins, G. B. Viswanathan and H. L. Fraser, "Precipitation of grain boundary α in a laser deposited compositionally graded Ti-8Al-xV alloy—an orientation microscopy study," *Acta. Mater.*, 52, 377–385 (2004).

27. J. I. Qazi, B. Marquardt, and H. J. Rack, "High strength metatable beta-. titanium alloys for biomedical applications," *JOM*, 56(11), 49 (2004).

28. R. Banerjee, S. Nag, S. Samuel, and H. L. Fraser, "Laser Deposited Ti-Nb-Zr-Ta Orthopaedic Alloys," *J. Biomedical Mater. Res.*, 78A (2), 298, (2006).

29. Y. Ohmori, T. Ogo, K. Nakai, and S. Kobayashi, "Effects of omega phase precipitation on beta to alpha, alpha' transformations in a metastable beta titanium alloy," *Mater. Sci. Eng.*, A312, 182 (2001).

30. T. Ahmed, M. Long, J. Silvestri, C. Ruiz, and H. J. Rack, "A new low modulus, biocompatible titanium alloy," *Titanium 95: Science and Technology*, ed. P. A. Blekinsop, W. J. Evans, and H. M. Flower, Institute of Metals, London, 1760 (1995).

31. X. Tang, T. Ahmed, and H. J. Rack, "Phase transformations in Ti-Nb-Ta and Ti-Nb-Ta-Zr alloys," *J. Mater. Sci.*, 35, 1805 (2000).

32. R. E. Reed-Hill and R. Abbaschian, *Physical Metallurgy Principles*, 3rd edition, PWS Publishing Company, Boston, MA, 284–285 (1994).

33. R. Banerjee, P. C. Collins, and H. L. Fraser, "Phase evolution in laser-deposited titanium-chromium alloys," *Metall. Mater. Trans A*, 33, 2129 (2002).

34. L. Thair, U. Kamachi Mudali, R. Asokamani, and Baldev Raj, "Influence of microstructural changes on corrosion behaviour of thermally aged Ti-6Al-7Nb alloy," *Mater. Corros.*, 55 (5), 358 (2004).

35. H. Zitter and J. Plenk, "The electrochemical behavior of metallic implant materials as an indicator of their biocompatibility," *J. Biomed. Mater. Res.*, 21, 881 (1987).

36. S. Samuel, S. Nasrazadani, S. Nag, and R. Banerjee, manuscript under preparation (2009).

37. http://srdata.nist.gov/xps/

38. M. Long and H. J. Rack, "Subsurface deformation and microcrack formation in Ti–35Nb–8Zr–5Ta–O(x) during reciprocating sliding wear," *Mat. Sci. And Eng.*, C 25(3), 382–388 (2005).

39. M. Long and H.J. Rack, "Friction and surface behaviour of selected titanium alloys during reciprocating-sliding motion," *Wear*, 249, 158 (2001).

40. S. J. Li, R. Yang, S. Li, Y. L. Hao, Y. Y. Cui, M. Niinomi, and Z. X. Guo, "Wear characteristics of Ti-Nb-Ta-Zr and Ti-6Al-4V alloys for biomedical applications," *Wear*, 257, 869 (2004).

41. V. Ocelik, D. Mathews, and J. Th. M. De Hosson, "Sliding wear resistance of metal matrix composite layers prepared by high power laser," *Surf. Coat. Tech.*, 197, 303 (2005).

42. R. Banerjee, P. C. Collins, A. Genc, and H. L. Fraser, "Direct laser deposition of *in situ* Ti–6Al–4V–TiB composites," *Mater. Sci. Eng. A*, 358, 343 (2003).

43. R. Banerjee, P. C. Collins, and H. L. Fraser, "Laser Deposition of In Situ Ti–TiB Composites," *Advanced Engineering Materials*, 4(11), 847 (2002).

44. S. Samuel, S. Nag, T. Scharf, and R. Banerjee, "Wear Resistance of Laser-Deposited Boride Reinforced Ti-Nb-Zr-Ta Alloy Composites for Orthopedic Implants," *Mater. Sci. Eng. C* 28(3), 414 (2007).

45. M. N. Gardos, "Magneli phases of anion-deficient rutile as lubricious oxides. Part II. Tribological behavior of Cu-doped polycrystalline rutile (TinO2n-1)," *Trib. Lett.*, 8, 79 (2000).

10

FUNCTIONALLY GRADED ALL CERAMIC HIP JOINT

Omer Van der Biest, Guy Anné, Kim Vanmeensel, and Jef Vleugels

Department of Metallurgy and Materials Engineering, Katholieke Universiteit Leuven, Kasteelpark Arenberg 44, 3001 Heverlee, Belgium

Contents

10.1 Overview   324
10.2 Introduction Materials for Hip Implants   325
10.3 Ceramics for Total Hip Joint Replacement   327
     10.3.1 Alumina Implants   327
     10.3.2 Zirconia Implants   327
     10.3.3 Zirconia Toughened Alumina   328
     10.3.4 Ceramic Coatings on Metal Implants   329
     10.3.5 Functionally Graded Ceramics for Hip Components   330
10.4 Electrophoretic Deposition As a Shaping Technique for
     FGM Biomaterials   331
10.5 EPD of FGM Discs   332
     10.5.1 Introduction   332
     10.5.2 Mathematical Model to Predict the Composition Profile of
         FGM Discs   333
     10.5.3 Controlled Processing of FGM Discs   335
     10.5.4 Properties of FGM Discs   338
10.6 Ball-Heads and Cup Inserts Made by EPD   339

Advanced Biomaterials: Fundamentals, Processing, and Applications, Edited by Bikramjit Basu, Dhirendra S. Katti, and Ashok Kumar
Copyright © 2009 The American Ceramic Society

        10.6.1 Introduction   339
        10.6.2 E-Field Calculations for Electrode Design   340
        10.6.3 Shaping of Homogeneous and FGM Acetabular Cup Inserts   340
   10.7 Sintering and Microstructural Evaluation   344
        10.7.1 Introduction   344
        10.7.2 Sintering Kinetics of Al_2O_3, ZrO_2 and Their Composites   345
        10.7.3 Optimization of Grain Size of Al_2O_3 Composites   346
        10.7.4 Observation of Processing Defects in FGM Materials   348
   10.8 Conclusions   351
   10.9 Future Perspectives   352
        Acknowledgments   353
        References   353

10.1 OVERVIEW

Many materials are used in medicine for a variety of applications ranging from total replacement of hard tissues (such as bone plates, pins, joint, dental implants, and so on), repair, diagnostic or corrective devices (such as pacemakers, heart valves, and so on). Not only the mechanical properties are important, but also the material should be biocompatible with the human body and stable for a long period. Due to their excellent properties such as high strength, biocompatibility, and stability in physiological environments, ceramics are investigated as bone substitute materials. In this way, ceramic components have been used for total hip joint replacement components in Europe since the early 1970s. Alumina and zirconia monoliths are mainly used for these components. However, zirconia can undergo low temperature degradation in aqueous environment.

Current research is focusing on increasing the strength and wear resistance, meanwhile reducing the size and extending the lifetime of ceramic components. This chapter will briefly review the present state-of-the-art with respect to ceramic material development for total hip joint replacement (THR). In addition to ceramic monoliths, ceramic composites such as zirconia-toughened alumina and other alumina matrix composites are currently investigated. Another possibility to increase the strength is to use components based on alumina and zirconia with a functionally-graded composition. The latter possibility has been the focus of the authors' research and will be described in some detail. The composition gradient can be established during shaping by means of electrophoretic deposition (EPD) to obtain a pure alumina surface region and a homogeneous alumina/zirconia composite core with intermediate continuously graded regions to generate thermal residual stresses after sintering. The gradient profiles are designed to obtain maximum compressive surface stresses and minimum tensile stresses in the core of the component to increase the strength and wear resistance compared to pure alumina components. Practical aspects of this new production technology will be described, including the method to control the composition gradient, the electric field calculations necessary to design the electrodes, drying, and the sintering conditions.

10.2 INTRODUCTION MATERIALS FOR HIP IMPLANTS

Some 30 years ago, a revolution in medical care began with the successful replacement of tissues. Two alternatives are possible, transplantation or implantation. Transplantation belongs to the realm of surgery. Implantation involves the replacement of tissues by the development or modification of man-made materials to interface with living host tissue, that is, implants made of biomaterials. Material scientists have investigated metals, polymers, ceramics, as well as composites, as biomaterials for hard and soft tissues. Important issues in the development of biomaterials are the interfacial stability with host tissues, appropriate properties as close as possible to bone, and a minimum of wear debris generation.

Ceramics used for repair, reconstruction, and replacement of human tissue are called bioceramics. When any artificial material is implanted into the body, it will cause some reaction with the host tissue. Bioceramics exhibit four possible tissue /implant interactions [Hench and Ethridge, 1982]: toxic, when the tissue dies due to chemical leaching from the ceramic; biologically inert, when tissues form a non-adherent fibrous capsule around the implant surface; bioactive, in case the tissues chemically bond with the implant surface; and dissolution of the implant, when the implant surface dissolves allowing tissues to refill the space previously occupied by the implant.

Bioceramics have become a diverse class of biomaterials, presently including three basic types: bioinert high strength ceramics; bioactive ceramics which form direct chemical bonds with bone or even with soft tissue of a living organism; and bioresorbable ceramics that actively participate in the metabolic processes of an organism [Thamaraiselvi and Rajeswari, 2004]. Alumina (Al_2O_3), zirconia (ZrO_2) and carbon are bioinert. Bioactive glass and calcium phosphate ceramics such as hydroxyapatite are bioactive and bioresorbable depending on their composition and structure. An overview of the applications for bioceramics is given in Table 10.1.

TABLE 10.1. Overview of Applications for Bioceramics

Bioceramic	Function	Tissue reaction
Zirconia	Artificial total hip, knee, bone screws and plates, dental crowns and bridges	Bioinert
Alumina	Artificial total hip, shoulder, elbow, wrist, bone screws, porous coatings for femoral stems	Bioinert
Carbon	Coatings on heart valves, blood vessel grafts, surfaces in dentistry	Bioinert
Calcium phosphates	Drug delivery, bone substitute, coatings for metal implants, stems, ocular implants	Bioactive, Bioresorbable
Bioactive glass	Bone cement filler, bioactive coating on implants	Bioactive, Bioresorbable
TiN	Coating on implants like artificial hip, dental and shoulder implants	Bioactive

Materials for load bearing implants such as hip or knee implants should be able to resist peak loads as high as ten times body weight and an average load of three times the body weight [Black, 1992]. Therefore, only bioceramics like Al_2O_3, ZrO_2 and their composites are considered as suitable ceramics for ball-heads and acetabular cup inserts (liners) in total hip joint replacement and will be discussed in this paper. Compared to metals and polymers, advantages of these ceramic implants are the excellent bioinertia, the extremely low wear rate and the reduced osteolysis. Other ceramics as SiC and Si_3N_4 have also an excellent hardness, mechanical strength and corrosion resistance, but have been much less investigated as biomaterials. Part of the reasons for this is their more complicated processing routes, in particular with respect to densification, where high temperature and—in the case of silicon nitrides—also high gas pressure is necessary. Noteworthy are the biomorphic silicon carbide ceramics which have inherited their microstructure and in particular their pore structure from the wood from which they have been prepared. Biomorphic SiC is fabricated by molten-silicon infiltration of carbon templates obtained by controlled pyrolysis of wood. The bioactivity of such a material coated also with a bioactive glass layer has been reported by Gonzalez et al. (2003). Silicon nitride has been another silicon based ceramic which has hardly been investigated with respect to its potential applications as biomaterial. The role of the surface finish of the materials on the proliferation of osteoblast cells on reaction bonded silicon nitride has been highlighted by Kue et al. (1999). In a more recent study by Neumann et al. (2006), the potential application of silicon nitride for a miniplate osteofixation system for the midface has been investigated. One of the conclusions was that Si_3N_4 ceramics showed a good biocompatibility outcome both *in vitro* and *in vivo*.

In the early 1970s, ceramic components for total hip joint replacements (THR) were introduced. The hip joint consists of a ceramic ball-head attached to a metal stem and an acetabular ceramic or polyethylene insert, which is attached to a metallic cup, as illustrated in Figure 10.1. Today, more than 350,000 ceramic components for total hip joint replacement have been implanted.

In general, the material combinations for the femoral head–acetabular cup pair comprise metal-metal, metal-polyethylene, ceramic-polyethylene and ceramic-ceramic combinations. The currently used material combinations are summarized in Figure 10.1. The metal-polyethylene and ceramic-polyethylene couplings are still considered to be the most suitable in most cases. The wear rates and the consequent risks of loosening of the implant are proportional to the time and motorial activity. In fact, for elderly or barely active patients, the use of polyethylene must not be considered a limitation. The alternative ceramic-ceramic and metal-metal solutions are chosen for patients with a high motorial activity and it is stated that ceramic-ceramic couplings are appropriate in almost 20% of cases, while metal-metal couplings only in five percent of all cases. Indeed metal-metal bearings carry the risk that the released metal ions and debris may cause (among other potential negative effects) allergic reactions leading at least to discomfort to the patient. Because of the long-term biocompatibility of the debris

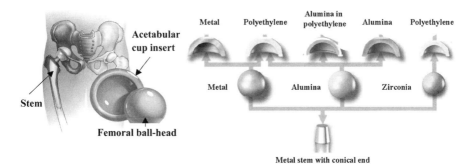

Figure 10.1. Components for total hip replacement and current material combinations for total hip replacement [CeramTec, 2002].

produced by the wearing action, the ceramic-ceramic coupling should be preferred for young, heavy and active patients.

10.3 CERAMICS FOR TOTAL HIP JOINT REPLACEMENT

10.3.1 Alumina Implants

The first ceramic ball-heads were made of Al_2O_3, which today is still the most commonly-used ceramic. Alumina has a very good corrosion resistance, which is most important in biomedical applications [Black, 1992]. The hardness is very high, resulting in a very low wear rate. In fact, when testing the current generation of pure alumina ball heads and acetabular cups in a hip joint simulator, it becomes very hard to characterize the wear either from the loss of any material from the mating surfaces or by collecting the wear debris. The elastic modulus is 396 GPa, providing rigid and non-deformable implants [Willmann, 1996]. To obtain high strength Al_2O_3 (>450 MPa), high purity alumina is used with a very low concentration of sintering additives (<0.5 wt %) because the residual glass phase on the grain boundaries can degrade and mechanical strength will be lost. A reduction in grain size improves drastically the strength and therefore very small grain size and a narrow grain size distribution are essential. The average grain size of current medical grade alumina is 1.4 µm. To limit grain growth, Al_2O_3 is doped with MgO (<0.5 wt %). Despite these favorable properties, alumina is brittle [Kingery, 1976], which is a disadvantage compared to zirconia.

10.3.2 Zirconia Implants

The first ball-head made out of tetragonal zirconia polycrystalline (TZP) material was introduced by Christel et al. [Christel et al., 1988]. Until recently, about 25% of the total number of hip implant operations per year in Europe were performed with TZP [Cordingley et al., 2003]. Whereas the flexural strength of medical grade Al_2O_3 is in the range of 500–580 MPa, that of ZrO_2 is two to three times higher

TABLE 10.2. Overview of Mechanical Properties of Femur Bone, Al_2O_3 and ZrO_2

Properties	Femur [Currey, 1984]	Alumina	Zirconia
Density (g/cm^3)		≥3.97	>6.00
Tensile strength (MPa)	121	>500	900–1200
Hardness (GPa, HV$_{10}$)	0.37	22	12
Toughness (MPa · m$^{1/2}$)		4	5–10
Compressive strength (MPa)	167	4100	2000
E-modulus (GPa)	17–18	380	210

(>1500 MPa) [Clarke et al., 2003], also the fracture toughness is much higher (Table 10.2). The higher fracture toughness is of importance in femoral heads due to the tensile stress induced by the taper fit of the femoral stem [Cordingley et al., 2003]. Therefore, smaller ball-heads are possible with TZP compared to Al_2O_3.

Most of the zirconia implants are stabilized with two to three mol % Y_2O_3 [Cales et al., 1994], in order to stabilize the tetragonal ZrO_2 phase at room temperature. The high toughness of these ceramics is related to transformation toughening, that is, the stress-induced martensitic transformation of the tetragonal to monoclinic ZrO_2 in the vicinity of a propagating crack tip, resulting in a local volume expansion of three to four percent that results in compressive stresses inhibiting crack propagation [Hannink et al., 2000].

However, there is a major concern about the hydrothermal degradation of ZrO_2 at room temperature. The low temperature degradation (LTD) of Y-TZP involves a spontaneous transformation of the tetragonal phase when ageing in water, resulting in the formation of microcracks at the surface and a decrease of the mechanical properties [Sato et al., 1985]. Whether LTD will occur or not depends on the environment with which the material is in contact. The presence of water is an essential prerequisite. Also the composition, the microstructure, and the processing route of the material as well as any possible thermal activation play a role. Therefore, the grain size of the t-ZrO_2 grains, the Y_2O_3 content, the Y_2O_3 distribution, density, surface roughness and purity are important parameters in the possible degradation process [Piconi and Maccauro, 1999]. It has to be noted that ageing effects of ZrO_2 in a water or salt solution can differ from ageing in bovine serum. To avoid ageing of ZrO_2, several approaches have been proposed such as reducing the initial grain size, coating the implant surface with a stable layer of cubic ZrO_2, replacing the Y_2O_3 stabilizer by CeO_2, the addition of small amounts of SiO_2, the addition of small amounts of alumina, and the use of ZrO_2 composites [Clarke et al., 2003].

10.3.3 Zirconia Toughened Alumina

ZrO_2 and Al_2O_3 have both disadvantages, that is, the brittleness of Al_2O_3 and the risk of hydrothermal degradation in ZrO_2. To avoid these problems, a good alternative is composites in which ZrO_2 particles are embedded in an Al_2O_3 matrix.

These composites are commonly known as zirconia-toughened alumina (ZTA). In the case of a stabilized zirconia matrix reinforced with alumina particles, that is, alumina-toughened zirconia (ATZ), the risk of hydrothermal degradation remains.

In ZTA with eight-to-fifteen vol. % ZrO_2, the favorable properties of Al_2O_3 can be maintained since ZTA is nearly as hard as pure Al_2O_3. The ZrO_2 may induce extra toughening and leads to a smaller grain size in the composites since a homogeneous distribution of small ZrO_2 particles acts as grain growth inhibitor for Al_2O_3 grains during sintering [Konsztowicz and Langlois, 1996]. In ZTA composites, the ZrO_2 addition can take the unstabilized or the Y_2O_3-ZrO_2 form. The primary difference between these two forms of the ZTA system is that the former relies on microcrack toughening [Hannink et al., 2000; Rühle et al., 1987] whereas the latter has transformation toughening as the primary toughening mechanism [Hannink et al., 2000; Green et al., 1989].

The toughness of ZTA composites with unstabilized ZrO_2 addition can be improved by the processing of Al_2O_3-ZrO_2 nanocomposites [De Aza et al., 2002]. In this way, a larger amount of tetragonal ZrO_2 grains is present in the alumina matrix and contributes to the transformation toughening mechanism [De Aza et al., 2002]. It should be clear, however, that spontaneous transformation of the unstabilized ZrO_2 grains can only be avoided when the grain size is kept below a critical maximum value. A colloidal processing technique to establish this was recently developed by Schehl et al. [Schehl et al., 2002].

Another option to increase the strength of ZTA ceramics is to incorporate platelets into the matrix. The addition of whiskers is not allowed because they constitute a health risk, which can be avoided when platelets are grown *in situ* during sintering. Belmonte et al. [Belmonte et al., 1993] developed zirconia-toughened alumina with *in situ* formed plate-like shaped calcium and strontium hexaluminates with enhanced mechanical properties. It was found that plate-like shape hexaluminates as reinforcing phase are formed upon addition of 0.1–1 vol. % of strontium. In this way, Burger et al. [Burger, 1998] developed a ZTA material grade for biomedical applications, containing 25 vol. % Y-TZP. Cr_2O_3 was added to enhance the hardness of the alumina. The biomaterial has a tensile strength of 1150 MPa and a fracture toughness of 8.5 MPa m$^{1/2}$ [Rack and Pfaff, 2000].

10.3.4 Ceramic Coatings on Metal Implants

To avoid the brittleness of ceramic ball-heads, a metallic ball-head can be coated with a ceramic coating like TiN or DLC (diamond-like carbon). The idea is to combine the hardness of TiN or DLC with the good mechanical properties of the metallic ball-heads. It was found, however, that the beneficial properties like a reduced wear of DLC coatings in air or in vacuum are not present in bovine serum [Hauert, 2003]. TiN coatings have a very good biocompatibility and high hardness, reducing wear. The bioactivity of TiN promotes the formation of calcium phosphate phases with adhesion strength, forming a promising alternative for plasma sprayed hydroxyapatite coatings on titanium alloy stems [Piscanec et al.,

2004]. A review of the coatings commercially available for metal-PE joints has been given by Piconi et al. (2004).

A procedure often adopted for commercial hip joint implants is to coat parts of the metallic femoral stem by a porous hydroxyapatite coating in order to improve the bonding between implant and bone. This is usually done by plasma spraying; see L. Sun et al. (2001) for a review. Other ceramics and coating methods are being investigated.

10.3.5 Functionally Graded Ceramics for Hip Components

The concept of functionally graded materials (FGM) originates from the observation that many components only need to posses a certain property locally while elsewhere another often irreconcilable property is required by the design. To increase the strength of ceramic ball-heads, the concept of functionally-graded materials can be used to develop ceramic Al_2O_3/ZrO_2 graded composites. The potential of this bioinert system follows from the properties of Al_2O_3 (low wear rate, high hardness) and ZrO_2 (high strength, high toughness).

Due to the difference in thermal expansion coefficient of Al_2O_3 and ZrO_2, residual stresses are developed during cooling from the sintering temperature, which can strongly influence the mechanical properties like strength and toughness. Compressive surface stresses in the outer alumina layer will have a beneficial effect on the wear resistance [Katti, 2004].

The design of the composition gradient has to be in such a way that it generates compressive stresses at those places that are loaded under tensile stress. To obtain a beneficial effect on the strength and tribological properties of the component, compressive stresses at the surface of the component have to be generated. A correct design of the gradient from the point of view of thermal stresses is therefore of primary importance [Toschi et al., 2003; Gasik et al., 2003].

Figure 10.2 shows the concept of FGM ball head, which has been investigated. Note that all outer surfaces of the ball head as well as the acetabular cup consist of a mm thick layer of pure alumina. The zirconia is only present in the interior and is not exposed to the environment so that LTD will not be an issue.

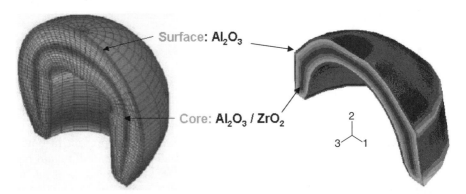

Figure 10.2. Schematic of an Al_2O_3/ZrO_2 FGM ball-head and liner. [Anné, 2005a].

Amongst the different methods to process functionally-graded materials (FGM), electrophoretic deposition (EPD) is explored here to process complex-shaped FGM hip prosthesis components. During EPD, particles having acquired an electric charge in the liquid in which they are suspended are forced to move toward one of the electrodes by applying an electric field and forming a coherent deposit on it. The deposit takes the shape imposed by this electrode. Hence, after drying and removal from the electrode, a shaped green ceramic body is obtained. Firing this green body results in the ceramic component.

10.4 ELECTROPHORETIC DEPOSITION AS A SHAPING TECHNIQUE FOR FGM BIOMATERIALS

In order to produce a FGM by conventional powder processing, a green body of powders containing the desired phase gradient is first fabricated. After formation, this green body is densified by sintering. A wide range of powder processes can be used to obtain a gradient, including common powder metallurgy and colloidal (wet) processes [Anné et al., 2006a]. Whereas only discrete layers can be made by dry powder processing, continuous gradients can be made by colloidal processes. Among the different colloidal processing techniques, electrophoretic deposition is very promising because it is a fairly rapid, low-cost process for the fabrication of ceramic coatings, monoliths, composites, laminates, and functionally graded materials varying in thickness from a few nanometers to centimeters [Cordingley et al., 2003].

Electrophoretic deposition (EPD) is a two-step process (Figure 10.3). In a first step, particles having acquired an electric charge in the liquid in which they are suspended, are forced to move towards one of the electrodes by applying an electric field to the suspension (electrophoresis). In a second step (deposition), the particles collect at one of the electrodes and form a coherent deposit on it.

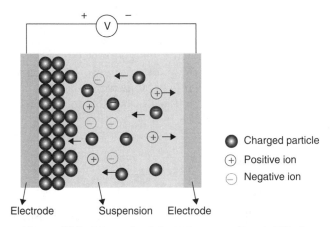

Figure 10.3. Schematic of the EPD process. [Anné, 2005a].

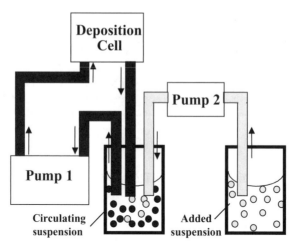

<u>Figure 10.4.</u> Schematic of the electrophoretic deposition set-up. [Anné, 2005a].

Since the local composition of the deposit during the EPD process is directly related to the composition of the suspension at the moment of deposition, the EPD technique allows processing of functionally graded materials with a continuous gradient in composition by judiciously adjusting the suspension composition in time (Figure 10.4).

The deposit takes the shape imposed by the deposition electrode. Hence, after drying and removal from the electrode, a shaped green ceramic body is obtained. Firing this green body results in the ceramic component. In general, the only shape limitation is the feasibility of removing the deposit from the electrode after deposition. In practice, complex geometries like femoral ball-heads and cup inserts require an appropriate design of the counter electrode in order to generate a constant electric field at the surface of the deposition electrode. The design of the most suitable counter electrodes needs to be supported by electrical field calculations using finite element analysis (section 10.6.2).

For the EPD of complexly shaped components, a relatively high suspension stability is necessary, since the powder particles should not immediately sediment. Because the particles require an electric charge for electrophoresis, electrostatic stabilization is essential. In this work, most of the work was carried out with a stable suspension based on methyl ethyl ketone with n-butylamine and nitrocellulose [Anné et al., 2006b] although it is also possible to work with suspensions based on ethanol [Popa et al., 2005].

10.5 EPD OF FGM DISCS

10.5.1 Introduction

In order to experimentally verify the maximum allowable tensile stress level in the core to prevent spontaneous transformation of the tetragonal ZrO_2 phase and

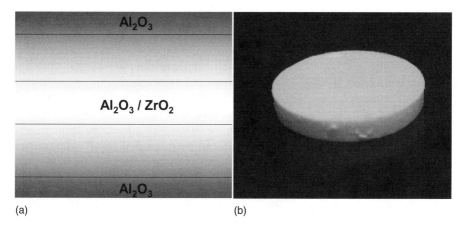

Figure 10.5. Schematic illustration of the desired Al₂O₃/FGM/ZrO₂-Al₂O₃/FGM/Al₂O₃ profile (a) and a sintered FGM disc made by EPD (b). [Anné, 2005a].

the achievable compressive stresses at the surface of the FGM cup inserts and ball-heads, FGM discs are processed by EPD and analyzed. The gradient profiles are comparable to those to be generated in the hip-prosthesis components. The plates are also used for the densification studies and for property assessment so that the effects of the gradient on the overall strength and wear resistance can be determined. Discs with a thickness >5 mm and a diameter >36 mm after sintering are processed. The sintering and microstructural evaluation of the Al_2O_3/ZrO_2 FGM components is discussed in section 10.6.

Flat discs with a symmetric or semi-symmetric gradient profile, going from a pure Al_2O_3 surface layer to a homogeneous ZrO_2/Al_2O_3 composite core with intermediate graded zones are made by means of EPD (Figure 10.5).

The procedure for depositing functionally graded discs by EPD, involves:

1. The development of a suitable suspension for EPD, as discussed above.
2. The design and construction of a cell with the proper dimensions.
3. The development of a mathematical model to predict the composition profile of the FGM discs.
4. The processing of a green FGM disc, according to the mathematical model.
5. Drying of FGM discs.
6. Sintering.

10.5.2 Mathematical Model to Predict the Composition Profile of FGM Discs

Vandeperre [Vandeperre et al., 2000] developed a kinetic model to predict the current and deposition kinetics in EPD. Put et al. further developed this model to predict the composition profile in a one sided gradient as well as for semi-symmetrically graded plate-shaped components [Put et al., 2003]. The prediction of the concentration profiles are based on the description of the deposition yield by means of the effective charge of the suspended powder particles, Q_{eff}, the electrophoretic mobility, μ, and the specific conductivity of the solvent, σ_{liq}. Although this model predicts the yield during EPD well, the parameters Q_{eff}, σ_{liq} and μ are fitted parameters rather than real physical values.

If different powders i are present in the suspension, the deposition yield of each powder on the deposition electrode can be described by [Biesheuvel and Verweij, 1999]:

$$\frac{dy_i}{dt} = E S f_i \mu_i c_i \frac{\phi_{di}}{\phi_{di} - \phi_{si}} \tag{10.1}$$

with $\dfrac{dy_i}{dt}$, the deposition rate of powder i on the electrode (g/s)

E, the electric field strength (V/m)

μ_i, the electrophoretic mobility of powder i (m^2/V.s)

c_i, the concentration i of powder i in suspension (g/cm^3)

f_i, factor for powder i which takes in account that not all powder brought to the electrode is incorporated in the deposit

S, the surface area of the deposition electrode (m^2)

ϕ_{di} concentration (vol. %) of the powder in the deposit

ϕ_{si} concentration (vol. %) of the powder in the suspension

The concentration $c_{i,t}$ of powder i at time t is a function of the powder mass in the suspension and the suspension volume at $(t-1)$ and the change in mass and volume during Δt:

$$c_{i,t} = \frac{M_{i,t-1} + \Delta M_{i,\Delta t} - \int_{t-1}^{t} \frac{dy_i}{dt} dt}{V_{t-1} + \Delta V_{\Delta t}} \tag{10.2}$$

With $M_{i,t-1}$ the mass of powder i in suspension at time $(t-1)$ (g)

$\Delta M_{i,\Delta t}$ the change in mass of powder i by adding or removing suspensions between $(t-1)$ and t (g)

V_{t-1} the total volume suspension at time $(t-1)$ (cm^3)

$\Delta V_{\Delta t}$ change in suspension volume between $(t-1)$ and t (s)

The total amount of powder deposited (ΔY_{tot}) during Δt is given by:

$$\Delta Y_{tot} = \sum_i \int_{t-1}^{t} \frac{dy_i}{dt} dt \tag{10.3}$$

If the powder i is a mixture of different components X_j, the wt% of component X_j in the deposited layer Δd is given by:

$$X_j(wt\%) = \frac{1}{\Delta Y_{tot}} \sum_i X_{i,j} \int_{t-1}^{t} \frac{dy_i}{dt} dt_i \qquad (10.4)$$

with $X_{i,j}$ wt% of component j in powder i.

The thickness increase of the deposited layer Δd during Δt is given by:

$$\Delta d = \frac{\Delta Y_{tot}}{\rho} \qquad (10.5)$$

With ρ the green density as a function of the local composition if the composition as a function of green thickness is desired or with ρ the theoretical density for the local composition if the composition as a function of sintered thickness is wanted.

At time t, the thickness d of the disc is:

$$d(t) = \int_0^t \Delta d \, dt \qquad (10.6)$$

By means of equations 10.1 through 10.6, the concentration profile in an FGM disc can be predicted provided that the factor $f_i\mu_i$ is determined for the individual powder particles by experiments on the pure powder i [Anné, 2005b]. This is proven in the next paragraph for symmetrical Al_2O_3/Y-ZrO_2 FGM discs.

10.5.3   Controlled Processing of FGM Discs

The starting materials are 3 mol% Y_2O_3 co-precipitated ZrO_2 powder (Daiichi HSY-3U, 3 mol% Y_2O_3 co-precipitated) and α-Al_2O_3 powder (Baikowski grade SM8). A MEK (Acros, 99%) with 10 vol.% n-butylamine (99.5%, Acros) and 1 wt% nitrocellulose (Aldrich, 435058-250 g) solution is used as suspension medium.

The set-up for the graded plates, schematically presented in Figure 10.4, is composed of a suspension flow-through deposition cell, a suspension circulation system driven by pump one, a mixing cell where two suspensions are mixed by a magnetic stirrer, and a suspension supply system to add a second suspension to the circulating suspension in the mixing cell at a controlled rate. The distance between the flat disc shaped electrodes ($\phi = 43$ mm) is 35 mm.

For the deposition of a semi-symmetrical disc, a 175 ml starting suspension I containing 70 g/l Al_2O_3 is pumped through the deposition cell by peristaltic pump one at a rate of 2.5 ml/s. After 100 s of deposition, 125 ml of suspension II with 135 g/l of an Al_2O_3/ZrO_2 (70 vol. % Al_2O_3) mixture is added to the circulating suspension by pump two. After 570 s, the addition of suspension II is completed. During the subsequent step, the suspension is circulated for 630 sec without any further additions. Afterwards, 140 ml of suspension III with 150 g/l Al_2O_3 is added

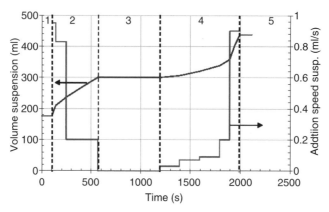

Figure 10.6. The amount of circulating suspension (ml) and the addition rate (ml/s) of suspension II and III as a function of time during EPD of a graded Al_2O_3/ZrO_2 disc. [Anné, 2005a].

for 800 sec. In the last step, the remaining suspension is circulated for 120 sec. During all the described steps, EPD is continued in the deposition cell. The addition speed of suspension II and III by pump two is varied in such a way that the wanted concentration profile was obtained in both gradient zones. The addition speed of suspension II and III, which is computer-controlled, and the amount of circulating suspension as a function of time is given in Figure 10.6.

After EPD, the powder deposits are removed and dried. After at least one day of drying in air, the green bodies were sintered for one hour at 1550 °C in air. Sintered cross-sectioned discs are ground, polished and thermally etched for 30 minutes in air at 1350 °C for microstructural analysis. The compositional change is measured on polished cross-sectioned samples using semi-quantitative electron probe micro-analysis (JEOL Superprobe 733).

The measured composition profile on a sintered cross-sectioned FGM plate, is presented in Figure 10.7, together with the predicted composition profile according to the model of section 10.5.2, revealing an excellent correlation between the experimentally measured and the predicted profile.

The FGM profile however is not perfectly symmetrical since only 91 vol. % Al_2O_3 is deposited in the final step of EPD. Reaching 100 vol. % Al_2O_3 is possible at this end, but the circulating suspensions needs to be changed and this complicates the process. Only limited bending is observed after sintering of the disc.

Based on stress calculations, the FGM profile given in Figure 10.7, results in the highest compressive stresses in the outer surface layer of the FGM discs and the lowest tensile stresses in the core of the disc. The thermally-etched microstructures at different locations in the cross-sectioned FGM plate are shown in Figure 10.8.

The ZrO_2 (white) and Al_2O_3 (grey) phases can be clearly differentiated in the microstructure. The ZrO_2 phase is well dispersed in the Al_2O_3 matrix in the gradient parts and the core of the FGM. No agglomerates and defects were observed in the sintered FGM disc. The Al_2O_3 grain growth limiting effect of the presence of the ZrO_2 phase is clearly illustrated by comparing the alumina grain size in the homogeneous pure alumina outer layer with all other regions in the FGM.

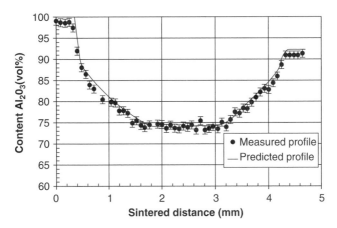

Figure 10.7. Measured and predicted FGM profile of Al_2O_3/ZrO_2 FGM disc. [Anné, 2005a].

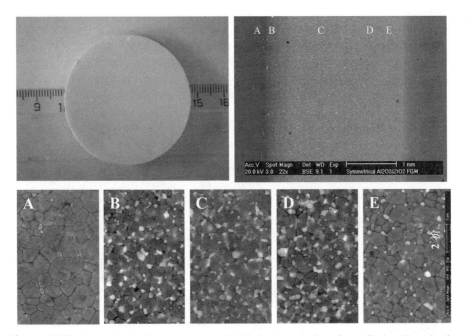

Figure 10.8. General overview and some detailed micrographs of specific locations in the FGM disc. [Anné, 2005a].

10.5.4 Properties of FGM Discs

One of the main advantages of FGM materials is the influence of residual stresses on the properties of the component. A correct design of a composition gradient can generate compressive stresses at those places that are loaded under tensile stress during operation. In this way, the strength of FGM materials can be higher than that of the homogeneous material.

To study the FGM effect on the strength, biaxial strength measurements are performed on homogenous and Al_2O_3/ZrO_2 FGM discs with a diameter of 35 mm after sintering one hour at 1550 °C and hot isostatic pressing (20 minutes at 1390 °C at 140 MPa Ar pressure) to ensure full density. The composition profile is given in Figure 10.7. Hard machining is performed to obtain plan-parallel surfaces; 0.5 mm is removed from the pure Al_2O_3 surface, which resulted in a compressive stress of 170 ± 30 MPa on this surface. A biaxial (ring-on-ring) test is used according ISO 6474. Whereas an average strength of 288 MPa is reached with a Weibull modulus of $m = 9$ for the pure Al_2O_3 disc, the strength of the ground Al_2O_3/ZrO_2 FGM discs is much higher. A mean strength of 513 MPa was reached with a Weibull modulus of $m = 12$ (Figure 10.9.)

The beneficial effect of the compressive stresses in functionally graded alumina–zirconia composites on their wear and friction behavior during sliding in water is shown in Figure 10.10. The FGM discs in this study were prepared by sequential slip casting [Novak and Beranič, 2005]. The results, which are compared to results from homogeneous alumina, show that with increasing residual compressive stresses in the samples of functionally graded material (FGM) the wear is strongly reduced. As a consequence of reduced crack formation and debris detachment from the surface (due to increased residual compressive stress) the tribochemical layer became thinner, with fewer topographical irregularities at the surface. This increases the role of the tribochemical actions compared to the mechanical wear, which beneficially affects the tribological performance in water [Novak et al., 2007].

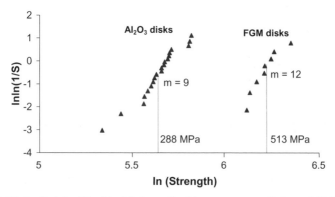

Figure 10.9. Weibull plot of the biaxial strength of homogeneous Al_2O_3 and Al_2O_3/ZrO_2 FGM discs [Anné, 2005a]; S is the probability of survival.

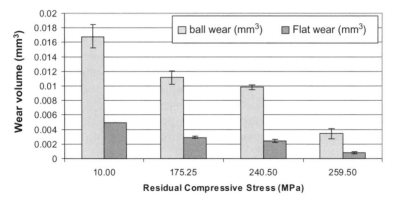

ball wear (mm³) ■ Flat wear (mm³)

Figure 10.10. Ball on flat wear data: alumina ball on alumina flat showing the clearly improved wear resistance due to compressive stresses in the surface layer of the flat. Residual stresses in flat measured by XRD.

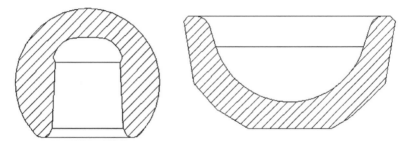

Figure 10.11 Schematic cross-sections of a ball-head with a diameter of 28 mm and a corresponding acetabular cup insert. [Anné, 2005a].

10.6 BALL-HEADS AND CUP INSERTS MADE BY EPD

10.6.1 Introduction

During EPD, the deposit takes the shape imposed by the deposition electrode. For processing complex shapes, the only shape limitation is the feasibility to remove the deposit from the electrode after deposition. The deposition electrode has therefore the shape of the outer surface of the acetabular cup insert and of the ball-head (Figure 10.11) and consists for the latter of an upper and lower part, allowing removal of the EPD deposit. Complex geometries like femoral ball-heads and cup inserts require appropriate design of the counter electrode in order to generate a constant electric field at the surface of the deposition electrode. The design of the most suitable counter electrodes needs, therefore, to be supported by electric field calculations using finite element analysis and is discussed in the next section 10.6.2.

10.6.2 E-Field Calculations for Electrode Design

Since the electric field drives the transport and deposition of powder particles, a uniform electric field is necessary at the deposition electrode in order to obtain a deposit that follows the contours of the electrode. A non-uniform electrical field will make electrophoretic deposition uncontrollable because a linear relation exists between the deposition rate and the local electric field strength at the electrode for MEK with n-butylamine based suspensions (see Equation 10.1).

For the electric field calculation, Poisson's equation in a conductive medium is used:

$$\lambda \nabla^2 U = 0 \tag{10.7}$$

With λ, the specific resistance (Ωm) of the medium and U, the electrical potential (V). The material properties are given in Table 10.3.

A voltage of 100V is applied between the electrodes. The resistance of the deposit is thought to be the same as for the suspension as was shown in [Anné et al., 2006c] for methyl ethyl keton with n-butylamine. To calculate the electric field distribution inside the EPD cell, finite element analysis is performed using ANSYS 7. An element type for 2-D solids with thermal and electrical conductive capability (PLANE67) is chosen. This element has four nodes with two degrees of freedom, temperature and voltage, at each node.

Electric field calculations are shown here for the counter-electrodes of the acetabular cup insert. Two results in the optimization step are shown in Figure 10.12 for spherical counter-electrodes with different diameter and position in the cell. A perfect uniform electrical field at the deposition electrode is not possible due to the specific shape of the outer surface of the acetabular cup insert. To solve this problem of non-uniform electrical field, an insulating ball-shaped PTFE cap is placed between the deposition electrode and the spherical counter-electrode. In this (rotating) cap, small holes are made to conduct the current. The size of the holes is determined by the local E-field strength to allow uniform deposition (Figure 10.13).

10.6.3 Shaping of Homogeneous and FGM Acetabular Cup Inserts

Rigid positioning devices are needed so that the electrodes can be centered and positioned very accurately with respect to each other in order to maintain a

TABLE 10.3. Resistance of the Materials Used in the Electric Field Calculations

Material	Resistance (Ωm)	Source
Stainless steel	0.3	PolyTechnisch zakboekje, Koninklijke PBNA nv., The Netherlands, 1998
Teflon	1.10^{20}	idem
MEK	7.10^5	From our own measurements

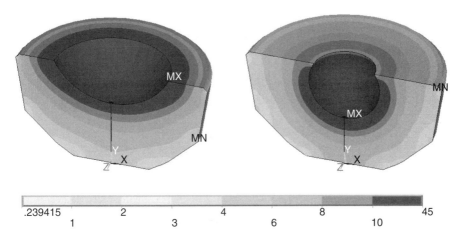

Figure 10.12. E-field strength calculation, performed in ANSYS 5.7, of the electrodes to process the cup insert. [Anné, 2005a].

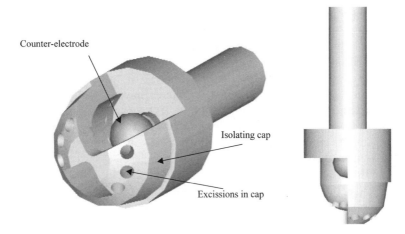

Figure 10.13. Counter-electrode with insulating cap in which well-defined holes are made for EPD of acetabular cup inserts. [Anné, 2005a].

uniform electrical field. Therefore, automatic rigid positioning devices were designed and constructed to prepare ball-heads and acetabular cup inserts.

The EPD process was fully automated. The displacement of the counter-electrode, the voltage, and the speed of the pumps can be programmed as a function of time. Additionally, the current and suspension conductivity is logged during the EPD process.

Since the procedures for the production of ball-heads has been described elsewhere [Anné et al., 2006d], the procedures for acetabular cup inserts are described here in some detail. The acetabular cups are deposited on an electrode that has the shape of the outer surface of the cup insert. The counter electrode has the shape of a ball and is positioned in the centre of the deposition electrode.

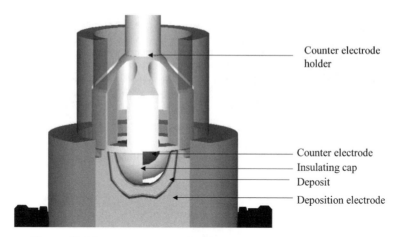

Counter electrode
holder

Counter electrode
Insulating cap
Deposit
Deposition electrode

Figure 10.14. Electrode set-up for EPD of cup inserts. [Anné, 2005a].

To prevent irregular deposition at the counter electrode, an insulating PTFE cap is placed (Figure 10.14) in-between the deposit and the counter-electrode. In this insulating cap, small excisions are made to conduct the current in order to maintain the E-field, as already explained in section 10.6.2. During EPD, this insulating cap is rotated.

For the EPD of the cup inserts, a sequence of three counter-electrodes is used (Figure 10.15). These counter-electrodes have the shape of a sphere (diameter = 18 mm) with a different insulating PTFE cap. The procedure to EPD FGM cup inserts is similar to that for the ball-heads. Homogeneous as well as FGM cup inserts could be successfully produced with a good surface finish, as shown in Figure 10.16.

For FGM acetabular cup inserts, a 135 ml starting suspension I, containing 222 g/l Al_2O_3, is pumped through the deposition cell (see Figure 10.4) by a peristaltic pump one at a rate of two ml/s. The counter-electrode is a ball-shaped electrode with a large insulating cap, positioned in the middle of the cell (step one of Figure 10.15). After $300s$ of deposition at 120 V, 90 ml of suspension II with 222 g/l of an Al_2O_3/ZrO_2 (45 vol. % Al_2O_3) mixture is added to the circulating suspension by pump two (Figure 10.4) at a constant speed during $340s$, creating a gradient in the deposit composition (step two of Figure 10.15). Subsequently, the suspension is circulated for $1800s$ without any further additions (step three of Figure 10.15). Afterwards, 100 ml of the circulating suspension is removed and the insulating cap is replaced with a smaller insulating cap II. 65 ml of suspension III with 230 g/l Al_2O_3 was added at a constant speed for $350s$ to the circulating suspension (step four of Figure 10.15). In the final step (step five of Figure 10.15), the counter-electrode is replaced with a smaller insulating cap III and the whole suspension is replaced with 50 ml of suspension IV with a solids loading of 200 g/l Al_2O_3 and EPD is continued for $500s$ to form the pure outside alumina layer.

Drying is performed in air without crack formation due to the more homogeneous thickness of the cup insert compared to the ball-heads. For the latter, drying

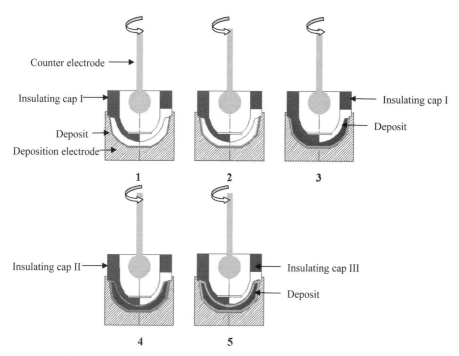

Figure 10.15. Sequence of three different electrode insulation caps for the processing of a FGM cup insert in five steps. Step 1: deposition of the outer pure alumina layer. Step 2: deposition of gradient layer. Step 3: deposition of inner Al_2O_3/ZrO_2 composite up to the insulating cap. Step 4: insulating cap is changed and the second gradient layer is deposited up to the insulating cap. Step 5: insulating cap is changed and a pure alumina layer is deposited up to the insulating cap. [Anné, 2005a].

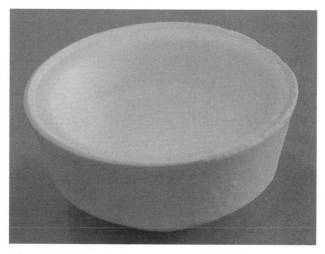

Figure 10.16. FGM cup insert, made by EPD. [Anné, 2005a].

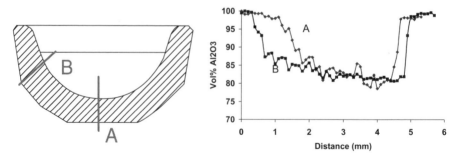

Figure 10.17. Schematic of a cup insert with indicated measured composition profile positions. [Anné, 2005a].

proved to be a severe problem. This is attributed to the strongly variable cross-section (thickness) of the part. The solution for the drying problem of the ball-heads was finally found by applying a colloidal isopressing technique. In this developed drying technique, the solvent is pressed out of the green body under isostatic pressure. For this purpose, the wet ball-head is packed in a plastic bag and placed in a cold isostatic press. To absorb the solvent, a dry plaster mould is inserted in the inner hole of the ball-head. Alternatively, solvent absorbing paper is inserted in the plastic bag around the ball-head. Under the influence of pressure (five MPa), a small part of the solvent, contained in the ball-head, is pressed into the plaster thereby reducing the residual amount of solvent in the ball-head below the critical level. The isostatic pressure prevents crack formation in the deposit during drying, allows a rapid solvent removal and increases the green strength. This drying technique is based on a colloidal forming technique, developed by Yu et al. [Yu et al., 2001].

Quantitative EPMA analyses are performed on polished cross-sections of sintered FGM cups (Figure 10.17). The measurements are performed from the outer to the inner surface of the cup insert. The different positions for profile measurements are schematically presented in Figure 10.17. These positions are chosen because of the wider FGM profile at position A and the sharpest profile at position B.

10.7 SINTERING AND MICROSTRUCTURAL EVALUATION

10.7.1 Introduction

The green EPD powder compacts need to be densified after drying. The powder compacts are sintered by means of pressureless sintering in air using conventional heating. Al_2O_3 and ZrO_2 and their composites are densified by means of solid state sintering. All densification is achieved through changes in particle shape, without particle rearrangement or the presence of liquid. Solid state diffusion is the predominant mass transport. The basic driving force for sintering is a decrease in the total free energy of powder compacts. The first step towards the goal of reduced energy is pores to be eliminated from the system because the specific surface energy of pores is larger than the grain boundary energy. Grain growth is driven by surface energy and the process of grain boundary elimination often begins before the process of pore elimination is completed. Discontinuous grain growth, that is, a few grains growing at a very large rate at the expense of all other grains, should be avoided since as a result pores are entrapped within the grains and such pores can not be eliminated. An optimal sinter cycle has to be applied to reach fully dense ceramics and to ensure that the grain size of the Al_2O_3 remains below two μm to obtain high strength [Willmann, 1996; ISO 6474].

Densification of graded materials is a challenge because cracks and crack-like defects are often observed in ceramic multi-layers as a result of mismatch stresses [Cheng and Raj, 1989; Hillman et al., 1996; Cai et al., 1997a; Cai et al., 1997b; Cai et al., 1998]. These mismatch stresses originate from the difference in sintering rate (densification kinetics) and thermal expansion coefficients [Hillman et al., 1996].

In the FGM components, similar defects as reported in literature [Cheng and Raj, 1989; Hillman et al., 1996; Cai et al., 1997a; Cai et al., 1997b; Cai et al., 1998] were detected when a too-large zirconia concentration difference between the surface layer and core was present. The critical composition in the core of FGM Al_2O_3/ZrO_2 discs was investigated to prevent defects during the sintering cycle.

10.7.2 Sintering Kinetics of Al_2O_3, ZrO_2 and Their Composites

The addition of ZrO_2 to Al_2O_3 has an effect on the densification behavior and the grain size development of the matrix. To study the differences on the densification behavior, the shrinkage of Al_2O_3, ZrO_2 and Al_2O_3/ZrO_2 (80 vol. % Al_2O_3) dry pressed samples (cold isostatically pressed at 300 MPa) is recorded as a function of temperature by means of a high temperature dilatometer (Netsch 402C) in air at a heating rate of 3 °C/min.

The experimental densification curves are plotted in Figure 10.18, as a function of the sintering temperature. The densification of the pure ZrO_2 material starts at lower temperatures than for the two-phase and the Al_2O_3 material. Furthermore, the curve of the pure ZrO_2 reaches a plateau at temperatures above 1500 °C and the sintered material is approaching the theoretical density.

During the first stage, densification in the ZrO_2 material is faster than in the two-phase and Al_2O_3 material. In the intermediate stage, the gradient of the densification curve is steeper for the two-phase material than for pure Al_2O_3. The two-phase material densifies faster during this stage. At the end of the final stage, the total shrinkage is larger for the two-phase material than for pure Al_2O_3. The larger densification shrinkage of the pure ZrO_2 and Al_2O_3/ZrO_2 can be explained by the lower green density compared to the pure Al_2O_3.

The addition of ZrO_2 to the Al_2O_3 matrix does not only influence the densification behavior, but also the grain size of the Al_2O_3 matrix (Figure 10.19). The

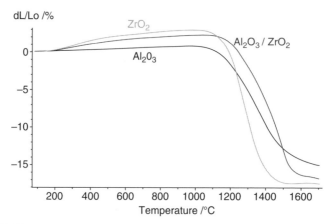

Figure 10.18. Dilatometer curves for Al_2O_3, ZrO_2 and their 80 vol. % Al_2O_3 composite.

ZrO_2 particles in the two-phase material are mainly located at the grain boundaries and at the grain boundary edges of the alumina grains. However, there are also some zirconia particles present that are embedded in relatively large alumina grains. These particles were initially located at grain boundaries and become intergranular by grain boundary migration of the Al_2O_3 phase. Figure 10.19 reveals that the average grain size of the alumina grains in the homogeneous Al_2O_3 material is larger than that of the two-phase material. In the latter, the grain growth in the alumina matrix is inhibited by the presence of the secondary ZrO_2 phase, due to pinning of the Al_2O_3 grain boundaries, enhancing grain boundary diffusion over grain boundary migration.

10.7.3   Optimization of Grain Size of Al_2O_3 Composites

Among the mechanical properties that change drastically with a reduction in grain size is the strength [Helbig, 2000]. The strength-grain size relationship for hot-pressed Al_2O_3 is given in Figure 10.20. It is clear that the strength is decreasing with increasing grain size and therefore, the grain size for the Al_2O_3 is desired to be smaller than $2\,\mu m$.

Temperature, soaking time, and heating rate influence densification and coarsening. The influence of soaking time and temperature is investigated on EPD powder compacts of Al_2O_3, ZrO_2 and a 50/50 (vol. %) Al_2O_3/ZrO_2 composite. The samples were sintered in air in the tube furnace of a TGA (Cahn TG-171) at three different temperatures (1450, 1550 and 1650°C) with three soaking times (one, 30 and 60 minutes). The specimens were heated at 20°C/min to 700°C and at 10°C/min to the sintering temperature. For sintering at 1650°C, heating between 1600 and 1650°C was done at 5°C/min. Cooling was performed at 20°C/min > 1000°C and 10°C/min < 1000°C. Afterwards, the samples were cross-sectioned, polished, and thermally etched for 30 minutes at 1350°C in air for SEM

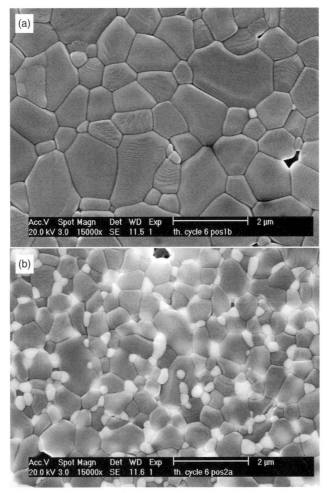

Figure 10.19. Microstructures of pure Al$_2$O$_3$ (a) and an Al$_2$O$_3$/ZrO$_2$ (80 vol. % Al$_2$O$_3$) composite sintered for one hour at 1500 °C. [Anné, 2005a].

investigation. On the resulting micrographs, image processing was performed to determine the grain size by the linear intercept method.

The grain size versus time and temperature for the sintered Al$_2$O$_3$ samples is given in Figure 10.21. At a sinter temperature of 1450 and 1550 °C, the average grain size hardly changes as a function of time and is 1.5 µm and 2.35 µm for 60 minutes soaking time, respectively. A sinter temperature of 1650 °C gives much larger grains (>5 µm, Figure 10.22) and severe coarsening was observed after one hour at 1650 °C (Figure 10.21). From the Al$_2$O$_3$ grain size point of view, a sinter cycle of one hour at 1550 °C was found to be the best, resulting in near full density of the ZrO$_2$-Al$_2$O$_3$ (50/50) composite (Figure 10.23).

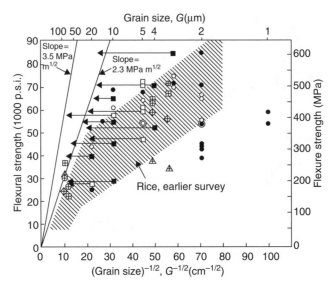

Figure 10.20. Strength-grain size relationship for alumina: circles indicate failure where homogeneous microstructures are involved, squares where exaggerated grains were present. Symbols with crosses represent specimens ground after hot pressing [Rice, 1997].

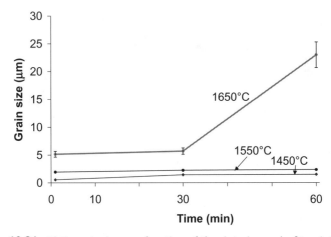

Figure 10.21. Al_2O_3 grain size as a function of the sintering cycle. [Anné, 2005a].

10.7.4   Observation of Processing Defects in FGM Materials

Al_2O_3/ZrO_2 FGM discs, made by EPD as described in section 10.5, are sintered for one hour at $1550\,°C$. The heating and cooling rate is $3\,°C/min$. After sintering, cross-sections are analyzed by scanning electron microscopy (SEM-FEG FEI XL-30) and the composition profiles are measured by means of EPMA.

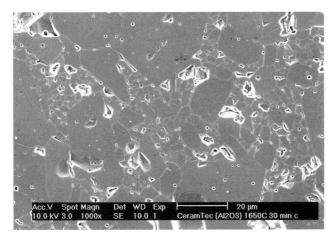

<u>Figure 10.22.</u> Microstructure of pure Al$_2$O$_3$ sintered for 30 minutes at 1650°C. [Anné, 2005a].

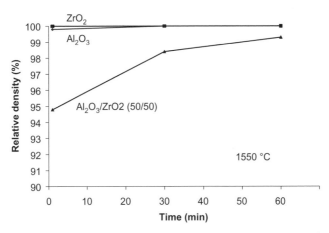

<u>Figure 10.23.</u> Evolution of the density of Y-ZrO$_2$, Al$_2$O$_3$ and 50/50 (vol. %) composite at 1550°C as a function of time. [Anné, 2005a].

Figure 10.24 gives an overview of the composition profiles of graded Al$_2$O$_3$/ZrO$_2$ discs, leading to transverse cracks after sintering (Figure 10.25). These cracks are not observed when the Al$_2$O$_3$ content in the core of the graded plate is ≥75 vol. %, indicating that a too large composition difference between surface layer and the core gives internal defects. There is no quantitative dependence found between the inter-crack distance and the composition profile. Mostly, the distance between two cracks is a few millimeters, but the number of cracks increases with the ZrO$_2$ content in the core of the plates.

Microstructural investigation reveals that these cracks are perpendicular to the surface (Figure 10.25) and are only present in the ZrO$_2$ rich core and not in

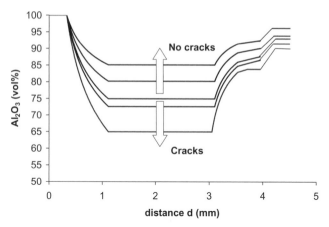

Figure 10.24. Concentration profiles of graded EPD Al_2O_3/ZrO_2 FGM discs. When the ZrO_2 concentration of the core exceeds 25 vol. %, transverse defects are observed. [Anné, 2005a].

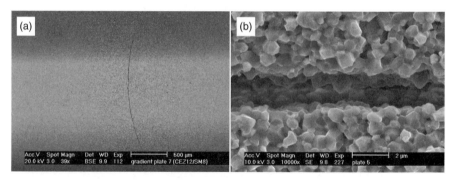

Figure 10.25. Typical transverse crack in a symmetrically graded plate with 50 vol. % Al_2O_3 in the core (a) and a detailed micrograph of a transverse crack surface. [Anné, 2005a].

the pure Al_2O_3 layer. The crack opening displacement of most cracks is smaller than 5 μm. From a micrograph of the crack surface (Figure 10.25b), it is clear that the crack surface is a clear fracture surface and not a sintered surface.

Hillman et al. [Hillman et al., 1996] observed similar defects in symmetrical laminates with Al_2O_3/ZrO_2 layers at the surface and a ZrO_2 central layer. They found the coexistence of two distinct classes of defects, that is, cracks with a large opening displacement (>30 μm) and cracks with a small opening displacement (<2 μm). It was suggested that defects originated from differential shrinkage during drying, and that the subsequent densification opened up the defects and produced cracks with a large opening. The surfaces of this type of crack have smooth round grains identical to that of a free surface of a densified body. Finer cracks are thought to be caused by the sintering process. Because the crack opening in Figure 10.25 is relatively small (<5 μm), the transverse cracks in the FGM discs can be assigned to the sintering cycle.

Cai et al. [Cai et al., 1997a; Cai et al., 1997b] discussed the embryonic stage of a sinter crack as observed in Figure 10.25. They found regions of low density and cavitational defects in $Al_2O_3/ZrO_2/Al_2O_3$ laminates. These defects are most susceptible to residual (tensile) stresses during cooling in the core, due to the higher CTE of zirconia. These regions of lower density (pores) must have formed as a result of the tensile stress that develops during the differential shrinkage during densification between the Al_2O_3 and the Al_2O_3/ZrO_2 layers. The pores then act as pre-existing flaws for the generation of thermal expansion mismatch cracks during cooling via linkage of the pores and cavitational defects.

Eliminating transverse cracks in literature is mostly done by decreasing the overall shrinkage of the composites. This is done in two different manners: decreasing the composition difference between the different layers [Hillman et al., 1996; Cai et al., 1997a], or adjusting the green density of the different layers [Novak, 2005] Another possibility is to decrease the cooling and heating rate during sintering [Cai et al., 1997a]. The mismatch stresses during the heating cycle are decreased by the viscous nature of the FGM material. The sintering mismatch stress is proportional to the mismatch sintering rate. Reduced cracking under slow cooling rate is probably due to the relaxation of residual stresses during the initial period of cooling. Cai et al. [Cai et al., 1997a] proposed, therefore, a cooling rate of $1\,°C/min$ at high temperature. A decreased cooling rate of $1\,°C/min$, however, did not remove the sinter defects in the authors' work. The cracks are also too large to remove by a hot isostatic pressing cycle.

Therefore, a minimum Al_2O_3 content of 75 vol. % in the homogeneous composite core of the FGM discs was considered as a critical design criterion to avoid the formation of transverse cracks.

10.8 CONCLUSIONS

Because the average life span of humans is drastically increasing and the need for spare parts begins at about 60 years of age, biomaterials for prosthesis components need to last for 20 years. The excellent performance of specially-designed bioceramics that have survived the harsh clinical body environment condition, represents one of the most remarkable accomplishments of ceramic research, development, production, and quality assurance during the past 25 years. Of special interest is the all-ceramic total hip joint replacement. Alumina and zirconia are mainly used for the bearing components. However, zirconia can undergo low temperature degradation in aqueous environment and alumina is brittle and has a limited strength. Further progress has been achieved by the development of zirconia-toughened aluminas (ZTA).

The very promising concept has been investigated in this work to combine the best properties of ZrO_2 and Al_2O_3 ceramics in a FGM, allowing to generate compressive stresses at the component surfaces, thus increasing the strength further.

A composition gradient in alumina and zirconia was engineered to obtain a pure alumina surface region and a homogeneous alumina/zirconia core with intermediate continuously graded regions allowing to generate thermal residual compressive stresses on the surface after sintering. It has been shown here that functionally graded Al_2O_3/ZrO_2 ball-heads and acetabular cup inserts can be processed by electrophoretic deposition (EPD). In order to experimentally verify the sintering behavior of complex FGM components, five millimeters thick Al_2O_3/ZrO_2 FGM discs were processed by EPD and analyzed. For this purpose a mathematical model to predict the composition profile was established. Defect-free Al_2O_3/ZrO_2 FGM discs with a diameter of more than 35 millimeters and a thickness of more than five millimeters were successfully produced.

A sequence of counter-electrodes was necessary to EPD complex shaped FGM components. The design of the counter-electrodes was supported by electrical field calculations to generate a constant electric field at the surface of the deposition electrode. To obtain deposits with a shape different from the deposition electrode, the deposit was allowed to grow up to the counter-electrode.

After deposition, the wet green ball-heads and acetabular cup inserts had to be removed from the electrode and dried. For the ball-shaped components, the drying step was very critical due to the inhomogeneous thickness of the component. For drying these components, a colloidal isopressing procedure was developed, whereby the solvent was pressed out of the green body under an isostatic pressure. In contrast, no such special procedure was needed for the acetabular cups, which have relatively uniform thickness.

After drying, the green EPD powder compacts were sintered by pressureless sintering in air. The sintering kinetics were studied and an optimal sinter cycle (one hour at $1550\,°C$) was found to ensure that the grain size of the Al_2O_3 grains remains below $2\,\mu m$. Al_2O_3/ZrO_2 FGM discs with pure Al_2O_3 at the surface, a homogeneous Al_2O_3/ZrO_2 core and graded interlayers contain internal defects when the zirconia content in the core exceeds 25 vol. %.

10.9 FUTURE PERSPECTIVES

Whereas the research summarized above has shown the feasibility of incorporating a functional gradient in hip joint components by EPD, further development of the process is necessary to implement it on an industrial scale, to further optimize the different steps in the processing in order to minimize processing defects, and to verify performance of the actual components in terms of load-bearing capability and wear resistance.

The commercial introduction of advanced alumina composites in hip prosthesis is presently ongoing. A zirconia toughened and platelet reinforced alumina is presently available from Ceramtec A.G. under the trade name BIOLOX delta [Merkert 2003]. This material is also a candidate for other prostheses such as knee prostheses where the material also sees a very high load. Its long term reliability has been documented. The functionally graded material concept could also be applied to these alumina composites by increasing internally the zirconia content in order to induce compressive stresses on the surface of the components.

With respect to the production technology for FGM material, electrophoretic deposition has the advantage that a specifically designed continuously changing composition gradient can be introduced into the component. However, electrophoretic deposition is mainly used for the application of coatings and is not yet implemented as a routine production route for bulk samples in the ceramic industry. An unpublished design study by a team of mechanical engineering and materials engineering students at K.U. Leuven indicated that it would be possible to produce the FGM ball-heads by EPD at a production cost of about five Euro. Sequential slip casting is an alternative technology that has some industrial base but one that will suffer from a rather low production rate. Other production techniques for FGMs remain to be investigated.

The FGM concept is also being investigated for other applications in biomaterials, where a gradual transition in the property of a material is necessary, rather than a sharply defined boundary: gradients in composition in order to prevent delamination of coatings; gradients in porosity and in bioactivity; graded scaffolds in tissue engineering; and others.

ACKNOWLEDGMENTS

Work supported by the GROWTH program of the Commission of the European Communities under project contract No. G5RD-CT2000-00354, the Fund for Scientific Research Flanders under project No. G.0180.02. and the Research Fund K. U. Leuven under project GOA/2008/07.

REFERENCES

Anné G, Vleugels J, Van der Biest O. 2006a. Functionally graded ceramics. In: Low IM, editor, Ceramic-matrix composites: Microstructure, properties and applications. 575–596. Cambridge, United Kingdom: Woodhead Publishing Limited. p. 575–596 (ISBN 1 85573 942 9 [ISBN-13: 978 1 85573 942 0]).

Anné G, Vanmeensel K, Neirinck B, Van der Biest O, Vleugels J. 2006b. Ketone-amine based suspensions for electrophoretic deposition of Al_2O_3 and ZrO_2. J. European Ceramic Society 26: 3531–3537.

Anné G, Vanmeensel K, Van der Biest O, Vleugels J. 2006c. Origin of the potential drop over the deposit during electrophoretic deposition. J. Amer. Ceram. Soc. 89 (3): 823–828.

Anné G, Vanmeensel K, Vleugels J, Van der Biest O. 2006d. "Electrophoretic deposition as a novel near net shaping technique for functionally graded biomaterials," Key Engineering Materials 314: 213–218.

Anné G. 2005a. "Electrophoretic deposition as a near net shaping technique for functionally graded biomaterials," Ph. D. Thesis, K.U. Leuven, Faculty of Engineering Sciences, ISBN 90-5682-633.

Anné G, Vanmeensel K, Vleugels J, Van der Biest O. 2005b. "A mathematical description of the kinetics of the electrophoretic deposition process for Al_2O_3 based suspensions," *Journal of the American Ceramic Society* 88: 2036–2039.

Belmonte M, Sanchez-Herencia AJ, Moreno R, Miranzo P, Moya JS, Tomsia AP. 1993. *In situ* formation of CA6 platelets in Al_2O_3 an Al_2O_3/ZrO_2 matrices. *J. de phys IV. Colloque C7.* Supplement au J. de Phys. III 3.

Biesheuvel PM, Verweij H. 1999. Theory of cast formation in electrophoretic deposition. *Journal of the American Ceramic Society* 82 (6): 1451–1455.

Black J. 1992. Biological Performance of Materials, 2nd ed. New York: Marcel Dekker.

Burger W. 1998. Umwandlungs- und platelet-verstärkte aluminiumoxidmatrixwerkstoffe. Teil 2. Keram. *Zeitschrift* 50: 18–22.

Cai PZ, Green DJ, Messing GL. 1997a. Constrained densification of alumina/zirconia hybrid laminates. 1. Experimental observations of processing defects. *Journal of the American Ceramic Society* 80 (8): 1929–1939.

Cai PZ, Green DJ, Messing GL. 1997b. Constrained densification of alumina/zirconia hybrid laminates. 2. Viscoelastic stress computation. *Journal of the American Ceramic Society* 80 (8): 1940–1948.

Cai PZ, Green DJ, Messing GL. 1998. Mechanical characterization of Al_2O_3/ZrO_2 hybrid laminates. *Journal of the European Ceramic Society* 18 (14): 2025–2034.

Cales B, Stefani Y, Lilley E. 1994. Long term *in vivo* and *in vitro* aging of a zirconia ceramic used in orthopaedy. *J. Biomed. Mater. Res.* 28: 619–624.

CeramTec. 2002. *Biolox©Forte—The gold standard in ceramics.* Brochure of the company CeramTec.

Cheng TN, Raj R. 1989. Flaw generation during constrained sintering of metal-ceramic and metal glass multilayer films. *Journal of the American Ceramic Society* 72 (9): 1649–1655.

Christel P, Meunier A, Dorlot JM, Crolet JM, Witvoet J, Sedel L, Boutin P. 1988. Biomechanical compatibility and design of ceramic implants for orthopaedic surgery. *Ann NY Acad. Sci.* 523: 234–256.

Clarke IC, Manaka M, Green DD, Williams P, Pezzotti G, Kim YH, Ries M, Sugano N, Sedel L, Delauney C, Ben Nissan B, Donaldson T, Gustafson GA. 2003. Current status of zirconia used in total hip implants. *The Journal of Bone and Joint Surgery* 85-A (4): 73–84.

Cordingley R, Kohan L, Bebissan B, Pezzotti G. 2003. Alumina and zirconia bioceramics in orthopaedic applications. *Journal of the Australasian Ceramic Society* 39 (1): 20–28.

Currey JD. 1984. The mechanical adaptations of bones. Princeton University Press.

De Aza AH, Chevalier J, Fantozzi G, Schehl M, Torrecillas R. 2002. Crack growth resistance of alumina, zirconia and zirconia toughened alumina ceramics for joint prostheses. *Biomaterials* 23: 937–945.

Gasik MM, Zhang B, Van der Biest O, Vleugels J, Anné G, Put S. 2003. Design and fabrication of symmetric FGM plates. *Materials Science Forum* 423–425: 23–28.

Gonzalez P, Serra J, Liste S, Chiussi S, Leon B, Perez-Amor M, Martinez-Fernandez J, De Arellano-Lopez AR, Varela-Feria FM. 2003. New biomorphic SiC ceramics coated with bioactive glass for biomedical applications. *Biomaterials* 24: 4827–4832.

Green DJ, Hannink RHJ, Swain MV. 1989. Transformation toughening of ceramics. Boca Raton, FL: CRC Press.

Hannink RH, Kelly PM, Muddle BC. 2000. Transformation toughening in zirconia-containing ceramics. *Journal of the American Ceramic Society* 83 (3): 461–487.

Hauert R. 2003. A review of modified DLC coatings for biological applications. *Diamond and Related Materials* 12 (3–7): 583–589.

Helbig J. 2000. Wet processing of nanosized ceramic particles. Dissertation for the degree of Doctor of Technical Science, Zürich.

Hench LL, Ethridge EC. 1982. Biomaterials, An Interfacial Approach. New York: Academic Press.

Hillman C, Suo ZG, Lange FF. 1996. Cracking of laminates subjected to biaxial tensile stresses. *Journal of the American Ceramic Society* 79 (8): 2127–2133.

ISO 6474. 1994. Implants for surgery—Ceramic materials based on high purity alumina. 1994.

Katti K. 2004. Biomaterials in total joint replacement. *Colloids and Surfaces B: Bio-interfaces.* 39: 133–142.

Kingery WD, Bowen HK, Uhlmann DR. 1976. Introduction to Ceramics. New York: John Wiley & Sons.

Konsztztowicz KJ, Langlois R. 1996. Effects of heteroflocculation of powders on mechanical properties of zirconia-alumina composites. *J. Mater. Sci.* 31: 1633–1641.

Kue R, Sohrabi A, Nagle D, Frondoza C, Hungerford D. 1999. Enhanced proliferation and osteocalcin production by human osteoblast-like MG63 cells on silicon nitride ceramic discs. *Biomaterials* 20: 1195–1201.

Merkert P. 2003. Next Generation Ceramic Bearings, Proceedings 8th International CeramTec Symposium, Stuttgart. See also the Ceramtec website.

Neumann A, Unkel C, Werry C, Herborn C, Maier H, Ragoß C, Jahnke K. 2006. Prototype of a silicon nitride ceramic-based miniplate osteofixation system for the midface, *Otolaryngology–Head and Neck Surgery* 134: 923–930.

Novak S, Beranič S. 2005. Densification of step graded Al_2O_3-ZrO_2 composites. *Materials Science Forum* 492–493: 207–212.

Novak S, Kalin M, Lukas P, Anne G, Vleugels J, Van Der Biest O. 2007. The effect of residual stresses in functionally graded alumina–ZTA composites on their wear and friction behaviour. *Journal of the European Ceramic Society* 27 (1): 151–156.

Piconi C, Maccauro G. 1999. Review: Zirconia as a ceramic biomaterial. *Biomaterials* 20: 1–25.

Piconi C, Maccauro G, Muratori F. 2004. Ceramic Coatings in Metal-PE Joints: Where Are We Now? Proceedings 9th International CeramTec Symposium, Stuttgart. See also the Ceramtec website.

Piscanec S, Ciacchi LC, Vesselli E, Comelli G, Sbaizero O, Meriani S, De Vita A. 2004. Bio-activity of TiN-coated implants. *Acta Materiala* 52: 1237–1245.

Popa AM, Vleugels J, Van der Biest O. 2005. Suspension development for colloidal shaping of Al_2O_3-ZrO_2 FGM's. *Materials Science Forum* 492–493: 777–782.

Put S, Vleugels J, Van der Biest O. 2003. "Gradient profile prediction in functionally graded materials processed by electrophoretic deposition," *Acta Materialia* 51 (20): 6303–6317.

Rack R, Pfaff HG. 2000. A new ceramic material for orthopaedics. Proceedings 5th International CeramTec Symposium, Stuttgart. Ed. G. Willmann, K. Zweymüller p. 141–145.

Rack R, Pfaff HG. 2001. Long-term Performance of the Alumina Matrix Composite Biolox delta, Proceedings 6th International CeramTec Symposium, Stuttgart. Ed. G. Willmann, K. Zweymüller p. 103–108.

Rice RW. 1997. Review Ceramic tensile strength-grain size relations: grain sizes, slopes, and branch intersections. *J. Materials Science* 32: 1673–1692.

Rühle M, Evans AG, McMeeking RM, Charalambides PG, Hutchinson JW. 1987. Microcrack toughening in alumina/zirconia. *Acta Metall.* 35 (11): 2701–2710.

Sato T, Ohtaki S, Endo T, Shimada M. 1985. Transformation of yttria-doped tetragonal ZrO_2 polycrystals by annealing under controlled humidity conditions. *Journal of the American Ceramic Society* 68 (12): C320–C322.

Schehl M, Diaz LA, Torrecillas R. 2002. Alumina nanocomposites from powder-alkoxide mixtures. *Acta Materiala* 50 (5): 1125–1139.

Sun L, Berndt CC, Gross KA, Kucuk A. 2001. Review: Material Fundamentals and Clinical Performance of Plasma Sprayed Hydroxyapatite Coatings. *J. Biomedical Materials Research* 58 (5): 570–592.

Thamaraiselvi TV, Rajeswari S. 2004. Biological Evaluation of Bioceramic Materials—A Review Trends. *Biomaterials & Artificial Organs* 18 (1): 9–17.

Toschi F, Melandri C, Pinasco P, Roncari E, Guicciardi S, de Portu G. 2003. Influence of residual stresses on the wear behaviour of alumina/alumina-zirconia laminates. *J. Am. Ceram. Soc.* 86: 1547–1553.

Van der Biest O, Vandeperre LJ. 1999. Electrophoretic deposition of materials. *Annual Review of Materials Science* 29: 327–352.

Vandeperre L, Put S, Van Der Biest O. 2000. Constant current and constant voltage-electrophoretic deposition of alumina, Ceramic Transactions: in Innovative Processing and Synthesis of Ceramics, Glasses, and Composites IV, vol. 115, ed Narottam Bansal, J.P. Singh.

Willmann G. 1994. Development in medical-grade alumina during the past two decades. *Journal of Materials Processing Technology* 56 (1–4): 168–176.

Willmann G. 1996. Development in medical-grade alumina during the past two decades. *Journal of Materials Processing Technology* 56: 168–176.

Yu BC, Lange FF. 2001. Colloidal isopressing: A new shape-forming method. *Advanced Materials* 13 (4): 276–280.

11

MEDICAL DEVICES BASED ON BIOINSPIRED CERAMICS

Pío González[1], Julián Martínez-Fernández[2],
Antonio R. de Arellano-López[2], and Mrityunjay Singh[3]

[1]*Departamento de Física Aplicada, ETSII, University of Vigo, Campus
Lagoas-Marcosende, 36310 Vigo, Spain*
[2]*Departamento de Física de la Materia Condensada-ICMSE, University of
Seville, Av. Reina Mercedes, Seville, Spain*
[3]*Ohio Aerospace Institute, Ceramics Branch, NASA Glenn Research Center,
Cleveland, Ohio*

Contents

11.1 Overview	358
11.2 Introduction	359
11.3 Bioinspired SiC Based Ceramics	360
11.3.1 Processing	360
11.3.2 Microstructure, Phase and Element Distribution	365
11.3.3 Reaction-Formation Mechanisms	370
11.3.4 Mechanical Properties	374
11.3.5 Optimization of Mechanical Properties by the Biomimetic Structure	381

Advanced Biomaterials: Fundamentals, Processing, and Applications, Edited by Bikramjit Basu,
Dhirendra S. Katti, and Ashok Kumar
Copyright © 2009 The American Ceramic Society

11.4 Bioinspired Ceramics Coated with Bioactive Materials   384
    11.4.1 Hydroxyapatite and Substituted Apatites   385
    11.4.2 Bioactive Glasses   386
    11.4.3 Coating Deposition Techniques   387
    11.4.4 Physico-Chemical Properties of the Hydroxyapatite and
           Substituted Apatite Coatings   389
    11.4.5 Physico-Chemical Properties of the Bioactive
           Glass Coatings   392
11.5 Biocompatibility Studies for Medical Applications   396
    11.5.1 *In Vitro* Cytotoxicity Test   396
    11.5.2 *In Vitro* Cell Attachment and Proliferation Tests   398
    11.5.3 *In Vivo* Biocompatibility Studies   400
11.6 Conclusions   401
    Acknowledgments   403
    References   403

11.1 OVERVIEW

Today biomedical devices are essential for improving human health and quality of life. Now that biomaterials have been optimized with the aim to minimise rejection by the host organism, they have entered a new stage in which they can be designed with bioactive properties, exchanging stimuli with the surrounding tissue and inducing specific cellular reactions. Man-made material solutions should now take inspiration from the most complex naturally organised chemical and biological structures, taking advantage of the knowledge that nature has been optimizing for over millions of years.

This chapter introduces the development of innovative bioinspired materials, based on silicon carbide ceramics coated with bioactive materials, as new biomedical devices. The bioinspired silicon carbide is fabricated via the pyrolysis and infiltration of natural wood-derived preforms; further, the technological process is completed with the deposition of a bioactive coating by laser techniques. The result is a new generation of light and high-strength ceramic products that mimic the natural structure of the bone tissues, incorporating the unique property of interconnected porosity, which allows the internal growth of tissue and favours angiogenesis. To further improve the fixation and osteointegration performance, the bioinspired ceramics are coated with a bioactive layer of hydroxyapatite, substituted apatites or silica-based glasses. Both material properties and deposition methods are reported.

In vitro biocompatibility studies demonstrate that the biological response of this ceramic product is similar to titanium controls, and *in vivo* implantation experiments show how it gets colonized by the hosting bone tissue due to its unique interconnected hierarchic porosity. The excellent biocompatibility of these innovative bioinspired materials reported here enters a new stage of very promising light, porous, and metal-free devices for medical applications.

11.2   INTRODUCTION

In the last few decades, different types of materials have been produced and further improvements have been made for specific medical applications, such as metals (stainless steel, cobalt-chromium, titanium and alloys), ceramics (alumina, zirconia, graphite), polymers, and composites [Brunette, 2001; Helsen, 1998; Williams, 1992; Jones, 2001; Vallet-Regí, 2001; Kokubo, 1993; Ratner, 2004].

In particular, ceramic materials designed to be implanted into the human body have experienced an enormous evolution as a response to the medical needs of an ageing population. The so-called first generation of bioceramics was developed to fulfill the requirement of bioinertness that is a minimum interaction with the living tissues. The most representative materials are alumina (Al_2O_3) and zirconia (ZrO_2). Indeed, today high-density (3.9 g/cc), high-purity (>99.8%) alumina is still widely used in load-bearing hip prostheses and dental implants because of its excellent corrosion resistance, good biocompatibility, low coefficient of friction, high wear resistance, bending strength (550 MPa) and compressive strength (4500 MPa). Other clinical applications of alumina include knee prostheses, bone screws, alveolar ridge and maxillofacial reconstruction. Zirconia is also used as the articulating ball in total hip prostheses and its potential advantages are its lower modulus of elasticity and higher strength [Ratner, 2004].

In the 1980s, the second generation of ceramics was investigated with the aim of a favourable interaction with the body. Bioactive and reabsorbable ceramics are able to form a mechanically strong bond with the living tissues. The most significant materials are crystalline calcium phosphates, bioactive glasses and glass-ceramics clinically used for applications such as the bone tissue augmentation, bone cements or the coating of metallic implants.

Porous ceramics have also been developed due to their potential advantage to provide good mechanical stability given by the highly convoluted interface that develops when bone grows into the pores of the ceramic. Although the optimal type of porosity and degree of interconnectivity of pores is still uncertain, when pore sizes exceed 100 µm, bone will grow within the interconnecting pore channels near the surface and maintain its vascularity and long-term viability. Therefore, the porous ceramic serves as a structural scaffold for bone formation. Nevertheless, porous materials like hydroxyapatite are weaker than the equivalent bulk form in proportion to the percentage of porosity, so that as the porosity increases, the mechanical properties of the material decrease rapidly. This fact severely restricts the use of these low-strength porous ceramics to non load-bearing applications.

Today, the concept of tissue replacement is being substituted by tissue regeneration and, therefore, more demanding properties are required. The third generation of advanced ceramics is currently developed to be used as scaffolds and templates of cells or other biologically active substances (growth factors, hormones, and so on), able to induce regeneration and repair of living tissues. Major challenges still remain in the implant technology field in terms of development of light-weight, reliable, and durable ceramic implants with enhanced mechanical properties and better biological responses [Hench, 1993; Yamamuro, 1990]. The remarkable biomechanical properties of human tissues to be replaced or repaired are based in their hierarchic structure, which is an organized assembly of structural units at increasing size levels that provides optimum fluid transfer and self-healing [Sikavitsas, 2001]. The new generation of materials for medical implant must mimic the smart hierarchical structures presented in nature.

Bioinspired materials take advantage of the knowledge that nature has been optimising by evolution over millions of years. Advanced ceramics can now take inspiration from the most complex naturally organised chemical and biological structures. In this context, wood-based SiC ceramics (bioSiC) have been a matter of interest in the last decade [Ota, 1995; Byrne, 1998; Byrne 1997; Greil, 1998, 1998a, 1999a; Shin, 1999; Martínez, 2000, 2000a, 2003]. This bioinspired material is fabricated via the pyrolysis and infiltration of natural wood-derived preforms, have tailorable properties with numerous potential applications. The experimental studies conducted to date on the development of materials based on biologically derived structures indicate that these materials behave like ceramic materials manufactured by conventional approaches. These structures have been shown to be quite useful in producing porous or dense materials having various microstructures and compositions. To further improve the fixation and osteointegration performance, the bioinspired ceramics can be coated with a bioactive layer of hydroxyapatite, substituted apatites, or silica-based glasses.

This chapter shows that a new generation of bioderived ceramics can be developed and successfully used as a base material for medical implants, because they mimic the natural structure of bone. *In vivo* implantation experiments demonstrate the excellent biocompatibility of this new material, and how it gets colonized by the hosting bone tissue due to its unique interconnected hierarchic porosity. Specific plant species can be used as templates on which innovative transformation processes, acting at molecular level, can modify the chemical composition maintaining the original biostructure. Utilizing these transformation processes and building on the outstanding mechanical properties of the starting lignocellulosic templates, it is possible to develop light-weight and high-strength scaffolds for bone substitution with a suitable structure-morphology for optimum biomechanical performance, which opens the door to a whole new generation of biomedical applications.

11.3   BIOINSPIRED SiC BASED CERAMICS

11.3.1   Processing

The melt infiltration method to produce biomimetic SiC-based ceramics follows the general flow chart in Figure 11.1. The final SiC product resembles the hardwood and softwood structures, shown in Figure 11.2 [Wheeler, 2001]. Therefore, a porous ceramic with a specified structure and density can be made by choosing the appropriate wood precursor.

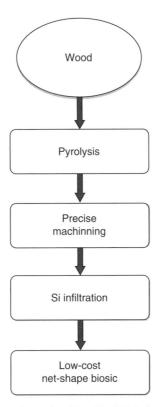

Figure 11.1. Schematic of the bioSiC fabrication process.

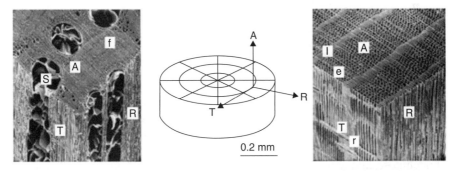

Figure 11.2. Microstructure of a ring-porous hardwood (left) and softwood (right).39 Noted features are planes perpendicular to the axial (A), radial (R), and tangential (T) directions, sap channels (s), fiber cells (f), rays (r), earlywood (e), and latewood (l).

These wood pieces are dried at 100 °C for a few hours and pyrolyzed in argon atmosphere with well-controlled heating and cooling ramps up to 1100 °C to create carbonaceous performs that mimic the wood microstructure (Figure 11.3). Typically in all kind of woods, approximately 75 ± 5% of the starting weight of the

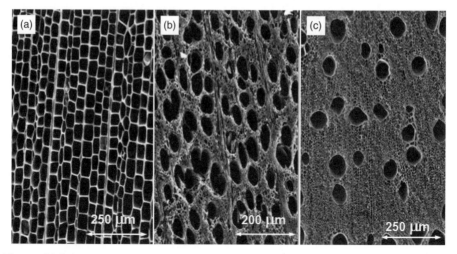

Figure 11.3. Microstructure of different types of natural wood-derived carbon performs: (a) pine, (b) beech, and (c) eucalyptus.

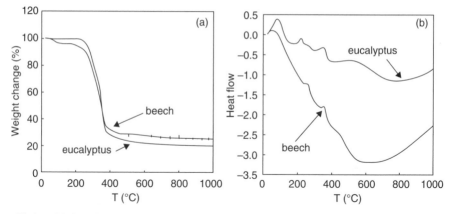

Figure 11.4. DSC and TGA curves for (a) maple and (b) mahogany during the pyrolysis.

natural original material is lost during the pyrolysis, mainly in the form of water vapor and other volatiles. Volume is reduced at the same time by about $60 \pm 5\%$.

Wood consists of three major macromolecular constituents, namely cellulose, hemicellulose, and lignin. Typically, half of the dry weight of wood is cellulose, and hemicellulose and lignin consists of other half (~25% each). The exact amount of these constituents changes with the specific nature and type of wood. The overall pyrolysis process of wood has been studied by a number of investigators and summarized in a recent review publication [Sinha, 2000].

Figures 11.4a and 11.4b show typical thermogravimetric analysis (TGA) and differential scanning calorimetry (DSC) of pyrolysis up to 1000 °C [Singh, 2002]. There are similarities in the decomposition process. During the initial heating of the specimens, the removal of moisture starts around 100 °C and is completed around 170 °C. During the second step of weight loss, the decomposition of hemicellulose takes place at around 190–280 °C and volatile products are released (CO_2, CO, and other organics vapors). In the temperature range of 280–500 °C, major weight loss takes place due to the decomposition of cellulose and lignin. The decomposition of lignin increases above 300 °C and it results in a rapid increase in carbon content of the material. Typically, the majority of the decomposition is completed by 500 °C, and minimal weight loss occurs afterwards. The major weight loss events are shown in DSC curves, which exhibit the endothermic and exothermic nature of the reactions. Although the TGA curves for different wood species are quite similar in their nature, the DSC curves may show slight differences due to differences in the chemical contents.

The pyrolyzed preforms were infiltrated with silicon under vacuum. Generally, the infiltration time and temperature depends on the melting point of the infiltrants and dimensions and properties of the preforms. For silicon, infiltration at 1450 °C for 30 minutes is adequate. The subsequent SiC formation reaction is spontaneous and exothermic [Singh, 2000; Martínez, 2000; Singh, 2003; Arellano-López, 2004; Greil, 1998].

The theoretical density of graphite is 2.16 g.cm^{-3} [Phule, 2002]. From the density of the carbon templates and the SiC density of Si-free final products, it was also possible to estimate, with linear correlation of $r^2 = 0.97$, that [Varela, 2002]:

$$\rho_{SiC} = (2.8 \pm 0.4)\rho_C \qquad (11.1)$$

and then:

$$\rho_{SiC} \approx 1.75\rho_{Wood} \qquad (11.2)$$

Reproducible microstructures and good properties can be obtained with carbon template pore sizes >5 µm. Final SiC materials are Si/SiC composites, with some unreacted C (Figure 11.5). To minimize the amount of unreacted C, which is deleterious for mechanical properties, an excess amount of Si over the stoichiometric amount is always necessary (20–100%), with the excess amount increasing as the typical pore size of the template increases. The reaction to form SiC results in a volume expansion which decreases the pore size and closes off some of the smaller pores compared to the C preforms, but the overall structure of the precursor wood is retained (Figure 11.6). The melt infiltration method allows good control of the shape and density of the final product by choosing the appropriate wood [Varela, 2002; Singh, 2002].

Nitric acid (HNO_3) and hydrofluoric acid (HF) can be used to remove the excess unreacted silicon, typically filling the larger pores. After etching away the excess silicon, a porous silicon carbide skeleton remains (Figure 11.7). An important advantage of this process is the possibility to tune the density of this material in a wide range (1.1–2.5 g.cm^{-3}). Its density is very low in comparison with the literature values of the theoretical density of SiC (3.21 g.cm^{-3}) and both medical-grade Ti (4,51 g.cm^{-3}) and Ti-alloy (4,42 g.cm^{-3}) [Mangonon, 1999].

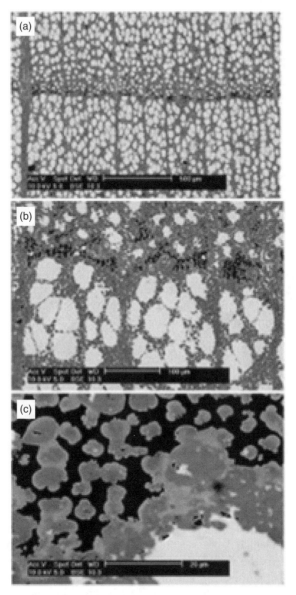

Figure 11.5. Sections (r/t) of beech-based bioSiC, observed in scanning electron microscopy using backscattered detectors, showing the distribution of SiC, Si, and C under increasing magnification (a), (b) and (c).

One of the advantages of the biomorphic SiC fabrication process, that make it give total freedom to obtain complex shapes, is that the final shape of the ceramic parts is machined on the carbon perform (there is no shape change during melt infiltration). This net-shaped process involves a soft material in an inter-

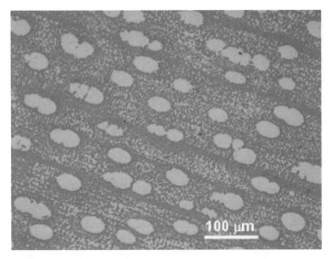

Figure 11.6. Optical micrographs showing the microstructure of silicon carbide made from maple.

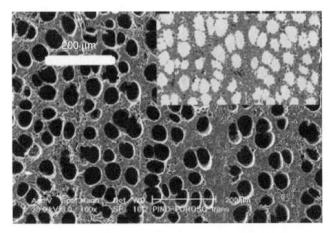

Figure 11.7. Porous SiC fabricated by chemical etching of Si from the Si/SiC composites (upper right corner). Original wood is beech.

mediate step, offers great flexibility and a wide range of possibilities for the fabrication of complex shapes (Figure 11.8). It allows efficiently producing precision complex parts with fewer operations and setups, reducing cost, waste, and delivery times.

11.3.2 Microstructure, Phase and Element Distribution

The main variables distinguishing different species of woods are the types, sizes, and distribution of cells. Due to seasonal growth rate changes, these variables also

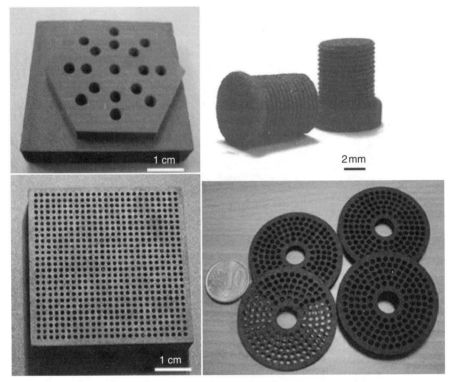

Figure 11.8. Complex shapes in bioSiC fabricated from different wood precursors.

differ within the same specific species [Panshin, 1980]. Woods can be classified into hardwoods (angiosperms) and softwoods (gymnosperms) based upon whether the trees produce covered or uncovered seeds. As shown in Figure 11.2, the microstructures of hardwoods and softwoods can also be used to distinguish the two groups due to the presence or absence of certain cell types. Hardwoods contain four types of cells: fiber cells, which serve as mechanical support, and rays, sap channels (tracheae), and long tubular cells, which serve to transport and store food. On the other hand, softwoods are comprised almost completely of long tubular cells (tracheids). Growth rings are formed due to the changing growth rate of the wood through different seasons in a year. The repeated transition from early wood, which is composed of larger pores, to latewood, which is composed of smaller pores, results in the distinct rings visible on the macroscopic scale. By convention, the axial direction runs parallel to the elongated pores, the radial direction is perpendicular and crosses the growth rings at right angles, and the tangential direction is orthogonal to the axial and radial directions. A further classification of hardwood microstructures divides them into two classes. Woods with a uniform distribution of cells are called diffuse-porous woods (poplar, beech, and so on), and woods with a bimodal distribution of cells are called ring-porous woods (sapele, red oak, mahogany, eucalyptus and so on).

Figures 11.9a and 11.9b shows SEM micrographs of carbon precursors. In hardwoods, the pores typically follow a bimodal distribution, with small pores with diameters ranging from 4 μm to 10 μm and large pores ranging from 30 μm to 200 μm, depending on the precursor [Singh, 2000; Martínez, 2000; Singh, 2003; Arellano, 2004]. The microstructure of the porous carbon performs are shown in Figures 11.9a and 11.9b in two different directions, respective to tree growth. There is a wide variation in the microstructure and density of the carbonaceous performs, due to the structural differences within a wood sample and between various types of wood. The variation of preform microstructure and properties can be utilized to produce final materials with controlled composition and phase morphologies. The perform density and microstructure control the composition and microstructure of final materials.

Figure 11.10 shows the principal aspects of the microstructure in bioSiC, as well as the main phases observed [Zollfrank, 2004; Zollfrank, 2005; Varela, 2005; Arellano-López, 2007; Varela, 2007]. As seen in the XRD in Figure 11.10a, both Si and SiC are crystalline in bioSiC, while the carbon precursors are amorphous. In the SEM micrographs in Figure 11.10b (1,2,3) crystalline Si is seen in brighter contrast. Crystalline SiC is seen as darker grey, and presents a bimodal grain size distribution consisting on both micron-sized grains (μ-SiC) and nanometersized grains (n-SiC), as seen in TEM pictures (4 and 5). Finally, unreacted amorphous C is seen as black. SEM/EDS micrograph (6) confirms these observations.

Micron-size SiC grains are formed in the walls of sap channels (large channels with diameter over 5 μm). In small channels, where Si is usually depleted in the reaction because micron-sized SiC grains closed the pores, nano-sized SiC grains can be observed between the large SiC grains and the unreacted carbon. These n-SiC grains are found forming rosettes in certain places, which is typical of diffusion-controlled growth, while μ-SiC grains are faceted, which is typical of solution-precipitation-controlled growth. Both unreacted Si and C areas can be found, normally separated by a SiC layer that prevents them from reacting with each other.

The previous observations make it possible to distinguish two reaction methods, depending on the diameter of the channels in the carbon preform. In both cases, molten Si penetrates through the carbon preform by capillarity and reacts with the solid C spontaneously and exothermically. If the channel is large and Si is abundant, Si-C groups are formed in Si solution until it saturates and μ-SiC grains precipitate. In the small channels, the process is similar but the large μ-SiC grains that precipitate close the pores. Under these conditions, the Si must diffuse through the previously formed SiC to react with the carbon perform. Thus, nanometer-sized SiC grains are formed in a process controlled by diffusion.

Concerning the chemical composition of these ceramics, EDS analyses show that this biomorphic material is a composite of a SiC skeleton with small amounts of unreacted Si and C. Recent studies conclude that the residual silicon does not present adverse physiological effects in the body; Si is safely excreted through the urine and no accumulation was found distributed in the major organs [Lai, 2002]. Table 11.1 shows the XRF and XPS analyses of the three SiC types [González,

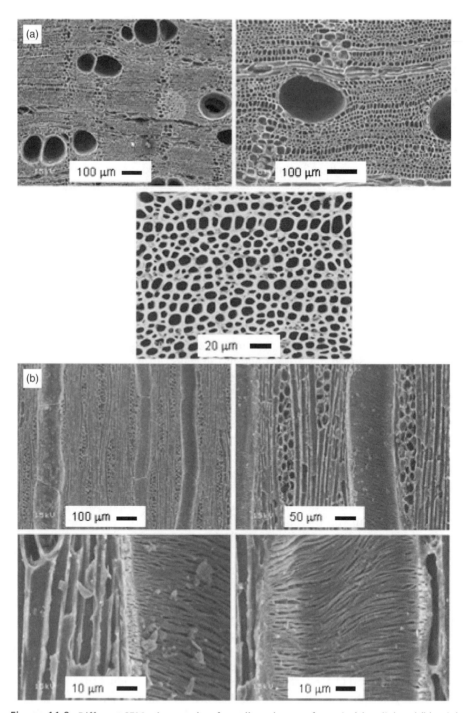

Figure 11.9. Different SEM micrographs of sapelly carbon preforms in (a) radial and (b) axial directions.

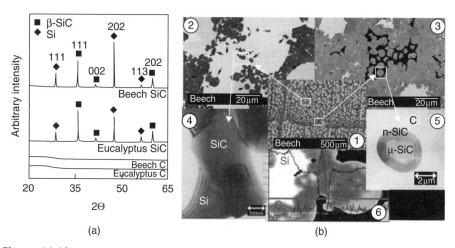

(a) (b)

Figure 11.10. (a) XRD spectra showing the crystalline phases present in the C preforms and bioSiC materials. (b) SEM, TEM micrographs and EDS composite showing different aspects of bioSiC microstructure.

TABLE 11.1. Chemical Composition Measured by XRF and XPS of Bio-SiC Obtained from Beech, Sapelly and Eucalyptus. The Presence in the Bio-SiC of the Corresponding Elements is Indicated by X

	Bio-SiC type					
	Beech		Sapelly		Eucalyptus	
Element	XRF	XPS	XRF	XPS	XRF	XPS
Al	X		X	X	X	X
B				X		X
C	X	X	X	X	X	X
Ca	X	X	X	X	X	X
Cr					X	
Cu	X		X		X	X
Fe	X		X		X	
K	X		X		X	
La					X	
Mn					X	
N		X		X		X
Na	X		X		X	X
O		X		X		X
P	X		X		X	
S	X		X		X	
Si	X	X	X	X	X	X
Ti	X		X		X	
Zn					X	

TABLE 11.2. Release Test of Bio-SiC (mg/l)

Element	SBF	Beech	Sapelly	Eucalyplus
Al	0.014	0.007	0.005	0.004
Ca	93	104	97.8	86.4
Cu	0.01	0.375	0.097	0.166
Fe	<0.005	<0.005	<0.005	<0.005
P	37.1	32.4	33.8	32.3
S	4.62	6.33	5.3	4.5
Si	0.369	5.76	4.69	0.829
Ti	<0.005	<0.005	<0.005	<0.005

2004]. The elements identified by both techniques are marked in grey. The measurements reveal the majority presence of Si and C. Small amounts of Ca were found in all samples and, in some cases, Al, Cu and Na. Other trace elements were also identified in very low concentrations.

The biocompatible behaviour of this material has been tested by soaking the SiC ceramics in Simulated Body Fluid. Table 11.2 shows the ICP-MS analyses of the SBF fluids after one-week immersion of the Bio-SiC materials [González, 2004]. The SBF element concentrations used as reference values are also shown. Only weak signals related to the release of Si and Cu until reaching concentration values in the order of ppm were observed. Most of the elements remain unchanged within experimental error. Therefore, it can be concluded that no important dissolution rate of these materials is observed and no adverse physiological effects in the body are expected.

The biomorphic SiC selected to be used as medical implant must have microstructural features similar to the ones of the cortical bones. In particular it will be important and adequate partial pore orientation and porous continuity; sufficient pore volume (typically 50% to 70%); micropores of approximately 10 µm in diameter for cell adhesion; macropores with diameters larger than 100 µm for cell penetration, tissue ingrowth, and vascularisation [Gauthier 1998, Black 1998]. The bimodal hard woods microstructures are very promising because they can fulfil these requirements, in particular the beech, sapelly and eucalyptus precursors.

11.3.3 Reaction-Formation Mechanisms

Molten Si infiltrates into the porous preform by effect of the capillary pressure [Bhagat, 1994; Gern, 1997; Greil, 2001; Sangsuwan, 1999]. Jurin's law establishes that the maximum height a liquid can penetrate inside a capillary is:

$$h_{\max} = \frac{2\sigma\cos\theta}{rg\rho} \qquad (11.3)$$

Where σ is the surface tension of the liquid, r is the capillary radius, θ the contact angle, g is gravity's acceleration, ρ the liquid's density and h_{max} is the maximum height of the liquid inside the capillary. To describe the dynamical aspects of the liquid's infiltration in the tubular capillary a laminar flow is assumed, so Poiseuille's law can be applied, giving:

$$t = \frac{8\eta}{r^2 \rho g}\left[h_{max} \ln\left[\frac{h_{max}}{h_{max}-h}\right] - h \right] \tag{11.4}$$

Where η is the liquid's viscosity, t is the time and h the height of the liquid inside the capillary. With these results, an estimation of the maximum infiltration height can be done using the physical properties of molten Si [Gern, 1997; Gerwien, 1986; Grabmaier, 1981]. A carbon preform with a mean pore diameter of 5 μm can be infiltrated with liquid Si up to approximately 25 m high. Clearly the infiltration process is very fast. For instance, a carbon preform with pore diameters ranging from 5 μm to 100 μm will be infiltrated in less than two seconds. Although the large channels are infiltrated faster than small ones (due to viscosity effects), the capillary pressure is much larger in the small channels, so because a large channel is connected to some small channels (see Figure 11.9), these will extract liquid Si from the large one until a pressure equilibrium is reached.

Most authors agree in the existence of an initial phase where the surface carbon is dissolved in the liquid Si and then is nucleated as SiC in the carbon surface. The latter growth of SiC can then be controlled by two different mechanisms. One of them is the diffusion of C and/or Si through the previously formed SiC, as described by Hon et al. [Hon, 1979; Hon, 1980], Fitzer and Gadow [Fitzer, 1985; Fitzer, 1986] and Zhou and Singh [Zhou, 1995]. The other possible process is the solution-precipitation of all the carbon present in the silicon, as described by Pampuch et al. [Pampuch, 1986; Pampuch, 1987]. Whether one mechanism or the other dominates will depend on the morphology of the carbon preform. On bulk, poreless carbon once the initial SiC layer is formed Si and/or C will have to diffuse through the SiC and this is a slow process, due to the low C and Si diffusion coefficients in SiC [Hon, 1979; Hon, 1979; Hong, 1980; Hong, 1981]. Typically, the formation of a 10 μm thick SiC layer takes about one hour at 1500 °C.

The β-SiC formation reaction follows first order kinetics, so the concentration of each phase can be modelled using:

$$[C_i] = [C_i^f] + ([C_i^0]-[C_i^f])\exp(kt) \tag{11.5}$$

Where k is the reaction constant of the SiC formation reaction and C_i is the concentration of phase i. C_i^f is the concentration of each phase for an infinite reaction time, which has to be introduced since Si is introduced in excess in the process, and C_i^0 is the initial concentration of phase i. Pampuch et al. studied the SiC formation process by reaction of bundles of C fibres 4–6 μm in diameter with liquid Si at 1422 °C and 1439 °C [Pampuch, 1986; Pampuch, 1987], and determined the reaction constant k using DTA analysis. They also estimated the reaction constant using diffusion data from Hon et al. [Hon, 1979; Hon, 1980] and assuming the reaction was controlled by diffusion through the SiC layer, concluding that the reaction had to be controlled by solution-precipitation of the C in the molten Si, as diffusion estimations gave much lower reaction rates than observed [Varela, 2007].

For porous carbon preforms with wall thickness smaller than 10 μm, the diffusion mechanisms play no significant role. Instead, the carbon is dissolved in the molten silicon and precipitated as silicon carbide near the carbon walls when the solution supersaturates. In the wood based carbon precursors used for bioSiC the carbon wall thickness is about 2 ± 1 μm, so the SiC formation should be exclusively controlled by solution-precipitation. However, as some of the channels in the preform have a diameter of the same range as the wall thickness, they can be closed as the SiC precipitates and thus coalesce with surrounding small channels, yielding an effective SiC layer that is significantly thicker, forcing a scenario where the SiC growth can only happen by a diffusion mechanism. This is also suggested by the presence of unreacted C in bioSiC (Figures 11.5 and 11.10).

In this scheme, the liquid Si must dissolve the cell walls of the carbon preform to form a solution which will then precipitate as micron-sized SiC grains. An estimation of the time required for the solution of the preform into the molten Si can be made using the Nerst-Noves-Whitney equation:

$$-\frac{dm_c}{dt} = \frac{DA(c_s - c_0)}{\zeta(t)} \tag{11.6}$$

In Equation 11.6 $-dm_c/dt$ is the carbon mass dissolved into the molten Si per unit time, D is the diffusion coefficient of carbon in liquid Si for a given temperature, A is the C-Si(L) contact surface, $\zeta(t)$ is the thickness of the solution layer, c_s is the carbon concentration and c_0 is the initial carbon concentration, which is zero as initially the molten Si contains no C. For this example's considerations and based on microstructural evidence, assume an initial wall thickness of one μm and suppose that the temperature is constant through the C/Si interface and its surroundings, due to the high thermal conductivity of molten Si [Bartlett, 1967]. Further, suppose that the carbon concentration at the interface is that of equilibrium at the reaction's temperature, that is, $c_s = c_e$ for all $t \geq 0$, being c_e the equilibrium concentration. Also, approximate $\zeta(t) \sim 4(Dt)^{\frac{1}{2}}$ [Crank, 1975]. Substituting into equation (4), one obtains:

$$\frac{-dm_c}{dt} = \frac{D(T)Ac_e}{4\sqrt{Dt}} = \frac{\sqrt{D(T)}Ac_e}{4\sqrt{t}} \tag{11.7}$$

Equation 11.7 make it possible to estimate the time needed to dissolve a with one μm-thick carbon wall as a function of temperature T. For these calculations c_e has been taken from the works of Scace [Scace, 1959] and D has been taken from [Gnesin, 1973]. It has been shown that the heat generated by the reaction can raise the temperature in the reaction zone by about 500 °C. This has been observed by Pampuch et al. [Pampuch, 1986; Pampuch, 1987] by Differential Thermal Analysis of the infiltration and reaction process of molten Si in a preform made of carbon fibres, and by Sangsuwan et al. [Sangsuwan, 1999]. Therefore, if the molten Si temperature is 1550 °C, then the process can reach 2000 °C inside the C preform. For this temperature, and considering a wall thickness of one µm, all the carbon of the wall is dissolved in about a minute.

A model for the formation of bioSiC based in the C-Si solubility [Kleykamp, 1993] has been proposed [Varela, 2007], as shown in Figure 11.11. If Si is majority, then a liquid solution of Si/SiC is formed and micrometric SiC is precipitated upon cooling or saturation of the solution. Wherever C is majority, there is no Si/C liquid interface and the SiC is formed by a diffusion process that yields nanosized SiC grains. Which scenario occurs depends mainly on the channel diameter.

In Figure 11.11a, the schematics of the SiC formation inside the large channels is shown, where liquid Si is majority. Liquid Si penetrates the carbon preform by capillary forces and because in the preforms the porosity is connected, the molten Si reaches all pores and channels. This process takes place in a few seconds, as has been previously shown. Silicon then reacts with the carbon preform forming Si-C groups dissolved in the liquid by corrosion of the carbon walls that surround the channels. As the walls are 1–2 µm thick, the amount of available C is small compared to the Si volume and C is quickly depleted. This process take about a minute as has been previously shown.

The solution process is aided by the heat generated during the reaction which in turn raises the liquid Si temperature and enhances the C solubility. The SiC/Si solution supersaturates for small C concentrations, producing the precipitation of SiC near the C walls, yielding SiC grains in the micron range. This is supported by the faceted morphology of the large SiC grains. The process ends when all the carbon is depleted and all SiC has precipitated.

If the channel diameter is comparable to the C wall thickness, then the pores can become closed by the precipitation of SiC. In that case, the SiC barrier prevents the complete reaction of the C preform in that zone, and so some unreacted C remains in the sample. The process in this scenario is schematized in Figure 11.11b. As happens when the channels are large, the Si infiltration occurs by means of capillary pressure. The liquid Si then reacts with the C in the perform, forming Si-C groups dissolved in the melt. Because there is more carbon than silicon, the solution is supersaturated earlier than in the previous case, and so micron-sized grains precipitate inside the channel and end up choking it. Up to now, the process is similar to the previous scenario and happens in the Si-rich part of the Si-C phase diagram. The Si is less and less available as the reaction takes place and so the system is displaced to the C rich part of the phase diagram. In this zone there is no solubility of Si into C so it is impossible for a solution-precipitation mechanism to occur. The only possibility available to the system is the formation of SiC by diffusion through the already formed SiC layer. At the SiC/C interface the grains have a size in the nanometre range because the kinetic of the reaction is extremely slow. For practical effects and considering the time

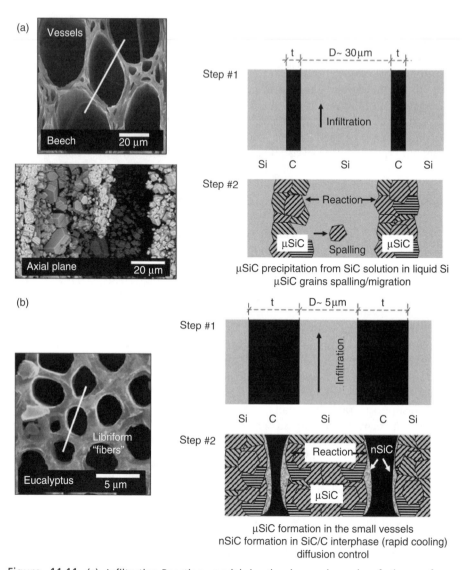

<u>Figure 11.11.</u> (a) Infiltration-Reaction model in the large channels of the preform. (b) Infiltration-Reaction model in the narrow channels of the preform.

the system is allowed to react in typical fabrication conditions, the microstructure is frozen in the first growth stage.

11.3.4   Mechanical Properties

The mechanical properties of biomorphic SiC have been extensively studied [Martínez, 2000; Martínez, 2003; Varela, 2001; Varela, 2002; Varela, 2002b; Singh,

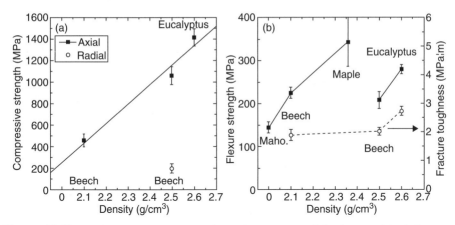

Figure 11.12. Ambient temperature mechanical properties of the biomorphic Si/SiC composites: (a) compressive strength; (b) flexure strength measured in four-point (solid lines and symbols) and fracture toughness (open circles and broken line).

2002; Presas, 2005; Presas, 2006; Kaul, 2006; Smirnov, 2003; Kardashev, 2005; Kardashev, 2006; Gutierrez-Mora, 2005]. This section presents the results more directly related to the use of this material as medical implant.

The mechanical properties of the biomorphic composites at ambient temperature are plotted as a function of density in Figure 11.12. [Presas, 2005]. The axial compressive strength (Figure 11.12a) of the Si/SiC composites was a linear function of the density, and this is in agreement with previous results on the compressive strength of biomorphic Si/SiC manufactured from pyrolyzed poplar and obeche [Singh, 2002], in which the porosity was also the main factor controlling the strength. Of course, the particular microstructure of the biomorphic composites, inherited from the precursor woods, was responsible for the anisotropy in the compressive strength along the axial and radial directions in beech (Figure 11.12a), and thus the oriented microstructure of the biomorphic composites provide optimized properties when loaded along the trunk axis. But the results indicate that the main factor controlling the axial compressive strength was the biomorphic density (or, inversely, porosity) rather than the actual precursor wood.

The behavior in bending and fracture is plotted in Figure 11.12b and shows that the strength and toughness of the beech-based biomorphic composite with low density (2.1 g/cm³) was similar to that of the beech- and eucalyptus-based materials with higher density (2.5–2.6 g/cm³). The flexure strength measured in four-point bending by Singh and Salem [Singh, 2002] on mahogany and maple-based biomorphic Si/SiC composites processed by the same technique is also included in Figure 11.12b. Maple and mahogany are also hardwoods and their C templates also present the typical bimodal pore structure. However, no free C was found in these biomorphic composites and their flexure strength was in good agreement with results in C-free low-density biomorphic Si/SiC composites processed from beech, taking into account the differences in density. The flexure strength of the high-density biomorphic composites processed from eucalyptus and beech was similar to that of the materials obtained from beech and mahogany, respectively, even though their density was significantly higher. The fracture surfaces were always very brittle, and little information on the fracture micromechanisms could be extracted from their analyses, although the most obvious reason for the better properties of the latter materials was the absence of residual C. Thus, the presence of residual C did not seem to influence significantly the compressive strength of biomorphic Si/SiC composites but it was clearly negative in bending. The bending strength of brittle materials—as opposed to compressive strength—is controlled by the presence of defects where cracks are nucleated. Regions containing amorphous residual C enhance the total volume fraction of these regions in the biomorphic composites and reduce the overall bending strength while its influence on the compressive strength was very limited.

The compressive strengths of the porous bioSiC (with Si removed) [Kaul, 2006] are considerable lower (decrease up to 60%) than those of fully dense bioSiC/Si (Figure 11.13) [Singh, 2002; Presas, 2005]. This is not surprising as the residual Si serves to reinforce the bioSiC.

The values measured here agree with compressive strength values for bioSiC/Si measured above the softening temperature of silicon [Varela, 2002; Martínez, 2003]. In addition to the influence of orientation on mechanical properties, precursor type, independent of porosity, appears to play a significant role. For a given porosity, SiC samples fabricated from diffuse-porous precursors have better mechanical properties than those fabricated from ring-porous precursors. In compression, failure is the result of accumulated damage. The lower compressive strength of ring-porous SiC cannot be explained only by the larger pores in these materials. The difference in strength between ring-porous and diffuse-porous SiC is hypothesized to be influenced by the amount of residual carbon.

It can be seen that for a given porosity ring-porous hardwoods tend to have a higher carbon content than that produced from diffuse-porous hardwoods in the final biomorphic SiC. In the diffuse-porous samples, residual carbon is generally 10 vol.% of the solid phase. However, this value ranges from five percent to 50% for ring-porous samples, and the amount of residual carbon tends to increase with decreasing porosity in the precursor. These measurements can be a consequence of SiC formation mechanism in the two types of porosity. To fully convert the carbon scaffold to SiC, the molten silicon must infiltrate all pores. In diffuse-porous preforms, the uniform distribution of sap channels allows for easier infiltration. In ring-porous samples, with a non-uniform distribution, there are areas of lower density where sap channels are present that are easily infiltrated as well as areas of higher density where only fiber cells are present that are not as easily infiltrated. The majority of the pores in ring-porous precursors are smaller fiber cells, so incomplete reaction is likely. Also from Table 11.2, it is evident that there is greater variability in the amount of residual carbon for the ring-porous than for the diffuse-porous SiC, which indicates that the residual carbon is not homogenously distributed in the material.

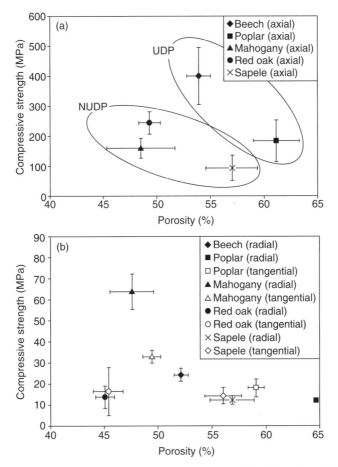

Figure 11.13. Compressive strength as a function of porosity for: (a) axial; and (b) tangential and radial orientations with UDP and NUDP bioSiC grouped in the axial plot (error bars equal one standard deviation).

Fracture toughness of porous bioSiC has a strong dependence on orientation and on porosity, as shown in Figure 11.14. Experiments show higher fracture toughness when cracks propagate in directions perpendicular to the axial direction and lower fracture toughness values for propagation in directions parallel to the axial direction. This dependence of fracture toughness on crack propagation direction can be explained by the orientation of the elongated anisotropic pores. Cracks propagating in directions parallel to the axial direction are able to propagate in preferred paths along these elongated pores. Cracks in transverse directions are forced to propagate along tortuous paths and across these elongated pores, which results in higher fracture toughness values. The fracture toughness of Si/SiC composites for crack propagation perpendicular to the axial direction are

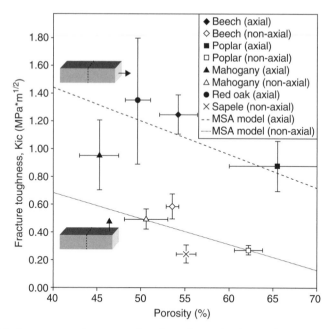

Figure 11.14. Fracture toughness as a function of porosity for cracks propagating perpendicular (axial) and parallel (non-axial, transverse) to the axial direction of bioSiC derived from several precursors (error bars equal one standard deviation and arrows refer to the axial direction). Values predicted by the MSA model for axial and transverse orientations are also shown by the dashed lines.

50–70% higher than the values measured on porous samples due to the presence of excess silicon, as expected [Presas, 2005].

The elastic moduli of porous bioSiC determined in compression in the axial and transverse directions are plotted as a function of porosity in Figures 11.15a and 11.15b [Kaul, 2006]. By grouping these data by the type of precursor (in this case, diffuse-porous and ring-porous), it is apparent that the axial stiffness of diffuse-porous SiC are more sensitive to porosity. Porous SiC is significantly stiffer in the axial direction than in transverse directions, in most cases by one order of magnitude. A similar trend as the compression strength.

Such behavior is typical of honeycomb materials where the transverse (or in-plane) strength and stiffness are controlled by cell-wall bending, whereas axial (or out-of-plane) strength and stiffness depend on compression of the cell walls. The elastic moduli reported here are about half that reported in the literature for biomorphic Si/SiC at room temperature [Singh, 2002; Smirnov, 2003; Kardashev, 2005; Kardashev, 2006]. This is not surprising as the unreacted silicon stiffens the composite.

Martínez et al. [Martínez, 2003] has compared the mechanical properties of biomorphic SiC with other siliconized SiC. Figure 11.16 shows the strength data for the reaction bonded SiC (RBSC), reaction formed SiC (RFCS), and BioSiC

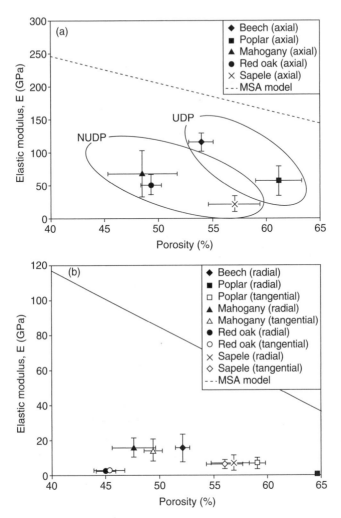

Figure 11.15. Elastic modulus as a function of porosity for: (a) axial; and (b) tangential and radial orientations with UDP and NUDP bioSiC grouped in the axial plot (error bars equal one standard deviation). Values predicted by the MSA model for both orientations are shown by dashed lines.

materials is plotted as relative strength, σ_c/σ_{ys} (where σ_c is the strength of the porous solid and σ_{ys} is the strength of the fully dense material), versus SiC volume fraction. The strength data of the fully dense sintered SiC, measured under the same experimental conditions, is taken from a previous work [Muñoz, 2002]. For every material, the average of the relative strength was taken, and the scatter is indicated with the error bars. The compressive strength of BioSiC was measured in the axial and radial orientation. It was up to six times larger when the compression was parallel to the axial direction, indicating the importance of the

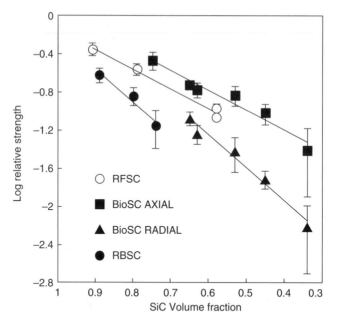

Figure 11.16. Plot of the relative strength versus the volume fraction of SiC for the siliconized SiC ceramics studied in this work. For every material, the average of the relative strength at different temperatures was taken. See text for further discussion.

orientation of the SiC cells on the high strength of the material. RFSC have a strength that is roughly the average of the axial and radial strength of BioSiC, and RBSC has a significant lower strength than the other two types of siliconized SiC. The curves of the axial BioSiC and RBSC (materials with the best and worse strength) are displaced roughly 20% on SiC content for the same strength.

In summary, the mechanical properties of biomorphic SiC with microstructure suitable of medical applications are very promising. The room-temperature compressive strength in the longitudinal (biological precursor growth) direction of sapelli-derived bioSiC is from 1160 ± 100 (s.d.) MPa to 210 ± 20 (s.d.) MPa, and in the radial direction is from 430 ± 50 (s.d.) MPa to 120 ± 10 (s.d.), depending on the amount of silicon removal, that can be controlled by thermal or chemical etching. These results compare positively with the compressive strength of a typical human cortical bone: 193 MPa in the longitudinal direction and 133 MPa in the radial direction [Gibson, 1973]. The absolute values of strength are in the same range that the lowest values of bioSiC, being their density range very similar (density range of cortical bone $1,6–2,0\,\mathrm{g.cm^{-3}}$) [Gibson, 1973]. The room temperature bending strength of bioSiC ranges from 430 ± 60 to 150 ± 20 MPa in the density range of 2.3 to $2.0\,\mathrm{g.cm^{-3}}$ [Presas, 2005]. Elastic modulus range from to 25 to 230 GPa depending on the amount of silicon removal [Smirnov 2003, Kaul 2006], so this property can be modelled close to the value of the elastic modulus of cortical bone ($15 \pm 5\,\mathrm{GPa}$) [Gibson, 1973]. The fracture toughness reach values between 2–$3\,\text{MPa(m)}^{1/2}$ [Presas, 2005], typical values for SiC ceramics already used in medical applications. The mechanical properties indicate that bioSiC ceramics are suitable materials for medical devices in terms of structural requirements as they present better strength than cortical bone and reasonable toughness. Moreover, taking into account the biomechanical requirements (density, elastic modulus, strain failure, porosity topology, and so on) of a particular type of bone in the body that should be repaired, biomorphic SiC ceramics can be tailored by an appropriate precursor selection.

11.3.5 Optimization of Mechanical Properties by the Biomimetic Structure

The models available in the literature for microstructure-strength dependence in porous materials can be classified under two main approaches: models for cellular materials (porosities over 70%) where the strength is mostly related with the bending strength of the cell walls [Gibson, 1988], and, models for systems with lower porosities, where it is assumed that the strength is only dependent of the minimum solid area perpendicular to the applied stress [Rice, 1996; Rice, 2000]. In the first case, mechanisms such as bending or crushing of individual cell walls may be active; in the second case, the behavior will be similar to that of a monolithic material with a certain detriment to the mechanical properties by the porosity.

The volume fraction of SiC on the materials studied in this work, and the microstructural observations, fit better with the assumptions of the minimum solid area approach, that is, the rather than as a cellular material. The limitations of the cellular model to study BioSiC strength data were already pointed out by Varela et al. [Varela, 2002]. In addition to the limitation to describe structures within our range of porosities, the cellular model cannot differentiate between the different topologies of the materials studied in this work. Results obtained will be discussed in terms of the effects of the porous topology on the minimum solid area of the system.

The porous structures can be modeled as formed by either stacking of particles with a certain degree of bonding (truncate shapes), or stacking of pores totally or partially enclosed by the solid web. The minimum solid area of a microstructure depends on the topology of the pores/particles composing the system, type of stacking, and the amount of porosity. In the case of stacking of regular particles, there is a maximum porosity limit after which the particles lose connectivity (and load carrying ability), and the structure has sectional cuts with zero solid area. For porosities under this value, the minimum solid area is calculated considering particles with truncated shapes. In the case of stacking of regular pores, the equivalent to the previous porosity limit define the transition from closed to connected porosity. A stacking of pores, then, can hold load in all the porosity range. The minimum solid area for close porosity is straight forward, and for connected porosity it is calculated considering pores with truncated shapes. The relative strength of a porous microstructure is equal to the relative minimum solid area in the direction perpendicular to the stress.

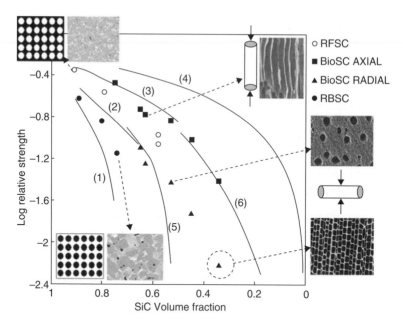

Figure 11.17. Theoretical values of the relative strength versus the volume fraction of SiC expected from the minimum solid area model, for ideal microstructures of (solid lines): spherical particles in rombohedral stacking (1), spherical particles in cubic stacking (2), spherical pores in cubic stacking (3), tubular pores aligned in the testing direction (4), cylindrical pores in random stacking perpendicular to testing direction (5), and square shaped tubular pores perpendicular to testing direction (6). The experimental values are also included. Each family of experimental values is connected with arrows (dashed lines) to drawings and micrographs of the ideal and real microstructures. See text for further discussion.

In Figure 11.17 [Martínez, 2003] it has been plotted, together with the experimental relative strength, the expected theoretical values for ideal microstructures composed of spherical particles in cubic stacking, spherical particles in rombohedral stacking, spherical pores in cubic stacking, tubular pores aligned in the testing direction, cylindrical pores perpendicular to testing direction in random stacking, and square shaped tubular pores perpendicular to testing direction [Rice, 1996; Rice, 2000]. The theoretical curves are slightly displaced to make the extrapolation to zero porosity of the experimental relative strength intersect the origin of these curves. The reason for this displacement is that the strength of the SiC contained in siliconized SiC may be different to the strength of the fully dense α-SiC used to calculate the relative strength.

In the case of reaction bonded silicon carbide (RBSC), the microstructure of SiC grains can be best modeled as a stacking of spherical particles. This ideal microstructure loses connectivity for porosities ranging from 26% to 52% depending on the type of stacking of the spherical particles. The strengths obtained in this work are located in-between these curves (curves one and two in

Figure 11.17). This approach explains the large decrease in strength of Cerastar RX. At these silicon contents, the contact sites are small enough to be fractured by the applied stresses, leading a deformation controlled by the flow of silicon.

The reaction formed silicon carbide (RFSC) microstructure can be modeled by a stacking of spherical pores (silicon regions), as it is generated from the silicon infiltration of a carbon preform with a sponge-like microstructure. Its strength is close to the curve expected for this ideal microstructure (curve three of Figure 11.17) although the experimental slope is a bit higher. The strength of BioSiC fabricated from mango wood (58% of SiC) is included together with the RFSC data, because it shows very little anisotropy due to its short longitudinal cells [Martínez, 2000].

The pores/channels in BioSiC have cylindrical/tubular shape, so this material must be modeled by a stacking of cylindrical/tubular pores. This implies that the behavior will be anisotropic and the strength in the axial and radial direction has to be different. It must be noted that the compressive strength of RBSC, RFSC, and BioSiC in the axial and radial direction, follow the same order in strength level as predicted by a stacking of spherical particles, spherical pores, cylindrical pores in the longitudinal and perpendicular direction, respectively (Figure 11.17).

In the case of axial compression of longitudinal tubular pores, the type of the stacking and shape of the tubular pores does not have influence on the theoretical strength (the strength is simply equal to the volume fraction). The experimental results are lower than the ones predicted by the model (curve four of Figure 11.17) and the slope of the experimental curve is slightly higher. There are several microstructural factors that can account for the differences with the idealized model:

1. The cells in biomorphic SiC are not perfectly aligned, which could promote some bending of the cell walls. This effect must be more important for the lower densities and could be partially responsible for the higher slope of the experimental curve.

2. The cell shape differs from a perfect cylinder. The walls present "defects" related with the nature of the precursors, as pores. Additionally, the separation between contiguous cells may not be flat.

3. There is a certain amount of radial channels, so the theoretical strength should be taken as an average of the strength of a solid with longitudinal tubular pores, and a small proportion of tubular pores oriented perpendicularly to the applied stress. This fact, may explain the differences in strength of the model and experimental values. In this regard, it is remarkable that microstructures like the one of BioSiC fabricated from *Cistus ladanifer* (rockrose), without radial channels, show a strength very close to the theoretical one (Figure 11.17, 75% SiC).

When the compression is done in the radial direction, the models predict a strong dependence with the type of stacking of the tubular pores and a slight dependence with their shape. In hard woods (higher densities) the distribution of pore size is bimodal and the packing of small pores around the big ones is random. The bimodal distribution of the pore size is the way nature reaches a high porosity, providing the necessary transfer of fluids for a particular vegetal species, and, at the same time keeping the wall thickness at adequate values. The strength of the BioSiC ceramics fabricated from these woods is close to that predicted by a random distribution of cylindrical pores (curve five of Figure 11.17).

However, for higher porosities, the random distribution of pores loses interconnection as reflected by the sudden decrease of strength in the curve five of Figure 11.17. At these lower densities the use of wall material available must be optimized, and compact packed structures like the one from pine are found. In pine wood, the number of neighbors is reduced to four and the cells have square shape. The radial strength of the BioSiC ceramics fabricated from pine wood is close to the expected values for an ideal cubic packing of tubular cells with square shape (curve six of Figure 11.17). The high scatter on the strength of BioSiC fabricated from pine wood, not found in other types of BioSiC ceramics (standard deviations of around 60% versus a typical 20%), can be explained by the high anisotropy of the strength between the axial and perpendicular direction, so small misalignments can have important consequences on the measured strength. This high anisotropy is also present within the plane perpendicular to the axial direction, where the strength is highly dependent on the orientation between compression direction and cell wall. The cells are stronger when compressed perpendicularly to the cell wall than at an angle. The distribution of the square cells forming rings in the tree, assures that any external force will be acting in the strongest orientation. Summarizing, as the density of the structures is reduced, the microstructure of these biomimetic SiC-based materials change to maintain a good strength value.

11.4   BIOINSPIRED CERAMICS COATED WITH BIOACTIVE MATERIALS

When bioinert materials, such as titanium, Co-Cr alloys, stainless steel, alumina, zirconia, and so on, are implanted into the body, a thin layer of fibrous tissue forms around them, leading to the encapsulation of the implant [Anderson, 2004]. The interface between prosthesis and its host tissue is especially susceptible to stress, and the mismatch in either biochemical or biomechanical factors can lead to interfacial deterioration and eventual failure. As the isolation of the implant from the body can have disastrous effects on some clinical applications, these implants require a periodical revision and, eventually, a replacement due to, among other factors, the lack of interaction with the receptor bone [Hench, 1993; Ratner, 2004].

To solve these problems and produce cementless devices with enhaced fixation and osteointegration performance, a new approach leading to the formation of a bond across the interface between the implant and the bone via chemical reactions has been attempted, the so-called bioactive bonding. The implant surface is often coated with bioactive ceramics, which is designed to elicit a specific biological response at the interface of the material, resulting in the formation of a bond between tissues and the material [Hench, 1993; Yamamuro, 1990]. This concept includes a large number of bioactive materials including hydroxyapatite [Darimont, 2002], glass ceramics [Andersson, 1990] and glasses [West, 1990], which have been successfully applied as coatings in metal prosthesis.

11.4.1 Hydroxyapatite and Substituted Apatites

Hydroxyapatite (HA), $Ca_{10}(PO_4)_6(OH)_2$, is the calcium phosphate biomaterial most frequently used due to its high biocompatibility and bond integration, being the material most similar to the mineral component of the bones. HA finds broad clinical applications in the repair of bone defects, the bone augmentation and in a variety of other areas in the muscoskeletal and dental fields not involving high loads. Its poor mechanical properties are the greatest impediment to its broader use in load-bearing applications in the human body. However, as HA is so similar to the receptor tissue, HA coatings have been widely applied in metallic implants in load-bearing orthopaedic applications [Hallab, 2004], improving dramatically the adhesion of these implants to the living bone tissue.

Despite HA being the main mineral component of the bone, its mineral phase cannot be described only as hydroxyapatite but also as a multi-substituted calcium phosphate, and, in fact, there has been an increasing interest in the production of enhanced HA materials, such as the silicon substituted hydroxyapatite (Si-HA) [Balas, 2003; Marques, 2001]. As a matter of fact, the role of Si during the mineralization that takes place at early stages of bone development is well known [Carlisle, 1970] and investigations on Si deficiency in the diet showed that it stands behind diseases like osteoporosis [Pérez-Granados, 2002].

The HA, being only osteoconductive, does not satisfy the criteria of an ideal bioactive material because HA resorbs very slowly and the dissolution products do not stimulate the genes in the osteogenic cells. Silicon-substituted HA coatings or scaffolds release small concentrations of silicon and calcium ions, which have been found to stimulate seven families of genes in osteoblasts, increasing proliferation and bone extracellular matrix production [Jones, libro 2005]. Genes are activated by small concentrations (less than 20 parts per million) of hydrated silicon ($Si(OH)_4$). Therefore, small amounts of silica (SiO_2) can be substituted for calcia (CaO) in synthetic hydroxyapatite. There is also enough experimental evidence of the improved bioactivity of the Si-HA when compared to the ordinary HA. *In vivo* experiments have shown that bone ingrowth in silica-substituted HA granules was significantly greater than that in phase-pure HA granules, the former being classified as an osteoproductive or regenerative material [Jones, 2005; Porter, 2003]. Therefore, it is clear that the production of coatings from this new material can be of interest to the medical industry.

11.4.2 Bioactive Glasses

Glasses, as a subclass of ceramics, constitute the most important group of non-crystalline solids. Glasses are amorphous materials that maintain a disordered atomic structure, characteristic of liquids of a very high viscosity, which behave like solids. The most common and technologically the most important group of glasses are the silicate glasses. Silicate glasses are made up of a network of tetra-hedra of four large oxygen ions with a silicon ion at the centre. Each oxygen is shared by two tetrahedra, giving the bulk composition of SiO_2. However, the basic silicate network can incorporate virtually all atoms of the periodic table of elements, and thus silicate glasses of numerous different compositions and properties can be obtained.

Special compositions of glasses containing the same compounds present in bones and tissue fluids (Na_2O, P_2O_5, CaO and SiO_2) are bioactive, which means that bioactive glasses have the ability to react chemically with living tissues, forming with them mechanically strong and lasting bonds [Hench, 1993; Yamamuro, 1990; Jones, 2001; Ducheyne, 1998]. Bioactive silica-based glasses are structurally based on tetrahedral units SiO_4^{4-}, where the central silicon atom with the external electronic configuration $3s^2 3p^2$ assumes a tetrahedral hybrid state sp^3 and contributes one electron to each bond. Consequently, two cases can occur; either:

1. each oxygen atom with electronic configuration $1s^2 2s^2 2p_x^2 2p_y^1 2p_z^1$ uses their two unpaired electrons in σ covalent bonds with two neighbour silicon atoms ("bridging oxygen," BO), or

2. each oxygen uses one unpaired electron in a σ covalent bond with the neighbour silicon atom, the other unpaired electron being available to ionic interaction with alkaline or alkaline-earth metals, the so-called network modifiers (Na^+, K^+, Ca^{2+}, Mg^{2+}, etc.), forming "non-bridging" oxygen (NBO) bonds [Galeener, 1979; Gaskell, 1991].

The presence of these cations results in a disruption of the continuity of the glass network. For this reason, NBOs play a key role in the bioactive response of these glasses [Serra, 2002]. After implantation, the surfaces of these materials in contact with body fluids give rise to the formation of a silica hydrogel layer that leads to subsequent crystallisation of the apatite-like phase. Hench et al. [Hench, 1972, 1993], proposed a theoretical model to explain the interfacial bonding mechanism of bioactive glasses in inorganic fluid environment.

The bioactivity process can be summarized in five steps:

1. rapid exchange of alkali or alkali-earth ions with H^+ or H_3O^+ from the solution;

2. loss of soluble silica in the form of $Si(OH)_4$ to the solution;

3. condensation and repolymerization of SiO_2-rich layer on the surface depleted in alkalis and alkaline-earth cations;

4. migration of Ca^{2+} and PO_4^{3-} groups to the surface through the SiO_2-rich layer forming a CaO-P_2O_5-rich film on top of the SiO_2-rich layer, followed by the growth of the amorphous CaO-P_2O_5-rich film by incorporation of soluble calcium and phosphorus from the solution;

5. crystallization of the amorphous CaO-P_2O_5 film by incorporation of OH^-, CO_3^{2}, or F^- anions from the solution to form a mixed hydroxy-carbonate-fluorapatite layer.

Melting and sol-gel are two well-known methods of producing glasses. The first bioactive melt-derived silicate glass was reported by Hench [Hench, 1972]. The synthesis process consisted of mixing the analytical grade precursors, such as $Ca(H_2PO_4)_2$, Na_2CO_3, $CaCO_3$, MgO and SiO_2, and melting them in a platinum crucible, in air, at 1500 °C for one hour, to ensure a good homogeneity and fining. Next, the product was quenched in water in order to produce a glass frit which was crushed and reduced to glass powder.

The synthesis process of sol-gel glasses [Vallet, 2001] consists of the hydrolysis and polycondensation of tetraethyl orthosilicate (TEOS) and triethyl phosphate (TEP), catalyzed by $Ca(NO_3)_2$. Next, the solution is introduced into a hermetically-sealed container where it is allowed to gel at room temperature and then aged at 60–70 °C for three days. Drying is carried out at 150 °C under high humidity conditions. The dried gel is then ground and sieved. Glass pieces are processed combining uniaxial and isostatic pressing and, then, exposed to a stabilization treatment carried out by heating at around 700 °C.

At present, the main clinical applications of bioactive glasses are in the middle ear surgery to replace ossicles damaged by chronic infection, in replacing the iliac crest and in vertebral surgery, periodontal repair, maxilofacial reconstruction and orthopaedic repair [Hench, 2005]. The production of bioactive glass films can also be of interest with a view to using them in coat load-bearing orthopaedic devices, since they improve dramatically the adhesion of the coated implants to the living bone tissue.

11.4.3 Coating Deposition Techniques

The coating of implants with bioceramic materials is a complex process. The clinical success of the coated implants is greatly determined by the quality and the endurance of the fixation at the interface, which largely depends on the purity, the particle size, the chemical composition, the thickness of the coating and the surface morphology of the substrate.

Different coating methods have been applied to the production of bioactive coatings, such as plasma spray [Dyshlovenko, 2006], biomimetic method [Tanahashi, 1994], magnetron sputtering [Thian, 2007], sol-gel [Vallet-Regí, 2001] and electroforetic deposition [Ducheyne, 1986]. Among them, pulsed laser deposition (PLD) is an attractive technique due to its unique advantages, such as good adhesion, possible deposition of materials with high melting-point, absence of contamination, possibility of preparing coatings in a reactive environment, ability

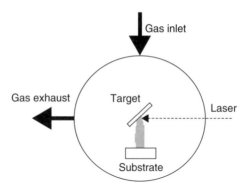

Figure 11.18. Detailed scheme of the experimental setup for the production of bioactive coatings.

to transfer the stoichiometry of very complex materials to the coating, and a fine control of the film properties [Cotell, 1993; Serra, 1995; Arias, 1998; González, 2003].

This technique is based on melting and vaporization of a starting material source with the required composition for obtaining the final coating. A high-power laser is used to ablate the target material, forming a plasma plume which is directed towards the substrate to be coated. The ablation process is carried out in vacuum or in a gas environment favouring the chemical reaction of the highly excited ablated particles with other gaseous precursors [Chrisey, 1994; Miller, 1998]. Several processing conditions, such as the substrate temperature, gas pressure and laser parameter influence the growth rate and the physico-chemical properties of the coatings which can be finely tuned.

Figure 11.18 depicts a typical experimental system for pulsed laser deposition. The target and the substrate are situated inside a high vacuum chamber equipped with a turbomolecular pump to ensure low base pressures. The chamber consists of a heatable substrate holder and a target rotation system to avoid the crater formation and, therefore, improve the homogeneity of the coating. Several measuring devices ensure the control of the processing pressure, gas flow and substrate temperature. The beam of an excimer or Nd:YAG laser is focussed onto the target through a transparent window, and its energy density and pulse repetition rate are also controlled.

The physical mechanisms involved in the different stages of the PLD process, which are quite complex [Chrisey, 1994; Miller, 1998], are the following:

1. interaction of the laser with the target, where the photons are absorbed by the target material leading to the evaporation of the material;
2. expansion of the ablated products, where an ablation plume is generated, consisting of a hot plasma at high pressure which expands in presence of ambient gases;

3. interaction of the plasma plume with the substrate, leading to a large number of gas phase collisions;
4. nucleation and growth of the coating on the substrate surface, which also involve many processes such as atomic deposition, re-evaporation, cluster nucleation and growth, species diffusion within the surface and cluster dissociation.

All these mechanism can be influenced by the experimental processing conditions and would influence the physicochemical properties of the coatings.

11.4.4 Physico-Chemical Properties of the Hydroxyapatite and Substituted Apatite Coatings

The pulsed laser deposition method has been successfully applied to the preparation of high quality crystalline HA coatings on Ti substrates [Cotell, 1993; Arias, 1997; Solla, 2005], enhancing greatly the film properties in comparison with those obtained by commercial techniques such as plasma spray [García-Sanz, 1997]. Also, silicon substituted apatite [Solla, 2007] coatings have been recently obtained by laser ablation.

Thin films of hydroxyapatite (HA) and Si substituted hydroxyapatite (Si-HA) were grown from ablation targets made with different mixtures of commercial carbonated HA and Si powder (0, 2.5, 5, 7.5 and 10% at.), in the presence of a water vapour atmosphere. The physico-chemical properties of the coatings and the incorporation of the Si into the HA structure were studied by Fourier Transform Infrared Spectroscopy (FTIR), X-Ray Diffraction (XRD) and X-Ray Photoelectron Spectroscopy (XPS).

Figure 11.19 shows the FTIR spectra of the coatings, exhibiting the presence of the main absorption bands corresponding to carbonated hydroxyapatite, being:

1. 1000–1200, 960 and 560 cm^{-1} attributed to asymmetric stretching, symmetric stretching and asymmetric bending vibrations of PO_4^{3-} groups respectively,
2. 1400–1500 and 875 cm^{-1} that are assigned to asymmetric stretching and bending vibration of CO_3^{2-} groups respectively, and
3. an absorption at 3575 cm^{-1} corresponding to the stretching vibration of the OH^- groups that are present in the HA structure.

With the progressive introduction of the amount of Si in the ablation target, many differences were observed in the IR spectra:

1. an intense reduction of the intensity of the OH^- stretching absorption band at 3575 cm^{-1},
2. an evident diminution of the intensity of the CO_3^{2-} asymmetric stretching,

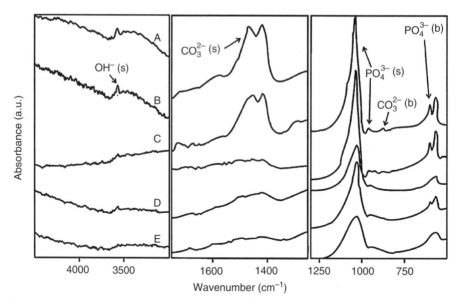

Figure 11.19. FTIR spectra divided in the main areas of interest of the following samples: A) HA (0% Si), B) HASi25 (2,5% Si), C) HASi50 (5% Si), D) HASi75 (7,5% Si) and E) HASi100 (10% Si). The target ablation was carried out with an ArF excimer laser (193 nm), operating at 175 mJ and a pulse repetition rate of 10 Hz. The films were deposited in a water vapour atmosphere (0,45 mbar), and the Si and Ti substrates were maintained at 460 °C during the film growth. From [Solla, 2007].

3. a peak at 940 cm^{-1} present in all the samples except the Si free one (HA), iv) a small shoulder at 690 cm^{-1} and,

4. a small peak at 670 cm^{-1} for samples with high Si content. These phenomena have been reported before by many authors [Gibson, 1999; Botelho, 2002; Arcos, 2004].

Figure 11.20 shows the XRD spectra of the HA, HASi50, and HASi100 coatings. All of the coatings produced exhibit a crystalline structure and present exactly the same reflection peaks as the reference coating of pure HA, thus it is clear that all the coatings have a hydroxyapatite structure and no secondary phases were formed due to the Si substitution. The only difference that arises is that, when the Si content is increased, XRD reflections become less intense. This phenomenon indicates a progressive loss of cristallinity along with the Si substitution, a fact that is coherent with the FTIR analysis aforementioned.

The chemical surface characterization of the Si-HA coatings was performed by XPS analysis which provides very useful information on the Si bonding environment. The quantification of the Si transferred to the coating from the initial ablation target is summarised in Table 11.3. It is clear that as the concentration of Si in the ablation target increases, the quantity of Si transferred to the coating

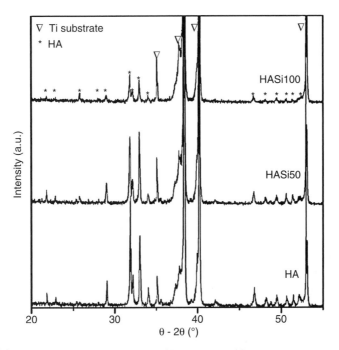

Figure 11.20. XRD pattern of different thin films deposited by PLD in a water vapour atmosphere. From [Solla, 2007].

TABLE 11.3. Quantified XPS Results for the Different Si-HA Coatings Obtained by PLD in a Water Vapour Atmosphere

Sample	Composition (at. %)				Binding energy (eV ± 0.2 eV)		
	Si	Ca	P	$Ca/(P + Si)$	Si_{2p}	Ca_{2p}	P_{2p}
HA	—	26.0	12.5	2.08	—	347.3	133.3
HASi25	1.6	25.8	11.2	2.01	100.9	347.3	133.2
HASi50	2.6	23.8	12.2	1.61	101.7	347.2	133.1
HASi75	2.8	24.7	12.3	1.63	101.4	347.5	133.5
HASi100	3.4	20.7	9.8	1.57	101.5	347.4	133.3

From [Solla, 2007].

increases as well, on the other hand, the quantities of Ca and P remain almost constant within the error range, the exception being a small decrease in the HASi100 sample.

Considering their binding energy, the energies of the Si_{2p}, Ca_{2p}, P_{2p} and O_{1s} peaks are all constant within the error range. The P_{2p} peak is centered at $133,3 \pm 0.2\,eV$, and the O_{1s} is at $531.1 \pm 0.2\,eV$ and $532.7 \pm 0.2\,eV$, the binding energies that can be assigned to apatite groups. The Si_{2p} energies around $101.6 \pm 0.2\,eV$

can be assigned to Si atoms present in an ortho-silicate group, SiO_4^{4-}. Most of the literature references of chemically-synthesised Si-HA show that since the SiO_4^{4-} groups occupy PO_4^{3-} sites, the commonly agreed mechanism is a subsequent substitution of PO_4^{3-} by SiO_4^{4-} groups [Gibson, 1999; Arcos, 2004].

On the other hand, there is evidence that when CO_3^{2-} groups are present in the HA structure, it is more accurate to talk about a competition between the CO_3^{2-} and SiO_4^{4-} groups for the PO_4^{3-} sites, rather than about a 1:1 substitution of phosphate by silicate [Marques, 2001]. Given that the percentage of P does not vary importantly with the Si substitution, and that FTIR results show an important decrease of the CO_3^{2-} groups in the coatings as the Si is incorporated, it can be stated that in this case and with the deposition technique, SiO_4^{4-} groups are preferentially displacing the CO_3^{2-} rather than the PO_4^{3-} groups, although substitution of phosphate by silicate may occur at some extent.

In fact, when the Ca and P values remain very stable from the HA pure to the HASi75 coating, the HASi100 sample has slightly lower values for these atoms, indicating that the phosphate by silicate substitution is gaining importance in this case. Another indicator that is very frequently used in the field of bioactive calcium phosphates is the Ca to P ratio (Ca/P), and its purpose is to be compared with the Ca/P ratio that is found in the mineral part of the bone (1.67). In the study of Si-HA this factor is replaced by the Ca/P+Si ratio [Gibson, 1999], and it is usually intended to remain the closest to the Ca/P ratio of the bone. On the other hand, it has been found that with this technique silicate groups are principally replacing carbonate instead of phosphate groups, and consequently the Ca/P+Si ratio grows with the Si incorporation as the quantity of P is not being altered.

11.4.5   Physico-Chemical Properties of the Bioactive Glass Coatings

Comprehensive works on bioactive glass coatings grown by Pulsed Laser Deposition (PLD) have been reported [D'Alessio, 1999; Serra, 2001; Liste, 2004a, 2004b]. The physico-chemical properties of the coatings should be carefully tuned by changing the processing conditions in order to obtain films with optimized properties and adequate biological response. To illustrate this fact, in this section, the dependence of the composition of the bulk glasses used as ablation targets on the properties and bioactivity of the bioactive glass coatings is reported.

Different compositions of bulk glasses (Table 11.4) in the system SiO_2-Na_2O-K_2O-CaO-MgO-P_2O_5-B_2O_3 have been used to grow bioactive coatings. Although the PLD coating technique allows the congruent transfer of the bulk glass composition to the coatings [Liste, 2004a, 2004b], FTIR and XPS analyses show important differences between the bulk and the film bonding configuration. Figure 11.21 shows the FTIR spectra of a typical bioactive glass target and the corresponding coating. In both cases, the main peaks of bioactive glass [González, 2002; Serra, 2002] are observed:

1. a band at 1000–1200 cm^{-1} assigned to the Si-O-Si asymmetric stretching vibration,

TABLE 11.4. Composition of Bioactive Glasses (wt%)

	Na_2O (wt%)	K_2O (wt%)	CaO (wt%)	P_2O_5 (wt%)	MgO (wt%)	B_2O_3 (wt%)	SiO_2 (wt%)
BG42	20	10	20	3	5	—	42
BG50	15	15	15	—	2	3	50
BG55	21	9	8	4	2	1	55
BG59	10	5	15	3	5	3	59

From [Liste, 2004b].

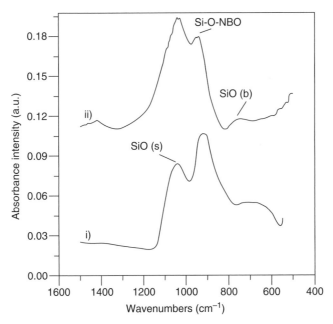

Figure 11.21. Typical FTIR spectra of i) bulk glass (BG50) used as ablation target and ii) the corresponding PLD coating. From [Liste, 2004b].

2. a weak band at around $750\,cm^{-1}$ associated to the Si-O-Si bending vibration, and
3. an additional band at $900–950\,cm^{-1}$, corresponding to the non-bridging silicon-oxygen groups (Si-O-NBO).

Two important variations in the IR bands can be remarked:

1. the peak associated to the Si-O-Si stretching vibration shifts to lower wavenumbers and its intensity increases, and
2. the band intensity assigned to the Si-O-NBO groups decreases.

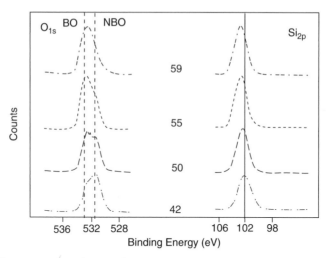

Figure 11.22. XPS spectra of O_{1s} and Si_{2p} photoelectrons for different bioactive glass coatings. From [Liste, 2004b].

These facts evidence the rearrangement of the coating silica network towards a more organized structure.

In order to clarify the chemical bonding of the bioactive glass coatings, X-ray induced Photoelectron Spectroscopy (XPS) analyses were carried out. The O_{1s} and Si_{2p} photoelectron spectra of different coatings are shown in Figure 11.22. The O_{1s} photopeak can be studied to provide useful information on the bonding states of the oxide ions in the silicate glasses. The curve fitting of the O_{1s} photoelectron spectrum shows two well-resolved peaks around 532 and 530 eV, associated with the bridging silicon-oxygen groups (BO) and non-bridging silicon-oxygen groups (NBO) respectively. When the silica content of the bioactive glasses is increased, two important effects are observed: variations in the intensity of the BO and NBO bands; and the shift of the binding energies of the photopeaks (O_{1s} and Si_{2p}) towards higher values.

These results are associated with a change in the chemical environment of the silica structural unit. The vitreous silica structure is formed by SiO_4 tetrahedra connected by BO groups. If network modifiers (Na^+, K^+, Ca^{2+} and Mg^{2+}) are added to the silica network, the peak intensity corresponding to BO groups decreases due to the formation of NBO groups. The ions induce structural changes leading to the breaking of Si-O-Si groups between adjacent tetrahedra. The charge is compensated by the formation of NBO groups which are associated with a nearby alkali or alkali earth ion.

Fourier Transform Infrared and X-ray Induced Photoelectron Spectroscopies show that the physico-chemical properties of the bioactive glass coatings grown by laser ablation can be finely tuned. Therefore, the reactivity of the glass coatings can be controled when they are exposed to physiological fluids. This fact is demonstrated [Liste, 2004b] by a comparative *in vitro* study of the bioactive behaviour

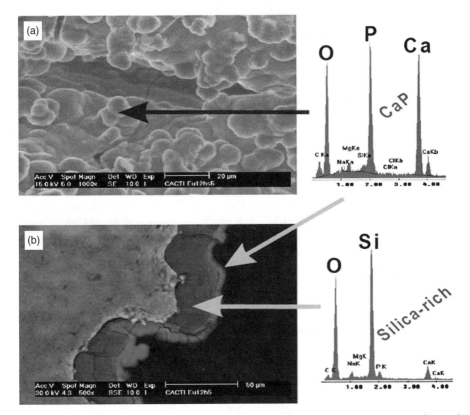

Figure 11.23. Typical SEM micrographs and EDS analyses of bioactive glass coating (BG42Y) on biomorphic SiC after immersion in SBF for 72 h. Longitudinal axis (a) and cross-section (b) images are shown. The coating processing conditions were: laser energy density 4.17 J/cm², repetition rate 10 Hz, substrate temperature 200 °C. From [Borrajo, 2006].

of the PLD-coatings and bulk glasses in simulated body fluid (SBF), with ion concentrations and pH nearly equal to those of human plasma [Kim, 2001], keeping the specimens in an incubator at 36.5 °C for 72 hours.

Figure 11.23 shows the products which originated after the immersion of beech-based SiC coated with a 30 µm glass coating. The SEM micrograph and EDS spectrum (Figure 11.23a) demonstrate the formation of a calcium phosphate (CaP) layer on the top of the coating. The presence of the silica-rich layer which corroborates the bioactivity of the PLD glass coatings deposited on biomorphic SiC is observed in the SEM cross-section (Figure 11.23b). This fact is the first sign of the possible bioactivity of this material *in vivo* [Borrajo, 2006].

SEM/EDS analyses of the *in vitro* tested bulk glasses and of the corresponding PLD coatings after immersion in SBF are shown in Figure 11.24. The bulk glasses present the three expected layers (CaP-rich, CaP-SiO₂ mixture and SiO₂-rich), which correspond to different phases of the chemical routes of the

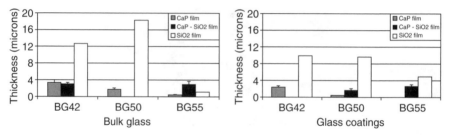

Figure 11.24. Thickness of CaP, CaP-SiO$_2$ and silica-rich layers of the bulk and the coatings of bioactive glasses. From [Liste, 2004b].

bioactivity process explained previously. When the silica content of the glass decreases, the thickness of the CaP-rich layer increases and, therefore, the glass bioactivity increases due to the presence of the network modifiers.

The coatings grown by PLD show a similar behaviour to the bulk glasses but two important differences can be observed: a decrease in the layer thickness and a shifting of the *in vitro* bioactivity behaviour with respect to the bulk glass. It should be noted that a similar bioactivity grade was found for the bulk BG50 and the coating BG42.

This phenomenon corroborates that the growth of thin film bioactive materials should be carefully controlled because their composition and bonding configuration play an important role in their bioactivity, which is a key factor for the development of biomedical products with an adequate biological response.

11.5   BIOCOMPATIBILITY STUDIES FOR MEDICAL APPLICATIONS

11.5.1   *In Vitro* Cytotoxicity Test

Testing for cytotoxicity is a good first step towards ensuring the biocompatibility of this innovative product for its application in biomedical devices. A negative result indicates that the material is either free of harmful extractables or contains a quantity of them insufficient to cause serious effects in isolated cells under exaggerated conditions. However, it is certainly not, on its own merit, evidence that a material can be considered biocompatible; it is simply a first step. On the other hand, a positive cytotoxicity test result can be taken as an early warning sign that a material contains one or more extractable substances that could be of clinical importance. In such cases, further investigation is required to determine the utility of the material.

The biological response of the human osteoblast-like cell line MG-63 (ATCC number CRL 1427) to different biomorphic SiC types and to SiC ceramics coated with bioactive materials has been determined [de Carlos, 2006; Borrajo, 2006]. The cells were regularly grown in EMEM (EBSS) culture medium supplemented with 2 mM glutamine, 1% non-essential amino acids and 10% foetal bovine serum (FBS), at 37 °C in a humidified atmosphere with 5% of CO$_2$.

The test on extracts was conducted by measuring the cellular activity in response to different concentrations of solvents extracted from the materials using the MTT cell proliferation assay. This test is a colorimetric assay system that measures the reduction of the yellow tetrazolium salt MTT (3-[4,5-dimethyl-tihazol-2-yl]-2,5-diphenyl tetrazolium bromide) into an insoluble purple formazan crystals by the mitochondrial enzyme succinate dehydrogenase, only present in viable cells. This cellular reduction involves the pyridine nucleotide cofactors NADH and NADPH. The formazan crystals formed were solubilized and the resulting coloured solution was quantified using a scanning multiwell spectrophotometer, with the absorbance values being proportional to the number of viable cells [Selvakumaran, 2005].

Extracts were prepared by rolling bioSiC pieces (coated and uncoated) in EMEM culture medium supplemented with 10% foetal calf serum for 90 hours at 37°C. Different concentrations of these extracts were incubated for 24 hours with MG-63 human osteoblast. Extracts obtained from Polyvinyl chloride discs and Thermanox plastic cover slips were used as positive and negative controls respectively. The extracts were diluted with EMEM to give 10, 20, 30, 50 and 100% of the original concentration.

MG-63 osteoblast-like cells were seeded at a concentration of 6×10^5 cells per mL, grown to confluent layers in 96-well tissue culture plates in a final volume of 0.1 mL of culture medium per well. The different concentrations of the extracts were incubated with cells for 24 hours. Four wells per substrate and extract concentration were used. After incubation, cellular activity was quantified by using the MTT assay as previously described.

Normalized solvent extraction tests summarize the MG-63 osteoblast-like cell activity after the incubation with different concentrations of the extracts obtained from uncoated biomorphic SiC ceramics and coated bioSiC ceramics with bioactive glass (Figure 11.25). Thermanox plastic cover slips were used as a negative control and PVC were used as a positive toxic control. A bulk bioactive glass and Ti6Al4V were used as references for the test. As can be seen, PVC extract (positive for cytotoxicity) reduced cell viability in a progressive manner for all tests, thus validating the solvent extraction method and dilution procedures.

In the solvent extraction test for uncoated samples (Figure 11.25a), the reference materials present an absorbance similar to Thermanox slips, which means the absence of cytotoxicity. All the extracts did not significantly affect the cellular activity at any of the concentrations tested, not even at 100% concentration. Only a slight detrimental effect was found for sapeli and eucalyptus wood ceramics for extract concentrations of 30 and 50% that disappears at 100% of extract concentration. Nevertheless, the differences fall within the statistical range. This result suggests that bioSiC is free of harmful extractable substances or has, at least, an insufficient quantity of it to cause serious effects in cell monolayers under *in vitro* culture conditions.

The same behaviour was found for the coated biomorphic SiC. Cells incubated in the bioactive glass-coated SiC ceramics extracts (Figure 11.25b) showed

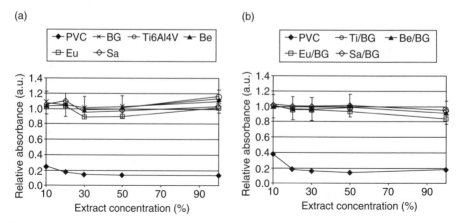

<u>Figure 11.25.</u> Relative cellular activity from the solvent extraction test for (a) uncoated bioSiC and (b) coated bioSiC with bioactive glass by PLD. PVC: positive toxic control; BG: bioactive glass, Ti6Al4V: titanium alloy; Be, Eu, Sa: beech, eucalyptus and sapelli; Ti/BG: Ti coated with bioactive glass; Be/BG, Eu/BG, Sa/BG: beech, eucalyptus and sapelli-based SiC ceramics coated with bioactive glass. From [Borrajo, 2006].

a proliferation rate similar to that of the Thermanox control and reference materials. The hydroxyapatite and Si-substituted apatite coated SiC extracts also did not affect cellular activity at any of the concentrations tested (not shown), their values being similar to the ones obtained with the Thermanox cytotoxic negative control. A slight decrease in cellular activity could be observed for the 100% concentration of the coated SiC ceramic extract, which was not over the significant limits.

There were no significant differences when the cellular attachment response of the cells to the wood-based biomorphic SiC ceramics, uncoated or coated with bioactive materiales (hydroxyapatite, Si-substituted apatite and bioactive glass), was compared to the one exhibited by reference materials Ti6Al4V and bulk bioactive glass. These facts demonstrate that bioinspired ceramics coated with bioactive materials do not have any negative effects on the activity of MG-63 osteoblast-like cells and this fact is very promising for biomedical applications.

11.5.2 *In Vitro* Cell Attachment and Proliferation Tests

The ability of bioSiC to sustain cell attachment and growth was assessed by seeding MG-63 human osteoblast-like cells on the material [de Carlos, 2006; Borrajo, 2006]. The attachment of the cells on beech, eucalyptus and sapelli-based biomorphic SiC ceramics coated with bioactive glass was compared by means of SEM (Figure 11.26). Provided that the same number of cells (10^5 cells/cm^2) has been seeded, the attachment of the cells occurs in the same way in all tested samples. None of the wood-based SiC ceramics, coated or uncoated, exhibited a higher rate of cell attachment and growth. The cells attached in the same efficient

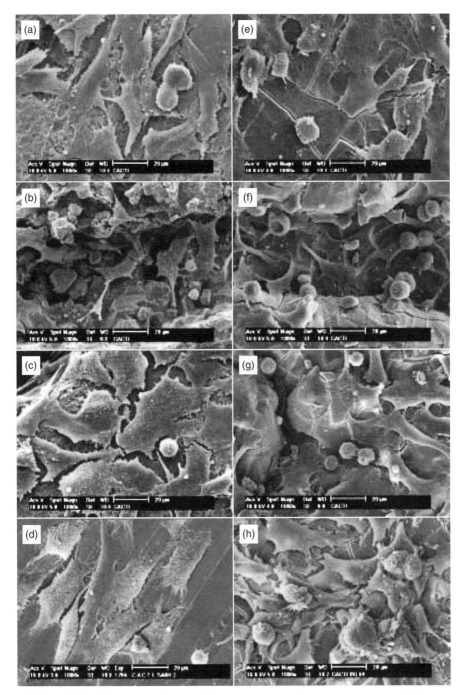

Figure 11.26. Scanning electron microscopy images showing the comparative attachment of MG-63 osteoblast-like cells six hours after seeding on uncoated (A, B, C) or bioactive glass-coated (E, F, G) beech (A, E), eucalyptus (B, F) and sapelli (C, G)—based biomorphic SiC ceramics, and on two reference materials, Ti6Al4V (D) and bioactive glass (H). Magnifications in all cases are 1000×. From [de Carlos, 2006].

manner to all parts of the ceramic pieces, including naturally occurring pores and channels present on axial (A and C, upper right angles) and longitudinal (B, F) sections of uncoated (A, B, C) or coated (E, F, G) samples. At this magnification (1000x), where cell details become more conspicuous, flattened and spread osteoblastlike cells were observed, which began to penetrate and colonise the inner surface of the existing pores. Rounded cells involved in cellular division events could be seen attached to the outer surface on the inside of the pores. After six hours, cells spread out, displaying a flat configuration and a normal morphology. Expansion of the cytoplasm was already visible and completely spread with, in many cases, the bulge of the nucleus and surface microvilli very apparent, with profusion of filopodia, as well as with larger cytoplasm extensions (lamellipodia). Neighbouring cells maintained physical contact with one another through cytoplasm extensions. No evidence of any major deleterious or cytotoxic responses was observed. The appearance of the MG-63 cells was the same as the one observed on two reference materials, namely Ti6Al4V (D) and bulk bioactive glass (H). Similar results were found for cell attachment and growth on biomorphic SiC ceramics coated with hydroxyapatite and silicon substituted apatite by seeding Saos-2 cells on the material.

11.5.3 *In Vivo* Biocompatibility Studies

To explore the potentials of the biomorphic silicon carbide and bioactive coatings for medical applications, *in vivo* biocompatibility studies were carried out [Borrajo, 2007; González, 2008]. Caution must be increased when comparing *in vitro* models to the multi-factorial and multi-cellular *in vivo* environment. Cells invariably behave differently *in vivo* due to the presence of other cell types, numerous cell signalling factors, the extracellular matrix and physiological differences in terms of mechanical stress, blood flow and 3D growth.

To assess the bioSiC as a biocompatible material, *in vivo* experiments by implantation in the femur condyles of twelve rabbits were carried out. The new bone growth on the periphery of bioSiC cylinders (3.9 mm diameter and 10 mm length) and inside the pores was evaluated and compared with titanium pieces implanted as controls. After 12 weeks of implantation, specimens for histological examination using Optical Microscopy were taken. Samples were fixed in formaldehyde solution, dehydrated by increasingly concentrated alcohols, infiltrated with and embedded in Technovit 7200 VLC, and processed by the cutting-grinding method. Final 30 μm sections were stained with Levai-Laczko staining technique.

Histological (Figure 11.27) examination showed the new bone formation around the implants and inside the SiC porous matrix, without the appearance of fibrous tissue on the bone-implant boundary and without any relevant inflammatory reaction. There were no significant differences between the bone density formed around the SiC implants and Ti controls (Table 11.5).

Additional analysis of SEM micrographs (Figure 11.28) showed the presence of trabecular bone in the central pores of the ceramics, reaching an average

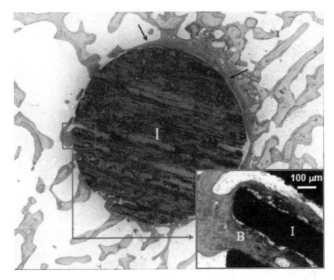

Figure 11.27. Optical images of the histological section of a bioSiC implant retrieved 12 weeks after implantation. At the periphery of the implant (I), the newly formed bone is in close contact with the bioSiC (arrows) and in continuity with the surrounding trabechular host bone. Inset: Newly formed bone (B) is growing inside the SiC porous matrix (I).

TABLE 11.5. Bone Density Evaluated on the Periphery of the BioSiC Implants Fabricated from Pine and Sapelli. Titanium Implants were Used as Reference Materials

	Bone density (mm²)					
Implant	1	2	3	4	5	Av.
Pine-SiC	0.48	0.48	0.41	0.49	0.36	0.45
Sapelli-SiC	0.42	0.27	0.34	0.32	0.15	0.31
Titanium	0.25	0.36	0.32	0.45	0.35	0.35

growth of 700 μm inside the implant. Different zones around the implant and inside the pores were identified as tissue in the first steps of the bone mineralization process by backscattering electron detection and Energy Dispersive X-Ray Spectroscopy (EDS) analysis. Ca/P ratio values close to those of trabecular bone were found. As the last step, the *in vivo* biocompatibility of biomorphic SiC was demonstrated.

11.6. CONCLUSIONS

This chapter introduces the development of an innovative bio-inspired product, based on silicon carbide ceramics coated with bioactive materials, as new

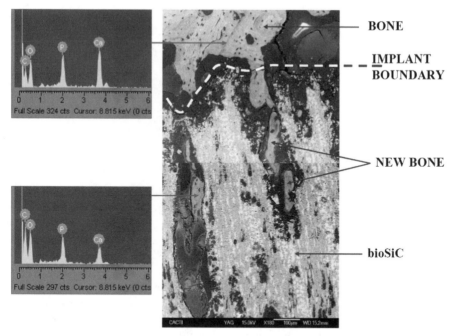

Figure 11.28. Typical cross-section SEM micrograph of a sapelli based SiC ceramics implanted for 12 weeks in rabbit femur. The porosity of the implant is colonized by the bone tissue with high concentrations of Ca and P (see EDS spectra).

biomedical devices. The complete technological process, from the production of the bio-derived silicon carbide and the bioactive coating deposition to *in vitro* and *in vivo* biocompatibility studies, is presented.

Bio-derived silicon carbide ceramics, fabricated from cellulose templates, are light, tough and high-strength materials that mimic the natural structure of the bone. The physico-chemical properties of the bioactive coatings can be tuned to provide the optimum reactivity in contact with the host tissues, improving the fixation and osteointegration.

This study demonstrates that this ceramic product, formed by the bioSiC and the bioactive coating, presents a good biological response, being similar to titanium controls but additionally, it incorporates the unique property of interconnected porosity, which is colonized by the bone tissue.

The versatility of the SiC fabrication process and the coating deposition method opens the door to a whole new generation of metal-free implants for biomedical applications. In particular, to solve problems of degenerative disc diseases, bioinspired SiC is being investigated for the fabrication of intersomatic vertebral cages for posterior fusion surgery of the lumbar column with the purpose to immobilize spinal segments and in an attempt to obtain a higher fusion rate, restore disc height and indirectly decompress neural structures.

Further studies on the design of highly performing bioinspired materials from marine precursors (such as algae and marine plants) are carrying out. These new inspirational templates are interesting for the development of novel bioceramics with adequate microstructures for highly porous tissue-engineered scaffolds.

Finally, the focus should be on advanced bioactive scaffolds enabling internal growth of tissue and the site specific delivery of bioactive signalling factors (temperature, pH, concentration, internal stimuli, etc). The approaches should include issues such as drug delivery devices, remodelling of large bone defects and improved tissue-biomaterial interface.

ACKNOWLEDGMENTS

The authors would like to express their deepest gratitude to B. León, J. Serra, S. Chiussi, A. de Carlos, F. Muñoz, M. López, J.P. Borrajo, S. Liste, E. Solla, V. Castaño, J. Rodiño, N. Miño F. M. Varela Feria and J. Ramirez Rico. The financial sup-port of the Spanish administration (projects MAT2004-02791, PGIDIT03TMT30101PR, PGIDT05PXIC30301PN, MAT 2006-13005 and PETRI 2006-0658) is gratefully acknowledged.

REFERENCES

Anderson JM. 2004. Inflammation, wound healing and the foreign-body response. In: Ratner BD, Hoffman AS, Schoen FJ, Lemons JE, editors. Biomaterials science: An introduction to materials in medicine. 2nd eds. London: Elsevier. p 302–304.

Andersson ÖH, Karlsson KH. 1990. Development of bioactive glasses and glass-ceramics. In: Yamamuro T, Hench LL, Wilson J, editors. 1990. Handbook of bioactive ceramics. Boca Raton, FL: CRC Press. p 143–153.

Arcos D, Rodríguez-Carvajal J, Vallet-Regí M. 2004. Silicon incorporation in hydroxylapatite obtained by controlled crystallization. Chem. Mater. 16: 2300–2308.

Arellano-López AR, Martínez Fernández J, Varela Feria FM, Sepúlveda RE, López Robledo MJ, Llorca J, Pastor JY, Presas M, Faber KT, Kaul VS, Pappacena KE, Wilkes TE. 2007. Processing, microstructure and mechanical properties of SiC-based ceramics via naturally derived scaffolds. In: Tandon R, Wereszczak A, Lara-Curzio E, editors. Mechanical Properties and Performance of Engineering Ceramics and Composites II. New Jersey: Wiley and Sons. p 635–650.

Arellano-López AR, Martínez-Fernández J, González P, Domínguez C, Fernández-Quero V, Singh M. 2004. Biomorphic SiC: a New Engineering Ceramic Material. International Journal of Applied Ceramic Technology 1: 95–100.

Arias JL, García-Sanz FJ, Mayor MB, Chiussi S, Pou J, León B, Pérez-Amor M. 1998. Physicochemical properties of calcium phosphate coatings produced by pulsed laser deposition at different water vapour pressures. Biomaterials 19:883–888.

Arias JL, Mayor MB, García-Sanz FJ, Pou J, León B, Pérez-Amor M, Knowles JC. 1997. Structural analysis of calcium phosphate coatings produced by pulsed laser deposition at different water-vapour pressures. J. Mater. Sci. Mater. Med. 8: 873–876.

Balas F, Pérez-Pariente J, Vallet-Regí M. 2003. *In vitro* bioactivity of silicon-substituted hydroxyapatites. J. Biomed. Mat. Res. A 66: 364–375.

Bartlett RW, Nelson WE, Halden FA. 1967. Influence of Carbon Transport Kinetics on Solution Growth of Beta-Silicon Carbide Crystals. J. Electrochem. Soc. 114: 1149–1154.

Bhagat RB, Singh M. 1994. Modeling of infiltration kinetics for the *in-situ* processing of inorganic composites. In: Singh M and Lewins D, editors. In-Situ Composites: Science and Technology. The Minerals, Metals and Materials Society. Pittsburgh: CSA. p 135–148.

Black J, Hastings G. 1998. In: Handbook of Biomaterial Properties. London: Chapman & Hall.

Borrajo JP, González P, Serra J, Liste S, Chiussi S, León B, de Carlos A, Varela-Feria FM, Martínez-FernánDez J, de Arellano-López AR. 2006. Biomorphic Silicon Carbide Ceramics Coated with Bioactive Glass for Medical Applications. Materials Science Forum 514–516: 970–974.

Borrajo JP, Serra J, González P, León B, Muñoz FM, López M. 2007. *In vivo* evaluation of titanium implants coated with bioactive glass by pulsed laser deposition. J. Mater. Sci.: Mater Med DOI 10.1007/s10856-007-3153-z.

Botelho CM, Lopes MA, Gibson IR, Best SM, Santos JD. 2002. Structural analysis of Si-substituted hydroxyapatite: Zeta potential and X-ray photoelectron spectroscopy. J. Mat. Sci. Mat. Med 13: 1123–1127.

Brunette DM, Tengvall P, Textor M, Thomsen L (eds.). 2001. Titanium in medicine. Berlin: Springer.

Byrne CE, Nagle DE. 1996. Carbonized Wood and Materials Formed Therefrom. US Patent 6051096 and US Patent 61224028 (1998).

Byrne CE, Nagle DE. 1997. Cellulose-derived Composites. A New Method for Materials Processing, Mat. Res. Innovat. 1: 137–145.

Carlisle EM. 1970. Silicon: a possible factor in bone calcification. Science 167: 279–280.

Chrisey DB, Hubler GK. 1994. Pulsed laser deposition of thin films. New York: John Wiley & Sons.

Cotell CM. 1993. Pulsed laser deposition and processing of biocompatible hydroxylapatite thin films. Applied Surface Science 69: 140–148.

Crank J. 1975. The mathematics of diffusion. Oxford: Clarendon Press.

D'Alessio L, Teghil R, Zaccagnino M, Zaccardo I, Ferro D, Marotta V. 1999. Pulsed laser ablation and deposition of bioactive glass as coating material for biomedical applications. Appl. Surf. Sci. 138–139: 527–532.

Darimont GL, Cloots R. 2002. *In vivo* behaviour of hydroxyapatite coatings on titanium implants: a quantitative study in the rabbit. Biomaterials 23: 2569–2575.

de Carlos A., Borrajo JP, Serra J, González P, León B. 2006. Behaviour of MG-63 osteoblast-like cells on wood-based biomorphic SiC ceramics coated with bioactive glass. J. Mater. Sci: Mater. Med. 17: 523–529.

Ducheyne P, Van Raemdonck W, Heughebaert JC, Heughebaert M. 1986. Structural analysis of hydroxyapatite coatings on titanium. Biomaterials 7: 97–103.

Ducheyne P. 1998. Stimulation of biological function with bioactive glass. MRS Bulletin, November: 43–49.

Dyshlovenko S, Pawlowski L, Roussel P, Murano D, Le Maguer A. 2006. Relationship between plasma spray operational parameters and microstructure of hydroxyapatite coatings and powder particles sprayed into water. Surface and Coatings Technology 200: 3845–3855.

Wheeler E. 2001. In: Jurgen Buschow KH (ed.).Wood: Macroscopic Anatomy, in Encyclopedia of Materials: Science and Technology. New York: Elsevier. p 9653–9658.

Fitzer E, Fritz W, Gadow R. 1985. Development of Silicon-Carbide Composites. Chem. Ing. Tech. 57: 737–746.

Fitzer E, Gadow R. 1986. Fiber-Reinforced Silicon-Carbide. Am. Ceram. Soc. Bull. 65: 326–335.

Galeener FL. 1979. Bands limits and the vibrational spectra of tetrahedral glasses. Physical Review B 19: 4292–4297.

García-Sanz FJ, Mayor MB, Arias JL, Pou J, León B, Pérez-Amor M. 1997. Hydroxyapatite coatings: A comparative study between plasma-spray and pulsed laser deposition techniques. J. Mater. Sci. Mater. Med. 8: 861–865.

Gaskell PH. 1991. Models for the structure of amorphous solids. In: Zarzycki J, editor. Glass and Amorphous Materials. Materials Science and Technology. Weinheim: VCH. p 175–274.

Gauthier O, Bouler JM, Aguado E, Pilet P, Daculsi G. 1998. Macroporous biphasic calcium phosphate ceramics: influence of macropore diameter and macroporosity percentage on bone ingrowth. Biomaterials 19: 133–139.

Gern FH, Kochendorfer R. 1997. Liquid silicon infiltration: Description of infiltration dynamics and silicon carbide formation. Composites Part A—Applied Science and Manufacturing 28: 355–364.

Gerwien ML. 1986. In: Warucke R, editor. Gmelin Handbook of Inorganic Chemistry (8th Edition). Berlin: Springer-Verlag.

Gibson IR, Best SM, Bonfield W. 1999. Chemical characterization of silicon-substituted hydroxyapatite. J. Biomed. Mater. Res. 44: 422–428.

Gibson LJ, Ashby MF. 1988. Cellular Solids: Structure & Properties. 2nd ed. Cambridge: Cambridge University Press.

Gnesin GG, Raichenko AI. 1973. Kinetics of the liquid-phase reactive sintering of silicon carbide. Poroshkovaya Metallurgiya 5: 35–43.

González P, Borrajo JP, Serra J, Chiussi S, León B, Martínez-Fernández J, Varela-Feria FM, de Arellano-López AR, de Carlos A, Muñoz FM, López M, Singh M. 2008. A New Generation of Bio-derived Ceramic Materials for Medical Applications. Journal of Biomedical Materials Research: Part A DOI: 10.1002/jbm.a.31951.

González P, Serra J, Liste S, Chiussi S, León B, Pérez-Amor M, Martínez-Fernández J, De Arellano-López AR, Varela-Feria FM. 2003. New biomorphic SiC ceramics coated with bioactive glass for biomedical applications. Biomaterials 24: 4827–4832.

González P, Serra J, Liste S, Chiussi S, León B, Pérez-Amor M. 2002. Ageing of pulsed laser deposited bioactive glass films. Vacuum 67: 647–651.

González P, Borrajo JP, Serra J, Liste S, Chiussi S, León B, Semmelmann K, de Carlos A, Varela-Feria FM, Martínez-FernánDez J, de Arellano-López AR. 2004. Extensive

Studies on Biomorphic SiC Ceramics Properties for Medical Applications. Key Engineering Materials 254–256: 1029–1032.

Grabmaier J, Ciszek TF. 1981. Silicon. Berlin: Springer-Verlag.

Greil P. 2001. Biomorphous ceramics from lignocellulosics. J. Eur. Ceram. Soc. 21: 105–118.

Greil P, Lifka T, Kaindl A. 1998. Biomorphic Cellular Silicon Carbide Ceramics from Wood: I. Processing and Microstructure. J. Eur. Ceram. Soc. 18: 1961–1973.

Greil P, Lifka T, Kaindl A. 1998a. Biomorphic Cellular Silicon Carbide Ceramics from Wood: II. Mechanical Properties. J. Eur. Ceram. Soc. 18: 1975–1983.

Greil P. 1999a. Near Net Shape Manufacturing of Ceramics. Mater. Chem. Phys. 61: 64–68.

Gutierrez-Mora F, Goretta KC, Varela-Feria FM, Arellano López AR, Martínez Fernández J. 2005. Indentation Hardness of Biomorphic SiC. International Journal of Refractories, Metals and Hard Materials 23: 369–374.

Hallab NJ, Jacobs JJ, Katz JL. 2004. Orthopedic applications. In: Ratner BD, Hoffman AS, Schoen FJ, Lemons JE, editors. Biomaterials science: An introduction to materials in medicine. 2nd eds. London: Elsevier. p 526–555.

Helsen JA, Breme HJ, editors. 1998. Metals as Biomaterials. Biomaterials Science and Engineering Series. New York: John Wiley & Sons.

Hench LL, Splinter RJ, Alen WC, Greenlee TK. 1972. Bonding mechanisms at the interface of ceramic prosthetic materials. J. Biomed. Mater. Res. 5: 117–141.

Hench LL, Wilson J, editors. 1993. An introduction to bioceramics. Singapore: World Scientific.

Hench LL. 2005. Repair of skeletal tissues. In: Hench LL, Jones JR, editors. Biomaterials, artificial organs and tissue engineering, Cambridge: CRC Press. p. 126–127.

Hon MH, Davis RF, Newbury DE. 1980. Self-Diffusion of Si-30 in Polycrystalline Beta-SiC. J. Mater. Sci. 15: 2073–2080.

Hon MH, Davis RF. 1979. Self-Diffusion of C-14 in Polycrystalline Beta-SiC. J. Mater. Sci. 14: 2411–2421.

Hong JD, Davis RF, Newbury DE. 1981. Self-Diffusion of Si-30 in Alpha-SiC Single-Crystals. J. Mater. Sci. 16: 2485–2494.

Hong JD, Davis RF. 1980. Self-Diffusion of C-14 in High-Purity and N-Doped Alpha-SiC Single-Crystals. J. Am. Ceram. Soc. 63: 546–552.

Jones JR. 2001. Biomedical materials for new millennium: perspective on the future. Mat. Sci. & Technol. 17: 891–900.

Jones JR. 2005. Scaffolds for tissue engineering. In: Hench LL, Jones JR, editors. Biomaterials, artificial organs and tissue engineering, Cambridge: CRC Press. p. 204–209.

Kardashev BK, Burenkov Y, Smirnov BI, de Arellano-Lopez AR, Martinez-Fernandez J, Varela-Feria FM. 2005. Internal Friction and Young's Modulus of a Carbon Matrix for Biomorphic Silicon Carbide Ceramics. Physics of the Solid State 47: 886–890.

Kardashev BK, Smirnov BI, de Arellano-Lopez AR, Martinez-Fernandez J, Varela-Feria FM. 2006. Elastic and anelastic properties of SiC/Si ecoceramics. Materials Science and Engineering A 428: 225–232.

Kaul VS, Faber KT, Sepúlveda R, de Arellano López AR, Martínez-Fernández J. 2006. Precursor selection and its role in the mechanical properties of porous SiC derived from Wood. Materials Science and Engineering A 428: 225–232.

Kim HM, Miyazaki T, Kokubo T, Nakamura T. 2001. Revised Simulated Body Fluid. Key Eng. Mat. 192–195: 47–50.

Kleykamp H, Schumacher G. 1993. The Constitution of the Silicon-Carbon System. Ber. Bunsen-Ges Phys. Chem. 97: 799–805.

Kokubo T, Tanahashi M, Yao T, Minoda M, Miyamoto T, Nakamura T, Yamamuro T. 1993. Bioceramics 6: 327.

Lai W, Garino J, Ducheyne P. 2002. Silicon excretion from bioactive glass implanted in rabbit bone. Biomaterials 23: 213–217.

Liste S, González P, Serra J, Borrajo JP, Chiussi S, León B, Pérez-Amor M, García-López J, Ferrer FJ, Morilla Y, Respaldiza MA. 2004a. Study of the stoichiometry transfer in pulsed laser deposition of bioactive silica-based glasses. Thin. Solid. Films. 453 –454: 219–223.

Liste S, González P, Serra J, Serra C, Borrajo JP, Chiussi S, León B. 2004b. *In Vitro* Bioactivity Study of PLD-Coatings and Bulk Bioactive Glasses. Key Engineering Materials 254–256: 355–358.

Mangonon PL. 1999. The Principles of Materials Selection for Engineering Design. 1st ed. Upper Saddle River, New Jersey: Prentice-Hall.

Marques PAAP, Magalhaes MCF, Correia RN, Vallet-Regí M. 2001. Synthesis and characterisation of silicon-substituted hydroxyapatite. Key Engineering Materials 192–195: 247–250.

Martínez Fernández J, Muñoz A, de Arellano López AR, Varela Feria FM, Domínguez-Rodríguez A, Singh M. 2003. Microstructure-mechanical property correlation in siliconized silicon carbide ceramics. Acta Materialia 51: 3259–3275.

Martínez-Fernández J, Varela-Feria FM, Singh M. 2000a. High temperature compressive mechanical behavior of biomorphic silicon carbide ceramics. Scripta Materialia 43: 813–818.

Martínez-Fernández J, Varela-Feria FM, Domínguez Rodríguez A, Singh M. 2000. Microstructure and thermomechanical characterization of biomophic silicon carbide-based ceramics. In: H. Mostaghaci, editor. Environment Conscious Materials— Ecomaterials. Canadian Institute Mining Metallurgy Petroleum. p. 733–740.

Miller JC, Haglund RF. 1998. Laser ablation and desorption. San Diego: Academic Press.

Muñoz A, Martínez Fernández J, Singh M. 2002. J. Europ. Ceram. Soc. 22: 2719–2725.

Ota T, Takahashi M, Hibi T, Ozawa M, Suzuki H. 1995. Biomimetic Process for Producing SiC Wood. J. Am. Ceram. Soc. 78: 3409–3414.

Pampuch R, Bialoskorski J, Walasek E. 1987. Mechanism of Reactions in the Si + C System and the Self-Propagating High-Temperature Synthesis of Silicon-Carbide. Ceram. Int. 13: 63–68.

Pampuch R, Walasek E, Bialoskorski J. 1986. Reaction-Mechanism in Carbon Liquid Silicon Systems at Elevated-Temperatures. Ceram. Int. 12: 99–106.

Panshin AJ, deZeeuw C. 1980. Textbook of Wood Technology. New York: McGraw-Hill.

Pérez-Granados AM, Vaquero MP. 2002. Silicon, aluminium, arsenic and lithium: Essentiality and human health implications. J. Nutr. Health. Aging 6: 154–162.

Phule PP, Askeland DR. 2002. The Science and Engineering of Materials. New York: Wadsworth Publishing.

Porter AE, Patel N, Skepper JN, Best SM, Bonfield W. 2003. Comparison of *in vivo* dissolution processes in hydroxyapatite and silicon-substituted hydroxyapatite bioceramics. Biomaterials 24: 4609–4620.

Presas M, Pastor JY, Llorca J, de Arellano López AR, Martínez-Fernández J, Sepúlveda R. 2005. Mechanical Behavior of Biomorphic Si/SiC Porous Composites. Scripta Materialia 53: 1175–1180.

Presas M, Pastor JY, Llorca J, de Arellano-López AR, Martínez-Fernández J, Sepúlveda R. 2006. Microstructure and Fracture Properties of Biomorphic SiC. International Journal of Refractory, Metals and Hard Materials 24: 49–54.

Ratner BD, Hoffman AS, Schoen FJ, Lemons JE, editors. 2004. Biomaterials science: An introduction to materials in medicine. 2nd ed. London: Elsevier.

Rice RW. 2000. Porosity of Ceramics. New York: Marcel Dekker Inc.

Rice RW. 1996. Evaluation and extension of physical property-porosity behaviour with minimum solid area models. J. Mat. Sci. 31: 102–118.

Sangsuwan P, Tewari SN, Gatica JE, Singh M, Dickerson R. 1999. Reactive infiltration of silicon melt through microporous amorphous carbon preforms. Metal Mater Trans A 30: 933–944.

Scace RI, Slack GA. 1959. Solubility of Carbon in Silicon and Germanium. J. Chem. Phys. 30: 1551–1555.

Selvakumaran J, Jell G. 2005. A guide to basic cell culture and applications in biomaterials and tissue engineering. In: Hench LL, Jones JR, editors. Biomaterials, artificial organs and tissue engineering, Cambridge: CRC Press. p. 225–226.

Serra J, González P, Chiussi S, León B, Pérez-Amor M. 2001. Processing of bioglass coatings by excimer laser ablation. Key Engineering Materials 192–195: 635–638.

Serra J, González P, Liste S, Chiussi S, León B, Pérez-Amor M, Ylänen HO, Hupa M. 2002. Influence of the non-bridging oxygen groups on the bioactivity of silicate glasses. J. Mat. Sci. Mat. Med. 13: 1221–1225.

Serra P, Palau J, Varela M, Esteve J, Morenza JL. 1995. Characterization of hydroxyapatite laser ablation plumes by fast intensified CCD-imaging. Journal of Materials Research 10: 473–478.

Shin DW, Park SS, Choa YH, Niihara K. 1999. Silicon/Silicon Carbide Composites Fabricated by Infiltration of a Silicon Melt into Charcoal. J. Am. Ceram. Soc. 82: 3251–3256.

Sikavitsas VI, Temenoff JS, Mikos AG. 2001. Biomaterials and bone mechanotransduction. Biomaterials 22: 2581–2593.

Singh M, Martínez–Fernández J, de Arellano–López AR. 2003. Environmentally Conscious Ceramics (Ecoceramics) from Natural Wood Precursors. Current Opinions on Solid State & Material Science 7: 247–254.

Singh M, Salem JA. 2002. Mechanical properties and microstructure of biomorphic silicon carbide ceramics fabricated from wood precursors. Journal of the European Ceramic Society 22: 2709–2717.

Singh M. 2000. Environment conscious ceramics (ecoceramics). Ceram. Sci. Eng. Proc. 21: 39–44.

Sinha S, Jhalani A, Ravi MR, Ray A. 2000. Modeling of pyrolysis in wood: a review. J. Solar Energy Society of India 10: 41–62.

Smirnov BI, Burenkov YA, Kardashev BK, Varela Feria FM, Martínez Fernández J, de Arellano-López AR. 2003. Temperature Dependences of Young's Modulus of Biormophic Silicon Carbide Ceramics. Physics of the Solid State 45: 482–485.

Solla EL, Borrajo JP, González P, Serra J, Liste S, Chiussi S, León B, Pérez-Amor M. 2005. Plasma assisted pulsed laser deposition of hydroxylapatite thin films. Appl. Surf. Sci. 248: 360–364.

Solla EL, Borrajo JP, González P, Serra J, Liste S, Chiussi S, León B, García López J. 2007. Study of the composition transfer in the pulsed laser deposition of silicon substituted hydroxyapatite thin films. Applied Surface Science, doi:10.1016/j.apsusc.2007.02.116.

Tanahashi M, Yao T, Kokubo T, Minoda M, Miyamoto T, Nakamura T, Yamamuro T. 1994. Apatite coating on organic polymers by a biomimetic process. J. Am. Ceram. Soc. 77: 2805–2808.

Thian ES, Huang J, Best SM, Barber ZH, Bonfield W. 2007. Silicon-substituted hydroxyapatite: The next generation of bioactive coatings. Materials Science and Engineering C 27: 251–256.

Vallet-Regí M. 2001. Ceramics for medical applications. J. Chem. Soc., Dalton Trans. 2: 97–108.

Varela-Feria FM., Ramírez-Rico J, de Arellano-López AR, Martínez-Fernández J, Singh M. 2007. Reaction-Formation Mechanisms and Microstructure Evolution of Biomorphic SiC. Accepted in *J. Mat. Science*.

Varela-Feria FM, Ramírez-Rico J, Martínez-Fernández J, de Arellano-López AR, Singh M. 2005. Infiltration and Reaction-Formation Mechanism and Microstructural Evolution of Biomorphic SiC Fabricated by Si-Melt Infiltration. Ceramic Transactions 177: 93–101.

Varela-Feria FM, Martínez-Fernández J, de Arellano López AR, Singh M. 2002b. Precursor Selection for Properties Optimization in Biomorphic SiC Ceramics. Ceramics Engineering Science Proceedings 23: 681–685.

Varela-Feria FM, Martínez–Fernández J, de Arellano–López AR, Singh M. 2002. Low Density Biomorphic Silicon Carbide: Microstructure and Mechanical Properties. Journal of the European Ceramic Society 22: 2719–2725.

Varela-Feria FM, López Pombero S, Martínez-Fernández J, de Arellano López AR, Singh M. 2001. Creep Resistant Biomorphic Silicon-Carbide Based Ceramics. Ceramics Engineering Science Proceedings 22: 135–145.

West JK, Clarck AE, Hall MB, Turner GE. 1990. *In vivo* bone-bonding study of bioglass-coated titanium alloy. In: Yamamuro T, Hench LL, Wilson J, editors. 1990 Handbook of bioactive ceramics. Boca Raton, FL: CRC Press. p 161–166.

Williams DF, editor. 1992. Medical and Dental Materials. Materials Science and Technology, vol. 14. New York: VCH Publishers Inc.

Yamamuro T, Hench LL, Wilson J, editors. 1990. Handbook of bioactive ceramics. Boca Raton, FL: CRC Press.

Zhou H, Singh RN. 1995. Kinetics Model for the Growth of Silicon-Carbide by the Reaction of Liquid Silicon with Carbon. J. Am. Ceram. Soc. 78: 2456–2462.

Zollfrank C, Sieber H. 2004. Microstructure and Phase Morphology of Wood Derived. Biomorphous SiSiC-Ceramics. J. Eur. Ceram. Soc. 24: 495–506.

Zollfrank C, Sieber H. 2005. Microstructure evolution and reaction mechanism of. Biomorphous SiSiC ceramics. J. Am. Ceram. Soc. 88: 51–58.

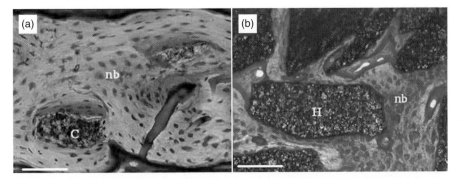

Figure 2.14. Histological micrographs showing carbonate apatite granule (A) and sintered hydroxyapatite (HAP) granule (B) 12 weeks after implantation in rat calvaria (toluidine blue staining). Bar = 100 μm. C: carbonate apatite; H: sintered HAP; nb: new bone; pb: parietal bone. The sizes of the carbonate apatite and HAP granules before implantation were similar.

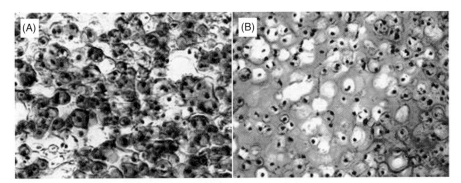

Figure 6.1. Histological analysis of chondrocytes photoencapsulated in PEG hydrogels with 15% macromer after 8 weeks *in vitro*. A. Stained with Safranin-O which stains proteoglycans red and B. Stained with Masson trichrome which stains collagen blue (×200).

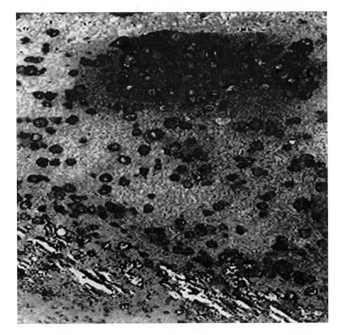

Figure 6.4. Toluidine blue stain of C/GP gel with 30 lg BP demonstrated an abundance of chondrocytes encompassed by a territorial cartilagenous matrix. (10×)

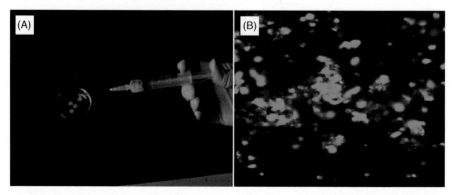

Figure 6.5. A. Demonstrates the injectability of the hdyrogel using a 21 guage needle. B. Human foreskin fibroblast cells encapsulatedin chitosan-ammonium hydrogen phosphate thermogels after 3 days in culture. Cells stained green (live cells) and cells stained red (dead cells).

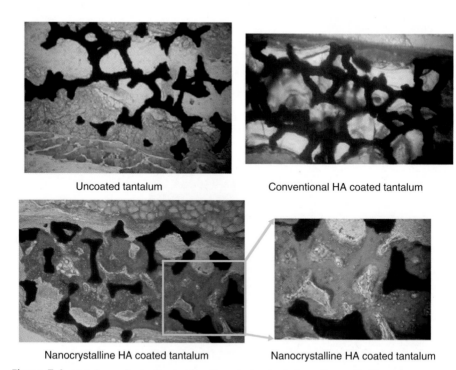

Uncoated tantalum   Conventional HA coated tantalum

Nanocrystalline HA coated tantalum   Nanocrystalline HA coated tantalum

Figure 7.4. Histology of rat calvaria after 6 weeks implantation of uncoated tantalum, conventional HA coated tantalum and nanocrystalline HA coated tantalum. Greater amounts of new bone formation occurs in the rat calvaria with implanting nanocrystalline HA coated tantalum compared to uncoated and conventional HA coated tantalum. Red represents new mineralized bone and blue represents unmineralized tissue. Adapted and redrawn from [131].

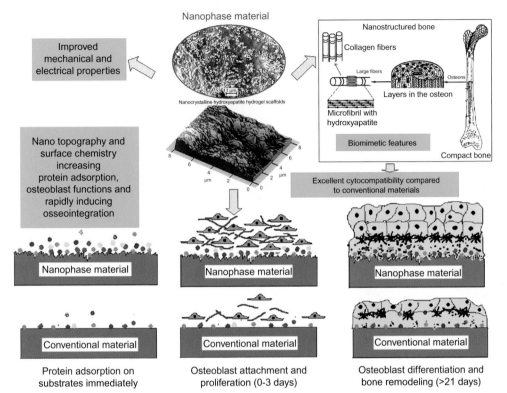

Figure 7.13. Schematic illustration of the proposed mechanism of the superior properties of nanomaterials over conventional materials to improve orthopedic applications. Compared to conventional micron-scale materials, nanomaterials have enhanced mechanical, cytocompatibility and electrical properties, which make them suitable for orthopedic and bone tissue engineering applications. The nano and bioactive surfaces of nanomaterials mimicking bones can promote greater amounts of protein adsorption and efficiently stimulate more new bone formation than conventional materials. Redrawn from [135–137].

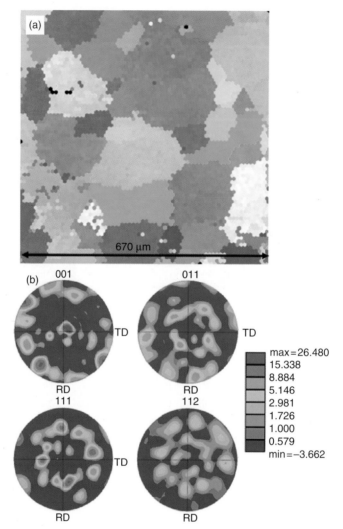

Figure 9.7. (a) Pseudo-colored OIM map from the cross-section of the tensile-tested LENS™ deposited TNZT sample viewed parallel to the tensile axis. The β grains are clearly visible in this map. (b) {001}, {011}, {111}, and, {112} β pole figures from the same sample exhibiting a strong <001> texture. [Rajarshi Banerjee et al. *Laser Deposited Ti-Nb-Zr-Ta Orthopedic Alloys* (J. Bio. Mater. Res., 78A (2), 2006), 298.]

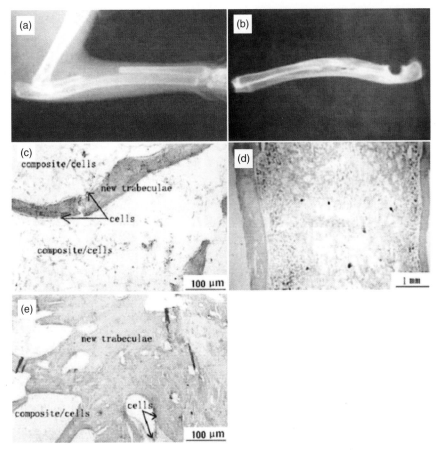

Figure 16.4. Results of nano-HA/collagen/PLA composite scaffold in a rabbit model. (See text for full caption.)

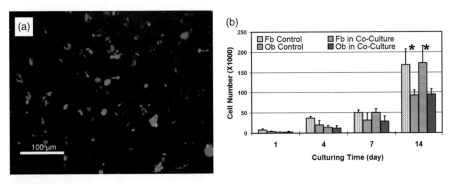

Figure 17.2. Effects of Heterotypic Cellular Interactions on Cellular Phenotypes. (See text for full caption.)

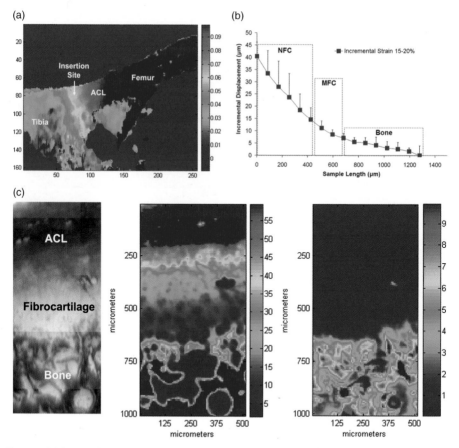

Figure 17.3. Structure-Function Relationship at the Ligament-to-Bone Insertion Site. (See text for full caption.)

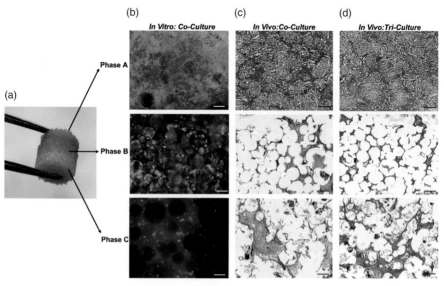

Figure 17.4. Biomimetic Multiphasic Scaffold for Interface Tissue Engineering: Design, *In Vitro* and *In Vivo* Testing. (See text for full caption.)

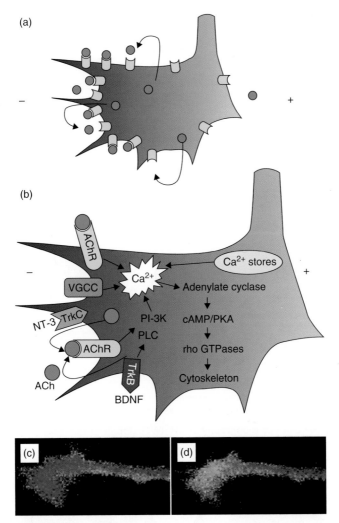

(a)

(b)

AChR

Ca²⁺ stores

Ca²⁺

VGCC

Adenylate cyclase

NT-3 TrkC

PI-3K

cAMP/PKA

PLC

AChR

rho GTPases

TrkB

Cytoskeleton

ACh

BDNF

(c)

(d)

Figure 18.5. Growth cone changes due to an EF (McCaig et al. 2005). Used with permission from The American Physiological Society.

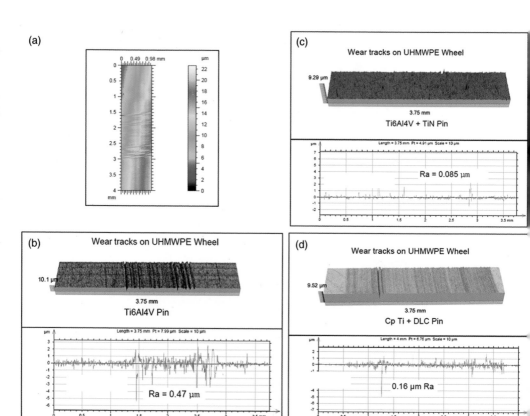

Figure 21.4. Wear surface topography of UHMWPE (initial surface finish 0.15 μm Ra typical) against bare metal and coated counter faces. (See text for full caption.)

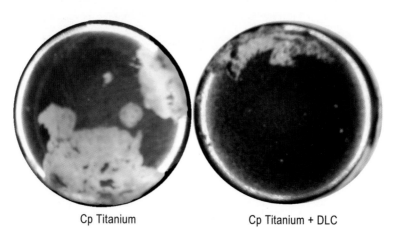

Cp Titanium Cp Titanium + DLC

Figure 21.11. Thrombus deposits on the material surfaces during the *in vivo* blood compatibility experiments. (See text for full caption.)

12

IONOMER GLASSES: DESIGN AND CHARACTERIZATION

Artemis Stamboulis and Fei Wang

University of Birmingham, Metallurgy and Materials, Edgbaston, Birmingham, UK

Contents

12.1 Overview   411
12.2 Introduction   412
12.3 Ionomer Glass Compositions   414
12.4 Design   415
12.5 Structure of Ionomer Glasses   417
    12.5.1 Structural Characterization of Ionomer Glasses by Solid State
        MAS-NMR Spectroscopy   418
12.6 Crystallization of Ionomer Glasses   423
12.7 Cation Substitution in Ionomer Glasses   427
12.8 Conclusions and Future Perspectives   429
    Acknowledgments   429
    References   429

12.1 OVERVIEW

Ionomer glasses are an important type of glasses used for the formation of glass polyalkenoate cements (glass ionomers), a popular type of white dental fillings,

Advanced Biomaterials: Fundamentals, Processing, and Applications, Edited by Bikramjit Basu, Dhirendra S. Katti, and Ashok Kumar
Copyright © 2009 The American Ceramic Society

the setting of which is based on an acid–base reaction. The acid attacks and degrades the glass structure, releasing metal cations that cross-link the carboxyl groups on the polyacrylic acid chains, forming a cement with a microstructure consisting of reacted and unreacted glass particles that are embedded in a poly-salt matrix. Although the main application of glass polyalkenoate cements is in dentistry, these cements may have potential as bone cements eliminating a lot of problems associated with conventional acrylic cements. The development of ionomer glasses is therefore an important part of current research in this area as the structure and the properties of the glass would influence the application range of glass polyalkenoate cements. There are several types of ionomer glasses that have been developed since the discovery of glass polyalkenoate cements by Wilson and Kent in the late 1960's. The most common type of ionomer glasses is fluorine containing aluminosilicate glasses.

This chapter will give an overview of what has been achieved until today in this area and will focus on the design and structural characterisation of fluorine containing alumino-phospho-silicate ionomer glasses. The chapter starts with an introduction to the subject, which is followed by a brief description of Zachariasen's Random Network Theory and Lowenstein's glass formation rules based on which the ionomer glasses were designed. The chapter continues with a review on the structural characterisation including original results from the author's own studies the last four years based on advanced multinuclear solid state MAS-NMR spectroscopy. The chapter closes with a reference to the crystal-lisation behaviour of ionomer glasses and recent work on the cation substitution and its effect on the structure of glasses.

12.2   INTRODUCTION

Glass ionomer cement or glass poly-alkenoate cement is a dental cement produced by mixing a powder prepared from a calcium alumino-silicate glass with an aqueous solution of poly-acrylic acid. The calcium alumino-silicate glass that usually contains fluoride ions is called an *ionomer* glass. Glasses for this application generally contain 20–36 wt.% SiO_2, 15–40% Al_2O_3, 0–35% CaO, 0–10% $AlPO_4$, 0–40% CaF_2, 0–5% Na_3AlF_6 and 0–6% AlF_3 [1]. During the setting reaction of the cement, the ionomer glass provides the ions that leach from the glass as a result of glass surface dissolution under the polymeric acid attack that leads eventually to the polymer chains cross-linking as shown in Figure 12.1 [2].

Glass ionomer cements were first described by Alan Wilson and Brian Kent in 1971 and presented a natural extension to the zinc polycarboxylate cements that became available in the late 1960s [3–8]. The first commercial dental cements were launched in 1975. Their mechanical properties were far more inferior compared to the materials available today [8, 9]. The glass component in dental cements is of an alumino-silicate type containing Ca and fluoride ions. The glasses can be made by mixing the appropriate oxides and fusion of ingredients in the temperature range of 1200 °C to 1590 °C, depending on the composition. The final

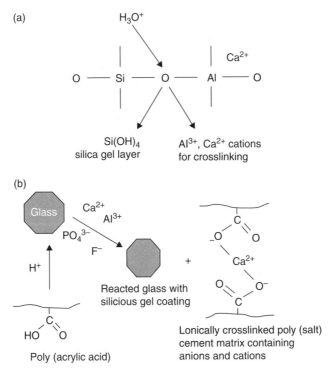

Figure 12.1. Schematic illustration of A: acid degradation of an alumino-silicate network and B: setting reaction in a glass ionomer cement [2].

form is usually a coarse glass frit that results from the quenching of the melt either onto a metal plate and then into water or directly into water. The glass is then ground further by dry milling in a ball mill or a gyro mill to a particle size less than 45 μm for a filling grade cement or less than 15 μm for a fine grained lutting cement. The main criterion for the design of the glasses is their basic character that would compensate for the low acidity of polyacrylic acid. Often, the reactivity of the glasses needs to be reduced by etching of the glass particles with 5% aqueous acetic acid or annealing of the glass at temperatures in the range of 400 °C to 600 °C depending on the composition. There is a large number of ionomer glass compositions that have been studied as cement formers. An important advantage of the ionomer glasses is that under appropriate heat treatments, they crystallise into an apatite phase that makes the glass-ceramics biocompatible and promising for use in restoring and replacing hard tissues in orthopaedic and dental fields. Hill et al. developed a series of glasses that crystallise into needle-like fluorapatite and mullite phases that interlock with each other giving rise to high fracture toughness values [10, 11].

This chapter aims to give an overview of the structure of ionomer glasses starting from the design of the glasses and finishing with the characterisation emphasising advanced techniques used to elucidate the presence of complex species within the glass network.

12.3   IONOMER GLASS COMPOSITIONS

Four main types of ionomer glasses have been used for cement forming:

1. Alumino silicate glasses, that have been mainly studied by Wilson and co-workers [4, 5, 12] in the early 1970's and are based on the systems SiO_2-Al_2O_3-CaO or SiO_2-Al_2O_3-CaF_2;
2. Aluminoborate glasses studied by Combe et al. [13–15] based mainly on the system Al_2O_3-B_2O_3-ZnO-ZnF_2;
3. Zinc silicate glasses based on the systems CaO-ZnO-SiO_2 or Al_2O_3-ZnO-SiO_2 and
4. Alumino-phospho-silicate glasses based on the system SiO_2-Al_2O_3-P_2O_5-CaO-CaF_2.

Among the glasses with interesting properties were the aluminoborate glasses formulated by Combe et al. [14]. These glasses can undergo hydrolysis in the presence of aqueous environment, which can be controlled by appropriate heat treatments resulting in controlled reactivity of the glass ionomer cements and enhancing compressive strength [13, 15]. However, the reported compressive strengths were not comparable to aluminosilicate glass based ionomer cements and therefore the aluminoborate glasses were abandoned for cement formation [8]. Zinc silicate glasses were investigated by Hill and co-workers [16, 17] and the resulting glass ionomer cements exhibited high strength. The main characteristic of the glass compositions was that in contrast to the aluminosilicate glasses, the ratio of Al/Si was not an important factor to determine the reactivity of the glasses. Depending on the role of zinc in the glass network whether it was a network modifier or an intermediate oxide, the network connectivity of the glass determined its reactivity and cement forming ability. According to Nicholson [8] these cements were very weak for clinical dental applications and as they could degrade by hydrolysis, the glasses did not prove to be successful substitutes for alumino-silicate glasses. However, Boyd et al. [17] recently reported that there is a great potential for the glasses to be used for bone cement formation. Especially when aluminium is considered a potent neuro-toxin promoting cellular oxidation, zinc-silicate glasses may have a positive effect *in vivo*, increasing the DNA of osteoblasts, which would result in increased bone mass. Furthermore, zinc is important for the function of the immune system and has been recognised as an antibacterial agent. All these factors make zinc-silicate glasses interesting materials that could be used for aluminium-free-cement formation.

In order to serve the purpose of this chapter, the authors will concentrate on the design and characterisation of the fluorine containing alumino-phospho-silicate glasses, which is the most important type of ionomer glasses used today for commercial glass ionomer cements.

12.4 DESIGN

The models for glass structures today are all based on the original ideas of Zachariasen and are grouped under the general term of Random Network Theory, although Zachariasen's first approach did not use the term random but vitreous network, instead. Zachariasen's rules were formed initially to explain the glass formation and were not intended to be used as a discussion of structural models. However, the rules expanded through wide usage and empirical observations into a set of rules for formulating models of glass structures. Table 12.1 summarises Zachariasen's rules, stating the conditions for the formation of a continuous 3D glass network with no indication, however of the degree of long range order, together with three modified rules for more complex glass systems [18, 19].

The model itself states that glass consists of random assemblies of SiO_4 tetrahedra that are linked in the corners to form chains. The simplest composition that is capable to form a glass network must consist only of such tetrahedra. This type of structure, however, would be resistant to an acid attack due to its neutral electron charge. By aluminium inclusion, the behaviour of the glass can be altered as aluminium provides only three positive charges and therefore, according to Loewenstein's rules [20], aluminium is forced to take up a four-fold coordination $[AlO_4]^{5-}$ creating a deficiency of positive charge in the aluminosilicate network, which means that a negative surplus charge resides in each SiO_4 tetrahedron (Figure 12.2). The negative charge can be compensated by cations like Ca^{2+}, Na^+, Mg^+ or Al^{3+} that can play the role of the glass network modifier.

Loewenstein's rules restrict the formation of the glass network in that, whenever two tetrahedra are linked by one oxygen bridge, the centre of only one of them can be occupied by aluminium, whereas the other centre must be occupied by silicon or another small ion of four or more electrovalence, like phosphorus. Similarly, whenever two aluminium ions are neighbours to the same oxygen anion

TABLE 12.1. Zachariasen's Rules for Glass Formation (Random Network Theory)

1. Each oxygen atom is linked to no more than two cations
2. The oxygen coordination number of the network cation is small
3. Oxygen polyhedra share only corners and not edges or faces
4. At least three corners of each oxygen polyhedra must be shared in order to form a 3D network
5. The samples must contain a high percentage of network cations which are surrounded by oxygen tetrahedral of triangles
6. The tetrahedral or triangles share only corners with each other
7. Some oxygens are linked only to two network cations and do not form further bonds with any other cations.

[19].

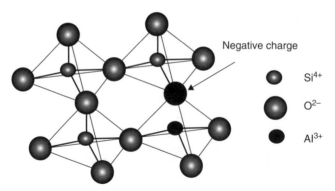

Figure 12.2. Structure of tetrahedral $[SiO_4]^{4-}$ with a Si/Al substitution ($[AlO_4]^{5-}$) yielding a negative surplus charge [74].

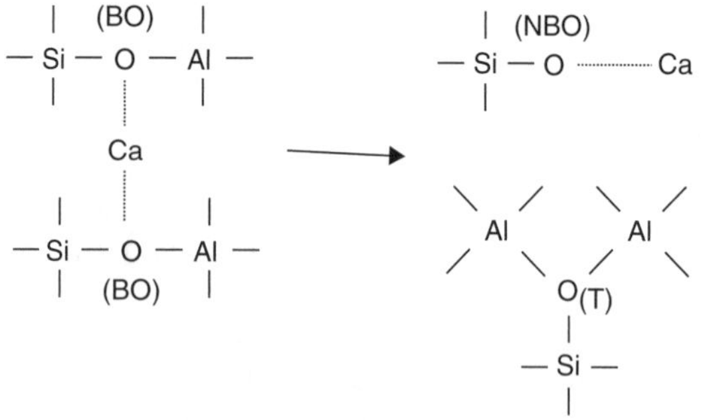

Figure 12.3. Cartoon of transformation of bridging oxygen (BO) to non-bridging oxygen (NBO) [21].

at least one of them must have a coordination number higher than four, that is, five or six, towards oxygen. The Al/Si ratio plays also an important role in the glass composition. The substitution of Si^{4+} by Al^{3+} can only happen up to a limit of 1:1 ratio, above which aluminium is no longer forced to adopt the tetrahedral coordination. All oxygens in the alumino-silicate glass network are bridging oxygens (BO). Inclusion of species such as CaO in the glass leads to the development of non-bridging oxygens (NBO). Stebbins and Zhu [21] reported the transformation of BO to NBO in simple aluminosilicate glass structures. They considered that if all Al remains as AlO_4 tetrahedra the new structural unit should be a tricluster notated as T in Figure 12.3.

On the other hand, if AlO_5 and AlO_6 are formed, the tricluster oxygen may itself behave as an NBO. CaO is considered therefore to be a network modifier as opposed to the network formers silicon and aluminium. However, aluminium can easily play both roles adopting a six-fold coordination and forcing the creation of sites in the glass structure, where additional oxygen atoms need to be present.

12.5 STRUCTURE OF IONOMER GLASSES

The glass compositions that will be described in this section are based mainly on the system SiO_2-Al_2O_3-P_2O_5-CaO-CaF_2. The properties of the glasses depend directly on the alkali content as well as the aluminium to silicon ratio and the fluorine content. Phosphorus also plays a role in the glass structure as the ratio of calcium to phosphorus determines the stoichiometry of the glass referenced to that of apatite. The structure of the glass as well as the composition, are very important parameters for the setting in glass polyalkenoate cements.

E. De Barra, S.G. Griffin and R.G. Hill [2, 22, 23] investigated the role of alkali metal ions, phosphate content and Al/Si ratio on the mechanical properties of glass polyalkenoate cements. The Al/Si ratio of the studied fluoro-phospho-alumino-silicate glass was not found to have a significant influence on the properties of glass polyalkenoate cements. One explanation is that phosphorus charge balances the aluminium within the glass network reducing the number of Al-O-Si bonds available for acid hydrolysis. Hill et al. [22] introduced another possible mechanism for glass hydrolysis that of P-O bonds hydrolysis, especially in the case of glasses with high phosphorus content or in the case of glasses that have undergone amorphous phase separation. In the case of simple alumino-silicate glasses (Figure 12.1a) the removal of charge balancing cations after the acid attack will lead to hydrolysis of Si-O-Al bonds in the glass network and the subsequent formation of a silica gel layer around the remaining glass particles and the release of Al^{3+} and Ca^{2+} available for crosslinking.

In the case of phosphorus containing alumino-silicate ionomer glasses on the other hand, the lack of alkali earth charge balancing cations because of the presence of Al-O-P bonds in the glass network will lead only to the release of aluminium and phosphorous in the glass network and the formation of a depleted glass layer instead. Hydrolysis of Si-O-Al bonds does not occur in this case. It is important to note, that it is likely that phosphate groups would compete with carboxylate groups for aluminium and calcium ions thereby inhibiting the cross-linking reaction in the cement matrix (Figure 12.1b). In the case of low phosphorus content the setting and working times were extended, whereas at higher content, the compressive strength and Young's modulus of the cement decreased. Introducing an alkali ion such as sodium would generally decrease the cement properties as sodium ions released from the glass disrupted the crosslinking reaction in the polysalt matrix. However, this would also depend on the cement formulation (powder to polymer liquid ratio) as well as the amount of sodium in the glass composition.

Most interesting however, is the role of fluorite in the glass structure and the mechanical properties of the resulting polyalkenoate cements [1, 24, 25]. Figure 12.4 illustrates the role of fluorine in the glass network. Whereas calcium disrupts the glass network forming NBO's and charge balancing the charge deficient AlO_4 tetrahedra, fluorine replaces BO's with non-bridging fluorine, thus facilitating melting of the glass at lower temperature and the acid attack during the setting reaction in the cement [12, 26, 27]. Furthermore, addition of fluorite increases the

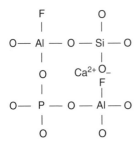

Figure 12.4. Schematic illustration showing the structural role of calcium and fluorine in ionomer glasses. The calcium ions disrupt the glass network forming non-bridging oxygens as well as charge balancing charge deficient AlO_4 tetrahedra. Fluorine replaces bridging oxygens and forms non-bridging fluorines [24].

reactivity of the glasses resulting in shorter working and setting times but leading to increased Young's modulus and compressive strength of cements. On the other hand, fracture toughness of cements is not influenced significantly by the addition of fluorite in the glass composition [24].

Generally, fluorine has two major roles in the glass structure. Firstly, it lowers the refractive index of the glass and enables a match to the polysalt matrix giving rise to optically translucent cements, a property of particular importance for anterior restorations at the front of the mouth, where the appearance of the cement is critical and secondly, it results in fluorine complexes present in the polysalt matrix that lead to fluoride release from the set cement that has a caries inhibitory role. Furthermore, Wood and Hill [28] observed a significant reduction in the glass transition temperature by increasing the fluorine content in a series of ionomer glasses of the composition $2SiO_2\text{-}Al_2O_3\text{-}(2\text{-}x)CaO\text{-}xCaF_2$. The reduction was attributed to the replacement of BOs by non-bridging fluorines reducing the network connectivity and allowing network motion at a lower temperature. However, recent MAS-NMR (Magic Angle Spinning Nuclear Magnetic Resonance) studies [29] showed that the above explanation was only partly true.

12.5.1 Structural Characterization of Ionomer Glasses by Solid State MAS-NMR Spectroscopy

Solid state MAS-NMR spectroscopy is a powerful technique to study the structure of complex amorphous and crystalline solid materials. For nuclei with spin $I = 1/2$, high resolution MAS-NMR spectra allow the observation of narrow lines by removing effects of dipolar and chemical shift anisotropies. This provides structural information on the local surroundings of nuclei in different environments. MAS-NMR of abundant quadrupolar nuclei, on the other hand, can provide some structural information for complex structures with the analysis of the isotropic chemical shift, the quadrupolar interaction, and their respective distributions. The half-integer spins $I > 1/2$ are subjected to strong quadrupolar interactions among the $2I$ allowed transitions and the central one $(+1/2, -1/2)$ is usually observed. The broadening of the central transition comes primarily from the second-order quadrupole interaction, which is not completely averaged to zero by the magic angle spinning (MAS) [30]. This produces an anisotropic line which shape depends on the site symmetry and width on the magnitude of the electric field gradient around the site. In MAS–NMR spectroscopy, the resolution and sensitivity when quadrupolar nuclei are studied, is often limited because of the inherent distribution of the quadrupolar coupling interactions, PQ, in disordered materials. It is well known that most anisotropic interactions to which non-quadrupolar nuclei are subject are effectively eliminated by MAS. However, MAS alone is incapable of completely narrowing the peaks of half integer quadrupolar nuclei such as ^{27}Al (I = 5/2). The effect of the second order quadrupolar coupling is a broadening of the peak to lower frequency relative to the isotropic chemical shift. Therefore, by employing high magnetic field there is an increase in Larmor frequency, v_0, which provides greater frequency dispersion in chemical shifts and decreases the second order quadrupolar effect on the nuclei [31].

In the case of ionomer glasses, the useful information obtained from a MAS-NMR experiment is mainly information on the coordination states of the elements in study, the local bonding environment and the information on the next nearest neighbours to the elements in study. The authors will refer only to information obtained from ^{27}Al, ^{31}P, ^{29}Si and ^{19}F MAS-NMR experiments. MAS-NMR studies [29] of a series of glasses based on the composition 2SiO$_2$-Al$_2$O$_3$-(2-x) CaO-xCaF$_2$ showed that the increase in the fluorine content resulted in the formation of F-Ca(n) species (Figure 12.5) around –150 ppm where n is the number of Ca around a fluorine atom. These species bonded ionically with only one NBO in the glass compared to the fluorine free glass where Ca^{2+} ionically bonded with two or possibly more NBOs. Consequently, the glass network became disrupted and at high fluorine contents replacement of NBOs by non-bridging fluorine occurred. In this case aluminium in five- and six-fold coordination state appeared, as reported by Stebbins et al. [32] and Stamboulis et al. [31], and that can be related to the appearance of significant amount of Al-F-Ca(n) species in the ^{19}F MAS-NMR spectra.

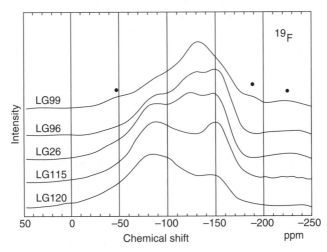

Figure 12.5. ^{19}F MAS-NMR spectra for a series of ionomer glasses. Spinning side bands are indicated by • [35].

A systematic study of fluorine containing ionomer glasses by Stamboulis and Hill [29, 33–36] using MAS-NMR spectroscopy gave a lot of information on the structural role of fluorine in these glasses. Various authors proposed in the past that fluorine was present either as fluorite clusters [36] or bound to silicon as Si-F [37] or, as reported recently [32, 38–43], bound to aluminium as Al-F type species. Hill et al. [42] suggested that Si-F bonds were not present in a glass composition based on $2SiO_2$-Al_2O_3-CaO-CaF_2 but instead fluorine was bound to Al as Al-F rather than being present as CaF_2 clusters. Kohn et al. [38] and Zeng and Stebbins [40] found evidence of the presence of aluminium in five- and six-fold coordination in fluoro-aluminosilicate glasses but no evidence for the presence of Si-F bonds for the specific glass compositions. However, they concluded that in fluoro-alumino-silicate glasses the formation of Si-F bonds if present could be significant. The latter probably depends strongly on the glass composition as well as the fluorine content. Specifically, Stamboulis et al. [35] in a recent study in glasses of the general composition $4.5SiO_2$-$3Al_2O_3$-$1.5P_2O_5$-$(5-x)$CaO-$xCaF_2$ where $x = 0$–3, reported that Si-F-Ca(n) species were clearly present in the high fluorine containing glasses. Figure 12.5 shows the ^{19}F MAS-NMR spectra of the above series of glasses. The lower fluoride containing glasses (LG120 and LG115) showed a peak with two maxima at -90 and -150 ppm suggesting that fluoride was preferentially associated with Ca i.e., F-Ca(n) and with both calcium and aluminium i.e., Al-F-Ca(n). The higher fluoride containing glasses LG26, LG96 and LG99 with $x = 2.0, 2.4$ and 3, respectively, showed the formation of an additional peak at -125 ppm that increased in intensity with increasing fluoride content.

Zeng and Stebbins [40] had reported that in fluoro-alumino-silicates a signal from Si-F-Ca(n) groups could occur in the range of -123.4 to 134.5 ppm. Therefore, it is possible that in low fluoride containing glasses, the Si-F-Ca(n) species could be present in small amounts but could be largely hidden by overlapping peaks. On the other hand, high fluorine containing glasses showed clearly that Si-F-Ca(n) species increased significantly with fluorine content. Similar glasses based on the composition $2SiO_2$-Al_2O_3-$(2-x)CaO$-$xCaF_2$ were studied by Stamboulis et al. [29] and the ^{19}F MAS-NMR spectra showed two peaks at -150 and -90 ppm attributed to Al-F-Ca(n) and F-Ca(n) species, respectively. There was no evidence of any Si-F-Ca(n) species present even at high fluoride contents (Figure 12.6). In all glasses however, it was observed that Al-F-Ca(n) species increased with fluoride content.

Figure 12.7 shows the relative proportion of four- Al(IV), five- Al(V) and six- Al(VI) fold coordinated aluminium as a function of fluoride content in a series of glasses based on the composition $4.5SiO_2$-$3Al_2O_3$-$1.5P_2O_5$-$(5-x)CaO$-$xCaF_2$.

It is worth noticing that the proportion of Al(IV) decreased linearly with fluoride content of the glass, whereas the proportion of Al(V) increased with fluoride content up to $x = 1$ and was almost kept constant between $x = 1$ and 3, but the proportion of Al(VI) increased with higher fluoride contents ($x \geq 1$). The peaks corresponding to both Al(IV) and Al(VI) in the ^{27}Al MAS-NMR spectra (Figure 12.8) shifted slightly to a more negative direction with increasing fluoride content

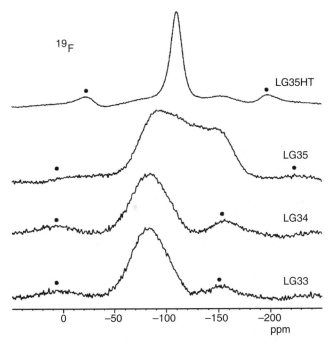

Figure 12.6. ^{19}F MAS-NMR spectra of alumino-silicate glasses of the composition $2SiO_2$-Al_2O_3-$(2-x)CaO$-$xCaF_2$; LG33 ($X = 0.25$), LG34 ($X = 0.5$), LG35 ($X = 1.0$) and heat treated LG35 (LG35HT) (spinning side bands are marked as •) [29].

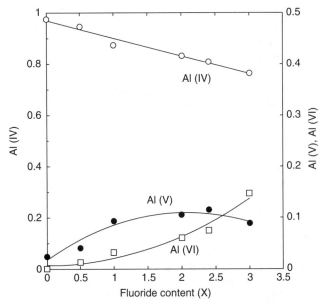

Figure 12.7. Relative proportion of Al(IV), Al(V) and Al(VI) as a function of fluoride content in the ionomer glasses [35].

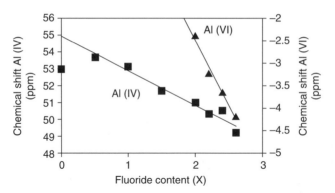

<u>Figure 12.8.</u> Al(IV) and Al(VI) peak positions plotted as a function of fluoride content in the glass [35].

but there was no effect from the presence of fluoride on the peak position of Al(IV) species at low fluoride contents.

At high fluoride contents ($x > 0.5$), there was significant influence of fluoride on the peak position and a consistent reduction in the peak values corresponding to Al(VI). Similar reduction was observed in $2SiO_2$-Al_2O_3-$(2-x)CaO$-$xCaF_2$ glasses providing evidence to support the existence of Al-F bonds being present in both Al(IV) and Al(VI) species. It was suggested by Stamboulis et al. [35] that the aluminium species in a series of glasses based on the composition $4.5SiO_2$-$3Al_2O_3$-$1.5P_2O_5$-$(5-x)CaO$-$xCaF_2$ can be represented by $[AlO_xF_y]^{n-}$ where $x = 3$-6, $y = 6$-x and n = charge of the total complex with Al(IV), Al(V) and Al(VI) present. These species had previously been postulated by Youngman et al. [43] by ^{19}F-^{27}Al cross-polarisation. However, since Al(V) and Al(VI) were present in small quantities within the glass in study, the dominant species should be $[AlO_3F]^-$. On the other hand, the formation of Al(V) and Al(VI) at high fluorine contents might not be due only to the presence of Al-F complexes but also due to the fact that the presence of fluoride limited the ability of calcium to perform its charge balancing functions within the glass compositions as a result of forming F-Ca(n) type species. Therefore, there might be insufficient Ca^{2+} and F-Ca^+ to charge balance aluminium and maintain it in four-fold coordination and consequently aluminium will take higher coordination states. However, there was no evidence that calcium was coordinated entirely by fluorine but in the contrary calcium might be still also involved with NBOs and other oxygen species. In addition, it is worth noticing that the glass preparation involved quenching, which may had resulted in structures present in the melt to "freeze." Often, in the melt aluminium takes higher than four coordination states and it is possible that Al(V) and Al(VI) were "frozen" during glass quenching. Another explanation for the presence of higher than four-fold coordinated aluminium species in the glasses might be the observation by Kirkpatrick and Brow [44] that in Na-alumino-silicate glasses with Al/P ratio <1, the aluminium speciation was mostly IV and VI. The Al/P ratio might play a role on the aluminium speciation, however, in the glass compositions studied by Stamboulis and Hill the Al/P ratio was >1.

12.6 CRYSTALLIZATION OF IONOMER GLASSES

Another interesting aspect in the characterisation of ionomer glasses is the study of the crystallisation mechanism. Ionomer glasses have been studied for applications as bone substitutes in both orthopaedic and dental fields. The resulting glass ceramics exhibit excellent mechanical properties and good osteo-conductivity [45–50].

The exact amount of fluorite in an ionomer glass composition has a dramatic effect on the nucleation and the crystallisation behaviour of the glasses. This effect is not only a result of the stoichiometric considerations of crystal formation but also of the network disrupting role of fluorine within the glass network. Addition of fluorite, whilst not altering the basicity of the glass, leads to increased disruption of the glass network and other effects as mentioned above. An interesting composition is the apatite stoichiometric composition where Ca/P = 1.67 and particularly the resulting glass-ceramics after appropriate heat treatments, which crystallise to two main phases: apatite and mullite. Apatite–mullite glass-ceramics based on SiO_2-Al_2O_3-P_2O_5-CaO-CaF_2 glasses were developed by Hill and co-workers [10, 11, 51]. The glasses based on the general composition $4.5SiO_2$-$3Al_2O_3$-$1.5P_2O_5$-(5-x)CaO-xCaF_2 where x is between zero and three, crystallised to fluorapatite (FAP) and mullite on appropriate heat treatments. Both the apatite and mullite phases had a needle like habit and interlocked with each other giving rise to high fracture toughness values. Differential scanning calorimetry (DSC) and X-ray diffraction analysis [11] showed two crystallisation temperatures that decreased with CaF_2 content and corresponded to $Ca_5(PO_4)_3F$ (fluorapatite, FAP) and $3Al_2O_3$-$2SiO_2$ (mullite) phases, respectively, while the fluorine free glass exhibited two crystallisation temperatures corresponded to β-$Ca_3(PO_4)_2$ (β-calcium phosphate) and $CaAl_2Si_2O_8$ (anorthite), respectively. MAS-NMR was used successfully in the past to characterise phosphorus containing aluminosilicate glasses as well as their crystallisation process [51–57]. Stamboulis, Hill and Law used multinuclear ^{27}Al, ^{29}Si, ^{31}P and ^{19}F MAS-NMR experiments in order to characterise the crystallisation process of glass ceramics based on $4.5SiO_2$-$3Al_2O_3$-$1.5P_2O_5$-(5-x)CaO-xCaF_2.

The mechanism of apatite crystal nucleation in these glass-ceramics was thought to occur as a result of prior *amorphous phase separation* (APS) or *glass-in-glass phase separation*. The amorphous phase separation has been under investigation for many years for different glass systems. Glass often appears homogeneous but if one looks closer on the glass microstructure on a scale of a few hundred atoms, glass is not as homogeneous as a perfect crystal or a liquid solution. There are two processes leading to the development of inhomogeneous glass microstructure. The first one is the crystallisation or devitrification, where definite crystals nucleate and grow from a supercooled liquid mass and the second one is based on the theory that crystallites are not microcrystals but they possess distorted lattices and have definite chemical composition that is determined by the phase equilibrium diagram of the glass composition. In the simplest situation, the glass is considered to be a liquid that undergoes demixing as it cools. If the two

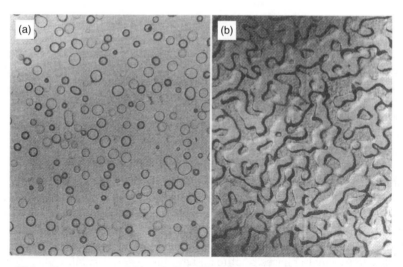

Figure 12.9. Microstructure of (a) soda lime silica glass heated at 740 °C for 7.25 h(14,000×) showing nucleated droplet phase separation, and (b) "Vycor" glass heated at 700 °C for 5.5 h(24,000×) showing spinodal decomposition [60].

phases are liquid, then the phase separation is called liquid-liquid immiscibility. The immiscibility can be stable or metastable, depending on whether the phase separation occurs at temperatures above the liquidus or below the liquidus, respectively. This metastable immiscibility is of great interest. There are two routes that lead to the formation of discrete phases by a metastable phase separation; the nucleation and growth mechanism [19, 58–61] and the spinodal decomposition [19, 60, 62]. Figure 12.9 shows the microstructure of a) a soda lime silica glass heated at 740 °C for 7.25 h showing nucleated droplet phase separation and b) a "Vycor" glass heated at 700 °C for 5.5 hours showing spinodal decomposition [60].

The differences between these two processes are clear. During the nucleation and growth mechanism the second phase composition does not change with time at constant temperature, the interface between phases retains the degree of sharpness during growth, the particle sizes and positions are randomly distributed and the second phase consists of spherical particles with very low connectivity. On the other hand, during spinodal decomposition, there is a variation of phase compositions with time until equilibrium compositions are reached, the interface between phases is diffuse and eventually sharpens, the second phase distribution is regular and characterised by geometric spacing and the second phase consists of non-spherical particles with high connectivity [60].

The view that crystallisation occurs via prior amorphous phase separation (APS) in ionomer glasses is evidenced by the optimum nucleation temperatures being close to the experimentally determined glass transition temperatures and the presence of two loss peaks in dynamic mechanical thermal analysis experiments on nucleated (phase separated) glasses [63]. The two loss peaks were thought to correspond to two different glass transition temperatures associated with the two glass phases present. One phase was calcium, phosphate and fluoride rich and crystallised to FAP and the other phase was aluminium and silicon rich and crystallised to mullite. Rafferty et al. [64] reported that the ionomer glasses studied showed the presence of sparse droplets (20–100 nm) dispersed in a matrix. The second phase droplets were spherical with clear interfaces, distributed randomly with no obvious connectivity, suggesting a phase separation mechanism involving nucleation and growth. The matrix, on the other hand, looked speckled. According to James [65], for some glass systems, the effective spinodal boundary may be depressed at low temperatures and the samples have to traverse a nucleation region before reaching the spinodal. The speckled matrix might occur because of the fine APS within the spinodal. Evidence of an APS mechanism that involved both prior nucleation and spinodal decomposition came later in time when Hill et al. [66] reported that a FAP glass–ceramic studied by a real-time small angle neutron scattering exhibited two characteristic scales of phase separation and underwent APS. Isothermal small angle neutron scattering (SANS) studies at 740 and 750 °C showed the same phenomena but without any change in the scattering after 30 and 12 minutes, respectively. This observation lead to the suggestion that further phase separation and crystal growth were restricted by the high glass transition temperature of the second glass phase. Figure 12.10 shows the schematic representation of the above suggestion on sub-micro-scale, where the size of FAP crystals was correlated with the size of the droplet phase suggesting, that FAP crystals did not grow beyond the boundaries of the droplet phase until the higher glass transition temperature of the second phase was reached. The above is important as similar ideas could be applied for glasses that could undergo APS on a nano-meter scale.

Real time neutron diffraction studies showed that crystallisation of FAP in ionomer glasses occurred first, followed by crystallisation of both FAP and mullite. Dissolution at higher temperatures and re-crystallisation during cooling occurred (Figure 12.10). The results showed that the volume fraction of FAP decreased during holding at 1200 °C and then FAP re-crystallised on cooling, suggesting that

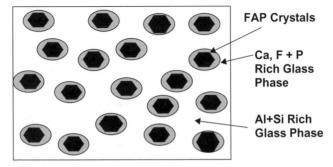

FAP Crystals

Ca, F + P
Rich Glass
Phase

Al+Si Rich
Glass Phase

Figure 12.10. Schematic of FAP crystal growth being inhibited by the droplet size. The size of FAP crystals is correlated with the size of the droplet phase, suggesting that FAP crystals do not grow beyond the boundaries of the droplet phase until the glass transition temperature of the second phase is reached [66].

the mechanism of coarsening of FAP involved dissolution of the small crystals and re-crystallisation of FAP on the remaining coarse crystallites. The mechanism, however, should have been controlled by the composition phase diagram and not the thermodynamic drive to reduce the surface energy.

Multinuclear MAS-NMR analysis in the ionomer glass-ceramics [67] verified APS occurring in the glass during heat treatments at three temperatures; the first crystallisation temperature Tp1, the second crystallisation temperature Tp2 and an intermediate temperature (Tp1 + Tp2)/2 half way between Tp1 and Tp2. As mentioned above, ^{27}Al MAS-NMR spectra showed, that Al(V) and Al(VI) were present in the glasses with increasing fluoride content. By heat treating the glasses, the above aluminium species disappeared and appeared again during crystallisation at Tp2. A typical example is shown in Figure 12.11 for a glass composition based on $4.5SiO_2$-$3Al_2O_3$-$1.5P_2O_5$-$(5-x)CaO$-$xCaF_2$ ($x = 2$) that was heat treated at Tp1, Tp(1 + 2)/2 and Tp2. The small Al(VI) peak, that appeared in the original glass decreased significantly with heat treatments and increased again when the glass was heat treated at Tp2.

A small but distinct peak appeared at about 39 ppm assigned by Dollase et al. to crystalline $AlPO_4$ [68]. ^{19}F MAS-NMR analysis showed that the two peaks in the original glass, that corresponded to F-Ca(n) species and Al-F-Ca(n) species decreased significantly with heat treatments (Figure 12.12).

Specifically, the F-Ca(n) species disappeared already during heat treatment at Tp1, indicating a contribution of F-Ca(n) to the formation of F-Ca(3) species, that correspond to crystalline FAP and appeared at ca -103 ppm. On the other hand, the Al-F-Ca(n) species decreased with heat treatments but they were present in the residual glass even at heat treatments to Tp2. Most of the Al-F-

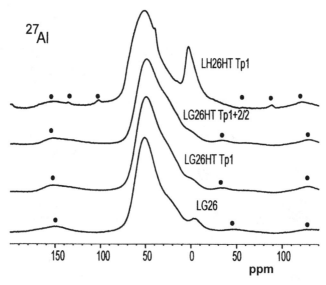

Figure 12.11. ^{27}Al MAS NMR spectra of $4.5SiO_2$-$3Al_2O_3$-$1.5P_2O_5$-$(5-x)CaO$-$xCaF_2$ glass composition, where $x = 2$; LG26 and LG26 heated treated to Tp1, Tp(1 + 2)/2 and Tp2 [67].

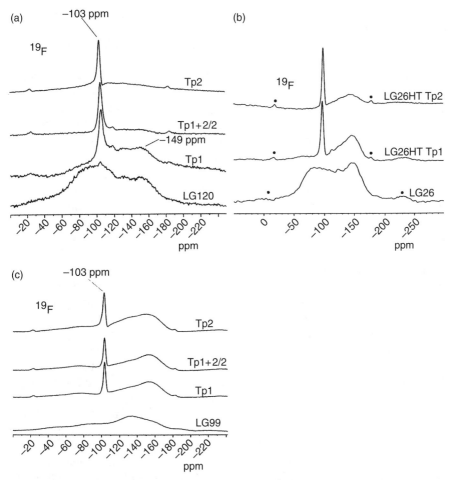

Figure 12.12. ^{19}F MAS-NMR spectra of some glasses based on $4.5SiO_2$-$3Al_2O_3$-$1.5P_2O_5$-$(5-x)$ CaO-xCaF$_2$; A) LG120(x = 0.5), B) LG26(x = 2) and C) LG99(z = 3.0) heat treated to Tp1, Tp(1 + 2)/2 and Tp2 [67].

Ca(n) species corresponded to Al(IV) species; however, an increase in Al(VI) at Tp2 indicated that there was an aluminium-silicon reach phase attributed to mullite, considering that in ^{29}Si MAS-NMR spectra the change of the chemical shift of the crystalline glass at Tp2 was due to the mullite formation of which aluminium is present as Al(VI).

12.7 CATION SUBSTITUTION IN IONOMER GLASSES

Often in dental and medical applications radiopacity is a very important aspect for materials selection. In glass polyalkenoate cements, the ionomer glasses used often contain strontium as a radiopaque agent [69]. Strontium has an ionic radius of 1.16 nm, close enough to that of calcium 0.94 nm and therefore, strontium can be substituted for calcium. Strontium not only can be substituted for calcium in the glass structure, but also in apatite structures. Solid solution of mixed calcium strontium hydroxyapatite and pure strontium hydroxyapatite were reported and produced from aqueous solutions [70]. Hill et al. [69], investigated the influence of substituting strontium for calcium on the structure and the nucleation and crystallisation behaviour of an apatite stoichiometric ionomer glass based on similar series of glasses as above. ^{27}Al MAS-NMR spectroscopy showed that the usual aluminium species present in a calcium glass were replaced by F-Sr(n) and Al-F-Sr(n) species in the strontium glass and mixed species in a calcium-strontium glass. But as expected, there was only a little influence on the glass structure. Significant influence of the substitution was observed, however, on the nucleation and crystallisation behaviour of strontium and mixed calcium-strontium glasses. Replacement of calcium by strontium promoted surface crystallisation of the apatite phase. Low strontium substitution resulted in a calcium fluorapatite phase being formed first, whereas higher strontium substitution resulted in a mixed calcium/strontium fluorapatite. Also, strontium substitution resulted in the formation of an anorthite phase instead of the mullite phase at Tp2. The crystallisation of anorthite was the result in the reduction in quantity of the apatite phase leaving increased quantities of calcium that subsequently would form anorthite. In the 100% strontium substituted glass the first phase was as expected pure strontium fluorapatite but the second phase was not an anorthite. XRD analysis gave a peak at about 7.5° 2 theta, which at the time was not identified [69]. However, further studies revealed that the second phase in the strontium ionomer glass was indeed a Sr-feldspar phase ($SrAl_2Si_2O_8$) most probably Sr-hexacelcian [71]. Generally, two main changes were observed in the strontium substituted glasses: strontium hindered apatite formation and inhibited bulk nucleation. The observed changes could be possibly attributed to the lower lattice energy of strontium fluorapatite as well as the possibility that strontium might have suppressed the amorphous phase separation (APS) that was observed in the calcium ionomer glasses [63].

A whole series of cation substitutions in the above ionomer glasses are being studied including Mg and Ba cation substitutions. The general observation is that the effect of cations on the structure and crystallisation of the ionomer glasses is strongly connected with the size of the cation. In Ba-substituted glasses, for example, the substitution did not seem to have a strong influence in the silicon and phosphorous environment of the glass. FTIR studies showed, however that Ba substitution can lead to a lower inter-tetrahedral angle in Si-O-Si and a less strained glass network [72]. The crystallisation process of the glasses is strongly influenced by the barium substitution; in low barium contents the main phases are calcium fluorapatite, mullite and some mixed barium-calcium fluorapatite, whereas in high barium contents, there is no fluorapatite forming but mostly a barium aluminosilicate phase together with crystalline $BaPO_4$ [73]. A lot more attention should be given to the cation substitution as morphologies and consequently the properties of ionomer glasses change.

12.8 CONCLUSIONS AND FUTURE PERSPECTIVES

There is a lot of work to be done in order to fully understand the structure and the mechanisms of glass formation and crystallisation in ionomer glasses. MAS-NMR spectroscopy has proved to be a powerful tool to elucidate the structure in these materials; however, other complimentary techniques should be used. Ionomer glasses have been used extensively in dental filling materials as glass fillers in glass ionomer cements and resin composites. However, the potential of the glasses has not yet been fully reached. Ionomer glass ceramics show good biocompatibility and bioconductivity and could potentially be used as bone substitutes for bone fixation. They also exhibit good mechanical properties and with some compositions the machinability of materials is excellent. The structural investigations as well as the crystallisation studies showed that certain compositions of fluorine containing ionomer glasses have the capability of being crystallised into a fluorapatite phase in the nanoscale leaving the material optically clear. This should be a very useful property for optoelectronics. On the other hand, the continuous development of new materials for dental applications reflects the need of new glass compositions. There is, therefore, a large scope for research and development in the area of ionomer glasses.

ACKNOWLEDGMENTS

The authors would like to thank Prof. Robert Hill of Queen Mary University of London for the long and useful discussions.

REFERENCES

1. K. Stanton and R. Hill, "The role of fluorine in the devitrification of $SiO_2 \cdot Al_2O_3 \cdot P_2O_5 \cdot CaO \cdot CaF_2$ glasses," *Journal of Materials Science*, vol. 35, pp. 1911–1916, 2000.
2. S. G. Griffin and R. G. Hill, "Influence of glass composition on the properties of glass polyalkenoate cements. Part I: influence of aluminium to silicon ratio," *Biomaterials*, vol. 20, pp. 1579–1586, 1999.
3. S. Crisp and A. D. Wilson, "Reactions in Glass ionomer cements: I. Decomposition of the Powder," *Journal of Dental Research*, vol. 53, pp. 1408–1413, 1974.
4. A. D. Wilson and B. E. Kent, "Dental Cements: Decomposition of the Powder," *Journal of Dental Research*, pp. 7–13, 1970.
5. A. D. Wilson and B. E. Kent, "A new translucent cement for dentistry," *British Dental Journal*, vol. 132, pp. 133–135, 1972.
6. B. E. Kent, B. G. Lewis, and A. D. Wilson, "The properties of glass ionomer cement," *British Dental Journal*, vol. 135, pp. 322–326, 1973.
7. S. Crisp, M. A. Pringuer, D. Wardleworth, and A. D. Wilson, "Reactions in Glass Ionomer Cement: II An infrared Spectroscopic Study," *Journal of Dental Research*, vol. 53, pp. 1414–1419, 1974.

8. J. W. Nicholson, "Chemistry of glass-ionomer cements: a review," *Biomaterials*, vol. 19, pp. 485–494, 1998.

9. A. D. Wilson, D. M. Groffman, and A. T. Kuhn, "The release of fluoride and other chemical-species from a glass-ionomer cement," *Biomaterials*, vol. 6, pp. 431–433, 1985.

10. R. Hill and D. Wood, "Apatite-mullite glass ceramics," *Journal of Materials Science*, vol. 6, pp. 311–318, 1995.

11. A. Rafferty, A. Clifford, R. Hill, D. Wood, B. Samuneva, and M. Dimitrova-Lukacs, "Influence of fluorine content in apatite-mullite glass ceramics," *Journal of the American Ceramic Society*, vol. 83, pp. 2833–2838, 2000.

12. A. D. Wilson, S. Crisp, H. J. Prosser, B. G. Lewis, and S. A. Merson, "Aluminosilicate Glasses For Poly-Electrolyte Cements," *Industrial & Engineering Chemistry Product Research And Development*, vol. 19, pp. 263–270, 1980.

13. A. D. Neve, V. Piddock, and E. C. Combe, "The effect of glass heat treatment on the properties of a novel polyalkenoate cement," *Clinical Materials*, vol. 12, pp. 113, 1993.

14. A. D. Neve, V. Piddock, and E. C. Combe, "Development of novel dental cements. I. Formulation of aluminoborate glasses," *Clinical Materials*, vol. 9, pp. 7, 1992.

15. A. D. Neve, V. Piddock, and E. C. Combe, "Development of novel dental cements. II. Cement properties," *Clinical Materials*, vol. 9, pp. 13, 1992.

16. M. Darling and R. Hill, "Novel polyalkenoate (glass-ionomer) dental cements based on zinc silicate glasses," *Biomaterials*, vol. 15, pp. 299, 1994.

17. D. Boyd, M. R. Towler, R. V. Law, and R. G. Hill, "An investigation into the structure and reactivity of calcium-zinc-silicate ionomer glasses using MAS-NMR spectroscopy," *Journal of Materials Science: Materials in Medicine*, vol. 17, 2006.

18. W. H. Zachariasen, "The atomic arrangements in glass," *Journal of the American Chemical Society*, vol. 54, pp. 3841–3851, 1932.

19. J. E. Shelby, *Introduction to Glass Science and Technology*: RSC paperbacks, The Royal Society of Chemistry 1997.

20. W. Lowenstein, "The distribution of aluminium in the tetrahedral of silicates and aluminates," *American Mineralogist*, vol. 39, pp. 92–96, 1954.

21. J. F. Stebbins and Z. Xu, "NMR evidence for excess non-bridging oxygen in an aluminosilicate glass," *Nature*, vol. 390, pp. 60–62, 1997.

22. S. G. Griffin and R. G. Hill, "Influence of glass composition on the properties of glass polyalkenoate cements. Part II: influence of phosphate content," *Biomaterials*, vol. 21, pp. 399–403, 2000.

23. E. De Barra and R. G. Hill, "Influence of alkali metal ions on the fracture properties of glass polyalkenoate (ionomer) cements," *Biomaterials*, vol. 19, pp. 495–502, 1998.

24. E. De Barra and R. G. Hill, "Influence of glass composition on the properties of glass polyalkenoate cements. Part III: influence of fluorite content," *Biomaterials*, vol. 21, pp. 563–569, 2000.

25. S. G. Griffin and R. G. Hill, "Influence of glass composition on the properties of glass polyalkenoate cements. Part IV: influence of fluorine content," *Biomaterials*, vol. 21, pp. 693–698, 2000.

26. A. D. Wilson and J. W. McLean, *Glass ionomer cement*. Chicago, IL: Quintessence Books, 1988.

27. R. G. Hill and A. D. Wilson, "Some structural aspects of glasses used in ionomer cements," *Glass Technology*, vol. 29, pp. 150–157, 1988.

28. D. Wood and R. G. Hill, "Structure-Property relationships in Ionomer Glasses," *Clinical Materials*, vol. 7, pp. 301–312, 1991.

29. A. Stamboulis, R. G. Hill, and R. V. Law, "Characterisation of the structure of calcium alumino-silicate and calcium fluoro-alumino-silicate glasses by magic angle spinning nuclear magnetic resonance (MAS-NMR)," *Journal of Non-Crystalline Solids*, vol. 333, pp. 101–107, 2004.

30. F. Angeli, T. Charpentier, P. Faucon, and J.-C. Petit, "Structural characterisation of glass from the inversion of ^{23}Na and ^{27}Al 3Q-MAS-NMR spectra," *Journal of Physics and Chemistry B*, vol. 103, pp. 10356–10364, 1999.

31. A. Stamboulis, R. G. Hill, and R. V. Law, "Structural characterization of fluorine containing glasses by F-19 Al-27 Si-29 and P-31 MAS-NMR spectroscopy," *Journal of Non-Crystalline Solids*, vol. 351, pp. 3289–3295, 2005.

32. J. F. Stebbins, S. Kroeker, S. K. Lee, and T. J. Kiczenski, "Quantification of five- and six-coordinated aluminum ions in aluminosilicate and fluoride-containing glasses by high-field, high-resolution Al-27 NMR," *Journal of Non-Crystalline Solids*, vol. 275, pp. 1–6, 2000.

33. A. Stamboulis, R. V. Law, and R. G. Hill, "Characterisation of commercial ionomer glasses using magic angle nuclear magnetic resonance (MAS-NMR)," *Biomaterials*, vol. 25, pp. 3907–3913, 2004.

34. R. G. Hill, A. Stamboulis, and R. V. Law, "Characterisation of fluorine containing glasses by F-19, Al-27, Si-29 and P-31 MAS-NMR spectroscopy," *Journal of Dentistry*, vol. 34, pp. 525–532, 2006.

35. S. Matsuya, A. Stamboulis, R. G. Hill, and R. V. Law, "Structural characterisation of ionomer glasses by multinuclear solid state MAS-NMR spectroscopy," *Journal of Non-Crystalline Solids*, vol. 353, pp. 237–243, 2007.

36. E. M. Rabinovich, "On The Structural Role of Fluorine In Silicate-Glasses," *Physics And Chemistry Of Glasses*, vol. 24, pp. 54–56, 1983.

37. D. Kumar, R. G. Ward, and D. J. Williams, "Effect of fluorides on silicates and phosphates," *Discussions of the Faraday Society*, vol. 32, pp. 147–154, 1961.

38. S. C. Kohn, R. Dupree, M. G. Mortuza, and C. M. B. Henderson, "NMR Evidence For 5-Coordinated And 6-Coordinated Aluminum Fluoride Complexes In F-Bearing Aluminosilicate Glasses," *American Mineralogist*, vol. 76, pp. 309–312, 1991.

39. T. J. Kiczenski and J. F. Stebbins, "Fluorine sites in calcium and barium oxyfluorides: F-19NMR on crystalline model compounds and glasses," *Journal of Non-Crystalline Solids*, vol. 306, pp. 160–168, 2002.

40. Q. Zeng and J. F. Stebbins, "Fluoride sites in aluminosilicate glasses: High-resolution F-19 NMR results," *American Mineralogist*, vol. 85, pp. 863–867, 2000.

41. J. F. Stebbins and Q. Zeng, "Cation ordering at fluoride sites in silicate glasses: a high-resolution F-19 NMR study," *Journal of Non-Crystalline Solids*, vol. 262, pp. 1–5, 2000.

42. R. Hill, D. Wood, and M. Thomas, "Trimethylsilylation analysis of the silicate structure of fluoro-alumino-silicate glasses and the structural role of fluorine," *Journal of Materials Science*, vol. 34, pp. 1767–1774, 1999.

43. R. E. Youngman and M. J. Dejneka, "NMR studies of fluorine in aluminosilicate-lanthanum fluoride glasses and glass-ceramics," *Journal of The American Ceramic Society*, vol. 85, pp. 1077–1082, 2002.

44. R. J. Kirkpatrick and R. K. Brow, "Nuclear-Magnetic-Resonance investigation of the structures of phosphate and phosphate-containing glasses—a review," *Solid State Nuclear Magnetic Resonance*, vol. 5, pp. 9–21, 1995.

45. C. M. Gorman and R. G. Hill, "Heat-pressed ionomer glass-ceramics. Part II. Mechanical property evaluation," *Dental Materials*, vol. 20, pp. 252, 2004.

46. R. D. Goodridge, D. Wood, C. Ohtsuki, and K. W. Dalgarno, "Biological evaluation of an apatite-mullite glass-ceramic produced via selective laser sintering," *Acta Biomaterialia*, vol. 3, pp. 221–231, 2007.

47. J. M. Walsh, R. G. Hill, A. Johnson, and P. V. Hatton, "Evaluation of Castable Apatite-Mullite Glass-Ceramics for Medical and Dental Applications," in *Materials for Medical Engineering, Euromat 99*, H. Stallfort and P. Revell, Eds., 2000.

48. C. O. Freeman, I. M. Brook, A. Johnson, P. V. Hatton, R. G. Hill, and K. Stanton, "Crystallization modifies osteoconductivity in an apatite-mullite glass-ceramic," *Journal of Materials: Materials in Medicine*, vol. 14, pp. 985–990, 2003.

49. K. T. Stanton and R. G. Hill, "Crystallisation in apatite-mullite glass ceramics as a function of fluorine content," *Journal of Crystal Growth*, vol. 275, pp. 2061–2068, 2005.

50. W. Hoeland, V. Rheinberger, and M. Schweiger, "Control of Nucleation in Glass Ceramics," *Philosophical Transactions: Mathematical, Physical and Engineering Sciences*, vol. 361, pp. 575–589, 2003.

51. A. Clifford, A. Rafferty, R. Hill, P. Mooney, D. Wood, B. Samuneva, and S. Matsuya, "The influence of calcium to phosphate ratio on the nucleation and crystallisation of apatite glass ceramics," *Journal of Materials Science: Materials in Medicine*, vol. 12, pp. 461–469, 2001.

52. J. M. Oliveira, R. N. Correira, M. H. Fernandes, and J. Rocha, "Influence of the Cao/MgO ratio on the structure of phase separated glasses: a solid sate ^{29}Si and ^{31}P MAS-NMR study," *Journal of Non-Crystalline Solids*, vol. 265, pp. 221–229, 2000.

53. G. Cody, B. Mysen, G. Saghi-Szabo, and J. A. Tossel, "Silicate phosphate interactions in silicate glasses and melts: Part I. A multinuclear (^{27}Al, ^{29}Si, ^{31}P) MAS-NMR and ab initio chemical shift shielding ^{31}P study of phosphorus speciation in silicate glasses," *Geochimica et Cosmochimica Acta*, vol. 65, pp. 2395–2411, 2001.

54. H. Grussaute, L. Montagne, G. Palavit, and J. L. Bernard, "Phosphate speciation in Na_2O-CaO-P_2O_5-SiO_2 and Na_2O-TiO_2-$P2O_5$-SiO_2 glasses," *Journal of Non-Crystalline Solids*, vol. 263 and 264, pp. 312–317, 2000.

55. M. J. Toplis and T. A. Schaller, "A ^{31}P MAS-NMR study of glasses in the system xNa_2O-$(1-x)Al_2O_3$-$2SiO_2$-yP_2O_5," *Journal of Non-Crystalline Solids*, vol. 224, pp. 57–68, 1998.

56. R. Dupree, D. Holland, M. G. Mortuza, J. A. Collins, and M. W. G. Lockyer, "Magic angle spinning NMR of alkali phospho-aluminosilicate glasses," *Journal of Non-Crystalline Solids*, vol. 112, pp. 111–119, 1989.

57. C. M. Moisescu, T. Hoche, G. Carl, R. Keding, C. Russel, and W. D. Heerdegen, "Influence of the Ca/P ratio on the morphology of fluorapatite crystals in SiO_2-Al_2O_3-CaO-P_2O_5-K_2O-F^- glass ceramics," *Journal of Non-Crystalline Solids*, vol. 289, pp. 123–134, 2001.

58. L. L. Burgner and M. C. Weinberg, "Crystal growth mechanisms in inorganic glasses," *Physics and Chemistry of Glasses*, vol. 42, pp. 184–190, 2001.

59. W. Hoeland, V. Rheinberger, and M. Frank, "Mechanisms of nucleation and controlled crystallisation of needle-like apatite in glass-ceramics of the SiO_2-Al_2O_3-K_2O-CaO-P_2O_5 system," *Journal of Non-Crystalline Solids*, vol. 253, pp. 170–177, 1999.

60. A. K. Varshneya, *Fundamentals of inorganic glasses*: Society of Glass Technology, 2006.

61. W. Haller and P. B. Macedo, "Origin Of Phase Connectivity In Microheterogeneous Glasses," *Physics And Chemistry Of Glasses*, vol. 9, pp. 153–155, 1968.

62. J. W. Cahn and R. J. Charles, "Initial Stages Of Phase Separation In Glasses," *Physics And Chemistry Of Glasses*, vol. 6, pp. 181–191, 1965.

63. A. Rafferty, R. Hill, and D. Wood, "Amorphous phase separation of ionomer glasses," *Journal of Materials Science*, vol. 35, pp. 3863–3869, 2000.

64. A. Rafferty, R. Hill, B. Kelleher, and T. O'Dwyer, "An investigation of amorphous phase separation, leachability and surface area of an ionomer glass system and a sodium-boro-silicate glass system," *Journal of Materials Science*, vol. 38, pp. 3891–3902, 2003.

65. P. F. James, *Glasses and Glass-ceramics*. London: Chapman and Hall, 1989.

66. R. Hill, A. Calver, A. Stamboulis, and N. Bubb, "Real time nucleation and crystallisation studies of a fluorapatite glass ceramics using small angle neutron scattering and neutron diffraction," *Journal of the American Ceramic Society*, vol. 90, pp. 763–768, 2007.

67. A. Stamboulis, R. G. Hill, R. V. Law, and S. Matsuya, "MAS-NMR study on the crystallisation process of apatite-mullite glass ceramics," *Physics and Chemistry of Glasses*, vol. 45, pp. 127–133, 2004.

68. W. A. Dollase, L. H. Merwin, and A. Sebald, "Structure of $Na_{3-3x}Al_xPO_4$ $x = 0$–0.5," *Journal of Solid State Chemistry*, vol. 83, pp. 140–149, 1989.

69. R. Hill, A. Stamboulis, R. V. Law, A. Clifford, M. R. Towler, and C. Crowley, "The influence of strontium substitution in fluorapatite glasses and glass ceramics," *Journal of Non-Crystalline Solids*, vol. 336, pp. 223–229, 2004.

70. F. C. M. Driessens and R. M. H. Veerbeck, *Biominerals*: CRC, 1990

71. F. Wang and A. Stamboulis, "Unpublished data," 2007.

72. F. Wang, A. Stamboulis, D. Holland, S. Matsuya, and A. Takeuchi, "Solid state MAS-NMR and FTIR study of barium containing aluminosilicate glasses," *Key Engineering Materials*, vol. 361–363, pp. 825–828, 2008.

73. F. Wang and A. Stamboulis, "Unpublished data."

74. J. Weitkamp, "Zeolites and catalysis," *Solid State Ionics*, vol. 131, pp. 175–188, 2000.

13

DESIGNING NANOFIBROUS SCAFFOLDS FOR TISSUE ENGINEERING

Neha Arya, Poonam Sharma, and Dhirendra S. Katti

Department of Biological Sciences and Bioengineering, Indian Institute of Technology Kanpur, Kanpur, India

Contents

	Abbreviations	437
13.1	Overview	438
13.2	Introduction	438
	13.2.1 Rationale for Tissue Engineering	438
	13.2.2 Importance of Scaffolds in Tissue Engineering	440
	13.2.2.1 Influence of Nanometer Scale Features of Scaffolds in Tissue Engineering	442
13.3	Methods of Nanofibrous Scaffold Synthesis	442
	13.3.1 Self Assembly	443
	13.3.2 Phase Separation	444
	13.3.3 Electrospinning	446
13.4	Polymers Used for Synthesizing Nanofibrous Structures Using the Electrospinning Technique	453
	13.4.1 Natural Polymers	453
	13.4.1.1 Proteins	454
	13.4.1.1.1 Collagen	454
	13.4.1.1.2 Gelatin	455
	13.4.1.1.3 Silk Fibroin	456

Advanced Biomaterials: Fundamentals, Processing, and Applications, Edited by Bikramjit Basu, Dhirendra S. Katti, and Ashok Kumar

    13.4.1.2 Carbohydrates 456
        13.4.1.2.1 Hyaluronic Acid (HA) 457
        13.4.1.2.2 Alginate 457
        13.4.1.2.3 Chitin and Chitosan 458
   13.4.2 Synthetic Polymers 459
    13.4.2.1 Poly(α-hydroxy) Esters 459
        13.4.2.1.1 Poly(Glycolic Acid) (PGA) 460
        13.4.2.1.2 Poly(Lactic Acid) (PLA) 460
        13.4.2.1.3 Poly(Lactic-Co-Glycolic Acid) (PLGA) 460
    13.4.2.2 Polycaprolactone (PCL) 461
    13.4.2.3 Polyurethanes (PU) 461
    13.4.2.4 Bacterial Polyesters 462
   13.4.3 Polymeric Blends 462
  13.5 Tissue Engineering Using Electrospun Nanofibrous Scaffolds 466
   13.5.1 Musculoskeletal System- An Introduction 466
   13.5.2 Tissues of the Musculoskeletal System that Have Been Engineered
     Using Electrospun Nanofibers 466
    13.5.2.1 Bone 466
        13.5.2.1.1 Potential Cell Sources for Bone
            Tissue Engineering 467
        13.5.2.1.2 Scaffolds for Bone Tissue Engineering 468
    13.5.2.2 Cartilage 471
        13.5.2.2.1 Potential Cell Source for Cartilage
            Tissue Engineering 472
        13.5.2.2.2 Scaffolds for Cartilage Tissue Engineering 472
    13.5.2.3 Skeletal Muscle 474
        13.5.2.3.1 Potential Cell Sources for Skeletal Muscle
            Tissue Engineering 475
        13.5.2.3.2 Scaffold for Skeletal Muscle Tissue Engineering 475
    13.5.2.4 Ligament and Tendon 476
        13.5.2.4.1 Potential Cell Sources for Ligament and Tendon
            Tissue Engineering 477
        13.5.2.4.2 Scaffold for Ligament and Tendon
            Tissue Engineering 478
 13.6 Conclusions and Future Directions 479
  Acknowledgments 481
  References 481

Abbreviations

ALP	Alkaline phosphatase (ALP)	PCL	Poly(ε-caprolactone)
ACI	Autologous chondrocyte implantation	PDLA	Poly(D-lactic acid)
		PDLLA	Poly(DL-lactic acid)
ACL	Anterior crucial ligament	PEG-PLA	Polyethylene glycol-polylactic acid
bFGF	Basic fibroblast growth factor	PEGDA	Poly(ethylene glycol)-diacrylate
BMP-2	Bone morphogenetic protein-2	PEO	Polyethylene oxide
		PEUU	Poly(ester urethane) urea
BSA	Bovine serum albumin	PGA	Poly(glycolic acid)
COMP	Cartilage oligomeric matrix protein	PHA	Poly-hydroxy alkanoates
		PHB	Poly-hydroxybutyrate
DCM	Methylene chloride	PHBV	Poly(3-hydroxybutyrate-co-3-hydroxyvalerate
DMF	N, N-dimethyl formamide		
ECM	Extra cellular matrix	PHV	Poly-hydroxyvalerate
EVOH	Poly(ethylene-co-vinyl alcohol)	PLA	Poly(lactic acid)
		PLCL	Poly(l-lactide-co-caprolactone)
FBCs	Fetal bovine chondrocytes		
FDA	Food and Drug Administration	PLGA	Poly(lactide-co-glycolide)
		PLGA/NHA	Poly(lactide-co-glycolide)/nano-hydroxyapatite
FHA	Fluor-hydroxyapatite		
GA	Glycolic acid	PLLA	Poly(L-lactic acid)
GAGs	Glycosaminoglycans	PLLA-CL	Poly(l-lactide-co-ε zyxoneonefivexyz-caprolactone)
GBR	Guided bone regeneration		
GFs	Growth Factors		
GTA	Glutaraldehyde	PLLA/PCL	Poly(L-lactic acid)/polycaprolactone
GTPase	Guanosine tri phosphatase		
HA	Hyaluronic acid	PVP	Poly(vinyl pyrolidine)
HA	Hydroxyapatite	PU	Polyurethanes
HA-DTPH	Hyaluronic acid 3,3'-dithiobis- (propanoic dihydrazide)	QCh	Quaternised chitosan
		RGD	Arginine-Glycine-Aspartic acid
HFP	1,1,1,3,3,3 Hexafluoro-2-propanol	TCPS	Tissue culture polystyrene
		TEGDA	Triethylene glycol diacrylate
HGF	Hepatocyte growth factor		
HLF	Human ligament fibroblast	TFE	2, 2, 2-trifluoroethanol
hMSCs	Human bone marrow derived mesenchymal stem cells	TGF ß1	Transforming growth factor ß1
		THF	Tetrahydrofuran
LA	Lactic acid	TIPS	Thermally induced phase separation
MCL	Medial collateral ligament		
MSCs	Mesenchymal stem cells	μm	Micrometer
MDSCs	Muscle-derived stem cells	nm	Nanometer
PA	Peptide-amphiphiles	2D	Two-dimensional
PAN	Poly(acryl nitrile)	3D	Three-dimensional

13.1   OVERVIEW

The currently available approaches for the treatment of organ and tissue loss include organ transplantation, surgical reconstruction, and implantation of synthetic devices that can perform the functions of the damaged organs. Shortcomings of the aforementioned methods such as donor site morbidity, limited tissue availability, and immune rejection have led to the development of alternate strategies such as tissue engineering. Tissue engineering strategies generally involve the use of biodegradable scaffolds as a transient extracellular matrix (ECM), cells and growth factors to create functional tissue replacements. Biomimetics of the extracellular matrix involve the development of fibers that have diameters in the micrometer to nanometer range to match the collagen fibers, and glycosaminoglycans/proteoglycans present in the natural milieu of tissue. Of the various techniques used for the synthesis of micro/nanofibrous scaffolds, electrospinning has emerged as a simple and robust method. This chapter discusses the different techniques used for the synthesis of electrospun nanofibers, polymeric materials that have been used to synthesize nanofibers using electrospinning, as well as their applications as scaffolds in musculo-skeletal tissue engineering.

13.2   INTRODUCTION

13.2.1   Rationale for Tissue Engineering

The human body is robust and elegant machinery whose maintenance is a continuous effort primarily in the form of repair processes. With ageing, the repair processes reduce and thereby lead to gradual wear of tissue. However, tissue loss/damage mostly occurs due to other reasons, such as trauma and disease. Current treatment options for tissue loss include drug therapy, artificial implants, and organ transplantation. Drugs can relieve patients from pain and can potentially help in the healing process. However, the drug treatment is often symptomatic and hence temporary, and at best can be used to enhance damaged tissue repair when tissue loss is not significant. In the event that tissue loss is substantial, treatment turns to tissue replacement strategies. The current approaches for organ or tissue replacement include tissue grafting from one site of the patient's body to another (autograft); from a donor of the same species (allograft), or; from donor of another species (xenograft) [1,2]. Although these therapeutic modalities can potentially improve the quality of human life, they are still limited by certain complications and shortcomings. For example, use of autografts is associated with donor site morbidity and limited tissue availability, whereas allografts pose the risk of disease transfer. Xenografts, though available in sufficient quantities, are associated with problems of humoral rejection and transfer of diseases of animal origin, specifically animal viruses [2]. Other strategies involving artificial implants have several shortcomings, such as the potential to evoke adverse immune response, structural failure over a period of time, and compromised physiological activity of the native tissue [3]. Therefore, there is a need for alternative strategies to overcome the shortcomings associated with the aforementioned approaches [3].

Tissue engineering has emerged as a potential approach to overcome the shortage of tissues and organs by combining a biodegradable scaffold [as a temporary extracellular matrix (ECM)] and cells to create functional tissue replacements. Tissue engineering [3] has been defined as: "The application of the principles and methods of engineering and life sciences toward the fundamental understanding of structure-function relationships in normal and pathological mammalian tissue and the development of biological substitutes to restore, maintain, or improve tissue function [4,5]."

The development of a biological substitute for the restoration of tissue function can involve multiple steps. The major stages involved in any tissue engineering approach can be classified as:

(1) Identification and isolation of a suitable source of cells;
(2) *in vitro* or *ex-vivo* expansion of cells to generate appropriate numbers;
(3) design of a scaffold/device to either carry cells and/or encapsulate growth factors (GFs);
(4) uniform seeding of cells onto or into the scaffold/device;
(5) appropriate culture of the seeded cells; followed by
(6) *in vivo* implantation of the engineered construct [6] (Figure 13.1).

Thus cells and scaffolds, with or without growth factors, together hold a promise for both *in vitro* regeneration of neo-tissue and *in vivo* regeneration of damaged tissue. Functional restoration for a large number of tissues is currently under investigation. Of these, the musculoskeletal tissues such as bone, cartilage, muscle and tendon have received increased attention [7].

All tissues/organs consist of tissue specific cells which are present in a well-defined manner within a complex structural and functional network of molecules that form the extracellular matrix. The variation in ECM composition and contents along with the respective cell type governs the diverse properties and function of each tissue and organ [8]. In addition, ECM is also a key component during dynamic events of tissue such as growth, development, repair, and regeneration. It acts as a reservoir for signaling molecules, which in turn have the potential to guide cell fate processes. Therefore, cells and ECM molecules along with GFs can be considered as the most important components for tissue regeneration.

One can follow two strategies for tissue repair or regeneration: First, cell-based therapy, wherein desired cell types can be injected directly into the defect site, and, second, scaffold-based tissue regeneration wherein a scaffold (artificial ECM) in combination with cells and/or GFs is used for tissue regeneration [9]. Cell therapy has played an important role in tissue repair including autologous chondrocyte implantation (ACI), and the commercially available carticel [10,11,12]. However, tissues have three-dimensional (3D) structure that prompts

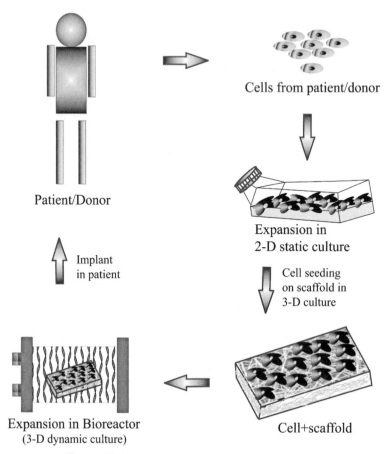

Patient/Donor

Cells from patient/donor

Expansion in
2-D static culture

Implant
in patient

Cell seeding
on scaffold in
3-D culture

Expansion in Bioreactor
(3-D dynamic culture)

Cell+scaffold

Figure 13.1. Important stages in tissue engineering.

the use of a guiding template and framework (scaffold) to facilitate 3D cell growth. Thus, in the second approach, cells are expanded in culture, seeded onto a guiding framework and allowed to grow and eventually re-implanted in the host [9]. Herein the guiding framework or the scaffold is a critical component as all human cells grow in a planer fashion in two-dimensional culture, whereas on a scaffold (that is, on a 3D structure) they will tend to grow to the shape of the scaffold, thereby providing the essential three dimensionality to the tissue.

13.2.2 Importance of Scaffolds in Tissue Engineering

One of the central objectives of tissue engineering is to create a 3D structure that can mimic the native ECM until cells seeded within the scaffold synthesize *de novo* ECM. This 3D structure acts as a template for cell attachment and tissue development. The ECM-mimicking scaffolds are normally constructed out of biomaterials [13] that could be synthetic, such as ceramics, and polymers or natural materials, such as proteins and carbohydrates (see section on synthetic and natural polymers for more details)[14]. In order for the cells to experience a native environment, the synthetic scaffold must comply with specific requirements in terms of physical (including 3D architecture), chemical, mechanical and surface properties. Some of the desirable characteristics of a scaffold include [15,16]:

1. The material used to synthesize scaffolds should be biodegradable and the rate of degradation should be coupled to rate of tissue regeneration.
2. Both the bulk biomaterial and its degradation products should be non-toxic (biocompatible) and the degradation products should preferably be metabolized in the body.
3. The scaffold should have high surface area-to-volume ratio to enable maximal cell seeding.
4. The scaffold should be porous so as to permit the migration of cells in all three dimensions.
5. The pores should be interconnected, with a pore network that enables appropriate transport of nutrients, metabolites and regulatory molecules to and from the cells within the matrix.
6. The material must meet the mechanical requirements of the tissue at the site of implantation.
7. The 3D scaffold should be physically and chemically stable and easy to sterilize.
8. The scaffold should possess the ability to carry bioactive molecules such as growth factors and deliver the same at an appropriate rate at the site of interest.
9. The scaffold should have a physicochemical structure that promotes cell fate processes such as cell adhesion and migration.

Practically, it would be very difficult to meet all the aforementioned criteria for scaffold design. Therefore, the approach most often followed is to achieve as many criteria as is essential/detrimental for a specific application. The choice of technique for scaffold fabrication depends on the application, the type of biomaterial used for scaffold synthesis, and the environment in which the scaffold would be implanted.

The behavior of cells seeded on a scaffold is influenced by the chemical [17] as well as the physical properties of a scaffold [18,19,20]. The chemical properties of the scaffold majorly control the biocompatibility and biodegradability of the scaffold. Chemical properties and hence biodegradation/biocompatibility can be modulated by using a combination of synthetic and natural polymers [21]. On the other hand, the influence of physical properties of scaffold on cell behavior has not been extensively studied. Several studies evaluating the importance of geometry of a scaffold in the regulation of cell fate behavior have been reported recently [22,23,24]. Cells behave differently when cultured on a 3D scaffold than on a 2D (two dimensional) substrate. For example, chondrocytes maintain their phenotype when cultured on a 3D scaffold, but dedifferentiate to a fibroblastic cell type when cultured on a 2D substrate [25]. This provides a rationale for fabrication of scaffolds with 3D architecture, adequate porosity, and interconnectivity of pores. A potential constraint of using a 3D scaffold could be limited diffusion of nutrients and gases [26]. This can potentially be overcome by providing dynamic culture conditions to cells. Use of bioreactors can provide physiological levels of nutrient media transport, and mechanical stimuli for improved cell growth during construct development [26,27].

13.2.2.1 *Influence of Nanometer Scale Features of Scaffolds in Tissue Engineering.* The topography of the scaffolding surface plays an important role in terms of cell behavior [28]. Previous studies have already demonstrated the response of cells to micrometer range topographies such as grooves/ridges [29,30] and their ability to distinguish between different topographies [31]. The fibers present in the ECM and basal lamina possess diameter in the nanometer scale. One of the approaches for scaffold design is a biomimetic approach wherein the incorporation of nanoscale features in the scaffold architecture provide for closeness to the native environment [32]. It has been demonstrated that nanoscale features support better cell growth/response as compared to microscale surface features [33,34]. In connective tissue, the structural protein fibers, such as collagen, are the building blocks of natural ECM and they have a hierarchical structure with the fiber diameters ranging from 50–500 nm [35]. Since cells are accustomed to nanometer scale topographies present in the native ECM, the design strategies of scaffolds have recently involved mimicking these nanoscale features of ECM component [36].

Several studies have demonstrated that incorporation of nanoscale features in the scaffold elicit diverse cell behavior, ranging from changes in cell adhesion, cell motility, cell orientation to surface arrangement of cytoskeleton components [37,38]. The changes are even seen at the transcriptional level, as there is modulation in the intracellular signaling pathways that regulate cell activity and gene expression [39,40]. There is always an exchange of information between ECM, cytoskeleton and nucleus. Soluble mediators bind to integrin receptors on the cell surface which in turn stimulates the receptor mediated signaling, including the activation of kinase pathway, lipid pathway and specifically Rho GTPases, Rho, Rac, and Cdc42 [37,41]. Studies conducted in the past have demonstrated that the cells retained their morphology and shape on nanofiber matrices and there was a comparative increase in the production of ECM components by the cells [39,42]. Thus, for tissue engineering, the need is to mimic the native ECM at nanoscale in order to recapitulate the organization and function of native tissue.

13.3   METHODS OF NANOFIBROUS SCAFFOLD SYNTHESIS

Several novel fabrication techniques have been developed to process biodegradable and bioresorbable materials into 3D polymeric scaffolds [43]. Fiber bonding

[44], solvent casting and particulate leaching [45], membrane lamination [46], melt molding [47], *in-situ* polymerization [48], freeze drying [49], gas-foaming processing [50], extrusion [51], 3D printing [52] and polymer foams [53] are some of the techniques that have been explored for the synthesis of a porous 3D scaffold. As stated earlier, ECM is composed of nanoscale components that provide structure as well as guidance to cells. Thus, tissue engineers desire to develop nanofiber-based scaffolds that would essentially mimic the native ECM and favor the cell fate processes in the direction of tissue development/regeneration. Fibrous scaffolds have been synthesized by three methods, namely: self assembly, phase separation, and electrospinning. These three methods offer nanoscale dimensions in fibrous form along with the architecture that have potential to be used as an artificial ECM [54].

This section will briefly describe self assembly and phase separation techniques and will focus on electrospinning and its applications in tissue engineering.

13.3.1   Self Assembly

Also known as self organization, self assembly is the reversible process of formation of structured patterns from components of a pre-existing system that are not associated with structure/order [55]. The native ECM or the cellular microenvironment not only provides physical support but also provides ligands for cell attachment thereby facilitating cell fate processes such as cell adhesion, migration and differentiation [36]. Self assembly can be used to create scaffolds with well-defined 3D architecture at the nanometer scale to facilitate cell adhesion, consequential function and hence tissue regeneration [56]. Self assembly has been reported in multiple natural processes, such as during nucleic acid synthesis and protein synthesis, with these assembles mostly being governed by non-covalent interactions, such as ionic, Van der Waals, and hydrophobic interactions, as well as hydrogen bonds [57]. Taking cues from these natural processes, Hartgerink et al. reported the self assembly of peptide-amphiphiles [PA] for the formation of nanofibers. They demonstrated the mineralization of hydroxyapatite directed by self-assembled collagen fibers, thereby mimicking the hierarchical structure of bone. In their studies, the alkyl chain length and peptide amino acid composition was varied to allow for the synthesis of nanofibers with varying morphology, surface chemistry and bioactivity [58,59] (Figure 13.2). Further, Hosseinkhani et al. reported the synthesis of hepatocyte growth factor (HGF)-loaded, self-assembled PA nanofibers. Their results demonstrated enhanced vascularization in mice models following the subcutaneous injection of PA along with HGF, which was due to sustained release of the growth factor, as compared to the positive control (HGF only) [60].

An advantage associated with the process of self assembly is that it can be performed under physiological conditions without the usage of any harmful organic solvents, thereby making the technique more amicable for *in vivo* applications. Despite the ability to synthesize fibers having diameters in the nanometer scale, the process of self assembly remains a relatively complicated process and is

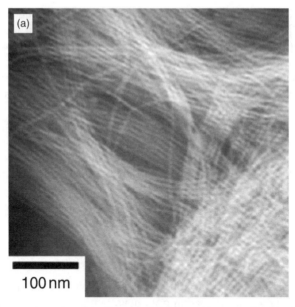

Figure 13.2. Tranmission Electron Micrograph of nanofibers synthesized by self assembly of peptide amphiphiles (negatively stained with phosphotungstic acid.) Reprinted from Hartgerink JD, Beniash E, Stupp SI. Peptide-amphiphile nanofibers: A versatile scaffold for the preparation of self-assembling materials. Proc Nat Acad Sci 2002;99(8):5133–5138. Copyright © 2002 National Academy of Sciences. USA. Reprinted with permission of the National Academy of Sciences, USA.

still limited by low productivity [61]. Further, the process is limited to the use of components of peptide origin only.

13.3.2 Phase Separation

Another method that has been used for the synthesis of nanofibrous scaffolds is phase separation [62]. This technique encompasses the following steps:

1. In this method, the polymer of interest is first mixed with a solvent.
2. The mixture is then allowed to undergo gelation (phase separation) at low temperatures.
3. The solvent is then extracted by immersing the gel into water, leaving behind pores in the gel.
4. The gel is then frozen.
5. It is then freeze-dried under a vacuum to obtain a porous nanofibrous structure.

Gelation plays a critical role in the formation of fibrillar matrix structure. Further, gelation temperature also controls the porous morphology of the matrix.

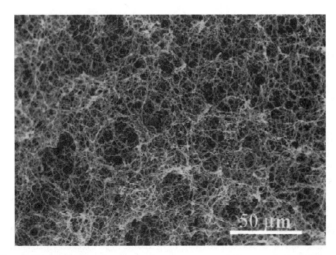

Figure 13.3. Scanning Electron Micrograph of PLLA scaffolds synthesized from 2.5% (w/v) PLLA/THF solution at a gelation temperature of 8 °C by phase separation. Reprinted from Ma PX, Zhang R. Synthetic nano-scale fibrous matrix. 1999;46(1):60–72. Copyright © 1999 J Wiley. Reprinted with permission of John Wiley & Sons Inc.

Nanofibrous poly(L-lactic acid) (PLLA)] scaffolds with high porosity (98.5%) have been synthesized by Ma and Zhang [62] (Figure 13.3). They demonstrated the gelation behavior of PLLA in different solvents as well as at variable temperatures; with gelation occurring readily in tetrahydrofuran (THF) and below 17 °C and platelet like structure at higher temperatures due to crystal nucleation and growth process. In another study, Hua et al. synthesized PLLA scaffolds with an interconnected porous structure by liquid-liquid phase separation of ternary PLLA-water-dioxane solution [63]. The synthesized scaffolds resulted in effective cell penetration and demonstrated potential in cartilage tissue engineering. Yang et al. synthesized highly porous and fibrous PLLA matrices [64] that resembled the natural ECM in the body with fiber diameter ranging from 50 nanometer(nm) to 350 nm. They demonstrated the differentiation of nerve stem cells on these nanofibrous PLLA scaffolds and hence their potential use of PLLA matrix in nerve tissue engineering.

Thermally-induced phase separation (TIPS) has been recently used extensively for the synthesis of interconnected and porous membranes. In this technique, homogenous polymer solution prepared at a higher temperature is converted into two phases (polymer rich phase and polymer lean phase) by changing the temperature [65]. Huang et al. used TIPS to synthesize poly(lactide-co-glycolide)/nano-hydroxyapatite (PLGA/NHA) scaffolds. Their results demonstrated enhanced mesenchymal stem cell (MSC) growth and proliferation on regular and highly interconnected porous PLGA/NHA scaffolds {100–150 micrometers (μm)} as compared on PLGA only scaffolds thereby establishing the potential of TIPS synthesized PLGA/NHA scaffolds in bone tissue engineering [66].

The advantage of the phase separation technique is that it is a relatively simple technique that is not equipment intensive. In addition, a highly-porous structure can be obtained with control over the mechanical properties of the nanofibrous matrix and batch to batch consistency can be easily maintained [62]. However, a disadvantage of this technique can be limited control on the internal architecture of the nanofibrous matrix [67].

13.3.3   Electrospinning

Electrostatic spinning (electrospinning) is the synthesis of fibers of diameter ranging from 10 nm to 10 μm or larger by drawing it from a polymer solution under the influence of electrostatic forces [68,69]. The concept of electrospinning is more than 100-years-old [70–76] and has regained the attention of researchers for the synthesis of nanofiber-based scaffolds for tissue engineering applications.

The apparatus for electrospinning (Figure 13.4) consists of a syringe which is the reservoir for holding the polymer solution, capillary/needle, high voltage power supply, grounded metallic collector (plate/mandrel), and a syringe pump (not shown in the figure) that pumps the polymer at a particular rate from the needle tip. The presence of a syringe pump is not mandatory when the syringe is placed in a vertical configuration, whereby the polymer solution is released from the capillary under the influence of gravity. Further, the collector can either be a grounded metallic plate that is stationary or a rotating cylinder, depending on the requirement of a non-woven mesh or aligned fibers, respectively.

During electrospinning, a polymer solution is taken in a glass syringe connected to a metallic needle. The polymer solution by virtue of its viscosity/surface

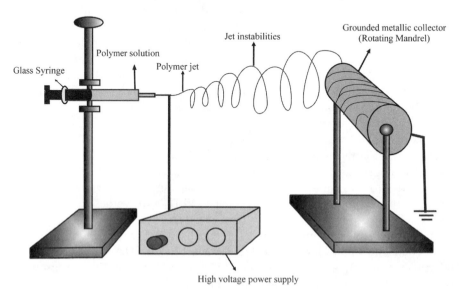

Figure 13.4. Schematic of the electrospinning technique.

tension produces a hemispherical meniscus at the tip of the capillary/needle. A high voltage is then applied between the needle and a grounded metallic plate that causes the induction of charges on the hemispherical droplet at the capillary tip. Mutual charge repulsion (coulombic repulsion) on the meniscus of the polymer solution induces a force that is initially balanced by the surface tension of the polymer. An increases in the voltage causes higher surface charges on the polymeric droplet and its elongation leading to the formation of a cone like structure called the Taylor cone [77]. With further increase in the voltage above a particular threshold, the repulsive forces overcome the surface tension forces and a jet ensues from the tip of the Taylor cone. The jet travels straight for a short distance and then undergoes bending instabilities that lead the jet to traverse a spiral path. During the course of movement of the jet to the collector plate, it thins due to solvent evaporation and stretching caused by bending instabilities [78]. Higher charges on the jet leads to increased elongation forces and hence reduced fiber diameter. The solidified polymeric nanofibers are deposited on the grounded metal plate in the form of a non-woven mesh (Figure 13.5).

Electrospinning has been extended from the phenomenon of electrostatic spraying (electrospraying). In electrospraying, charge is provided to a conducting liquid that splits mid-air, resulting in the formation of spray of fine particles following jet formation; hence, the process is termed as electrospraying [70,71]. When high molecular weight polymers are used instead of low molecular weight substance, the process leads to the formation of continuous fibers, and hence the

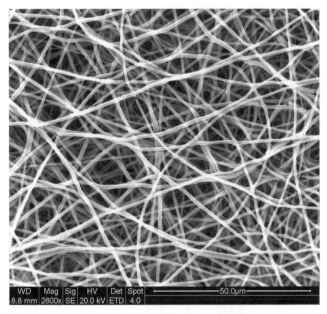

Figure 13.5. Scanning Electron Micrograph of PLGA nanofibers (non-woven mesh) synthesized by the electrospinning technique. (Unpublished data from the laboratory).

phenomenon is known as electrospinning. However, when charge is provided to low molecular weight polymeric solution, it results in the formation of nano-particles by the phenomenon of electrospraying [79].

Electrospinning is influenced by solution parameters namely viscosity, con-ductivity, and surface tension [80,81]; system parameters namely capillary diam-eter, electric potential at the tip, and the distance between the tip and the collection plate [77,82–85]; and ambient parameters like temperature and humidity in the electrospinning chamber [86].

(1) Solution parameters

    (a) **Solution viscosity** plays a key role in affecting fiber diameter and morphology. Low solution viscosities can lead to the formation of particles/beads whereas, higher solution viscosity, above a thresh-old yields fibers without beads [80]. Further, an increase in the solu-tion viscosity results in an increase in the fiber diameter. However, beyond an upper limit of viscosity, the solution dries at the nozzle, thereby preventing fiber formation.

    (b) **Conductivity** is another solution parameter that influences elec-trospinning by generation of repulsive forces on the polymeric jet. In general, a more conductive solution is easily drawn to form a jet during electrospinning. Conductivity on the polymeric droplet is governed by the type of polymer used and the solvent used to dissolve it.

        In a recent study, Choi et al. studied the influence of salts on nano-fibrous structure [87]. Their study indicates that increased charges on a polymer solution poly(3-hydroxybutyrate-co-3-hydroxyvalerate (PHBV) by addition of a salt benzyl trialkyl ammonium chloride led to increased elongation forces caused by self repulsion of similar charges that resulted in reduced fiber diameter. Therefore, increase in charges on a polymer solution can cause a significant reduction in fiber diameter.

    (c) **Surface tension** (closely linked to solution viscosity) plays an impor-tant role from the point of initiation of the process where it holds the hemispherical meniscus at the tip of the capillary. Surface tension is directed opposite to the electrostatic charges thereby determining the voltage threshold value responsible for jet formation. Excess sur-face tension encourages the formation of beads. Choice of solvent and polymer concentration can help alter surface tension and hence the formation of nanofibers/nanoparticles.

(2) System parameters

    (a) The **internal diameter of the needle** closely reflects the diameter of the base of the Taylor cone and hence the diameter of the jet issuing out of that Taylor cone. Katti et al. studied the influence of needle gauge (internal diameter of capillary) on the diameter of nanofibers and demonstrated a decrease in the average fiber diameter with reduction in needle diameter [82]. Hence, needle gauge can have a significant influence on the fiber diameter.

(b) **Voltage** plays a critical role in determining the fiber diameter. Since voltage is responsible for generation of charges on the polymeric droplet, an increase in voltage (or electric field strength) increases the charge density on the polymeric jet and hence repulsion. Higher charge repulsion causes an increased drawing effect on the polymer jet that leads to the formation of fibers with smaller diameter [77].

(c) **Electrospinning distance (distance between the tip of the capillary and the collector)** determines the time taken by the jet (path length) to reach the collector plate. Hence, the electrospinning distance can indirectly influence the length of the ejected jets' trajectory [83,84]. Decreased electrospinning distances prevent complete solvent evaporation, thereby leading to agglomeration of the fibers. It has been reported by Lee et al. [84] that with the increase in the electrospinning distance, the average fiber diameter increases, due to reduction in the effective field strength (per unit distance) and hence reduced thinning effect. However, in another study by Zhao et al. [85], it was observed that average fiber diameter decreased with increasing distance. It was discussed that the increase in the distance provides greater opportunity for the jet to split and elongate. Although the aforementioned studies [84,85] report contradictory results, it is intuitive to believe that an increase in electrospinning distance will lead to a decrease in nanofiber diameter. However, increase in electrospinning distance beyond a critical limit does not lead to the collection of fibers probably due to reduced influence of the electric field [85].

(3) Ambient parameters

(a) **Humidity** in the electrospinning environment affects fiber morphology to a great extent without influencing the fiber diameter. Increased humidity levels increase the pores on fiber surface, which ultimately coalesce to form non-uniform structures [86]. Humidity also determines the rate of solvent evaporation from the jet that deposits in form of fibers. High humidity levels interfere with solvent evaporation, hence fibers that would have otherwise dried in a controlled humidity environment would not dry completely in a high humidity environment.

Thus, the fiber diameter and morphology of the electrospun nanofibers can be altered by manipulating the solution, system and ambient parameters.

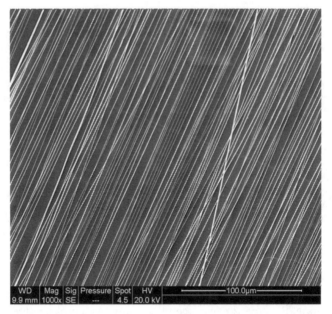

Figure 13.6. Scanning Electron Micrograph of aligned Polystrene nanofibers synthesized by the electrospinning technique. (Unpublished data from the laboratory).

As stated earlier, the electrospun nanofibers deposited on the grounded metal collector are in the form of a non-woven mesh. However, fibers can also be directed in a particular orientation to enable the synthesis of aligned fibers (Figure 13.6). ECM molecules in connective tissue like cartilage, ligament, and even skeletal muscle have a specific orientation, and hence aligned fibers can provide contact guidance for cells that can potentially direct their alignment along the length of the fibers [88]. This in turn can lead to desirable repair/regeneration of the tissue. Multiple methods have been reported for the alignment of fibers synthesized using the electrospinning technique [89–93]. One such method involves the use of a rotating mandrel in place of a grounded metal plate as the collector. In this method, when the linear velocity of the rotating mandrel matches that of the jet, fibers get deposited on the collecting substrate/ mandrel in a circumferential manner that generates aligned fibers (Figure 13.2). This method has been exploited by Mathews et al. for the alignment of collagen nanofibers [89]. Another method that has been reported for nanofiber alignment makes use of a needle as the counter electrode that serves to focus the entire set of fibers from the jet to a focusing electric field generated due to the sharp pin counter electrode. The counter electrode is mounted inside a rotating mandrel/drum. Therefore, the rotating mandrel along with the point counter electrode leads to the alignment of the nanofibers [90]. In another report, alignment has been obtained by using a rotating disc collector instead of a mandrel [91]. The bending instabilities result in the formation of a conical envelope that transforms into an inverted cone with the apex at the edge of the rotating disc. The sharp edge of the rotating disc is responsible for exerting a pulling force on the jet that leads to the assembly of nanofibers on the circumference of the disc in an aligned manner. Studies conducted in the past few years also state the influence of fiber alignment on ECM production. In one such study, Lee et al. reported the influence of fiber alignment on ECM production by human ligament fibroblast. Their results demonstrated that production of collagen on aligned fibers was greater when compared to that on non-aligned controls [92]. In another study, Xu et al. demonstrated the potential of biodegradable poly(L-lactic acid)/polycaprolactone (PLLA/PCL) scaffold using aligned fibers that matched the requirements of the middle layer in an artery. They observed orientation of smooth muscle cells along the length of the aligned fibers with enhanced adhesion and proliferation thus indicating the potential of the aligned nanofiber-based scaffold for application in blood vessel tissue engineering [93].

Apart from alignment, fiber diameter also plays a key role in gene expression. Supramolecular property of the ECM is defined by the composition of protein fibrils enmeshed within the hydrated network of glycosaminoglycans [94]. The nano-dimensioned fibers synthesized by electrospinning mimic this supramolecular property. However, smaller fiber size (diameter) reduces the expression of various genes involved in differentiation and migration due to less cellular attachment points [95]. These problems can be overcome by combining the microfibrous and nano-fibrous scaffolds in one system that would provide ECM like structures to the cells and the ability for cell attachment and guidance [95,96]. Another limiting factor in tissue engineering applications could be the cell seeding densities on electrospun nanofibers. This can potentially be overcome by spinning the matrix along with the cells to enable enhanced cellular densities, thereby improving functional connections between the cells [97]. Thus, electrospun nanofibers can serve as a potential scaffold in tissue engineering of ECM rich organs.

Variations in the process of electrospinning can be in terms of type of spinneret or collector plate. Coaxial electrospinning involves the synthesis of nanofibers with core-shell type geometry. This has been mostly exploited for the incorporation of water soluble growth factors that still remains a challenge in conventional electrospinning. Jiang et al. exploited this technique for the incorporation of water soluble bioactive agents, bovine serum albumin (BSA) and lysozyme within polyethylene glycol nanofibers with a shell of polycaprolactone (PCL) and demonstrated release of bioactive protein [98]. Researchers have also explored the possibility of increased rate of nanofiber production by employing multiple spinnerets [99]. Variations in collector plate, for example, stationary collector or rotating mandrel, determines fiber alignment and has been discussed earlier in this section.

Electrospinning is a relatively advantageous technique for scaffold production in comparison to self assembly and phase separation, as it is a one step technique and involves a simple experimental set-up. Further, it can be modulated to control the fiber diameter, morphology and density that can meet specific tissue

TABLE 13.1. Comparison of Processing Techniques for the Synthesis of Nanofibers

Features	Self assembly	Phase separation	Electrospinning
Ease of processing	No	Yes	Yes
Control on fiber diameter	No	No	Yes
Easy scale up	No	No	Yes
Advantages	• It can be performed without the use of any harmful organic solvents.	• Simple technique. • Not equipment intensive. • Highly porous scaffold with control over its mechanical properties. • Batch-to-batch consistency.	• One step technique. • Simple set-up, hence cost effective. • Can be modulated to control fiber diameter and alignment. • High porosity scaffold with interconnected pores. • Highly versatile in terms of variety of polymers.
Disadvantages	• Relatively complex. • Low productivity. • Limited to a few polymers only.	• No control over the internal architecture.	• Scaffolds have a miniscule three-dimensional profile. • Small pore size. • Use of high concentrations of organic solvent.

engineering requirements. In addition, the nanofibrous scaffolds generated by electrospinning have high porosities with interconnected pores [100]. Inspite of these advantages, nanofibers produced by conventional electrospinning are in the form of a non woven mesh with limited 3D profiles. Further, although porosities obtained can be large, the pore sizes obtained are relatively small when compared to matrix produced by other techniques. Table 13.1 provides a comparative analysis of the three techniques self assembly, phase separation, and electrospinning that have been discussed in this section.

Electrospinning has shown great potential in the field of biomedical sciences. Electrospun nanofibers have been used for the synthesis of scaffolds that have been applied for the engineering of multiple tissues such as cartilage, bone, muscle, ligament, nerve, skin and vasculature [88,92,101–105].

Further, these fibers have also been used for controlled delivery of drugs, proteins and nucleic acids [82,106,107]. Other areas of application include sensor devices [108], filtration [109], protective clothing [110], and electrical conductors [111] (Figure 13.7). Although there are number of applications of electrospun

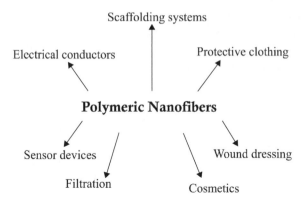

Figure 13.7. Potential applications of nanofibers using the electrospinning technique.

nanofibers, the discussion in this chapter is restricted to tissue engineering applications only, more specifically musculoskeletal tissue engineering.

13.4 POLYMERS USED FOR SYNTHESIZING NANOFIBROUS STRUCTURES USING THE ELECTROSPINNING TECHNIQUE

Instead of implanting permanent non-biodegradable devices within the body, there is a growing need to explore biodegradable implants that would coax the body for self repair/to regenerate. One of the main strategies in this direction is tissue engineering that involves the application of polymeric biomaterials, both biodegradable as well as non-biodegradable, as scaffolding systems. Degradation of polymeric devices (mainly by hydrolytic and enzymatic means) can be manipulated to match the regeneration rate of the specific tissue based on the rate of ECM generation of that tissue. This section discusses various polymers under the broad category of natural, that is, biologically derived and synthetic polymers.

13.4.1 Natural Polymers

There is a rapid increase in the use of natural polymers to make nanofibrous scaffolds. Natural polymers that have been used for scaffolding applications are either constituents of ECM or the chemical/physical mimics of ECM components that have been extracted from other living forms. ECM constituents have innate information for cell guidance, and thus can be advantageous if fabricated into nanofibrous scaffolds by electrospinning. Natural polymers have the advantage of being hydrophilic, biocompatible, with their degradation products being easily metabolized in the body. In addition, natural polymers have been demonstrated to enhance cell interaction and proliferation [112]. Therefore, natural polymers have been explored for the synthesis of nanofiber-based scaffolds for tissue engineering. Natural polymers that have been used for electrospinning can be broadly divided into two classes: protein based materials are used, that include collagen, gelatin, and silk; and carbohydrate like materials namely, chitin/chitosan, and alginate. This section briefly describes the electrospinning of these natural polymers.

13.4.1.1   Proteins. Proteins are a major category of natural polymers that are difficult to fabricate into fibrous forms [113]. This could be attributed to the complex macromolecular and 3D structure of proteins and the presence of strong intra- and/or inter-molecular bonding. Electrospinning has the capability to process protein polymers into nanofibrous scaffolds, with the use of different solvent system.

Successful attempts have been made to electrospin protein polymers from natural ECM components as well as proteins obtained from other organisms such as silk. Both fibrous and globular proteins have been electrospun into nanofibers, however, a discussion of all the proteins is beyond the scope of this chapter, hence, this discussion has been limited to some extensively studied proteins, namely collagen, gelatin, and silk.

13.4.1.1.1   COLLAGEN. Collagen is a major protein constituent of ECM of connective tissues, such as bone, tendon, ligament and cartilage [114]. At least 27 different types of collagen which differ in their structure, function, and location have been identified in mammalian tissues, of which collagen type I is the most abundant form [115].

All the collagen types share a common triple helical domain that has a characteristic primary structure, with repeated sequence of $(G-X-Y)_n$ units, where G is glycine, X is alanine or proline and Y is hydroxyproline [116]. Being a component of the natural ECM milieu, collagen has gained popularity in tissue engineering as a material for the synthesis of electrospun scaffolds [89,117].

Matthews et al. studied electrospinning of different collagen types such as collagen type I and type III into nanofibers [89]. Collagen type I nanofibers were obtained with an average diameter of 100 nm, and 1, 1, 1, 3, 3, 3 hexafluoro-2-propanol (HFP) was used as the solvent. An important observation made by authors was the presence of 67 nm banding pattern in the nanofibers which is a characteristic of collagen in its native form, thereby indicating that the process of electrospinning maintains the native structure of collagen. In another study, Shih et al. synthesized collagen type I nanofibers using HFP as the solvent system and studied the influence of collagen concentration on fiber diameter. Their results demonstrated an increase in fiber diameter with an increase in collagen concentration [39].

Collagen type II is a native constituent of articular cartilage. Hence, electrospinning of collagen type II could be a promising approach for *in vitro* cartilage tissue engineering. To validate this rationale, Shields et al. fabricated collagen type II scaffolds by electrospinning, and cross-linked the same with glutaraldehyde. The study demonstrated that although better mechanical properties were obtained for cross-linked scaffolds when compared to non cross-linked scaffolds, the mechanical properties of cross-linked scaffolds were less than that of native collagen type II fibers [117].

The drawback associated with collagen fibers is their rapid degradation in the physiological environment. This has been overcome by cross-linking of collagen fibers using cross-linkers such as glutaraldehyde, formaldehyde, epoxy compounds and zero length cross linkers such as carbodiimide [39,117,118]. Although the electrospun collagen fibers do not fully recapitulate the native collagen fibers, they still hold promise for tissue engineering applications.

13.4.1.1.2 GELATIN. Gelatin is a denatured form of collagen obtained by subjecting the collagen source (bone, tendon or skin) to acid or alkaline pretreatment [119]. It is a relatively inexpensive substitute for collagen. Being a derivative of collagen, it has a polypeptide nature and possesses RGD peptides required for cell adhesion. However, unlike collagen, gelatin contains multiple oligopeptides of diverse molecular weight. Use of gelatin in drug delivery applications [120], wound dressing applications and as a food additive has been known for many years [121,122]; however, its use as a biomaterial for electrospinning is relatively recent.

Gelatin is soluble in water at room temperature; however, gelatin contains ionizable groups that form hydrogen bonds in the aqueous environment that makes electrospinning of gelatin quite challenging. Being a biopolymer with strong polarity, gelatin needs to be dissolved in highly polar organic solvents to enable electrospinning. Huang et al. demonstrated the use of a highly polar solvent 2, 2, 2-trifluoroethanol (TFE) for electrospinning of gelatin [123]. Huang et al. also validated that the mechanical performance of gelatin nanofibers was influenced by the fiber diameter as well as fiber morphology. The finest fibrous mat without beads was obtained at a relatively higher concentration of gelatin and this mat exhibited better mechanical strength as compared to relatively thick but beaded fibers [123]. Ki et al. examined the stability of gelatin in formic acid, and hence, its effect on the morphology of electrospun gelatin nanofibers [124]. They reported the formation of gelatin fibers having diameters in the range of 70–170 nm with formic acid showing no significant effect on gelatin fibers [124].

The hydrophilicity of gelatin causes loss in physical integrity when exposed to water; hence, there is a need for cross-linking gelatin fibers to enhance their mechanical strength and stability for their use as scaffolding systems. Zhang et al. reported the electrospinning of gelatin nanofibers that were cross-linked post synthesis with glutaraldehyde vapours (GTA) at room temperature for three days. There results demonstrated that the cross-linked nanofibrous membranes maintained their structural integrity after being immersed in water for six days. Further, these membranes were non-cytotoxic and exhibited enhanced thermal stability and mechanical strength [125]. Hence, cross-linked nanofibers show potential to be used in tissue engineering applications.

13.4.1.1.3 SILK FIBROIN. Conventional silk is a natural protein derived from the cocoon of *Bombyx mori* (silk worms) [126]. Other forms of silk such as dragline silk are obtained from *N. clavipes* spiders. Silk obtained from cocoons as well as *N. clavipes* spiders has a desirable combination of biocompatibility, high mechanical strength, and even compressibility [127]. Silk obtained from all sources has been electrospun into nanofibers. Although silk fibers provide improved strength, the immune response elicited—due to sericin protein present on the outer layer of silk protein—has limited its use in tissue engineering applications. Purified silk fibroin, after the removal of sericin, retains all the attributes of silk fiber, while reducing its immunogenicity.

Zarkoob et al. [127] reported the electrospinning of silk obtained from both *N. clavipes* spider and the *B. mori* silkworm using HFP as the solvent. The electrospun silk nanofibers obtained were smaller in diameter than the whole fibers produced by nature (*B. mori*, 10–20 µm and *N. clavipes*, 2–5 µm) as well as from conventional spinning techniques. Silk fibers obtained by electrospinning can be observed by electron diffraction without the need for microtome or other destructive sample preparation procedures. Sukigara et al. [128] reported the use of formic acid as the solvent system for the fabrication of nanofibers of silk fibroin. The use of formic acid helps does not affect the structure of fibroin (which imparts mechanical strength to the silk fiber) that can potentially be lost when HFP is used as the solvent [128]. In continuation to this study, Ayutsede et al. studied the influence of the process of electrospinning on the structure, morphology and properties of silk fiber assemblies. This study demonstrated that the dissolution of silk fibroin in formic acid enhances β-sheet crystallization and hence reduces the hydrodynamic radius of the fibroin molecules that result in an increase in intramolecular hydrogen bonding of the fibroin, which in turn facilitates β-sheet formation in the electrospun fiber [129]. Therefore, formic acid might be a desirable solvent for electrospinning of silk.

Other fibrous proteins that have been electrospun into nanofibers include fibrin, elastin, and fibrinogen [129–133]. Successful attempts have also been made towards electrospinning of globular proteins such as hemoglobin and myoglobin [134].

13.4.1.2 Carbohydrates. Carbohydrates are biologically-produced materials, with carbon, hydrogen and oxygen $[C_x(H_2O)_y]$ as the building blocks. Polysaccharides are long chains of simple sugar units bonded together. Commercially available products include starch, cellulose and its derivatives (such as cellulose acetate, carboxymethyl cellulose, and methyl cellulose), sodium alginate, xanthan gum, dextran, carrageenan, and hyaluronic acid. The synthesis of carbohydrate nanofibers using electrospinning has been extensively explored.

Glycosaminoglycans (GAGs) are long unbranched polysaccharides containing a repeating disaccharide unit. They are negatively charged polycarboxylated molecules that are located primarily on the surface of cells and in the ECM [135]. The majority of GAGs in the body are linked to core proteins, forming proteoglycans, and have an important role in binding of growth factors, maintaining the sol-gel property and water holding capacity of ECM [136].

13.4.1.2.1 HYALURONIC ACID (HA). Hyaluronic acid is a non-sulphated GAG, made up of repeating disaccharide units β-1, 4-D-glucuronic acid and β-1, 3-N-acetyl-D-glucosamine. It is the simplest form of all the GAGs present in the ECM [137,138] and is unique in that it does not exist in bound form with protein, that is, as a component of proteoglycans. An important property of hyaluronan is its capacity to bind large amounts of water (1000-times its own weight). This property makes them excellent lubricators and shock absorbers [136]. Electrospinning of hyaluronic acid can be challenging because of high viscosity and surface tension of HA in solution even at low concentrations. To overcome the high viscosity of HA that is obtained even at low concentrations, a low molecular weight thiolated form of hyaluronic acid that is a 3,3′-dithiobis- (propanoic dihydrazide)-modified derivative (HA-DTPH) has been reported [139]. In a recent study, Ji et al. reported the electrospinning of a blend of HA-DTPH and poly (ethylene oxide) (PEO), wherein PEO was added to further reduce the viscosity of HA and hence allow for HA fiber (diameters ranging from 50 to 300 nm) formation using electrospinning. The HA-DTPH/PEO nanofibrous scaffolds were further treated with water to remove PEO from the scaffolds to achieve pure HA-DTPH scaffolds. Disulfide linkages were introduced during electrospinning of HA-DTPH/PEO solution. The electrospun nanofibers of HA-DTPH/PEO had poor mechanical properties and they were water soluble. Ji et al. further cross-linked the scaffold with poly (ethylene glycol)-diacrylate (PEGDA) as cross-linking agent. Cross-linking improved the mechanical strength of the scaffold [139].

Um et al. fabricated HA nanofibers using a new set up called electroblowing, wherein the HA solution was heated to reduce its surface tension and viscosity and electrospun using air blowing. The air blowing enhanced the rate of solvent evaporation and HA nanofibers in the range of 49–74 nm were obtained [140]. To overcome the problems associated with the high viscosity of HA, blends of HA and gelatin solution in DMF as the solvent have also been reported. This study demonstrated that blending of HA with gelatin and use of DMF as a solven reduced the viscosity of HA, thereby making it easy to electrospin [141]. The ability to electrospun HA via blending with other polymer or electroblowing has improved the possibility of synthesizing HA nanofibers, and as a consequence, its potential for being used as a scaffold in tissue engineering applications.

13.4.1.2.2 ALGINATE. Alginate is a linear polysaccharide obtained from marine brown algae or seaweeds. It is composed of (1–4) linked β-D-mannuronic acid (M units) and α-L-guluronic acid (G units) monomers along the polymer backbone [142]. The alginate molecule is a block copolymer with repeated M and G blocks or with regions of MG blocks and is naturally available as a sodium or calcium salt. Alginate is a non-toxic and immunologically inert polymer that bears a structural resemblance to GAGs and hence, has been extensively explored in tissue engineering applications [143,144]. Like other natural polymers, alginate is hydrophilic and water soluble at room temperature. However, its use as an electrospun non-woven fibrous scaffold is relatively recent, owing to the difficulty associated with its electrospinning. Electrospinning of alginate solution is relatively challenging as gelation of alginate occurs even at low concentrations and using very low solution concentration does not lead to fiber formation [145]. In addition, an increase in polymer concentration results in highly viscous solutions that are difficult to electrospin. In an attempt to control the viscosity of alginate solutions, Bhattarai et al. incorporated PEO in alginate solution along with a surfactant [146]. The results of their study demonstrated that alginate could be electrospun into nanofibers when blended with PEO. Electrospun alginate-based scaffolds are relatively easy to fabricate, process, and scale-up, and hence have been extensively explored as a biomaterial [145,146]. Alginate can be co-electrospun with multiple types of polymers to form more complex matrices, that would more closely mimic natural ECM, and hence has the potential for use in diverse tissue engineering applications [145,146].

13.4.1.2.3   CHITIN AND CHITOSAN. Chitin is a linear polysaccharide found in marine crustacean shells and the cell walls of bacteria and fungi [147]. It is the second most abundant natural polymer after cellulose [148] and has structural resemblance to GAGs, such as chondroitin sulfates and hyaluronic acid, due to which it has been considered as a biomaterial for tissue engineering scaffolds [149]. Chitosan is a deacetylated (40–98%) derivative of chitin with repeating units of β (1–4) 2-amino-2-deoxy-D-glucose and having a molecular weight in the range of 300 KDa to 2000 KDa [148]. Chitosan, owing to its relatively better solubility, has received more attention than chitin. However, like other natural polymers, electrospinning of chitosan has been a challenging task because of its polycationic nature in solution that leads to high viscosities.

Noh et al. studied the electrospinning of chitin with HFP as the solvent and their results demonstrated that both chitin microfibers and nanofibers could be synthesized using HFP as the solvent system [149].

Recently Geng et al., electrospun chitosan nanofibers using acetic acid as the solvent system. The rationale for the use of acetic acid is that it reduces the viscosity of chitosan solution and increases the net charge on the jet [150]. Li et al. investigated the effect of chitosan molecular weight on its ability to electrospin along with the effect of an additive (PVA) on fiber formation and morphology. The study demonstrated that the ability of chitosan to be electrospun into nanofibers increases with the decrease in molecular weight of chitosan in presence of NaOH [151].

Quaternised chitosan derivatives have been reported to possess better antibacterial properties thereby enhancing their potential use as a wound dressing material. Ignatova et al. studied electrospinning of quaternised chitosan (QCh) solutions with PVA, followed by photo cross-linking by triethylene glycol diacrylate (TEGDA). The electrospun QCh/PVA fibers had diameters in 60–200 nm range [152]. The study demonstrated that an increase in QCh content in QCh/PVA solution resulted in an increase in solution conductivity, thereby leading to a decrease in the diameter of the electrospun nanofibers [152].

Chitosan is thus expected to be of great value as a scaffold material for tissue engineering with the combination of biocompatibility, intrinsic antibacterial activity, ability to bind to growth factors, and ability to be processed in a variety of shapes [153].

Encouraging results obtained after electrospinning of a few natural polymers has provided researchers an opportunity to explore other natural polymers, as well as their blends with other natural or synthetic polymers. Although natural polymers are a better choice for the synthesis of scaffolds for tissue engineering, they are still limited in their applications because of certain concerns like depletion of natural resources, risk of potential pathogen transmission, elicitation of immune response, limited control on molecular weight, and consequential degradation and mechanical properties [154].

13.4.2   Synthetic Polymers

Synthetic polymers have an advantage over natural polymers in that they can be modified or tailored depending upon the requirement for a specific biomedical application. In addition, one can also circumvent the batch-to-batch variability in properties as well as the reduced availability (in some cases) that are associated with natural polymers. Since synthetic polymers allow for a greater degree of control on properties (physical and chemical), they are a more desirable source of raw materials for biomedical applications. For example, polymer modifications (physical/chemical) can be advantageous for the immobilization of bioactive agents that can be very useful in drug delivery and tissue engineering applications. Amongst the available synthetic polymers, the ones more suitable for tissue engineering applications are most often the degradable types. Within this subclass, hydrolytically degradable polymers are preferred over the enzymatically degradable polymers to avoid any patient-to-patient variation in degradation profiles when used as implants. This section discusses various synthetic hydrolytically degradable polymers that have been electrospun and applied in tissue engineering.

13.4.2.1   Poly(α-hydroxy) Esters. Poly(α-hydroxy) esters are a family of polymers that contain hydrolytically cleavable ester linkages in their aliphatic back-bone chain. These thermoplastic polymers can be synthesized by ring opening or condensation polymerization reactions, depending upon the monomers used [155,156]. The most common amongst the class of poly(α-hydroxy) esters are the Food and Drug Administration (FDA) approved poly(glycolic acid) (PGA), poly(lactic acid) (PLA) and poly(lactide-co-glycolide) (PLGA).

13.4.2.1.1   Poly(Glycolic Acid) (PGA). PGA, a polymer of glycolic acid (GA), is highly crystalline and degrades relatively faster within the body due to its hydrophilic nature. However, the rates of degradation depend on the molecular weight, size, and surface area of the scaffold made of PGA [157]. The degradation product of PGA is glycolic acid, which can at times be a limiting factor due to its acidic nature. Nevertheless, PGA is desirable in many biomedical applications such as surgical sutures due to its high tensile strength, biocompatibility and biodegradability [158]. High crystallinity of PGA limits its solubility in organic solvents, the only exception being highly fluorinated compounds such as 1,1,1,3,3,3 hexafluoro-2-propanol (HFP). Boland et al. used the aforementioned solvent system for successful electrospinning of PGA and obtained fibers in the range of 0.22 µm to 0.88 µm at concentrations of 67-mg/mL PGA concentration and 143-mg/mL PGA concentration, thereby demonstrating the dependence of fiber diameter on polymer concentration [159].

13.4.2.1.2   Poly(Lactic Acid) (PLA). A polymer of lactic acid (LA), PLA is well known for its hydrophobicity, biocompatibility and biodegradability. Even though it is a crystalline polymer like PGA, its hydrophobicity enables relatively slower degradation rates. Unlike PGA, PLA is soluble in a variety of organic solvents due to the presence of an additional methyl group that also renders its hydrophobicity. High mechanical strength of PLA favors its potential application in load bearing applications. The variation in properties of PLA (both physical and chemical) is due to the presence of methyl group on the alpha carbon of lactic acid. Thus, the possible variations are poly (L-lactic acid) (PLLA), poly(D-lactic acid) (PDLA) and poly(DL-lactic acid) (PDLLA). Poly(DL-lactic acid) (PDLLA) is amorphous with low mechanical strength as compared to the D- and L-forms of PLA. Dong et al. reported the synthesis of PDLLA fibers and demonstrated that N, N-dimethyl formamide (DMF) was a better solvent than acetone for the electrospinning of PDLLA [160]. In addition, they studied the role of an additive-triethylbenzylammonium chlorate (organic salt) and demonstrated that the fiber diameter decreased from 500 nm to 100–200 nm following the addition of an organic salt due to the increased conductivity of the solution [160].

13.4.2.1.3   Poly(Lactic-Co-Glycolic Acid) (PLGA). PLGA is a copolymer of LA and GA with its degradation rates and mechanical properties amenable for tailoring by altering the ratio of LA and GA. The rate of degradation of the copolymer can be decreased by increasing the glycolic acid content and can be increased by increasing the lactic acid content. PLGA is one of the most commonly used polymers in tissue engineering as it supports cell adhesion and proliferation, in addition to being biodegradable and biocompatible. A study by Katti et al. demonstrated the influence of various parameters like polymer solution concentration, orifice diameter, and voltage on the morphology and diameter of electrospun PLGA nanofibers using THF:DMF (1:1) as the solvent system [82].

In another study, Min et al. reported the influence of solvent system on the fiber diameter of electrospun PLGA nanofibers. Electrospinning of PLGA in polar HFP led to a smaller average fiber diameter (310 nm) as compared to fibers produced in the same concentration of a non-polar chloroform (760 nm) [161]. Similar results were reported by You et al. while studying the role of solvent polarity in influencing fiber diameter of PLGA, PLA and PGA [163]. They demonstrated that electrospun PLGA fibers using less polar chloroform as a solvent system had a average fiber diameter of 760 nm, whereas PGA and PLA fibers electrospun using polar HFP had average fiber diameter of 310 nm and 290 nm, respectively. In another study, Bashur et al. studied the influence of polymer solution concentration on the diameter of electrospun PLGA fibers [163]. They demonstrated an increase in fiber diameter with increase in polymer solution concentration with least average fiber diameter of 140 nm at 5% polymer concentration.

The degradation products of PLGA are LA and GA. The acidic end products decrease the pH of the microenvironment and this can adversely affect growth factor delivery in tissue engineering due to acid catalyzed degradation of the encapsulated/released protein [164]. Thus, there is a need to blend PLGA with other polymers to enable the use of PLGA nanofibers as protein delivery vehicles in tissue engineering applications.

13.4.2.2   *Polycaprolactone (PCL).*

PCL is a semicrystalline polymer that is synthesized by ring-opening polymerization of its monomer ε-caprolactone [165]. Apart from possessing excellent biocompatibility, it is a slow-degrading polymer with high mechanical strength and has been widely explored in the area of tissue engineering [166]. Lee et al. reported the synthesis of PCL nanofibers and studied the influence of solvent system on the morphology and diameter of electrospun PCL nanofibers [81]. The solvent systems studied were: methylene chloride (DCM), mixture of DCM and N, N-DMF, mixture of DCM and toluene. It was observed that with an increase in the content of DMF in the solvent system, surface tension and viscosity decreased while conductivity and dielectric constant increased, thereby leading to a decrease in the fiber diameter. Another group reported the synthesis of electrospun PCL nanofibers in DCM/methanol (7:3) solvent system [167]. Methanol was primarily used to increase the conductivity of the solution, which was further increased by addition of heparin to the spinning solution. The average fiber diameter decreased from 360 nm (without heparin) to 260 nm (with heparin).

13.4.2.3   *Polyurethanes (PU).*

Polyurethanes form a class of elastomeric polymers that have been explored for the synthesis of long-term implants with stable mechanical properties [168]. They have found applications in cardiac pace makers and vascular grafts since they possess excellent biocompatibility [168,169]. Electrospun PU nanofibers have been demonstrated to have potential for wound-dressing based applications. Khil et al. studied mixture of THF and DMF as the solvent system for the synthesis of electrospun PU nanofibers as wound-dressing materials [170]. It has been reported that THF as the solvent system leads to the production of unstable jets moving in all directions. Low flow rate of the polymer solution in THF leads to its drying at the needle tip, while higher flow rate produces larger diameter fibers. On the other hand, DMF as a solvent system causes production of droplets with intermediate fibers. Therefore, Khil et al. optimized the ratio of DMF:THF and demonstrated the production of PU fibers in the range of 250 to 300 nm [170] with DMF:THF in the ratio of 30:70 (v/v), thereby demonstrating that the solvent system can play a major role in the formation of defect-free fibers in the nanometer range.

13.4.2.4 Bacterial Polyesters. As the name suggests, these polyesters are synthesized by bacteria like *Bacillus megaterium, Wautersia eutropha*, and *Pseudomonas species* and are meant to provide the bacteria with a reserve house for carbon and energy. Bacterial polyesters mainly include the family of poly-hydroxy alkanoates (PHA) with the most well studied members being poly-hydroxybutyrate (PHB) and poly-hydroxyvalerate (PHV). Bacterial polyesters have been explored in tissue engineering due to their biocompatibility and biodegradability. Further, PHB and a copolymer of PHB and PHV-PHBV are potential candidates for long-term implants due to their slow degradability.

Synthesis of PHBV nanofibers by electrospinning has been reported by Choi et al. [87]. PHBV fibers were obtained in the range of 1–4 μm when chloroform was used as the solvent system. They further studied the influence of an additive-benzyl trialkylammonium chloride. This salt was soluble in chloroform and its addition caused a significant increase in the conductivity of the solution, thereby leading to increased elongation effects due to repulsion of similar charges on the polymer jet. These favorable factors led to a decrease in average fiber diameter to 1 μm. Further, since PHBV nanofibers electrospun with the salts had higher surface area to volume ratio as compared to PHBV fibers generated without the use of an additive, they degraded faster. In another study, Lee et al. reported the synthesis of electrospun PHBV using 2,2,2-trifluoroethanol as the solvent system and obtained fibers having average fiber diameter of 185 nm [171].

13.4.3 Polymeric Blends

Current state-of-the-art of design of many tissue engineering scaffolds demands the combination of properties offered by natural and synthetic polymers. Few synthetic polymers—for example, poly(α-hydroxyesters)—possess poor processability and release acidic products during their degradation. Further, synthetic polymers lack cell-recognition moieties, which are present in natural materials. Natural polymers, on the other hand, form a gel-like phase at low polymer concentration and a highly viscous solution at increased polymer concentrations, making it difficult to electrospin. Further natural polymers rapidly go into solution in hydrophilic conditions. Thus, hybrid materials that combine the properties of both natural and synthetic polymers are a potential alternative. The properties possessed by such hybrid polymers include improved mechanical properties, high processability, negligible batch-to-batch variability and also the specific recognition ability to elicit a favorable cell response. Blending of polymers is also performed to improve the electrospinnability of some polymers and hence their potential use in tissue engineering. Blends can be composed of two or more natural polymers, or two or more synthetic polymers, or a combination of natural and synthetic polymers.

Blends of natural polymers that are ECM mimics have found great potential in tissue engineering. Nevertheless, electrospinning of natural polymers can be challenging. For example, silk fibroin is a collagen mimic but is mostly composed of hydrophobic residues. Thus, blending of silk fibroin with a hydrophilic polymer would render its electrospinning relatively easy. Making use of this concept, Park et al. demonstrated the synthesis of electrospun nanofibers using silk and chitin blends. The presence of chitin increased the conductivity of the solution that led to the production of nanofibrous matrices with reduced diameters (340 nm–920 nm as compared to 1260 nm for pure silk fibers) [172].

Blends between synthetic polymers combine the properties of the individual polymers. Zong et al. evaluated the ability of biodegradable blends of PLGA and PEG-PLA [(poly(ethylene glycol)-poly(lactic acid)] in preventing postsurgical adhesions in a rat model [173]. PLGA/PEG-PLA electrospun membranes maintained a good 3D stability as compared to shrink-prone hydrophobic PLGA membranes when implanted in rats. Mo et al. exploited the properties of PLLA and PCL and demonstrated the potential of electrospun PLLA/PCL blends in tissue engineering applications. They varied the ratio of both the polymers, thereby modulating the degradation rate and, as a consequence, permeation rates of steroids [174].

Some of the natural polymers, such as gelatin, when dissolved in water cannot be processed by electrospinning because a colloidal solution is formed that in turn cannot be quickly volatilized during the process. Potential solutions either involve the use of volatile solvent systems or blending with synthetic polymers. Various volatile solvents have been studied for electrospinning of gelatin (see section on natural polymers) [124]. Using the second strategy of blending, Li et al. electrospun silk by blending it with polyethylene oxide (PEO), thereby generating a viscosity and surface tension suitable for electrospinning [102]. Further, Li et al. electrospun PLGA, gelatin and elastin together to form a nanofibrous matrix that maintained the properties of the individual polymers. PLGA was the synthetic manipulative component while gelatin and elastin were the natural components serving for the mechanical properties of the ECM as well as cell migration and cell attachment [175].

There are other synthetic polymers that have been electrospun into nanofibers and applied in the area of tissue engineering. However, describing all polymers is beyond the scope of this chapter and hence they have been enumerated in Table 13.2.

TABLE 13.2. Polymers Used in Electrospinning to Form Nanofiber, their Potential Application and the Type of Construct Used in Tissue Engineering

Polymer	Form of nanofiber used in tissue engineering	Type of construct	Application	Ref.
Cellulose	Non woven		Biomaterial	[176]
Chitosan	Non woven		Biomaterial	[177]
				[150]
	Non woven		Cartilage tissue engineering	[178]
Chitin	Non woven		wound healing and tissue regeneration *in vivo* study in rat.	[179]
	Non woven		Biomaterial	[180]
Collagen	Non woven		Bone tissue engineering	[39]
	Non woven, Cross linked		Blood tissue engineering	[133]
	Non woven		Blood tissue engineering	[89]
	Non woven		Wound dressing, Tissue regeneration	[181]
	Non woven		Cartilage tissue engineering	[101]
				[118]
	Non woven, blend with PEO		Wound dressing, Tissue regeneration	[182]
Fibrinogen	Non woven		Tissue regeneration	[131]
Gelatin	Non woven, biomaterial		Collagen substitute	[124]
	Non woven, Cross linked		Sutures, tissue regeneration	[125]
	Non woven, blend with PAN		Electric conductive scaffold, tissue regeneration	[183]
HA	Non woven		Cell encapsulation, tissue regeneration	[139]
PHBV	Non woven		Tissue regeneration	[184]
Silk	Non woven, silk fibroin		Biomaterial	[185]
Zein(corn protein)	Non woven		Biomaterial	[186]
EVOH	Non woven		Wound dressing, tissue regeneration	[187]

TABLE 13.2. *Continued*

Polymer	Form of nanofiber used in tissue engineering	Type of construct	Application	Ref.
PCL	Non woven		Wound dressing	[188]
	Non woven		Heparin delivery for vascular injury	[189]
	Non woven	Aligned, tubular-construct	Blood vessel scaffold	[190]
	Non woven, *in vivo* study in rat		Tissue regeneration	[191]
		Plain weave of porous filament	Tissue regeneration	[192]
	Non woven		Tissue regeneration	[193]
PEO	Non woven		Biomaterial	[77] [194]
	Non woven, PEG-heparin incorporated in fiber	bFGF binding	Functionalized tissue engineering	[195]
Phosphazene	Non woven		Tissue regeneration	[196]
PGA	Non woven		Tissue regeneration *in vivo* study in rat	[159]
	Non woven		Tissue regeneration	[193]
	Non woven, chitin blend	BSA coating	Tissue regeneration	[197]
PLA	Non woven		Tissue regeneration	[193]
	Non woven		Biomaterial	[160]
	Non woven		Tissue regeneration	[198]
		Aligned	Neural tissue engineering	[88]
P(LLA-CL)	Non woven		Vascular graft	[199]
		Aligned	Blood tissue engineering	[93]
	Non woven		Tissue Regeneration	[174]
PLGA		Tubular construct	Vascular tissue graft *in vivo* study in sheep	[200]
	Non woven		Tissue regeneration	[193]
	Non woven, PLGA and PLA–PEG block copolymer		Delivery vehicle, tissue regeneration	[201]
	Non woven, PEG-heparin incorporated in fiber		Functionalized tissue engineering	[195]
PU		Aligned	Ligament tissue engineering	[92]
PVA		Aligned, yarn made with PVP nanofibers	Biomaterial	[202]

13.5 TISSUE ENGINEERING USING ELECTROSPUN NANOFIBROUS SCAFFOLDS

13.5.1 Musculoskeletal System- An Introduction

Musculoskeletal injuries are by far the most common type of injury in sports and trauma. Recent data reports an increased occurrence of sports and trauma related musculoskeletal injuries and this rise can be partially attributed to increase in ageing population [203–205]. It is predicted that by 2020, there will be an increase in the global ageing population that is expected to lead to a sharp rise in the musculoskeletal disorders in both developed, as well as developing, parts of the world. This, in turn, could adversely affect the health care system and economy of nations at large [206,207].

Currently available data indicates that rheumatoid arthritis, osteoarthritis, osteoporosis, spine disorders and trauma related injuries and disabilities are the major musculoskeletal conditions that present a significant disease burden on society [208,209]. Treatment of musculoskeletal impairment has improved with the current clinical therapies and treatment options. Despite the advances in clinical research these strategies are limited in terms of improved repair and regeneration [210]. Therefore, tissue engineering strategies that aim to restore, maintain or improve tissue function provide an exciting alternative to the existing treatment modalities [211].

This section of the chapter limits itself to tissue engineering for musculoskeletal disorders, with a focus on the use of electrospun nanofibers as potential scaffolds for bone, cartilage, skeletal muscle, ligament, and tendon tissue-engineering.

13.5.2 Tissues of the Musculoskeletal System that Have Been Engineered Using Electrospun Nanofibers

13.5.2.1 Bone. After blood, bone is the second most frequently replaced tissue of the human body. Depending on the functional requirement of the body, bone tissue has different morphology. Being a dynamic tissue, bone has the ability to continuously remodel itself without leaving a scar [212]. This well-defined process of remodeling is governed by rapid mobilization of minerals and calcium phosphate deposition.

Bone homeostasis is attributed to the activities of three cell types:

1. **Osteoblasts-** They are the bone forming cells responsible for the synthesis of the ECM and regulation of its mineralization.
2. **Osteocytes-** They are the mature bone cells derived from osteoblasts and are responsible for maintaining bone tissue by enzyme secretion and blood–calcium homeostasis.
3. **Osteoclasts-** They have the ability to resorb fully mineralized bone tissue and are responsible for the controlled break down of bone tissue.

The matrix synthesized by osteoblasts consists of 25% organic matter (that includes cells), 5% water and 70% inorganic mineral (hydroxyapatite). A typical bone ECM predominantly consists of fibrillar type I collagen (about 100 nm in diameter) packed in bundles, thereby increasing the tensile strength of the tissue. Further, the bone hardness is maintained by the inorganic hydroxyapatite well dispersed within the collagen bundles. Bone regeneration and homeostasis is governed by the mechanisms of osteoinduction, osteoconduction, and osteogenesis:

1. **Osteoinduction** involves the recruitment of immature cells and their stimulation into osteoprogenitors. In the context of tissue engineering, osteoinduction is the major process of bone healing during fractures.
2. **Osteoconduction** involves the growth of bone on the surface. In terms of tissue engineering or other bone healing implants, it is the provision of scaffold for cells to migrate, differentiate and induce the process of bone formation.
3. **Osteogenesis** is the process of the formation of new bone by the bone cells, osteoblasts. It is the ability of the graft to produce bone by virtue of the cellular components.

Bone lesions/defects that are less than the critical size defect heal by conventional treatment methods. However, large defects (larger than the critical size defect) do not heal and hence need an appropriate treatment such as a bone graft or their substitute. Every year, 28.6 million Americans incur a musculoskeletal injury [213]. The current state-of-the-art for treatment of bone defects is via autografts, allografts, or xenografts. However, these strategies have been limited due to limited availability (autografts), immune rejection and potential for disease transfer (in case of allografts and xenografts).

Vascularised bone grafts are an alternative to the aforementioned methods. The presence of vasculature allows for improved resistance to infection and hence a better healing capacity. However, the disadvantages of donor site morbidity and multiple surgeries still stand [214].

Apart from these, metal and ceramic–based implants have been used as an alternative to tissue grafts. Metals have the ability to provide immediate mechanical strength at the site of injury but fail to totally integrate with the tissue at that site [215]. The bioactive ceramics that have found application in orthopaedics are hydroxyapatite, tricalcium phosphate and bioglass [216]. Although such grafts can show good osteoconduction and integration, they are limited by their brittle nature and, hence, may not be suitable for load-bearing applications. Therefore, tissue engineering has emerged as an exciting alternative to the aforementioned approaches.

13.5.2.1.1 Potential Cell Sources for Bone Tissue Engineering. Mesenchymal stem cells (MSCs), also known as bone marrow stromal cells, have been the cells of choice next only to autologous primary cells [217] that have been used to engineer mesenchymal tissues such as bone and cartilage. Under appropriate culture conditions, MSCs can be caused to differentiate into more mature cell types of mesenchymal origin such as osteoblasts, chondrocytes and myoblasts. Petite et al. demonstrated that MSCs seeded on coral scaffolds led to complete bone reconstitution in large bone defects of a sheep model [218]. Bone marrow fibroblasts of human and mouse origin have been demonstrated as potential sources in bone regeneration [219]. The usage of progenitor cells from other lineages, including mesodermal origin, has also been explored for bone tissue engineering applications [220–222]. Other sources like subcutaneous adipose tissue have been explored as additional sources for bone-tissue engineering [223,224]. In addition to these, pulp tissue of human teeth has also been exploited for the generation of MSCs for potential use in bone-tissue engineering [225].

13.5.2.1.2   SCAFFOLDS FOR BONE TISSUE ENGINEERING. The scaffold for bone tissue engineering should possess critical properties like porosity (pore size ranging from 200–900 μm), appropriate mechanical properties, and surface properties that facilitate cell adhesion and proliferation [215]. Since the ECM of bone is mostly composed of type I collagen fibrous network with hydroxyapatite (HA) well distributed in it, the mimic of ECM must resemble the properties of type I collagen and HA in combination. The approach of mimicking the ECM through scaffold designing has led the researchers to explore nanofibrous scaffolds synthesized using the electrospinning technique. Materials that mimic both the organic and the inorganic components of bone tissues have been electrospun. The inorganic component HA together with its fluoridates, fluor-hydroxyapatite (FHA), have shown potential as biomaterial for dental applications. Apart from possessing requisite mechanical strength, HA and FHA also stimulate positive osteoblast response. Kim et al. [226] demonstrated electrospinning of HA and FHA and synthesized nanofibers ranging from hundreds of nanometers to several micrometers (236 nm-1.55 μm) by modulating processing parameters (mainly the concentration of polymer solution). Further, FHA nanofibers demonstrated efficient fluorine release profile, thereby making them potential candidates for dental applications.

Natural polymers like silk have also been explored for bone tissue engineering primarily due to its inherent biocompatibility, slow-degradability and high mechanical properties. In a recent study, Li et al. demonstrated the synthesis of silk-PEO nanofibers using the electrospinning technique [102]. Highest calcium levels with improved bone formation were observed following 31 days of static culture of human bone marrow derived mesenchymal stem cells (hMSCs) on silk-PEO scaffolds containing bone morphogenetic protein-2 (BMP-2) and HA nanoparticles. The authors underscored the importance of the combination of nano-scale features offered by electrospun fibers and functional features provided by BMP-2 and hydroxyapatite, thereby demonstrating the potential of silk-PEO nanofibrous scaffolds in bone tissue engineering.

In addition to natural polymers such as silk and HA, a large number of synthetic polymers-based electrospun nano/micro-fibers have been studied for bone tissue engineering applications. One such polymer, polycaprolactone, has been explored in bone tissue engineering primarily due to its low costs, slow degradation and non-toxic nature. Yashimoto et al. studied the potential of PCL nanofibers in bone tissue engineering when seeded with human MSCs and cultured in rotary bioreactors [227]. Their results demonstrated hardening of cell-matrix constructs after a few days, thereby supporting mineralized tissue formation and demonstrating the potential of PCL nanofibers in bone regeneration.

In another study, Venugopal et al. synthesized electrospun biocomposite scaffolds composed of PCL, hydroxyapatite nanoparticles, and collagen in the ratio of 60:90:30 [228]. The rationale for the composition was that PCL provided mechanical strength; collagen (component of the natural ECM) supported cell proliferation; and HA promoted osteogenesis and bone mineralization. The results demonstrated an interconnecting porous structure (porosity-80%) with fiber diameter ranging from 189 ± 0.026 nm to 579 ± 272 nm that provided sufficient mechanical strength of 1.73 MPa and good osteoblast morphology along with an increase in proliferation (up to 35%) and mineralization (up to 55%) as compared to the controls. Therefore, this study demonstrated the potential of PCL, collagen and HA in bone-tissue engineering. In a more recent study, Catledge et al. synthesized a triphasic scaffold composed of a similar mixture (PCL: collagen:HA in a ratio of 50:30:20) with mean fiber diameter of 180 ± 50 nm closely resembling the collagen fiber in the ECM of bone [229]. The collagen counterpart played an important role in improving the stiffness of the scaffold as indicated by the elastic modulus (highest for collagen/HA: 3.9 GPa) and demonstrated the potential of the composite scaffold in bone-tissue regeneration.

Recent advances in technology have led scientists to develop a strategy of guided bone regeneration (GBR). In this approach, a membrane—when placed on a defected bone site—"guides" the growth of the new bone and at the same time prevents the in-growth of fibrous scar tissue into the grafted site. GBR has been mainly explored in periodontal surgery with success of both non-degradable implant and biodegradable membranes. Fujihara et al. reported the phenomenon of GBR on nanofibrous surfaces due to the enhanced cell response as compared to microfibrous surfaces [230]. Initial experiments by their group focused on the synthesis of GBR membranes composed of PCL nanofibers with calcium carbonate nanoparticles that promoted osteoconduction and served as bone-filling material. The GBR membrane, however, lacked the requisite tensile strength. In later studies, they provided a supporting PCL nanofibrous layer to the mechanically stable composite of electrospun PCL nanofibers and demonstrated its mechanical stability by stretching it to around 200% strain without physical disruption. Further, the authors demonstrated osteoblast proliferation on the PCL/CaCO3 composite nanofibers on GBR membranes thereby their potential in bone tissue engineering. Approximately at the same time, another type of composite electrospun PCL mats impregnated with calcium carbonate or HA particles were synthesized by Wutticharoenmongkol et al. [231]. They demonstrated an increase in fiber diameter with an increase in concentration of nanoparticles as well as the base PCl solution. Also, high concentration of nanoparticles led to improved tensile strength of the mats. Their further *in vitro* studies demonstrated the potential of PCL-HA mats as bone scaffolding material due to osteoblast-promoting activity of HA with no threat to osteoblasts and mouse fibroblasts.

Silica has also been investigated as a potential candidate for bone-tissue engineering as it possesses silanol groups that are essential for apatite formation, thus resembling bone [232]. Sakai et al. demonstrated the proliferation of osteoblasts on electrospun nanofibrous meshes of silica. It was the first study of its type that reported apatite formation and its morphology on electrospun silicate fibers thereby confirming the bone bonding ability essential for bone-tissue engineering.

In the recent past, there has been an effort to develop active ceramic-biodegradable polymer composites in bone-tissue engineering to overcome the brittleness of the ceramic component and low mechanical strength of the polymeric component. However, this can potentially lead to other problems, such as decreased affinity of hydrophilic ceramic for organic solvent and hydrophobic polymers, thereby resulting in poor/uneven dispersion of the ceramic component within the polymeric matrix. Hence, Kim and co-workers designed a novel composite system composed of uniformly dispersed hydroxyapatite powder in PLA solution. The use of a surfactant, 12-hydroxysteric acid ensured uniform distribution of HA powder within the PLA matrix [233]. Electrospun nanofibrous HA-PLA mesh composite demonstrated improved osteoblast attachment, spreading and proliferation. Further, they demonstrated higher alkaline phosphatase (ALP a phenotypic marker of bone forming cells) expression on composite scaffolds as compared to plain PLA scaffolds, thereby establishing their potential in bone regeneration.

Electrospun matrices generated by synthetic polymers have demonstrated advantages in terms of better cell adhesion and proliferation; however, their hydrophobic nature has limited their use in certain tissue engineering applications. Hence, there have been attempts to augment the hydrophilicity of these polymers by blending them with hydrophilic polymers. A study by Spasova et al. explored the possibility of imparting hydrophilicity to hydrophobic PLLA electrospun scaffolds by the incorporation of varying amounts of PEG, a hydrophilic polymer. Nanofibrous PLLA-PEG electrospun meshes were synthesized by varying the concentrations of PLLA as well as PEG and the applied field strength [234]. The PEGylated scaffolds demonstrated uniform cell adhesion (both osteoblasts and fibroblasts) on all electrospun meshes irrespective of PEG concentration. Furthermore, in long-term cultures, the authors reported the organization of osteoblast-like cells into tissue-like structures, particularly on scaffolds with the highest concentration of PEG (PLLA:PEG at weight ratio 70:30). This study indicates that the presence of a hydrophilic polymer could modulate the cell response, thereby resulting in controlled cell adhesion, and can play a key role in scaffold design for application in bone-tissue engineering.

In vivo bone regeneration using nanofiber-based scaffolds was demonstrated by Shin et al. who reported the osteogenic differentiation ability of MSCs seeded on PCL electrospun scaffolds in a rat model [235]. The initial differentiation of MSCs (isolated from rat bone marrow) on PCL matrices was performed in rotational oxygen permeable bioreactors for four weeks, followed by *in vivo* implantation in the omentum of a rat model. They demonstrated successful differentiation of MSCs into osteoblasts with laid down osteoids following four weeks of implantation. Further, characteristic mineralization and the presence of collagen type I throughout the harvested cellular constructs strengthened the potential for bone graft development from highly porous electrospun PCL nanofibers.

13.5.2.2 *Cartilage.*

Cartilage is a tough, elastic, and flexible connective tissue that comprises cells in combination with a fibrous network. It is an avascular, alymphatic, and aneural tissue with limited innate ability for repair and regeneration [236]. Cartilage in the human body exists as three types: fibrocartilage, elastic cartilage, and hyaline cartilage [237,238]. Hyaline cartilage is the predominant type of cartilage that coats the surface of articulating joints [35,136,239] and hence is referred to as articular cartilage. Healthy articular cartilage is a water rich tissue (60–85%) with the remainder being ECM (mainly collagen type II: 15–22% and proteoglycans 4–7%) and chondrocytes (2–5%). High water content enables cartilage to withstand the forces associated with joint loading. Chondrocytes are the only cellular component of normal cartilage. Although low in number, chondrocytes continuously remodel and organize the surrounding ECM in a unique and complex anisotropic structure [136].

Collagen type II is the predominant component of cartilage ECM and provides tensile strength, whereas macromolecules-like glycosaminoglycans (GAGs) produced by chondrocytes contribute to the viscoelastic property of cartilage. GAGs attached to protein molecules form proteoglycans that impart compressive strength to cartilage tissue [136,239]. Cartilage defects, irrespective of their origin, are not life-threatening, but result in debilitating affliction and gradual loss in mobility [240]. Statistical data indicates that the disorders linked with damaged cartilage have rapidly increased in the last century and are expected to affect a large section of the population worldwide in the future [3,203]. Currently available treatment options heavily rely on tissue grafts (autograft and allograft) or on artificial prosthetic joints. Although a fair degree of success has been achieved with these treatment methods, challenges such as limited availability and donor site morbidity (autograft), disease transmission, and immunogenic response (allograft) still remain [3]. Total joint replacement is a successful treatment in most severe cases of arthritis; however, the implant has a limited life span, with an average of 10–15 years [241,242].

When cartilage is damaged or injured, a cascade of events occurs to restore and repair the damaged tissue. Only full thickness defects that penetrate the subchondral bone elicit a healing response [243]. Furthermore, despite the elicitation of repair processes in full thickness defect, mechanically inferior fibrocartilage is formed [240]. Consequently, a sequential permanent loss of structure and function of cartilage occurs. Thus, there is a need for an alternative strategy that can promote cartilage tissue regeneration and restore normal functioning of the joint.

Cartilage is a relatively simple tissue, as it does not require vasculature for maintenance and consists of only a single cell type. Thus, it is well suited for tissue engineering, which involves an appropriate combination of scaffolds, cells and chemical cues (GFs) for structural and functional regeneration of cartilage [240].

As stated earlier, type II collagen and proteoglycans form a fibrous mesh and are the major constituents of the ECM of articular cartilage [35]. Thus, electrospun polymeric nanofibers that can mimic ECM constituents may have the potential to facilitate cartilage regeneration [36].

13.5.2.2.1 POTENTIAL CELL SOURCE FOR CARTILAGE TISSUE ENGINEERING. Transplantation of cells at the defect site is an approach that can provide a new cell population at the site of damage, which in turn can lead to ECM production *in vivo* [244]. Brittberg et al. reported a cell-therapy-based approach for repair of injured cartilage in human knee joints. Autologous chondrocytes were isolated from a healthy site (upper medial femoral condyle of the damaged knee), cultured *in vitro*, and then re-implanted at the damaged site [12]. Their results demonstrated that the defects treated with autologous chondrocytes were eventually filled with hyaline cartilage with a gradual reduction in disease symptoms [12]. Although autologous chondrocytes are promising candidates, they are available in limited numbers. Consequently allogenic cells were used for cartilage repair. Freed et al. reported the possible use of allogenic chondrocytic cells for *in vivo* application in rabbit cartilage repair; however, the regenerated subchondral bone was not similar to the native subchondral bone [245]. In spite of the potential for using chondrocytes from autologous and allogenic sources for cartilage regeneration, the limited number of chondrocytes (~2% of the total weight of cartilage) combined with dedifferentiation in monolayer expansion has led to the exploration of alternative cell source. Mesenchymal stem cells [MSCs] can be an attractive cell source for cartilage repair due to their multipotency, easy availability, and demonstrated capability of monolayer expansion [246,247]. Chemical cues/growth factors can enhance the chondrogenesis of MSCs [248,249]. Thus, they could be a promising cell source for cartilage tissue engineering.

13.5.2.2.2 SCAFFOLDS FOR CARTILAGE TISSUE ENGINEERING. The search for an optimal scaffold for cartilage tissue regeneration has resulted in the study of both synthetic and natural materials including natural constituents of ECM. Collagen type II, the major protein constituent of native ECM of articular cartilage has been studied for regeneration of cartilage [238]. Shields et al. explored the potential of electrospun collagen type II nanofibrous scaffolds for cartilage tissue engineering [101]. Their *in vitro* studies demonstrated the ability of chondrocytes to adhere, proliferate, and infiltrate into the scaffold matrix [101]. The results indicated that electrospun collagen type II scaffolds provide a native environment for growth of chondrocytes *in vitro* and an increase in fiber diameter had no effect on the proliferation of chondrocytes. The inefficient mass transfer of nutrients and oxygen in a thick scaffold in static culture can lead to necrotic zones in the interior of scaffolds. Application of dynamic seeding techniques is an effective strategy to overcome the problems associated with static culture and can enhance cell proliferation and ECM synthesis [101].

GAGs play an important role in maintaining chondrocyte cell morphology, differentiation, and function [180,250]. Two abundantly available natural polymers, chitosan and alginate, are GAG mimics that have been explored for nanofiber synthesis by electrospinning [251]. Bhattarai et al. reported the successful proliferation and growth of chondrocytes on both these polymers [146,178]. Alginate nanofibers were fabricated using PEO as an additive to reduce the viscosity of the pure alginate solution and hence enable electrospinning. Their *in vitro* studies demonstrated that cartilage chondrocyte-like cells (HTB-94) seeded on the alginate scaffold were viable and maintained their morphology and characteristic phenotype after 72 hours of culture [146]. Another advantage of electrospun nanofibrous scaffold over bulk alginate scaffolds is that they do not require any precoated adhesion proteins such as fibronectin or arginine–glycine–aspartic acid peptides [RGD] to facilitate cell adhesion [146]. Therefore, the aforementioned studies indicated that alginate nanofibers could be potential scaffolding system for cartilage tissue engineering.

In a similar study, Bhattarai et al. assessed the cellular compatibility of chitosan nanofibrous scaffolds using chondrocytes. Chondrocytes (HTB-94) seeded on chitosan/PEO nanofibrous membranes exhibited a rounded morphology that is a characteristic feature of chondrocytes [178]. In another study, Subramanian et al. reported an increased elastic modulus (2.25 MPa) of electrospun chitosan mesh in comparison to chitosan cast film (1.19 MPa) [252]. Their results demonstrated better cell attachment and proliferation with chondrocytes onto chitosan nanofibrous meshes when compared to chitosan cast film. Therefore, these results demonstrated the potential of chitosan nanofibrous matrices as scaffolds in cartilage tissue engineering.

Electrospun synthetic biodegradable polymers have also been explored as potential scaffolds for cartilage tissue engineering. Shin et al. [253] studied the potential of PLGA electrospun nanofibrous scaffolds in cartilage regeneration. This study demonstrated the effect of content ratio of two different polymers (lactic acid/glycolic acid ratio) of PLGA on degradation and mechanical strength of scaffold. In their studies, they reported that PLGA nanofibrous scaffolds degraded in four to seven weeks, which is suitable to support cell and tissue development *in vivo*. Further, they investigated the behavior of primary chondrocytes on electrospun PLGA nanofibers and the effect of intermittent hydrostatic pressure on cell-seeded scaffolds. Their results demonstrated that electrospun nanofibrous PLGA scaffolds were non-cytotoxic and promoted chondrocytic proliferation and enhanced synthesis of ECM components. In addition, application of intermittent hydrostatic pressure on cell-seeded scaffolds increased cell proliferation and synthesis of collagen and proteoglycan [253].

Li et al. [254] described the potential application of electrospun poly(ε-caprolactone) (PCL) nanofibers as scaffolds for cartilage tissue engineering. Fetal bovine chondrocytes (FBCs) cultured on these scaffolds displayed a rounded or spindle shaped morphology that is typical of chondrocytes in contrast to the flattened and spread fibroblast like morphology that was observed on the tissue culture polystyrene (TCPS) surface. Moreover, a 21-fold increase in cell growth and upregulation in gene expression of collagen type II confirmed the potential of PCL nanofibers in cartilage tissue engineering. In another study, Li et al. [255] studied the influence of electrospun PCL scaffolds on the behavior of MSCs. Their results demonstrated that the MSCs preserved their phenotype on PCL nanofibers and in presence of transforming growth factor ß1 (TGF ß1), MSCs seeded on PCL nanofibers differentiated into a chondrocytic phenotype.

Electrospun nanofibrous scaffolds mimic the dimensions of collagen fibrils present in the native ECM. These nanofibers maintain the phenotype of chondrocytes seeded on their surface. Studies have demonstrated that chondrocytes exhibit different proliferation rates on fiber having different diameters. Li et al. demonstrated a significant increase in production of cartilage specific markers such as collagen type II and type IX, aggrecan and COMP on the electrospun fibers having diameter in the nanometer scale (500–900 nm) as compared to the fibers having diameters in the micrometer range (15–20 μm) [251]. Thus, the results indicated that electrospun nanofibrous scaffolds provide a more conducive environment to chondrocytes as compared to microfibrous scaffolds.

The aforementioned studies demonstrated that electrospun nanofibers show potential for use as scaffolds in cartilage tissue engineering.

13.5.2.3 Skeletal Muscle.

Skeletal muscle is a type of striated muscle that comprises the single largest organ of the human body, forming 48% of the human body by mass. It is not only highly organized at the microscopic level (a requirement to perform function), but is also compartmentalized when observed macroscopically. Skeletal muscles are composed of bundles of well organized, dense myotubes that are packed in a parallel arrangement to form a muscle fiber. Each fibril in turn is a multi-nucleated cell derived from myoblasts. The extracellular matrix in skeletal muscle tissue comprises of glycoproteins, collagen (mainly type I and III) and proteoglycans. These extracellular components govern the response to tensile stress. In particular, collagen crosslinking and fibril organization largely determine muscle elasticity [256].

Defects in skeletal muscle make it incapable of responding to nervous control and can lead to various genetic disorders such as muscular dystrophy and spinal muscle atrophy [256]. Muscle structural anomalies can also result from trauma, from tumor ablation, and even from continuous denervation.

The functional restoration of lost skeletal muscle through free tissue transfer from near or distant sites, although common, has been the only alternative [257]. This method has received very limited success primarily due to donor site morbidity and functional loss. Hence, muscle tissue engineering has been explored as an exciting alternative.

13.5.2.3.1 POTENTIAL CELL SOURCES FOR SKELETAL MUSCLE TISSUE ENGINEERING. The diseases caused due to skeletal muscle injury have led to a considerable interest in skeletal muscle regeneration. During skeletal muscle regeneration, myoblasts undergo proliferation, differentiation, and fusion to form a multinucleated structure typical of muscle myofibril. These myofibrils then undergo a specific arrangement to form a functional muscle. High degree of functional and structural specialization in the adult skeletal tissue results in existence of terminally-differentiated cell populations that have lost the capacity to proliferate and to form new myofibrils during tissue repair. Thus, cell replenishment is attributed to a store house of undifferentiated cells, called satellite cells, present in close contact with the myofibrils [258]. Under normal conditions, the satellite cells remain quiescent and can be activated through signals that are secreted following cell damage. Satellite cells are termed as precursor cells, rather than stem cells, due to their ability to produce only a single lineage of cells unlike multipotent stem cells. However, the use of satellite cells in skeletal tissue repair has been limited due to the non-availability of a pure populations of these cells. Montarras et al. isolated satellite cells by flow cytometry using satellite cell specific markers. These cells, when grafted into muscles of nude mice that lacked dystrophin (a protein mutated in patients having Duchenne muscular dystrophy), led to fiber repair [259]. Satellite cells are the most characterized of all the muscle-derived stem cells (MDSCs). MDSCs exhibit varied degrees of pluripotency and can differentiate into osteogenic lineage, adipogenic lineage, chondrogenic lineage, or skeletal myogenic lineage, depending on the culture conditions [260]. Further, experimental studies have validated the potential use of myoblasts in muscle tissue engineering [261].

13.5.2.3.2 SCAFFOLD FOR SKELETAL MUSCLE TISSUE ENGINEERING. Appropriate functioning of tissue-engineered skeletal muscle requires the proper organization of myofibrils, intracellular calcium storage, and acetyl-choline receptors that are important for the functioning of the muscle. The orientation of muscle cells should be in a direction parallel to each other in order to produce force in a desired direction. Thus, the scaffold should allow/facilitate the orientation of muscle cells in a parallel fashion. In addition, the scaffold should be biocompatible, moldable to provide sufficient strength, and must possess a vascular component [262]. Levenberg et al. reported the vascularisation of engineered skeletal muscle tissue constructs using a three-dimensional multiculture system consisting of myoblasts, fibroblasts, and endothelial cells on biodegradable PLLA/PLGA scaffolds [263]. Their results demonstrated the presence of endothelial vessel network throughout the engineered muscle tissue *in vitro* and improved performance of the constructs *in vivo* (in a mouse model) following pre-vascularisation.

In previous tissue-engineering strategies, myoblasts have been seeded on fibrous meshes [264], gels [265], and in between artificial tendons [266] with limited success. Myoblasts seeded on fibrous meshes were unable to align themselves in parallel orientation, while those seeded on gels did not produce forces comparable to those of a normal human body. Therefore, to overcome this problem, approaches using contact guidance are being explored that would allow the movement of cells along a desired direction. Neumann and co-workers demonstrated alignment of myoblast in a single layer on parallel polypropylene fibers [267]. As discussed in a previous section, electrospinning offers the ability to produce aligned fibers, thus generating a scaffolding system that could find use in skeletal muscle tissue engineering. Riboldi et al. fabricated electrospun polyesterurethane microfibers and explored their potential in skeletal muscle tissue engineering [105]. The rationale for selecting polyesterurethane, a degradable block polymer, was primarily due to its *in vitro* and *in vivo* biocompatibility and elastomeric behavior. The results of their study demonstrated adherence and proliferation of murine C2C12 muscle progenitor cells following differentiation on microfibrous scaffolds as indicated by positive staining for myosin heavy chain expression. Further, an elastic modulus of ten MPa was obtained that was comparable to the elasticity of skeletal muscles. Thus, electrospun membranes show the potential to be explored as scaffolds for skeletal muscle tissue engineering.

13.5.2.4 *Ligament and Tendon.*

Ligaments and tendons are soft tissues that play an important role in musculoskeletal biomechanics. Ligaments connect bone to bone, whereas tendons connect muscles to bone. Both these tissues possess high tensile strength, which is a characteristic feature of load-bearing tissue [268].

Ligaments and tendons, like most other musculoskeletal tissue, have a hierarchical structure that affects their mechanical behavior [269]. In addition, ligaments and tendons can adapt to changes in their mechanical environment due to injury, disease, or exercise. Despite the similarity of function and metabolism, ligaments are relatively more active than tendons [270].

Well-suited for their functional role, ligaments are tough fibrous cords, composed of both collagen and elastic fibers. The elastic fibers allow the ligaments to stretch to some extent. Water constitutes 60% of the wet weight of ligaments. The remaining 40% is contributed by other major constituents of ligaments such as collagen, proteoglycans, glycoprotein, and elastin. This ground substance is the source of viscoelastic properties of ligament. Collagen type I and type III are the major constituents, of which type I and III account for 90% and 10% of the wet weight of ligaments [271–273].

Tendons are complex structures. ECM of tendon comprises of water (55% of the wet weight of tendons), proteoglycans (<1%), along with cells and type I collagen (85% of dry weight). Other collagens, such as collagen type III, V, XII, and XIV are present in very lesser quantities, while decorin is the predominant type of proteoglycan present in ECM of tendon.

Both ligaments and tendons have a complex structure, with a hierarchy of collagen fibers with specific orientation, which provides tensile strength to the tissue. The hierarchical organization consists of collagen molecules, fibrils, fibril bundles, and fascicles that run parallel to the long axis of the tissue. Fascicles have fibroblasts sparsely distributed and oriented along the direction of collagen fibers [274,275].

Structural components of ligaments and tendon are similar but their characteristics may differ. Fibroblasts structure and size varies in ligament and tendon. Even diameter of collagen fibril, ratio of collagen type I to type III may vary [276].

Ligaments surround joints and bind them together by acting as a connecting bridge between two bones. They help to strengthen and stabilize joints, permitting movement only in certain directions. Thus, any excessive movement of ligament or movement in wrong direction can result in ligament rupture and bone injury [277]. When the injury causes total detachment of the ligament from the bone, an insertion surgery is recommended. Untreated injuries lead to unstable joints and excessive load on cartilage, which may progress into osteoarthritis [278–280]. It is important to note that ligaments present in the same joint can differ from each other in terms of regenerative capacity [272,281] Medial collateral ligament (MCL) has better capacity to heal, whereas anterior crucial ligament (ACL), once ruptured, cannot undergo self-repair. Thus, ACL, if injured, leads to disability because of its poor healing capacity. This is primarily because of the lack of vasculature and limited availability of nutrients to the damaged tissue from synovial fluid (depending on the severity of injury) [272,281].

Autografts and allografts have been explored for the reconstruction of ACL [282]. Non-biodegradable grafts, and even collagen grafts, could not successfully repair and replace damaged ligaments as they were mechanically unstable and could not perform the biochemical and physiological function [283].

Unlike ACL, tendons have the capacity of self repair; however, when the defect is too large (that is, beyond self repair), partial or total replacement is the only available option [284].

The drawback associated with the aforementioned strategies has led to the implementation of tissue-engineering approaches for ligament and tendon repair.

13.5.2.4.1 POTENTIAL CELL SOURCES FOR LIGAMENT AND TENDON TISSUE ENGINEERING. Autologous tissue specific cells are the gold standard for cell therapy. Ligaments have a dense ECM and low population of cells makes their isolation difficult [285,286]. Therefore, alternative cell sources have been explored for ligament-tissue engineering. As stated in the previous sections, MSCs have the potential to differentiate into variety of cell types of mesenchymal lineage, and thus, are also capable of differentiating into ligament fibroblasts [287]. Wantanabe et al. demonstrated that when MSCs from transgenic rats were injected into MCL of wild type rat, MSCs migrated to the injury site of ligament in three days, and after 28 days of study, it was found that the MSCs had differentiated into MCL fibroblast-like cells following adaptation to the environment [288]. Previous studies have demonstrated that when MSCs were used for tendon repair, there was an increase in ultimate stress, modulus and strain energy density when transplanted in a collagen matrix [270]. MSCs have an added advantage of ease-of-expansion in cell culture. Thus, MSCs can be used as a potential cell source for ligament and tendon repair.

13.5.2.4.2 SCAFFOLD FOR LIGAMENT AND TENDON TISSUE ENGINEERING. In order to design a bioresorbable scaffold for supporting and guiding regeneration of ligament and tendon tissue, a number of design requirements have to be met. Scaffold should be able to promote alignment of the cells and withstand repetitive tensile loading, and should also promote the gradual growth of host ligament tissue. Electrospun nanofibrous scaffolds are currently being explored as potential scaffolds for ligament and tendon repair [280].

Courtney et al. recently reported the use of electrospun poly(ester urethane) urea (PEUU) in soft-tissue engineering. Their studies demonstrated that electrospun-PEUU nanofibers possess elastomeric property and can be well-aligned. This attribute can be used to make biomimetic scaffolds for mechanically anisotropic soft tissues [290].

In another study, Basher et al. studied the influence of PEUU mesh topography (fiber diameter and alignment) on cell growth and proliferation [287]. Their studies demonstrated that PEUU surfaces allowed for cell adhesion and proliferation. Further, the cells oriented themselves and were aligned in the direction of fiber orientation. Also, aligned nanofibers showed improved cell adhesion with increase in fiber diameter and was highest for fibers with the largest diameters. Thus, PEUU aligned nanofibers can be potential scaffolds for ligament tissue engineering [291].

Lee et al. studied the influence of fiber alignment and the effect of mechanical strain direction on the behavior of human ligament fibroblast (HLF). HLF on aligned polyurethane nanofibers (PU) exhibited normal spindle shape and oriented them along the length of the fiber. Collagen content was used as a parameter to study the effect of cyclic uniaxial strain on HLF behavior. It was observed that the cells aligned themselves in the direction of aligned nanofibers and exhibited 150-times more collagen production when uniaxial strain was applied in the direction of cell alignment (that is, longitudinal stretching) as compared to unstrained control when uniaxial strain was applied [92].

Using biomimetic approaches for designing scaffolds has been a popular method in tissue engineering. However, interphase tissue engineering has emerged as an interesting approach for subchondral defects, wherein the scaffold has two different phases that mimic cartilage and bone. ACL connects to subchondral bone through an interface wherein three distinct tissue regions—namely, ligament, cartilage and bone—work in an integrated way such that load is dissipated to bone with minimal stress on the interphase. Spalazzi et al. recently reported a study which suggests that multi-tissue regeneration on a single scaffold is possible through interphase tissue constructs. The study further suggests that it is possible to mimic the multi-tissue organization present at the native ligament-to-bone insertion site, and each phase of the triphasic construct could form the corresponding tissue in which it has been inserted [292]. Knitted microfibers are considered to possess better mechanical strength, while nanofibers have large surface area. Combination of nanofibers and microfibers can provide a novel scaffold for tissue engineering with enhanced properties. Hybrid nano-microfibrous scaffold were fabricated by electrospinning PLGA nanofibers on the surface of knitted microfibrous PLGA scaffold. Porcine bone marrow stromal cells seeded on these scaffolds demonstrated better cellular adhesion and proliferation as compared to the control. Increased production of ECM and specifically enhanced expression of collagen-I, decorin, and biglycan, was observed on nano-microfibrous scaffolds compared to control of only PLGA-knitted fibers. Thus, novel nano-microfibrous scaffolds could be a potential scaffold for ligament and tendon tissue engineering [96].

Therefore, electrospun nanofibrous constructs can be manipulated to form appropriate scaffolds for ligament tissue engineering.

Although there have not been any studies on the use of electrospun nanofibers for tendon repair, it is intuitive to believe that aligned nanofibrous scaffolds can serve as potential scaffolds for tendon tissue engineering as well [293]. Table 13.3 provides a summary of the electrospun scaffolds applied in tissue engineering.

13.6 CONCLUSIONS AND FUTURE DIRECTIONS

The field of tissue engineering is less than three decades old and the progress made has been impressive. With the advent of novel biomaterials and processing technologies for biomaterials, scaffolding systems have improved significantly in the recent past. The fabrication technique plays a very important role in determining the kind of scaffold generated. Amongst the nanostructured scaffolds, nanofibers have been the choice for scaffold development. These continuous fibers with diameters in the nanometer scale have advantages of possessing high porosity, and high surface area to volume ratio that enable the cells to perform their functions, while providing for appropriate nutrient and waste transfer. More importantly, they possess physical similarity to the native ECM components. Hence, they are being explored by tissue engineers throughout the world for the regeneration of a wide variety of tissues of the human body. Electrospinning has emerged as a simple and versatile technique for the generation of ultrathin fibers that can potentially mimic the ECM components of tissue, that is, native environment of the cell. Nanofibers have revolutionized the field of tissue engineering by providing ECM mimicking via a relatively easy fabrication method of electrospinning. Variants of electrospinning technique in terms of collector plate as well as spinneret are now being explored. For instance, co-electrospinning involves the synthesis of nanofiber with coating of another fiber on it and has been used for the synthesis of core-shell type nanofibers and incorporation of sensitive compounds such as growth factors in the core.

This chapter provided a brief understanding of the scaffolds synthesized by electrospinning technique and their role in musculo-skeletal tissue engineering. There is description of the state of the art of each musculo-skeletal tissue in terms of *in vitro* and *in vivo* studies. The process of development of a nanofiber based bio-mimetic scaffolds is still in its initial stages and has a long way to go before it can be made available commercially for clinical use.

TABLE 13.3. Application of Electrospun Nanofibers in Tissue Engineering

Type of tissue engineering	Polymer scaffold	Cell type	Group (and Reference)
Bone tissue engineering	Silk-PEO, Hydroxyapatite nanoparticles	Human bone marrow derived mesenchymal stem cells	Li et al. [102]
	Hydroxyapatite and fluor-hydroxyapatite	—	Kim and Kim [226]
	PLA, hydroxyapatite powder	Human osteoblast like MG63 cells	Kim et al. [233]
	PLGA, PEO	Human osteoblast like MG-63 cells	Spasova et al. [234]
	Polycaprolactone	Human mesenchymal stem cells (from bone marrow of neonatal Lewis rat)	Yashimoto et al.; Shin et al. [227,235]
	PCL, hydroxyapatite, collagen	Human fetal osteoblasts;	Venugopal et al. Catledge et al. [228,229]
	PCL, calcium carbonate nanoparticles and supporting PCL layer	Human osteoblast	Fujihara et al. Wutticharoenmongkol et al. [230,231]
	Silica	Human osteoblast like MG-63 cells	Sakai et al. [232]
Cartilage tissue engineering	Collagen type II	Adult human articular chondrocytes	Shields et al. [101], Barnes et al. [118]
	Alginate, PEO	Human chondrocyte-like cell line	Bhattarai et al. [146]
	Chitosan, PEO	Chondrocytes	Bhattarai et al. [178]
	Chitosan	Chondrocytes	Subramanian et al. [179]
	PLGA	Primary chondrocytes from porcine articular cartilage	Shin et al. [253]
	PCL	Fetal bovine chondrocytes; mesenchymal stem cells	Li et al. [254,255]
Skeletal muscle tissue engineering	PEU	C2C12, rat myoblasts, primary human satellite cells	Riboldi et al. [105]
Ligament and tendon tissue engineering	PEUU	—	Courtney et al. [290]
	PEUU	NIH 3T3 Fibroblast	Bashur et al. [291]
	Polyurethane	Human ligament fibroblast	Lee et al. [92]

ACKNOWLEDGMENTS

One of the authors, NA, would like to acknowledge Council for Scientific and Industrial Research, India for her research fellowship and PS would like to acknowledge AICTE for providing National Doctoral Fellowship. DSK would like to acknowledge Indian Institute of Technology Kanpur and Department of Science and Technology, India and Department of Biotechnology, India for the research grants received.

REFERENCES

1. Betz RR. Limitations of autograft and allograft: new synthetic solutions. Orthopedics 2002;25(5):561–570.
2. Zhong R, Platt JL. Current status of animal to human transplantation. Expert Opin Biol Ther 2005;5(11):1415–1420.
3. Langer R, Vacanti JP. Tissue engineering. Science 1993;260:920–926.
4. Nerem MR, Sambanis A. Tissue engineering: From biology to biological substitutes. Tissue Eng 1995;1(1):3–13.
5. Shieh SJ, Vacanti JP. State-of-the-art tissue engineering: From tissue engineering to organ building. Surgery 2005;137(1):1–7.
6. Langer R. Tissue engineering. Mol Ther 2000;1(1):12–15.
7. Noishiki Y. *In vivo* tissue engineering: dreams for the future. J Artif Organs 2000;3:5–11.
8. Han D, Gouma PI. Electrospun bioscaffolds that mimic the topology of extracellular matrix. Nanomed Nanotech Biol Med 2006;2:37–41.
9. Hutmacher DW, Cool S. Concepts of scaffold-based tissue engineering—the rationale to use solid free-form fabrication techniques. J Cell Mol Med 2007;11(4):654–669.
10. Cancedda R, Dozin B, Giannoni P, Quarto R. Tissue engineering and cell therapy of cartilage and bone. Matrix Biol 2003;22:81–91.
11. Jakob RP, Varlet PM, Gautier E. Isolated articular cartilage lesion: repair or regeneration. Osteoarth Cart 2001;9(Supplement A):S3–S5.
12. Brittberg M, Lindahl A, Nilsson A, Ohlsson C, Isaksson O, Peterson L. Treatment of deep cartilage defects in the knee with autologous chondrocyte transplantation. New Engl J Med 1994;331:889–895.
13. Kim BS, Mooney DJ. Development of biocompatible synthetic extracellular matrices for tissue engineering. Trends Biotechnol 1998;16:224–230.
14. Yang S, Leong KF, Zhaohui DU, Chua CK. The design of scaffolds for use in tissue engineering. Part I. Traditional Factors. Tissue Eng 2001;7(6):679–689.
15. Agrawal CM, Ray RB. Biodegradable polymeric scaffolds for musculoskeletal tissue engineering. J Biomed Mater Res 2001;55:141–150.
16. Ikada Y. In: Tissue engineering: fundamentals and applications. By Ikada Y. New York: Academic Press; 2006:1–90.
17. Lee JH, Jung HW, Kang IK, Lee HB. Cell behaviour on polymer surfaces with different functional groups. Biomaterials 1994;15:705–711.

18. Miot S, Woodfield T, Daniels AU, Suetterlin R, Peterschmitt I, Heberer M, van Blitterswijk CA, Riesle J, Martin I. Effects of scaffold composition and architecture on human nasal chondrocyte redifferentiation and cartilaginous matrix deposition. Biomaterials 2005;26(15):2479–2489.

19. Woodfield TBF, Miot S, Martin I, van Blitterswijk CA, Riesle J. The regulation of expanded human nasal chondrocyte re-differentiation capacity by substrate composition and gas plasma surface modification. Biomaterials 2006;27:1043–1053.

20. Bhardwaj T, Pilliar RM, Grynpas MD, Kandel RA. Effect of material geometry on cartilaginous tissue formation *in vitro*. J Biomed Mater Res 2001;57:190–199.

21. Frenkel SR, Cesare PE. Scaffolds for articular cartilage repair. Ann Biomed Engg 2004;32(1):26–34.

22. Lu L, Mikos AG. The importance of new processing techniques in tissue engineering. MRS Bulletin 1996;21(11):28–32.

23. Flemming RG, Murphy CJ, Abrams GA, Goodman SL, Nealey PF. Effects of synthetic micro- and nano-structured surfaces on cell behavior. Biomaterials 1999;20: 573–588.

24. Misra SK, Mohn D, Brunner TJ, Stark WJ, Philip SE, Roy I, Salih V, Knowles JA, Boccaccini AR. Comparison of nanoscale and microscale bioactive glass on the properties of P(3HB)/bioglass composites. Biomaterials 2008;29:1750–1761.

25. Yates KE, Allemann F, Glowacki J. Phenotypic analysis of bovine chondrocytes cultured in 3D collagen sponges: effect of serum substitutes. Cell Tissue Bank 2005;6(1):45–54.

26. Jackson DW, Lalor PA, Aberman HM, Simon TM. Spontaneous repair of full-thickness defects of articular cartilage in a goat model. J Bone Joint Surg 2001; 83:53.

27. Freed LE, Vunjak-Novakovic G. Culture of organized cell communities. Adv Drug Dev Rev 1998;33:15–30.

28. Tan J, Saltzman M. Topographical control of human neutrophil motility on micro-patterned materials with various surface chemistry. Biomaterials 2002;23:3215–3225.

29. Berry CC, Campbell G, Spadiccino A, Robertson M, Curtis ASG. The influence of microscale topography on fibroblast attachment and motility. Biomaterials 2004;25: 5781–5788.

30. Curtis A, Wilkinson C. Topographical control of cells. Biomaterials 1997;18:1573–1583.

31. Price RJ, Ellison K, Haberstroh KM, Webster TJ. Nanometer surface roughness increases select osteoblast adhesion on carbon nanofiber compacts. J Biomed Mater Res 2004;70A:129–138.

32. Dalby MJ, Riehle MO, Sutherland DS, Agheli H, Curtis ASG. Changes in fibroblast morphology in response to nano-columns produced by colloidal lithography. Biomaterials 2004;25:5415–5422.

33. Lavine M. Design for living. Science 2005;310:1131–1132.

34. Kwon IK, Kidoaki S, Matsuda T. Electrospun nano- to microfiber fabrics made of biodegradable copolyesters: structural characteristics, mechanical properties and cell adhesion potential. Biomaterials 2005;26:3929–3939.

35. Mow VC, Ratcliffe A, Poole AR. Cartilage and diarthrodial joints as paradigms for hierarchical materials and structures. Biomaterials 1992;13(2):67–97.

36. Stevens MM, George JH. Exploring and engineering the cell surface interface. Science 2005;310:1135–1138.

37. Roskelley CD, Srebrow A, Bissell MJ. A hierarchy of ECM-mediated signaling tissue-specific gene expression. Curr Opin Cell Biol 1995;7:736–747.

38. Wallner EI, Yang Q, Peterson DR, Wada J, Kanwar YS. Relevance of extracellular matrix, its receptors, and cell adhesion molecules in mammalian nephrogenesis. Am J Physiol Renal Physiol 1998;275:467–477.

39. Shih YRV, Chen CN, Tsai SW, Wang YJ, Lee OK. Growth of mesenchymal stem cells on electrospun type I collagen nanofibers. Stem Cells 2006;24:2391–2397.

40. Norman JJ, Desai T. Methods for fabrication of nanoscale topography for tissue engineering scaffolds. Ann Biomed Engg 2006;34(1):89–101.

41. Juliano RL, Haskill S. Signal transduction from the extracellular matrix. J Cell Biol 1993;120(3):577–585.

42. Sun T, Norton D, McKean RJ, Haycock JW, Ryan JA, MacNeil S. Development of a 3D cell culture system for investigating cell interactions with electrospun fibers. Biotechnol & Bioeng 2007;97:1318–1328.

43. Lanza RP, Langer R, Vacanti J. Principles of Tissue engineering. San Diego: Academic Press. 2000;p251–262.

44. Mikos AG, Bao Y, Cima LG, Ingber DE, Vacanti JP, Langer R. Preparation of poly(glycolic acid) bonded fiber structures for cell attachment and transplantation. J Biomed Mater Res 1993a;27:183–189.

45. Freed LE, Marquis JC, Nohria A, Emmanual J, Mikos AG, Langer R. Neocartilage formation *in vitro* and *in vivo* using cells cultured on synthetic biodegradable polymers. J Biomed Mater Res 1993;27(1);11–23.

46. Mikos AG, Sarakinos G, Leite SM, Vacanti JP, Langer R. Laminated three-dimensional biodegradable foams for use in tissue engineering. Biomaterials 1993b;14:323–330.

47. Thomson RC, Yaszemski MJ, Powers JM, Mikos AG. Fabrication of biodegradable polymer scaffolds to engineer trabecular bone. J Biomater Sci Polym Ed 1996;7(1):23–28.

48. Pezzotti G, Asmus SMF, Ferroni LP, Miki S. *In situ* polymerization into porous ceramics: a novel route to tough biomimetic materials. J Mater Sci Mater Med 2002;13:783–787.

49. Whang K, Thomas H, Healy KE. A novel method to fabricate bioabsorbable scaffolds. Polymer 1995;36:837–841.

50. Mooney DJ, Baldwin DE, Suh NP, Vacanti JP, Langer R. Novel approach to fabricate porous sponges of poly(D,L-lactic-co-glycolic acid) without the use of organic solvents. Biomaterials 1996;17:1417–1422.

51. Widmer MS, Gupta PK, Lu L, Meszlenyi RK, Evans GR, Brandt K, Savel T, Gurlek A, Patrick CW Jr, Mikos AG. Manufacture of porous biodegradable polymer conduits by an extrusion process for guided tissue regeneration. Biomaterials 1998;19:1945–1955.

52. Park A, Wu B, Griffith LG. Integration of surface modification and 3D fabrication techniques to prepare patterned poly(L-lactide) substrates allowing regionally selective cell adhesion. J Biomater Sci Polym Ed 1998;9:89–110.

53. Thomson RC, Yaszemski MJ, Powers JM, Mikos AG. Hydroxyapatite fiber reinforced poly(α-hydroxy ester) foams for bone regeneration. Biomaterials 1998;19:1935–1943.

54. Vasita R, Katti DS. Nanofibers and their applications in tissue engineering. Int J Nanomed 2006;1:15–20.

55. Whitesides GM, Boncheva M. Beyond molecules: self-assembly of mesoscopic and macroscopic components. Proc Natl Acad Sci USA 2002;99:4769–4774.

56. Kisiday J, Jin M, Kurz B, Hung H, Semino C, Zhang S, Grodzinsky AJ. Self-assembling peptide hydrogel fosters chondrocyte extracellular matrix production and cell division: Implications for cartilage tissue repair. Proc Natl Acad Sci USA 2002;99:9996–10001.

57. Hamley IW. Nanotechnology with soft materials. Angew Chem Int Ed 2003;42:1692–1712.

58. Hartgerink JD, Beniash E, Stupp SI. Self-assembly and mineralization of peptide-amphiphile nanofibers. Science 2001;294:1684–1688.

59. Hartgerink JD, Beniash E, Stupp SI. Peptide-amphiphile nanofibers: A versatile scaffold for the preparation of self-assembling materials. Proc Nat Acad Sci USA 2002;99(8):5133–5138.

60. Hosseinkhani H, Hosseinkhani M, Khademhosseini A. Tissue regeneration through self-assembled peptide amphiphile nanofibers. Yakhteh Med J 2006;8(3):204–209.

61. Ma Z, Kotaki M, Inai R, Ramakrishna S. Potential of nanofiber matrix as tissue-engineering scaffolds. Tissue Eng 2005;11(1/2):101–108.

62. Ma PX, Zhang R. Synthetic nano-scale fibrous extracellular matrix. J Biomed Mater Res 1999;46(1):60–72.

63. Hua FJ, Kim GE, Lee JD, Son YK, Lee SD. Macroporous Poly(L-lactide) Scaffold 1. Preparation of a macroporous scaffold by liquid–liquid phase separation of a PLLA–dioxane–water system. J Biomed Mater Res 2001;22:1053–1057.

64. Yang F, Murugana R, Ramakrishna S, Wang X, Ma YX, Wang S. Fabrication of nano-structured porous PLLAscaffold intended for nerve tissue engineering. Biomaterials 2004;25:1891–1900.

65. Witte P van de, Dijkstra PJ, Berg JWA van den, Feijen J. Phase separation processes in polymer solutions in relation to membrane formation. J Memb Sci 1996;117:1–31.

66. Huang YX, Ren J, Chen C, Ren TB, Zhou XY. Preparation and properties of poly(lactide-co-glycolide) (PLGA)/nano-hydroxyapatite (NHA) scaffolds by thermally induced phase separation and rabbit MSCs culture on scaffolds. J Biomater Appl 2007.

67. Buckley CT, Kelly KU. Regular scaffold fabricaton techniques for investigations in tissue engineering. Topics in Bio-mechanical engineering. P.J. Prendergast and P.E. McHugh (Eds.) 2004;147–166.

68. Li D, Xia Y. Electrospinning of nanofibers: Reinventing the wheel? Adv Mater 2004;16(14):1151–1170.

69. Bognitzki M, Czado W, Frese T, Schaper A, Hellwig M, Steinhart M, Greiner A, and Wendorff JH. Nanostructured fibers via electrospinning. Adv Mater 2001;13:70–72.

70. Lord Rayleigh X. London, Edinburgh, Dublin Philos Mag 1882;44:184.

71. Zeleny J. Instability of electrified liquid surfaces. Phys Rev 1917;10:1–6.

72. Taylor GI. Disintegration of water drops in an electric field. Proc R Soc London Ser A 1964;280:383–397.

73. Taylor GI, McEwan AD. The stability of horizontally fluid interface in a vertical electrical field. J Fluid Mech 1965;22:1–15.

74. Taylor GI. The force exerted by an electric field on a long cylindrical conductor. Proc R Soc London Ser A 1966;291:145–158.

75. Taylor GI. Electrically driven jets. Proc R Soc London Ser A 1969;313:453–475.

76. Formhals A. Process and apparatus for preparing artificial threads. US patent 1,975,504 1934.

77. Doshi J, Reneker DH. Electrospinning process and applications of electrospun fibers. J Electrostat 1995;35:151–160.

78. Reneker DH, Yarin AL, Fong H, Koombhongse S. Bending instability of electrically charged liquid jets of polymer solutions in electrospinning. J Appl Phy 2000;87(9): 4531–4547.

79. Arya N, Chakraborty S, Dube N, Katti DS. Electrospraying: A facile technique for the synthesis of chitosan based micro/nanoparticles. J Biomed Mat Res Part B; Appl Biomater 2009;88B:17–31.

80. Ramakrishna S, Fujihara K, Ganesh VK, Teo WE, Lim TC. Science and engineering of polymer nanofibers. In: Geckeler KE, Rosenberg E editors, Functional nanomaterials American Scientific Publishers 2005;113–151.

81. Lee KH, Kim HY, Khil MS, Ra YM, Lee DR. Characterization of nano-structured poly(ε-caprolactone) nonwoven mats via electrospinning. Polymer 2003;44:1287–1294.

82. Katti DS, Robinson KW, Ko FK, Laurencin CT. Bioresorbable nanofiber-based systems for wound healing and drug delivery: optimization of fabrication parameters. J Biomed Mater Res B: Appl Biomater 2004;70B:286–296.

83. Lee KH, Kim HY, La YM, Lee DR, Sung NH. Influence of a mixing solvent with tetrahydrofuran and N,N-dimethylformamide on electrospun poly(vinyl chloride) nonwoven mats. J Polym Sci Part B: Polym Phys 2002;40:2259–2268.

84. Lee JS, Choi KH, Ghim HD, Kim SS, Chun DH, Kim HY, Lyoo WS. Role of molecular weight of atactic poly(vinyl alcohol) (PVA) in the structure and properties of PVA nanofabric prepared by electrospinning. J Appl Polym Sci 2004;93:1638–1646.

85. Zhao S, Wu X, Wang L, Huang X. Electrospinning of ethyl–cyanoethyl cellulose/tetrahydrofuran solutions. J Appl Polym Sci 2004;91:242–246.

86. Casper CL, Stephens JS, Tassi NG, Chase DB, Rabolt JF. Controlling surface morphology of electrospun polystyrene fibers: effect of humidity and molecular weight in the electrospinning process. Macromolecules 2004;37:573–578.

87. Choi JS, Lee SW, Jeong L, Bae SH, Min BC, Youk JH, Park WH. Effect of organo-soluble salts on the nanofibrous structure of electrospun poly(3-hydroxybutyrate-co-3-hydroxyvalerate). International J Biol Macromol 2004;34:249–256.

88. Yang F, Murugan R, Wang S, Ramakrishna S. Electrospinning of nano/micro scale poly(L-lactic acid) aligned fibers and their potential in neural tissue engineering. Biomaterials 2005;26:2603–2610.

89. Matthews JA, Wnek GE, Simpson DG, Bowlin GL. Electrospinning of collagen nanofibers. Biomacromolecules 2002;3:232–238.

90. Sundaray B, Subramanian V, Natarajan TS, Xiang RZ, Chang CC, Fann WS. Electrospinning of continuous aligned polymer fibers. App Phy Lett 2004;84(7):1222–1224.

91. Theron A, Zussman E, Yarin AL. Electrostatic field-assisted alignment of electrospun nanofibers. Nanotechnology 2001;12:384–390.

92. Lee CH, Shin HJ, Cho IH, Kang YM, Kim IA, Park KD, Shin JW. Nanofiber alignment and direction of mechanical strain affect the ECM production of human ACL fibroblast. Biomaterials 2005;26:1261–1270.

93. Xu CY, Inai R, Kotaki M, Ramakrishna S. Aligned biodegradable nanofibrous structure: a potential scaffold for blood vessel engineering. Biomaterials 2004;25:877–886.

94. Lutolf MP, Hubbell JA. Synthetic biomaterials as instructive extracellular microenvironments for morphogenesis in tissue engineering. Nat Biotech 2005;23:47–55.

95. Tuzlakoglu K, Bolgen N, Salgado AJ, Gomes ME, Piskin E, Reis RL. Nano- and micro-fiber combined scaffolds: a new architecture for bone tissue engineering. J Mater Sci Mater Med 2005;16:1099–1104.

96. Sahoo S, Ouyang H, Goh JCH, Tay TE, Toh SL. Characterization of a novel polymeric scaffold for potential application in tendon/ligament tissue engineering. Tissue Eng 2006;12:91–99.

97. Nicholson AT, Jayasinghe SN. Cell electrospinning: A unique biotechnique for encapsulating living organisms for generating active biological microthreads/scaffolds. Biomacromol 2006;7:3364–3369.

98. Jiang H, Hu Y, Li Y, Zhao P, Zhu P, Chen W. A facile technique to prepare biodegradable coaxial electrospun nanofibers for controlled release of bioactive agents. J Cont Rel 2005;108:237–243.

99. Dosunmu OO, Chase GG, Varabhas JS, Kataphinan W, Reneker DH. Polymer nanofibers from multiple jets produced on a porous surface by electrospinning. Chapter 10: Polymer Nanocomposites.

100. Ramakrishna S, Fujihara K, Teo WE, Yong T, Ma Z, Ramaseshan R. Electrospun nanofibers:solving global issues. Materials Today 2006;9:40–50.

101. Shields JK, Beckman JM, Bowlin GL, Wayne J. Mechanical properties and cellular proliferation of electrospun collagen type II. Tissue Eng 2004;10(9–10):1510–1517.

102. Li C, Vepari C, Jin HJ, Kim HJ, Kaplan DJ. Electrospun silk-BMP-2 scaffolds for bone tissue engineering. Biomaterials 2006;27:3115–3124.

103. Chong EJ, Phan TT, Lim IJ, Zhang YZ, Bay BH, Ramakrishna S, Lim CT. Evaluation of electrospun PCL/gelatin nanofibrous scaffold for wound healing and layered dermal reconstitution. Acta Biomaterialia 2007;3:321–330.

104. Xua CY, Inaic R, Kotaki M, Ramakrishna S. Aligned biodegradable nanofibrous structure: a potential scaffold for blood vessel engineering. Biomaterials 2004;25:877–886.

105. Riboldi Sa, Sampaolesi M, Neuenschwander P, Cossu G, Mantero S. Electrospun degradable polyesterurethane membranes: potential scaffolds for skeletal muscle tissue engineering. Biomaterials 2005;26:4606–4615.

106. Zeng J, Aigner A, Czubayko F, Kissel T, Wendorff JH, Greiner A. Poly(vinyl alcohol) nanofibers by electrospinning as a protein delivery system and the retardation of enzyme release by additional polymer coatings. Biomacromol 2005;6(3):1484–1488.

107. Liang D, Luu YK, Kim K, Hsiao BS, Hadjiargyrou M, Chu B. *In vitro* non-viral gene delivery with nanofibrous scaffolds. Nucleic Acids Res 2005;33(19):e170.

108. Wang X, Drew C, Lee SH, Senecal KJ, Kumar J, Samuelson LA. Electrospinning technology: a novel approach to sensor application. J Macromol Sci Part A 2002; 39(10):1251–1258.

109. Gopal R, Kaur S, Feng CY, Chan C, Ramakrishna S, Tabe S, Matsuura T. Electrospun nanofibrous polysulfone membranes as pre-filters: particulate removal. J Memb Sci 2007;289:210–219.

110. Lee S, Obendorf SK. Developing protective textile materials as barriers to liquid penetration using melt-electrospinning. J Appl Polym Sci 2006;102:3430–3437.

111. Kim C, Yang KS. Electrochemical properties of carbon nanofiber web as an electrode for supercapacitor prepared by electrospinning. App Phy Lett 2003;83(6):1216–1218.

112. Coombes AGA, Verderio E, Shaw B, Li X, Griffin M, Downes S. Biocomposites of non-crosslinked natural and synthetic polymers. Biomaterials 2002;23:2113–2118.

113. Xie J, Hsieh YL. Ultra-high surface fibrous membranes from electrospinning of natural proteins: casein and lipase enzyme. J Mater Sci 2003;38(10):2125–2133.

114. Aigner T, Stove J. Collagens—major component of the physiological cartilage matrix, major target of cartilage degeneration, major tool in cartilage repair. Adv Drug Dev Rev 2003;55:1569–1593.

115. Brinckmann J, Notbohm H, Müller PK. Collagen: primer in structure, processing and assembly. Top Curr Chem 2005;247:1–6.

116. Brinckmann J, Notbohm H, Müller PK. Collagen: primer in structure, processing and assembly. Top Curr Chem 2005;247:7–33.

117. Shields KJ, Beckman MJ, Bowlin GL, Wayne JS. Mechanical properties and cellular proliferation of electrospun collagen type II. Tissue Eng 2004;10:1510–1517.

118. Barnes CP, Pemble CW, Brand DD, Simpson DG, Bowlin GL. Cross-linking electrospun type II collagen tissue engineering scaffolds with carbodiimide in ethanol. Tissue Eng 2007;13(7):1593–1605.

119. Rowlands AG, Burrows DJ, Rainville RF, Noble P. Gelatin and method of manufacture. US Patent 185441 2001.

120. Kallinteri P, Antimisiaris SG. Solubility of drugs in the presence of gelatin: effect of drug lipophilicity and degree of ionization. Int J Pharm 2001;221:219–226.

121. Baziwane D, He Q. Gelatin: the paramount food additive. Food Rev Int 2003;19(4): 423–435.

122. Djagny KB, Wang Z, Xu S. Gelatin: A valuable protein for food and pharmaceutical industries: review. Crit Rev Food Sci Neut 2001;41(6):481–492.

123. Huang ZM, Zhang YZ, Ramakrishna S. Electrospinning and mechanical characterization of gelatin nanofibers. Polymer 2004;45:5361–5368.

124. Ki CS, Baek HD, Gang KD, Lee KH, Um IC, Park YH. Characterization of gelatin nanofiber prepared from gelatin-formic acid solution. Polymer 2005;46:5094–5102.

125. Zhang YZ, Venugopal J, Lim CT, Ramakrishna S. Crosslinking of the electrospun gelatin nanofibers. Polymer 2006;47:2911–2917.

126. Padamwar MN, Pawar AP. Silk sericin and its applications: a review. J Scient Ind Res 2004;63(4):323–329.

127. Zarkoob S, Eby RK, Reneker DH, Hudson SD, Ertley D, Adams WW. Structure and morphology of electrospun silk nanofibers. Polymer 2004;45:3973–3977.

128. Sukigara S, Gandhi M, Ayutsede J, Micklus M, Ko F. Regeneration of Bombyx mori silk by electrospinning—part 1: processing parameters and geometric properties. Polymer 2003;44:5721–5727.

129. Ayutsede J, Gandhi M, Sukigara S, Micklus M, Chen HE, Ko F. Regeneration of Bombyx mori silk by electrospinning—Part 3: Characterization of electrospun nonwoven mat. Polymer 2005;46:1625–1634.

130. Bowlin GL, Wnek GE, Simpson DG, Lam P, Bruno S, Carr Jr ME. Electroprocessed fibrin-based matrices and tissues. US patent. 60270118, 2001.

131. McManus MC, Boland ED, Simpson DG, Barnes CP, Bowlin GL. Electrospun fibrinogen: Feasibility as a tissue engineering scaffold in a rat cell culture model. J Biomed Mater Res Part A 2006;81A(2):299–309.

132. McManus M, Boland E, Sell S, Bowen W, Koo H, Simpson DG, Bowlin G. Electrospun nanofiber fibrinogen for urinary tract tissue reconstruction. Biomed Mater 2007;2:257–262.

133. Buttafoco L, Kolkman NG, Buijtenhuijs PE, Poot AA, Dijkstra PJ, Vermes I, Feijen J. Electrospinning of collagen and elastin for tissue engineering applications. Biomaterials 2006;27:724–734.

134. Barnes CP, Smith JM, Bowlin GL, Sell AS, Tang T, Matthews JA, Simpson DG, Nimtz JC. Feasibility of electrospinning the globular proteins hemoglobin and myoglobin. Journal of Engineered Fibers and Fabrics 2006;1(2):16–29.

135. Stick RV. Glycoconjugates and glycobiology. In: Carbohydrates: the sweet molecules of life. By Robert V. Stick. New York, Academic Press, 2001:223–231.

136. Poole AR, Kojima T, Yasuda T, Mwale F, Kobayashi M, Laverty S. Cartilage biology. In: Brighton CT, editor in chief. Clinical orthopaedics and related research. Hagerstown, MD: Lippincott Williams and Wilkins, 2001:S26–S33.

137. Noble PW. Hyaluronan and its catabolic products in tissue injury and repair. Matrix Biol 2002;21(1):25–29.

138. Kakehi K, Kinoshita M, Yasueda S. Hyaluronic acid: separation and biological implications. J Chromatogr B Analyt Technol Biomed Life Sci 2003;797(1–2): 347–55.

139. Ji Y, Ghosh K, Shu XZ, Li B, Sokolov JC, Prestwich GD, Clark RA, Rafailovich MH. Electrospun three-dimensional hyaluronic acid nanofibrous scaffolds. Biomaterials 2006;27(20):3782–3792.

140. Um IC, Fang D, Hsiao BS, Okamoto A, Chu B. Electro-spinning and electro-blowing of hyaluronic acid. Biomacromolecules 2004;5(4):1428–1436.

141. Li J, He A, Han CC, Fang D, Benjamin S, Hsiao, Chu B. Electrospinning of hyaluronic acid(HA) and HA/gelatin Blends. Macromol Rapid Commun 2006; 27(2):114–120.

142. Gacesa P. Alginates. Carbohydrate Polymers 1988;8:161–182.

143. Loredo GA, Koolpe M, Benton HP. Influence of alginate polysaccharide composition and culture conditions on chondrocytes in three-dimensional culture. Tissue Eng 1996;2(2):112–115.

144. Glicklis R, Shapiro L, Agbaria R, Merchuk JC, Cohen S. Hepatocyte behavior within three-dimensional porous alginate scaffolds. Biotechnol Bioeng 2000;67(3):344–353.

145. Lu JW, Zu YL, Guo ZX, Hu P, Yu J. Electrospinning of sodium alginate with poly(ethylene oxide). Polymer 2006;47:8026–8031.

146. Bhattarai N, Li Z, Edmondson D, Zhang M. Alginate-based nanofibrous scaffolds: structural, mechanical, and biological properties. Adv Mater 2006;18:1463–1467.

147. Rhazi M, Desbrières J, Tolaimate A, Alagui A, Vottero P. Investigation of different natural sources of chitin: influence of the source and deacetylation process on the physicochemical characteristics of chitosan. Polymer Int 344. 2000;47(4): 337.

148. Kumar MNVR. A review of chitin and chitosan applications. React Funct Polymer 2000;46:1–27.

149. Noh KH, Lee WS, Kim JM, Oh JE, Kim KH, Chung CP, Choi SC, Park WH, Min BM. Electrospinning of chitin nanofibers: Degradation behavior and cellular response to normal human keratinocytes and fibroblasts. Biomaterials 2006;27:3934–3944.

150. Geng X, Kwon OH, Jang J. Electrospinning of chitosan dissolved in concentrated acetic acid solution. Biomaterials 2005;26:5427–5432.

151. Li L, Hsieh YL. Chitosan bicomponent nanofibers and nanoporous fibers. Carbo Res 2006;341:374–381.

152. Ignatova M, Starbova K, Markova N, Manolova N, and Rashkov I. Electrospun nanofibre mats with antibacterial properties from quaternised chitosan and poly(vinyl alcohol). Carbo Res 2006;341:2098–2107.

153. Atsushi M, Go K, Rikako K, and Junzo T. Preparation of chitosan nanofiber tube by electrospinning. J Nanosci Nanotech 2007;7(3):852–855.

154. Murugan R, Ramakrishna S. Nano-featured scaffolds for tissue engineering: a review of spinning methodologies. Tissue Eng 2006;12:435–447.

155. Bendix D. Chemical synthesis of polylactide and its copolymers for medical applications. Polym Degrad Stab 1998;59:129–135.

156. Ajioka M, Enomoto K, Suzuki K, Yamaguchi A. Basic properties of polylactic acid produced by the direct condensation polymerization of lactic acid. Bull Chem Sot Jpn 1995:68:2125–2131.

157. Park K, Shalaby WSW, Park H. Chemically-induced degradation. Biodegradable hydrogels for drug delivery. New York: CRC Press 1993;141–152.

158. Schmitt EE, Polistina RA. Surgical sutures. US patent 3297033, 1967.

159. Boland ED, Telemeco TA, Simpson DG, Wnek GE, Bowlin GL. Utilizing acid pretreatment and electrospinning to improve biocompatibility of poly(glycolic acid) for tissue engineering. J Biomed Mater Res Part B: Appl Biomater 2004;71B: 144–152.

160. Dong C, Duan B, Yuan X, Yao K. Electrospinning and morphology of ultrafine poly (D, L-lactide) fibers. J Biomed Res 2005;22:1245–1248.

161. Min B-M, You Y, Kim J-M, Lee SJ, Park WH. Formation of nanostructured poly(lactic-co-glycolic acid)/chitin matrix and its cellular response to normal human keratinocytes and fibroblasts. Carbo Polymers 2004;57:285–292.

162. You Y, Min B-M, Lee SJ, Lee TS, Park WH. *In vitro* degradation behavior of electrospun polyglycolide, polylactide, and poly(lactide-co-glycolide). J Appl Polym Sci 2005;95:193–200.

163. Bashur CA, Dahlgren LA, Goldstein AS. Effect of fiber diameter and orientation on fibroblast morphology and proliferation on electrospun poly(D,L-lactic-*co*-glycolic acid) meshes. Biomaterials 2006;27:5681–5688.

164. Weert M van de, Hennink WE, Jiskoot W. Protein instability in poly(Lactic-co-glycolic acid) microparticles. Pharm Res 2000;17(10):1159–1167.

165. Kricheldorf HR, Berl M, Scharnagl N. Poly(lactones). 9. Polymerization mechanism of metal alkoxide initiated polymerizations of lactide and various lactones. Macromolecules 1988;21:286–293.

166. Mondrinos MJ, Dembzynski R, Lu L, Byrapogu VKC, Wootton DM, Lelkes PI, Zhou J. Porogen-based solid freeform fabrication of polycaprolactone–calcium phosphate scaffolds for tissue engineering. Biomaterials 2006;27:4399–4408.

167. Luong-Van E, Grøndahl L, Chua KN, Leong KM, Nurcombe V, Cool SM. Controlled release of heparin from poly(ε-caprolactone) electrospun fibers. Biomaterials 2005;27:2042–2050.

168. Lamba NMK, Woodhouse KA, Cooper SL. Polyurethanes in biomedical applications. New York: CRC Press 1998;205–241.

169. Stokes K, Cobian L. Polyether polyurethanes for implantable pacemaker leads. Biomaterials. 1982;3:225–231.

170. Khil MS, Cha DI, Kim HY, Kim IS, Bhattarai N. Electrospun nanofibrous polyurethane membrane as wound dressing. J Biomed Mater Res B: Appl Biomater 2003; 67(2):675–679.

171. Lee IS, Kwon OH, Meng W, Kang IK, Ito Y. Nanofabrication of microbial polyester by electrospinning promotes cell attachment. Macromol Res 2004;12:374–378.

172. Park KE, Jung SY, Lee SJ, Min BM, Park WH. Biomimetic nanofibrous scaffolds: Preparation and characterization of chitin/silk fibroin blend nanofibers. Int J Biol Macromol 2006;38:165–173.

173. Zong X, Li S, Chen E, Garlick B, Kim KS, Fang D, Chiu J, Zimmerman T, Brathwaite C, Hsiao BS, Chu B. Prevention of postsurgery-induced abdominal adhesions by electrospun bioabsorbable nanofibrous poly(lactide-co-glycolide) based membranes. Ann Surg 2004;240:910–915.

174. Mo XM, Xu CY, Kotaki M, Ramakrishna S. Electrospun (PLLA-CL) nanofiber: a biomimetic extracellular matrix for smooth muscle cell and endothelial cell proliferation. Biomaterials 2004;25:1883–1890.

175. Li M, Mondrinos MJ, Chen X, Lelkes PI. Electrospun blends of natural and synthetic polymers as scaffolds for tissue engineering.Proceedings of the 2005 IEEE. Engineering in medicine and biology 27th annual conference. 5858–5861.

176. Kim CW, Kim DS, Kang SY, Marquez M, Joo YL. Structural studies of electrospun cellulose nanofibers. Polymer 2006;47(14):5097–5107.

177. Min BM, Lee SW, Lim JN, You Y, Lee TS, Kang PH, Park WH. Chitin and chitosan nanofibers: electrospinning of chitin and deacetylation of chitin nanofibers. Polymer 2004;45:7137–7142.

178. Bhattarai N, Edmondson D, Veiseh O, Matsen FA, Zhang M. Electrospun chitosan-based nanofibers and their cellular compatibility. Biomaterials 2005;26:6176–6184.

179. Subramanian A, Vu D, Larsen GF, Lin HY. Preparation and evaluation of the electrospun chitosan/PEO fibers for potential applications in cartilage tissue engineering. J Biomater Sci 2005;16(7):861–873.

180. Martino AD, Sittinger M, Makarand V, Risbud. Chitosan: A versatile biopolymer for orthopaedic tissue-engineering. Biomaterials 2005;26:5983–5990.

181. Rho KS, Jeong L, Lee G, Seo BM, Park YJ, Hong SD, Roh S, Cho JJ, Park WH, Min BM. Electrospinning of collagen nanofibers: Effects on the behavior of normal human keratinocytes and early-stage wound healing. Biomaterials 2006;27:1452–1461.

182. Huang L, Nagapudi K, Apkarian RP, Chaikof EL. Engineered collagen-PEO nano-fibers and fabrics. J Biomater Sci Polym Ed 2001;12(9):979–993.

183. Li M, Guo Y, Wei Y, MacDiarmid AG, Lelkes PI. Electrospinning polyaniline-contained gelatin nanofibers for tissue engineering applications. Biomaterials 2006; 27:2705–2715.

184. Kwon OH, Lee IS, Ko YG, Meng W, Jung KH, Kang IK, Ito Y. Electrospinning of microbial polyester for cell culture. Biomed Mater 2007;2:52–58.

185. Jeong L, Lee KY, Liu JW, Park WH. Time-resolved structural investigation of regen-erated silk fibroin nanofibers treated with solvent vapor. Int J Biol Macromol 2006;38: 140–144.

186. Miyoshi T, Toyohara K, Minematsu H. Preparation of ultrafine fibrous zein mem-branes via electrospinning. Polym Int 2005;54(8):1187–1190.

187. Kenawy ER, Layman JM, Watkins JR, Bowlin GL, Matthews JA, Simpson DG, Wnek GE. Electrospinning of poly(ethylene-co-vinyl alcohol) fibers. Biomaterials 2003; 24:907–913.

188. Bhowmick S, Fowler A, Warner SB, Toner M. Bio-active bandages. *NTC Project* 2005:F03-MD15.

189. Van LE, Grondahl L, Chua KN, Leong KW, Nurcombe V, Cool SM. Controlled release of heparin from poly(e-caprolactone) electrospun fibers. Biomaterials 2006; 27:2042–2050.

190. Teo WE, Kotaki M, Mo XM, Ramakrishna S. Porous tubular structures with con-trolled fibre orientation using a modified electrospinning method. Nanotechnology 2005;16:918–924.

191. Bolgen N, Menceloglu YZ, Acatay K, Vargel I, Piskin E. *In vitro* and *in vivo* degrada-tion of non-woven materials made of poly (epsilon-caprolactone) nanofibers pre-pared by electrospinning under different conditions. J Biomater Sci Polym Ed 2005;16:1537–1555.

192. Khil MS, Bhattarai SR, Kim HY, Kim SZ, Lee KH. Novel fabricated matrix via elec-trospinning for tissue engineering. J Biomed Mater Res Part B: Appl Biomater 2004;72B(1):117–124.

193. Li WJ, Cooper JA Jr, Mauck RL, Tuan RS. Fabrication and characterization of six electrospun poly(α-hydroxy ester)-based fibrous scaffolds for tissue engineering applications. Acta Biomater 2006;2(4):377–385.

194. Deitzel JM, Kleinmeyer JD, Hirvonen JK, Tan NCB. Controlled deposition of electro-spun poly(ethylene oxide) fibers. Polymer 2001;42:8163–8170.

195. Casper CL, Yamaguchi N, Kiick KL, Rabolt JF. Functionalizing electrospun fibers with biologically relevant macromolecules. Biomacromolecule 2005;6(4):1998–2007.

196. Bhattacharyya S, Lakshmi S, Bender J, Greish YE, Brown PW, Allcock HR, Laurencin CT. Preparation of poly [bis(carboxylatophenoxy) phosphazene] non-woven nanofiber mats by electrospinning. Mat Res Soc Symp Proc 2004; Vol. EXS-1.

197. Park KE, Kang HK, Lee SJ, Min BM, Park WH. Biomimetic nanofibrous scaffolds: preparation and characterization of PGA/chitin blend nanofibers. Biomacromole-cule 2006;7(2):635–643.

198. Bhattarai SR, Bhattarai N, Viswanathamurthi P, Yi HK, Hwang PH, Kim HY. Hydro-philic nanofibrous structure of polylactide; fabrication and cell affinity. J Biomed Mater Res Part A 2006;78A(2):247–257.

199. He W, Yong T, Teo WE, Zuwei, Ramakrishna S. Fabrication and endothelialization of collagen-blended biodegradable polymer nanofibers: potential vascular graft for blood vessel tissue engineering. Tissue Eng 2005;11(9/10):1574–1588.

200. Stitzel J, Liu J, Lee SJ, Komura M, Berry J, Soker S, Lim G, Dyke MV, Czerw R, Yoo JJ, Atala A. Controlled fabrication of a biological vascular substitute. Biomaterials 2006;27:1088–1094.

201. Luu YK, Kim K, Hsiao BS, Chu B, Hadjiargyrou M. Development of a nanostructured DNA delivery scaffold via electrospinning of PLGA and PLA–PEG block copolymers. J Control Rel 2003;89:341–353.

202. Pan H, Li L, Hu L, Cui X. Continuous aligned polymer fibers produced by a modified electrospinning method. Polymer 2006;47(14):4901–4904.

203. Rothman HR, Freeman MAR. The bone and joint decade 2000–2010 For prevention and treatment of musculoskeletal disease. J Arthoplast 1999;14(8).

204. Hart LE. Physical Activity and Risk of Musculoskeletal Injury. Clin J Sport Med 2002;12(3):196–197.

205. Krug EG, Sharma GK, and Lozano R. The global burden of injuries. Am J Public Health 2000;90(4):523–526.

206. Katz SI. Boning up for health: The national bone and joint decade. J Bone Min Res 2004;19(10).

207. Weinstein SL. 2000–2010: the bone and joint decade. J Bone Joint Surg 2000;82A:1–3 (Editorial.)

208. Yelin E, Herrndorf A, Trupin L, Sonneborn D. A national study of medical care expenditures for musculoskeletal conditions: The impact of health insurance and managed care. Arth Rheum 2001;44(5):1160–1169.

209. Spiegel DA, Gosselin RA, Coughlin RR, Joshipura M, Browner BD, and Dormans JP. The burden of musculoskeletal injury in low and middle-income countries: challenges and opportunities. J Bone Joint Surg Am 2008;90(4):915–923.

210. Gauthy R. Musculoskeletal disorders: Where we are, and where we could be. HESA newsletter 2005;27:22–27.

211. Roberts SJ, Howard D, Buttery LD, and Shakesheff KM. Clinical applications of musculoskeletal tissue engineering. Br Med Bull 2008 (ahead of print).

212. Sommerfeldt DW, Rubin CT. Biology of bone and how it orchestrates the form and function of the skeleton. Eur Spine J 2001;10:S86–S95.

213. Praemer A, Furner S, Rice DP. Musculoskeletal Conditions in the United States. Rosemont, IL, Am Acad Ortho Surg 1999;107–117.

214. Perry CR. Bone repair techniques, bone graft, and bone graft substitutes. Clin Orthop Rel Res 1999;360:71–86.

215. Salgado AJ, Coutinho OP, Reis RL. Bone Tissue Engineering: State of the art and future trends. Macromol Biosci 2004;4:743–765.

216. Lu L, Currier BL, Yaszemski MJ. Synthetic bone substitutes. Curr Opin Orthop 2000;11:383–390.

217. El-Amin SF, Lu HH, Khan Y, Burems J, Mitchell J, Tuan RS, Laurencin RS. Extracellular matrix production by human osteoblasts cultured on biodegradable polymers applicable for tissue engineering. Biomaterials 2003;24:1213–1221.

218. Petite H, Viateau V, Bensaïd W, Meunier A, Pollak C, Bourguignon M, Oudina K, Sedel L, Guillemin G. Tissue-engineered bone regeneration. Nat Biotech 2000;18: 959–963.

219. Krebsbach PH, Kuznetsov SA, Satomura K, Emmons, RV, Rowe DW, Robey PG. Bone formation *in vivo*: comparison of osteogenesis by transplanted mouse and human marrow stromal fibroblasts. Transplantation 1997;63(8):1059–1069.

220. Sun JS, Wu HYH, Lin FH. The role of muscle-derived stem cells in bone tissue engineering. Biomaterials 2005;26:3953–3960.

221. Katagiri T, Yamaguchi A, Komaki M, Abe E, Takahashi N, Ikeda T, Rosen V, Wozney JM, Fujisawa-Sehara A, Suda T. Bone morphogenetic protein-2 converts the differentiation pathway of C2C12 myoblasts into the osteoblast lineage. J Cell Biol 1994;127(6):1755–1766.

222. Lu HH, Kofron MD, El-Amin SF, Attawia MA, Laurencin CT. *In vitro* bone formation using muscle-derived cells: a new paradigm for bone tissue engineering using polymer–bone morphogenetic protein matrices. Biochem Biophys Res Commun 2003;305:882–889.

223. Weinzierl K, Hemprich A, Frerich B. Bone engineering with adipose tissue derived stromal cells. J Cranio-Maxillofacial Surg 2006;34:466–471.

224. Dragoo JS, Choi JY, Lieberman JR, Huang H, Zuk PA, Zhang J, Hedrick MH, Benhaim P. Bone induction by BMP-2 transduced stem cells derived from human fat. J Orthop Res 2003;21:622–629.

225. Scheer M, Richter I, Neugebauer J, Arnhold S. Bone tissue engineering from mesenchymal stem cells derived from human pulp tissue. J Cranio-Maxillofacial Surg 2006;34 Suppl. S1Abstracts, EACFMS XVIII Congress.

226. Kim HW, Kim HE. Nanofiber generation of hydroxyapatite and fluor-hydroxyapatite bioceramics. J Biomed Mater Res Part B: Appl Biomater 2006;77B:323–328.

227. Yoshimoto H, Shin YM, Terai H, Vacanti JP. A biodegradable nanofiber scaffold by electrospinning and its potential for bone tissue engineering. Biomaterials 2003; 24:2077–2082.

228. Venugopal J, Vadgama P, SampathKumar TS, Ramakrishna S. Biocomposite nanofibres and osteoblasts for bone tissue engineering. Nanotechnology 2007;18:1–8.

229. Catledge SA, Clem WC, Shrikishen N, Chowdhury S, Stanishevsky AV, Koopman M, Vohra YK. An electrospun triphasic nanofibrous scaffold for bone tissue engineering. Biomed Mater 2007;2:142–150.

230. Fujihara K, Kotaki M, Ramakrishna S. Guided bone regeneration membrane made of polycaprolactone/calcium carbonate composite nano-fibers. Biomaterials 2005;26: 4139–4147.

231. Wutticharoenmongkol P, Sanchavanakit N, Pavasant P, Supaphol P. Preparation and characterization of novel bone scaffolds based on electrospun polycaprolactone fibers filled with nanoparticles. Macromol Biosci 2006;6:70–77.

232. Sakai S, Yamada Y, Yamaguchi T, Kawakami K. Prospective use of electrospun ultrafine silicate fibers for bone tissue engineering. Biotechnol J 2006;1:958–962.

233. Kim HW, Lee HH, Knowles JC. Electrospinning biomedical nanocomposite fibers of hydroxyapaite/poly(lactic acid) for bone regeneration. J Biomed Mater Res 2006; 79A:643–649.

234. Spasova M, Stoilova O, Manolova N, Rashkov I. Preparation of PLLA/PEG nanofibers by electrospinning and potential applications. J Bioact Comp Poly 2007;22: 62–76.

235. Shin M, Yoshimoto H, Vacanti JP. *In vivo* bone tissue engineering using mesenchymal stem cells on a novel electrospun nanofibrous scaffold. Tissue Eng 2004;10(1/2): 33–41.

236. Benedek TG. A history of the understanding of cartilage. Osteoarthritis and cartilage 2006;14:203–209.

237. Calandruccio RA, Gilmer WA Jr. Proliferation, Regeneration, and Repair of Articular Cartilage of Immature Animals. J Bone Joint Surg Am 1962;44:431–455.

238. Eyre DR, Muir H. The distribution of different molecular species of collagen in fibrous, elastic and hyaline cartilages of the pig. Biochem J 1975;151(3):595–602.

239. Anthony A, Lanza R. Methods of tissue engineering. San Diego: Academic Press 2002. p1027–1040.

240. O'Driscoll WS. The healing and regeneration of articular cartilage. J Bone Joint Surg 1998;80-A(12):1795–1812.

241. March LM, Cross MJ, Lapsley H, Brnabic AJM, Tribe KL, Bachmeier CJM, Courtney BG, Brooks PM. Outcomes after hip or knee replacement surgery for osteoarthritis: A prospective cohort study comparing patients' quality of life before and after surgery with age-related population norms. Med J Australia 1999;171:235–238.

242. Katz J. Total joint replacement in osteoarthritis. Best Prac Res Clin Rheumatol 2003;20(1):145–153.

243. Hunziker EB. Articular cartilage repair: are the intrinsic biological constraints undermining this process insuperable? Osteoarth Cart 1999;7:15–28.

244. Fodor WL. Tissue engineering and cell based therapies, from the bench to the clinic: The potential to replace, repair and regenerate. Rep Biol Endocrinol 2003;1: 102–107.

245. Freed LE, Grande DA, Lingbin Z, Emmanual J, Marquis JC, Langer R. Joint resurfacing using allograft chondrocytes and synthetic biodegradable polymer scaffolds. J Biomed Mater Res. 1994;28:891–899.

246. Grande DA, Southerland SS, Manji R, Pate DW, Schwartz RE, Lucas PA. Repair of Articular Cartilage Defects Using Mesenchymal Stem Cells. Tissue Eng 1995;1(4):345–353.

247. Ahmed N, Stanford WL, Kandel RA. Mesenchymal stem and progenitor cells for cartilage repair. Skel Radiol. 2007;36(10):909–912.

248. Fibbe WE. Mesenchymal stem cells. A potential source for skeletal repair. Ann Rheum Dis 2002;61(2):29–31.

249. Caplan IA, Bruder PS. Mesenchymal stem cells: building blocks for molecular medicine in the 21st century. Trends Mol Med 2001;7(6):259–264.

250. Bayliss MT, Venn M, Maroudas A, Ali SY. Structure of proteoglycans from different layers of human articular cartilage. Biochem J 1983;209(2):387–400.

251. Li JW, Jiang YJ, Tuan RS. Chondrocyte phenotype in engineered fibrous matrix is regulated by fiber size. Tissue Eng 2006;12(7):1775–1785.

252. Subramanian A, Vu D, Larsen GF, Lin HY. Preparation and evaluation of the electrospun chitosan/PEO fibers for potential applications in cartilage tissue engineering. J Biomater Sci 2005;16(7):861–873.

253. Shin HJ, Lee CH, Cho IH, Kim YJ, Lee YJ, Kim IA, Park KD, Yui N, Shin JW. Electro-spun PLGA nanofiber scaffolds for articular cartilage reconstruction: mechanical stability, degradation and cellular responses under mechanical stimulation *in vitro*. J Biomater Sci Polym Edn 2006;17(1–2):103–119.

254. Li JW, Danielson KG, Alexander PG, Tuan RS. Biological response of chondrocytes cultured in three-dimensional nanofibrous poly(ε-caprolactone) scaffolds. J Biomed Mater Res Part A 2003;67A(4):1105–1114.

255. Li JW, Tuli R, Okafor C, Derfoul A, Danielson KG, Hall DJ, Tuan RS. A three-dimensional nanofibrous scaffold for cartilage tissue engineering using human mesenchymal stem cells. Biomaterials 2005;26:599–609.

256. Velleman SG. Role of the extracellular matrix in muscle growth and development.

257. Bach AD, Stem-Straeter J, Beier JP, Bannasch H, Stark GB. Engineering of muscle tissue. Clin Plast Surg 2003;30:589–599.

258. Mauro A. Satellite cells of skeletal muscle fibers. J Biochem Biophys Cytol 1961;9:493–498.

259. Montarras D, Morgan J, Collins C, Relaix F, Zaffran S, Cumano A, Partridge T, Buckingham M. Direct isolation of satellite cells for skeletal muscle regeneration. Science 2005;209:2064–2067.

260. Peng H, Huard J. Muscle derived stem cells for musculoskeletal tissue regeneration and repair. Trans Immunol 2004;12:311–319.

261. Saxena AK, Marler J, Benvenuto M, Willital GH, Vacanti JP. Skeletal muscle tissue engineering using isolated myoblasts on synthetic biodegradable polymers: Preliminary studies. Tissue Eng 1999;5(6):525–531.

262. Bach AD, Beier JP, Staeter JS, Horch RE. Skeletal muscle tissue engineering. J Cell Mol Med 2004;8(4):413–422.

263. Levenberg S, Rouwkema J, Macdonald M, Garfein ES, Kohane DS, Darland DC, Marini, van Blitterswijk CA, Mulligan RC, D'Amore PA, Langer R. Engineering vascularized skeletal muscle tissue. Nat Biotech 2005;23:879–884.

264. Saxena AK, Willital GH, Vacanti JP. Vascularized three-dimensional skeletal muscle tissue-engineering. Biomed Mater Eng 2001;11:275–281.

265. Wachem PB van, Brouwer LA, Luyn MJA Van. Absence of muscle regeneration after implantation of a collagen matrix seeded with myoblasts. Biomaterials 1999;20:419–426.

266. Dennis RG, Kosnik P. Excitability and isometric contractile properties of mammalian skeletal muscle constructs engineered *in vitro*. Cell Dev Biol Animal 2000;36:327–335.

267. Neumann T, Hauschika SD, Sanders JE. Tissue engineering of skeletal muscle using polymer fiber arrays. Tissue Eng 2003;9(5):995–1003.

268. Woo SLY, Thomas M, Saw SSC. Contribution of biomechanics, orthopaedics and rehabilitation: The past, present and future. Surg J R Coll Surg Edinb Irel 2004:25–136.

269. Duthon VB, Barea C, Abrassart S, Fasel JH, Fritschy D, Menetrey J. Anatomy of the anterior cruciate ligament. Knee Surg Sports Traumatol Arthrosc 2006;14:204–213.

270. Ikada Y. Animal and human trials of engineered tissue. In: Tissue Engineering: Fundamentals and applications By Ikada Y. Academic Press, 2006:129–137.

271. Goh JCH, Ouyang HW, Teoh SH, Chan CKC, Lee EH. Tissue-engineering approach to the repair and regeneration of tendons and ligaments. Tissue Eng 2003;9(1):S31–S44.

272. Doroski DM, Brink KS, Temenoff JS. Techniques for biological characterization of tissue-engineered tendon and ligament. Biomaterials 2007;28:187–202.

273. Gouelt F, Rancourt D, Cloutier R, Germain L, Poole AR, Auger FA. Tendons and ligaments. In: Lanza RP, Langer R, Vacanti J, editor. Principles of tissue Engineering. San Diego: Academic Press 2000;711–722.

274. Freeman JW, Woods MD, Laurencin CT. Tissue engineering of the anterior cruciate ligament using abraid twist scaffold design. J Biomech 2007;40:2029–2036.

275. Vunjak-Novakovic G, Altman G, Horan R, Kaplan DL. Tissue Engineering of Ligaments. Annu Rev Biomed Eng 2004;6:131–56.

276. Amiel D, Frank C, Harwood FL, Fronek J, Akeson WH. Tendons and ligaments: a morphological and biochemical comparison. J Orthop Res 1984;1:257–265.

277. Woo SLY, Debski RE, Zeminsk J, Abramowitch SD, ChanSaw SS, Fenwick JA. Injury and repair of ligaments and tendons. Annu Rev Biomed Eng 2000;2:83–118.

278. Milz S, Aktas T, Putz R, Benjamin M. Expression of extracellular matrix molecules typical of articular cartilage in the human scapholunate interosseous ligament. J Anatomy 2006;208(6):671–679.

279. Kannus P, Järvinen M. Posttraumatic anterior cruciate ligament insufficiency as a cause of osteoarthritis in a knee joint. Clin Rheumatol 1989;8:251–260.

280. Lohmander SL, Englund PM, Dahl LL, Roos EM. The long-term consequence of anterior cruciate ligament and meniscus injuries: osteoarthritis. Am J Sports Med 2007;35(10):1756–1769.

281. Martha MM, Spindler PK. Anterior cruciate ligament healing and repair. Sport Med Anthro Rev 2005;13(3):151–155.

282. Spindler KP, Kuhn JE, Freedman KB, Matthews CE, Dittus RS, Harrell FE Jr. Anterior cruciate ligament reconstruction autograft choice: bone-tendon-bone versus hamstring: does it really matter? A systematic review. Am J Sports Med 2004;32:1986–1995.

283. Lin VS, Lee MC, O'neal S, Mckean J, Sung KLP. Ligament tissue engineering using synthetic biodegradable fiber scaffolds. Tissue Eng 1999;5(5):443–451.

284. Tang JB. Tendon injuries across the world: treatment. Injury, 2006;37:1036–1042.

285. Woo SLY, Abramowitch SD, Kilger R, Liang R. Biomechanics of knee ligaments: injury, healing, and repair. J Biomech 2006;39:1–20.

286. Van EF, Saris DB, Riesle J, Willems WJ, Van Blitterswijk CA, Verbout AJ, Dhert WJ. Tissue engineering of ligaments: a comparison of bone marrow stromal cells, anterior cruciate ligament, and skin fibroblasts as cell source. Tissue Eng 2004;10(5–6):893–903.

287. Tuan RS, Boland G, Tuli R. Adult mesenchymal stem cells and cell-based tissue engineering. Arth Res Ther 2002;5(1):32–45.

288. Watanabe N, Woo SLY, Papageorgiou C, Celechovsky C, Takai S. Fate of donor bone marrow cells in medial collateral ligament after simulated autologous transplantation. Microsc Res Tech 2002;58:39–44.

289. Ge Z, Yang F, Goh JCH, Ramakrishna S, Lee EH. Biomaterials and scaffolds for ligament tissue engineering. J Biomed Mater Res 2006;77A:639–652.

290. Courtney T, Sacks MS, Stankus J, Guan J, Wagner WR. Design and analysis of tissue engineering scaffolds that mimic soft tissue mechanical anisotropy. Biomaterials 2006;27:3631–3638.

291. Bashur CA, Guelcher SA, Goldstein AS. Electrospun polymers for ligament tissue engineering. Proceedings of the IEEE 32nd Annual Northeast 2006.

292. Spalazzi JP, Doty SB, Moffat KL, Levine W, Lu HL. Development of controlled matrix heterogeneity on a triphasic scaffold for orthopedic interface tissue engineering. Tissue Eng 2006;12(12):3497–3508.

293. Huang D, Balian G, Chhabra A. Tendon Tissue Engineering and Gene Transfer: The Future of Surgical Treatment. J Hand Surg 2006;31(5):693–704.

14

DESIGN OF SUPERMACROPOROUS BIOMATERIALS VIA GELATION AT SUBZERO TEMPERATURES— *CRYOGELATION*

Fatima M. Plieva[1,2], Ashok Kumar[3], Igor Yu. Galaev[1], and Bo Mattiasson[1]

[1]*Department of Biotechnology, Lund University, SE-22100 Lund, Sweden*
[2]*Protista Biotechnology AB, SE-22370 Lund, Sweden*
[3]*Department of Biological Sciences and Bioengineering, Indian Institute of Technology Kanpur, Kanpur, India*

Contents

14.1 Overview	500
14.2 Introduction	500
14.3 Preparation of Supermacroporous Biomaterials through Cryogelation Technique	502
14.3.1 General Concept of Cryogelation	502
14.3.2 Parameters Influencing Cryostructuration (Cryogelation) of Polymeric Systems	504
14.3.2.1 Freezing Rate and Freezing Temperature	504
14.3.2.2 Concentration and Composition of Gel Precursors in the Initial Reaction Mixture	508
14.4 Preparation of Macroporous Gels (MGs) from Different Gel Precursors	513
14.4.1 Physically Cross-Linked MGs	513
14.4.2 Covalently Cross-Linked MGs	515

Advanced Biomaterials: Fundamentals, Processing, and Applications, Edited by Bikramjit Basu, Dhirendra S. Katti, and Ashok Kumar
Copyright © 2009 The American Ceramic Society

14.5 Characterization of MGs 516
   14.5.1 Pore Volume of MGs 516
   14.5.2 Characterization of Porous Structure Using Different
      Microscopy Techniques 518
14.6 Biomedical Application of MGs 522
14.7 Conclusion and Outlook 525
   Acknowledgments 525
   References 525

14.1 OVERVIEW

Design of supermacroporous polymeric materials with controlled porosity and gel surface chemistry is important in the field of biomaterials. The macroporous gels with a broad variety of morphologies are prepared using cryotropic gelation technique, meaning gelation at subzero temperatures (so-called *cryogelation*). The cryogelation technique allows for the formation of biocompatible macroporous materials with unique properties such as open and highly permeable porous structure, tissue-like elasticity, and excellent mechanical strength. Proper control over solvent crystallization (formation of solvent crystals) and rate of chemical reaction during the cryogelation allows for the reproducible preparation of macroporous polymeric materials with tailored properties.

14.2 INTRODUCTION

The development of new macroporous (with pore size above 1 μm) functional polymeric materials for biomedical applications is of great interest. Hydrophilic macroporous materials designed from natural and synthetic polymers are important in the field of biomaterials and used as matrices for controlled drug delivery, as wound dressing and as scaffolds for cell growth within the tissue engineering field [Cai et al., 2002; Chen et al., 1995; Hentze and Antonietti, 2002; Lai et al., 2003; Miralles et al., 2001; Peppas et al., 2000; Shapiro and Cohan, 1997]. An important approach to design the biomaterials is to involve the preparation of co-polymers with various functional groups that permit the attachment (grafting) of polymer chains with bioactive substances that can induce tissue in-growth. The biocompatible synthetic polymers as poly(2-hydroxyethyl methacrylate) (pHEMA) [Kaufman et al., 2006; Kroupova et al., 2006; Vijayasekaran et al., 2000], poly(ethylene glycol) (PEG) [Sannino et al., 2006; Sawhney et al., 1993] and poly(vinylpyrrolidone) (PVP) [Engström et al., 2006] were shown to be attractive for the development of biocompatible materials for drug delivery and tissue engineering. Among polysaccharides, alginate, chitosan and dextran have found various biomedical applications due to their bioavailability and biocompatibility [Ito et al., 2007; Lai et al., 2003; Levesque et al., 2005; Levesque and Shoichet, 2006; Mi et al., 2001; Miralles et al., 2001; Shapiro and Cohan, 1997].

There are different cross-linking approaches to design degradable hydrogels for biomedical applications [Hennik and Nostrum, 2002]. Biodegradable macroporous material prepared using synthetically adaptable cross-linkers offer a new tool in designing the drug delivery systems and in tissue engineering. The majority of biodegradable polymers belong to the polyester family. Among these poly(α-hydroxy acids) such as poly(lactic acid), PLA, poly(glycolic acid), PGA and their copolymers have been intensively used as synthetic biodegradable materials in a number of clinical applications [Gunatillake and Adhikari, 2003; Hasirci et al., 2001].

Design and manufacture of appropriate three dimensional (3D) scaffolds for a particular application are of key importance in tissue engineering. The fundamental properties of scaffolds are their biocompatibility, adequate degradation time, appropriate biodegradation rate (not too fast in a first stage of contact with cells and tissues) and proper porous microstructure. Depending on the tissue of interest and specific application, the requirements for the scaffold material differ. The materials should meet several requirements to be used as scaffolds for cell applications. The open porous structure and interconnectivity of macropores are needed for proper oxygen and nutrients delivery to cells, waste removal, vascularization and tissue in-growth [Peters and Mooney, 1997]. Typically, cell scaffolds should have a 3D porous structure and its porosity should be at least 90% in order to provide a high surface area for maximizing cell seeding and attachment [Cai et al., 2002]. Even the pore size is very type-specific. It is generally accepted that pore size should be in the range of 10–400 μm. Porosity can, however, adversely affect important mechanical characteristics of a polymer, requiring more complex material design. Pore size, shape, and surface roughness affect cellular adhesion, proliferation and phenotype. Cells can discriminate even the subtlest changes in topography, and they are most obviously sensitive to chemistry, topography, and surface energy [Burg et al., 2000]. Providing adequate mechanical support is a critical requirement. The porous scaffold should have a mechanical modulus in the range of soft tissues (0.4–350 MPa) [Hollister, 2005]. Scaffolds made using traditional polymer-processing techniques, such as porogen leaching or gas foaming, have maximum compressive module of 0.4 MPa [Hollister, 2005].

Classical approaches to synthesize the macroporous biomaterials include freeze-drying [O'Brien et al., 2004, 2005; Patel and Amiji, 1996; Wan et al., 2007; Yeong et al., 2007], porogenation [Wood and Cooper, 2001], microemulsion formation [Bennett et al., 1995], phase separation [Liu et al., 2000; Nam and Park, 1999] and gas blowing technique [Kabiri et al., 2003; Sannino et al., 2006]. Recently, the cryotropic gelation (cryogelation technique), implying the synthesis at subzero temperature, was intensively employed for the preparation of macroporous materials (known as *cryogels*) for biotechnological and biomedical applications [Lozinsky et al., 2002; Kumar et al., 2003; Dainiak et al., 2006; Plieva et al., 2007a].

In most cases, the macroporous biomaterials with well defined porous structure are produced through freeze-drying technique [Wan et al., 2007; Yeong et al., 2007] when the porosity is created by the sublimation of frozen solvent (most frequently, water or dioxane), and the polymer is concentrated in the thin walls of macropores. However, freeze-dried materials can be produced only as relatively thin objects, such as films, plates, or small beads [O'Brien et al., 2004]. Besides, the freeze-drying procedure is well-known to be a highly energy- and time-consuming process. However, the macroporous gels (*cryogels*) are prepared at moderately low temperatures and can be produced in any desirable shape, that is, blocks, rods, disks, beads and so on. The cryogels can be produced from practically any gel forming system with a broad range of porosity, from 0.1 to 200 μm [Lozinsky et al., 2002; Plieva et al., 2005, 2006a; Srivastava et al., 2007].

14.3 PREPARATION OF SUPERMACROPOROUS BIOMATERIALS THROUGH CRYOGELATION TECHNIQUE

14.3.1 General Concept of Cryogelation

Cryogels are formed as a result of cryogenic treatment (freezing, storage in the frozen state for a definite time, and defrosting) of low- or high-molecular-weight precursors, as well as colloid systems, all capable of gelling. Cryotropic gelation (or cryostructuration) is a specific type of gel-formation that takes place as a result of cryogenic treatment of the systems potentially capable of gelation. The essential feature of the cryogelation is compulsory crystallization of the solvent, which distinguishes cryogelation from chilling–induced gelation when the gelation takes place on decreasing temperature (as, for example, gelation of agarose or gelatin solutions on cooling, which proceeds without any phase transition of the solvent).

The processes of cryogelation have some unique characteristics:

1. Cryotropic gelation proceeds in a non-frozen liquid microphase existing in a macroscopically-frozen sample. At moderately-low temperature below the freezing point of solvent (often water), some part of solvent remains non-frozen. All reagents are concentrated in this non-frozen part (so-called non-frozen liquid microphase, NFLMP) where the chemical reaction or process of physical gelation proceeds with time.
2. Crystals of the frozen solvent grow until they merge and after melting leave behind the interconnected pores, thus playing a role of porogen. As the size and alignment of solvent crystals is varied to a large extent, the pores in the prepared cryogels are in the range of 1–200 μm.
3. Typically, the critical concentration of gelation (CCG) is decreased for cryogels as compared to the conventional gels prepared at room temperature due to the concentrating of reagents in NFLMP (so-called cryoconcentration).

The *cryogels* (referred here as macroporous gels, MGs) are synthesized in semi-frozen aqueous media where ice crystals perform as porogen and template the continuous interconnected pores after melting. Contrary to conventional gels (which are homophase systems where solvent is bound to the polymer network), the MGs are heterophase systems where solvent (water) is presented both inside interconnected pores and bound to the polymer network. Depending on the gel precursors and chemical reaction used, the micro- and macroporous structure of MGs can be varied to a large extent [Plieva et al., 2007a]. In fact, the cryogelation technique allows for the formation of biocompatible macroporous materials with unique properties such as open and highly permeable porous structure, tissue-like elasticity, and excellent mechanical strength of the MGs. It is somewhat difficult to achieve these properties with other techniques that are being used for the preparation of macroporous biomaterials.

The MGs are produced via gelation processes at subzero temperatures when most of the solvent is frozen while the dissolved substances (monomers or polymer precursors of a cryogel) are concentrated in small non-frozen regions (NFLMP), where the gel-formation proceeds. While all reagents are concentrated in NFLMP, some part of the solvent remains non-frozen and provides the solutes accumulated into NFLMP with sufficient molecular or segmental mobility for reactions to perform. An acceleration of chemical reactions performed in NFLMP compared to the chemical reaction in bulk solution is often observed within a defined range of negative temperatures [Lozinsky, 2002]. After melting the solvent crystals (ice in case of aqueous media), a system of large continuous inter-connected pores is formed (Figure 14.1).

Thus the shape and size of the crystals formed determine the shape and size of the pores formed after defrosting the sample. In general, the size of ice crystals depends on how fast the system is frozen, provided other parameters (such as

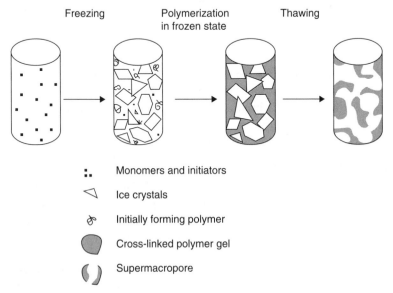

Freezing   Polymerization   Thawing
                  in frozen state

:. Monomers and initiators

◁ Ice crystals

ℰ Initially forming polymer

● Cross-linked polymer gel

( ) Supermacropore

Figure 14.1. Schematic presentation of the formation of macroporous gels. Reproduced from [Plieva et al., 2004b] with permission.

concentration of the dissolved substances, volume, and geometrical shape of the sample) remain the same [Lozinsky et al., 2002]. The pore size depends on the initial concentration of precursors in solution, their physicochemical properties and the freezing conditions [Plieva et al., 2005, 2006b, 2007a]. Specifically, cryogels differ from traditional gel materials due to the system of interconnected macropores (frequently enduring the cryogels with sponge morphology) and due to the structure of pore walls formed when a compulsory increase in polymer concentration in non-frozen regions (NFLMP) takes place (enduring the MGs with a relatively higher mechanical strength as compared to traditional gels with the same formal bulk concentration of the polymer). One of the principal differences of MGs compared to other macroporous materials (with the same range of pore size) is that the MGs possess tissue-like elasticity and withhold large deformations without being collapsed.

14.3.2 Parameters Influencing Cryostructuration (Cryogelation) of Polymeric Systems

Cryotropic gelation allows for the formation of polymeric materials with essentially different morphology compared to gels prepared in non-frozen media. Several parameters should be taken into account when preparing the polymeric materials at sub-zero temperatures. Two main processes, namely the chemical reaction (which proceeds in NFLMP) and solvent crystalization (which generate the interconnected pores) proceed in the semifrozen systems. In order to obtain a reproducible freezing pattern, a careful control of all experimental conditions is required. Many parameters influence the cryostructuration of polymeric systems, such as cooling (freezing rate), concentration and composition of gel precursors in the initial reaction mixture, thermal prehistory of the reaction mixture, sample size, the presence of nucleation agents, and so on.

14.3.2.1 Freezing Rate and Freezing Temperature. The cooling (freezing) rate is one of the crucial parameters to be controlled during the preparation of MGs. The lower the freezing rate (or the higher the freezing temperature), the bigger the size of growing ice crystals and, as a result, the cryogels with bigger pore size are prepared [Plieva et al., 2004a,b]. However, at high freezing temperature there is the risk that the solution to be frozen will be in an overcooled (supercooled) state. Overcooling (or supercooling) is defined as cooling below the initial freezing point of the water without forming ice crystals. This is a non-equilibrium, metastable state of water. The nucleation temperature of water is affected by both the cooling (freezing) rate, volume of the sample and the addition of a nucleation agent [Chen and Lee, 1998; Chen et al., 1999]. So the temperature should be low enough to securely freeze the reaction mixture. The faster the freezing (or the lower the freezing temperature), the more spontaneous nucleation is promoted, and the greater the number of crystals of smaller size [Lozinsky et al., 2002]. During freezing of an aqueous solution, one could distinguish at least three essential temperatures: the final freezing temperature, T_f (defined as temperature set in a low temperature thermostat); the solution freezing point temperature (T_{mc}) and actual initial solvent crystallization temperature (T_c). While the final freezing temperature (T_f) is programmed, both values (T_{mc} and T_c) are estimated from freezing curves. Analysis of the freezing curves (freezing thermograms) is highly instrumental for the determination of phase and structural changes during cooling and crystallization within a system [Akyurt et al., 2002; Liu and Zhou, 2003; Luyet, 1966]. In a typical freezing curve, an abrupt rise of temperature indicates the appearance of ice crystals and the corresponding temperature is T_c, while the maximum temperature induced by the released latent heat of crystallization is equal to T_{mc}.

The freezing curves obtained for the solution of monomers (acrylamide (AAm), N,N'-methylenebisacrylamide (MBAAm) and allyl glycidyl ether (AGE)) during the preparation of polyacrylamide MG (pAAm-MGs) at three different final freezing temperatures T_f of −12, −20 and −30 °C showed clearly the different phase state of the system under freezing [Plieva et al., 2006a] (Figure 14.2).

Overcooling up to −11 °C for two minutes was observed for the reaction mixture frozen at −12 °C followed by an abrupt rise of temperature indicating that initialized solvent crystallization at T_c about −11 °C. Once the critical mass of nuclei was reached (2.6 minutes after the reaction mixture was placed in the low temperature thermostat), the system nucleated at temperature T_{mc} about −2.5 °C, (Figure 14.2). After crystallization was completed, the temperature dropped slowly till the fixed T_f value of −12 °C was reached. A freeze-concentration process occurred as water was frozen out from the solution. The increase in viscosity of the unfrozen liquid phase hindered the further crystallization, which was over after about eight minutes (Figure 14.2). At lower final freezing temperatures (T_f −20 and −30 °C, respectively), the freezing thermograms revealed practically no overcooling with a small crystallization plateau near 0 °C. A small peak observed

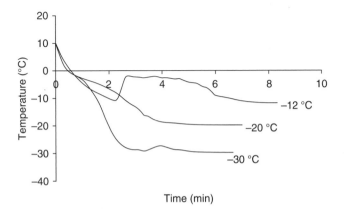

Figure 14.2. Thermograms for freezing aqueous solution of acrylamide monomers at −12, −20 and −30 °C in the presence of 1.2% initiating system (APS/TEMED). Reproduced from [Plieva et al., 2006a] with permission.

at about 3.3 minutes for the thermogram obtained at T_f −30 °C (a temperature which is below the eutectic point of about −20 °C for water/acrylamide system [Plieva et al., 2006a] indicated probably the complete crystallization of the liquid microphase that is not frozen at higher temperatures.

When freezing a dispersed system (as collagen dispersion), the amount of bound solvent (in addition to the free solvent) should be taken into account when choosing the freezing regime to provide the conditions for ice crystallization. Collagen (one of the most important extracellular matrix (ECM) proteins) is known to undergo gel formation on cooling at positive temperatures [Podorozhko et al., 2000]. The swelling of collagen particles in aqueous collagen dispersions in acidic and basic media governed the ratio of the amount of free solvent to that bound by protein, thus promoting the favorable conditions for the efficient non-covalent interactions and gel-formation of this protein. High swelling of collagen particles in dispersions in basic and especially in acidic medium was accompanied by irreversible change in the morphology of the dispersed particles [Podorozhko et al., 2000]. The freezing curves obtained for the 7.5% aqueous dispersions of collagen in acidic and basic media at final freezing temperature T_f of −25 °C showed how the temperature changed during the cooling of the system that contained both free and bound water (collagen dispersion in basic medium at pH 12) or only bound solvent (collagen dispersion in acidic medium at pH 3) (Figure 14.3).

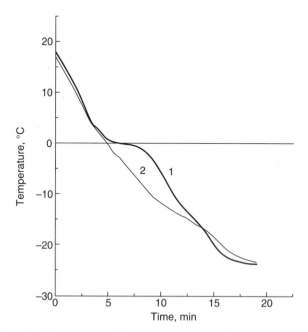

Figure 14.3. Freezing thermograms of 7.5% aqueous collagen dispersions at freezing temperature of −25 °C. Curve 1 for collagen dispersions at pH 12 and curve 2 for collagen dispersions at pH 3. Reproduced from [Podorozhko et al., 2000] with permissions.

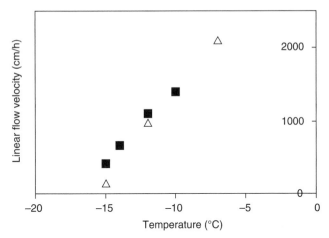

Figure 14.4. Linear flow velocity of water through supermacroporous monolithic cryogels prepared at different temperatures: plain-pAAm (open triangles), epoxy-pAAm (closed squares). The flow rate of water passing through the monolithic columns was measured at the constant hydrostatic pressure equal to 100 cm of water-column corresponding to a pressure of circa 0.01 MPa. For each sample the average of three measurements was taken. Reproduced from [Plieva et al., 2004a] with permission.

A crystallization plateau near 0 °C was observed for the system that contained both free and bound water (collagen dispersion at pH 12). The change of slope for the curve two (collagen suspension at pH 3) at a temperature of about −15 °C was treated as the freezing of the bound water [Podorozhko et al., 2000].

A different cooling (freezing) rate of the reaction mixture directly affected the porous properties of MGs. Namely, the pAAm MGs formed at different final freezing temperatures (T_f) had different flow resistances when they were produced as monolith columns [Plieva et al., 2004a]. The water flow resistance (estimated as water flow path through the cryogel monolith column at a given hydrostatic pressure equal to one meter of water column) decreased significantly when decreasing the freezing temperature (T_f) from −10 to −15 °C (Figure 14.4).

At lower freezing temperatures smaller ice crystals are formed, yielding smaller cross-section area of each macropore, and, therefore, flow resistance of the cryogel monolith increases. Besides, the gel fraction yield as well as compressive strength were decreased for the pAAm-MGs prepared at T_f of −30 °C (Table 14.1) [Plieva et al., 2006a].

The low gel fraction yield for the pAAm MGs prepared at T_f of −30 °C compared to that prepared at −12 °C was due to the quenching of the polymerization process when the system was completely frozen (no NFLMP remained) at temperatures below the eutectic point (which for AAm solution is about −18 °C). In agreement with high flow resistance of the pAAm-MGs prepared at T_f of −30 °C, scanning electron microscopy (SEM) analysis revealed no macroporous structure formed after polymerization at −30 °C [Plieva et al., 2006a].

TABLE 14.1. Properties of the pAAm-MGs Prepared at Different Temperatures

Temperature, °C	Gel fraction yield, %	Compressive strength, kPa	Watch flow at a pressure of 1 m, watch column, cm/h
−12	79 ± 4	28.3	310
−20	83 ± 3	29.2	215
−30	68 ± 4	21.0	30

Reproduced from [Plieva et al., 2006a] with permission.

14.3.2.2 Concentration and Composition of Gel Precursors in the Initial Reaction Mixture.

An increase in initial co-monomer concentration (when other conditions were identical) gives rise to increase in both polymer concentration in pore walls and the overall strength of macroporous gel material, but results in decrease in interconnectivity of macropores [Plieva et al., 2005]. The latter is due to lower amount of solvent, which is frozen out from the more concentrated initial solution and, as a consequence, smaller total volume of ice crystals forming the macropores. Pore size and thickness of pore walls in the MGs are controlled in a wide range by simply changing the monomer/macromonomer concentration in the feed and type of the cross-linker used [Plieva et al., 2006a,b,c]. The control of pore size also allows for optimizing the availability of the ligands coupled to polymer backbone for different biological targets. Depending on the potential application, one could, with the same technique, produce materials with large pores and porosity up to 90% (e.g., materials attractive as potential cell scaffolds) [Kumar et al., 2006a,b; Nilsang et al., 2007] or materials with smaller pores, thicker pore walls having sufficiently large interface for interacting with biomolecules and good mechanical properties (e.g., materials attractive as potential chromatographic adsorbents) [Dainiak et al., 2004; Plieva et al., 2004b, 2005].

Increasing the concentration of monomers from six to 15% during the preparation of pAAm-MGs resulted in decreasing the pore volume in the pAAm-MGs from 93 to 80% [Plieva et al., 2005]. The same was observed for the preparation of MGs from polymeric precursors as polyvinyl alcohol (PVA): the pore volume decreased from 91 to 84% when increasing the initial concentration of PVA from 3.5 to 8% [Plieva et al., 2006b]. Typically, the thickness of pore walls was increased and interconnectivity of pores was decreased at increasing the concentration of monomer or polymer precursors in the initial reaction mixture [Plieva et al., 2005; Plieva et al., 2006a,b]. The thickness of pore walls along with density of pore walls determine the macroscopic mechanical properties of the pAAm-MGs, while the pore size and pore wall density affect the accessibility of the ligands chemically bound to the polymer backbone [Plieva et al., 2005]. Despite increased density of MGs prepared from high monomer concentration, the MGs remained highly elastic. The load-displacement curves obtained for pAAm-MGs prepared from the feeds with 6, 10 and 15% monomer concentration, respectively, show typical behavior of the highly elastic materials (Figure 14.5) with extensive flexibility and

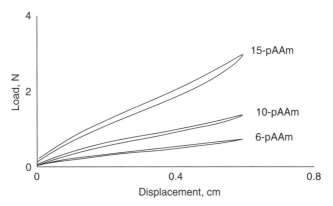

<u>Figure 14.5.</u> Load-displacement curves for pAAm MGs prepared from different concentration of monomers: 6% (6-pAAm), 10% (10-pAAm) and 15% (15-pAAm). Reproduced from [Plieva et al., 2007a] with permission.

shape-recover property against compression. Due to the elasticity and sponge-like morphology, most MGs can withstand large deformations and can be easily compressed up to 80% without getting mechanically damaged, whereas traditional polyacrylamide gels are easily destroyed even when deformed less than 30% [Plieva et al., 2006a]. The high elasticity of the MGs was efficiently exploited for the detachment of affinity-bound bioparticles through the mechanical deformation of the MGs [Dainiak et al., 2006; Galaev et al., 2007]. After releasing compression, the MGs immediately adopted initial shape. Due to the mechanical stability, the MG monoliths can be compressed repeatedly with no distortion of the porous structure. Increasing the concentration of monomers in the initial reaction mixture resulted in increasing the mechanical strength of MGs [Lozinsky, 2002; Plieva et al., 2006a; Srivastava et al., 2007].

Quite often the MGs prepared at subzero temperatures are more mechanically stable compared to the conventional gels prepared at ambient temperature from the same feedstock. The MGs prepared from 3wt% 2-hydroxyethylcellulose (HEC) solution through irradiation with UV-vis light at −30°C had the storage and loss moduli (G' and G'') orders of magnitude higher than those for the gel obtained from HEC solution irradiated at room temperature (Figure 14.6).

The reason is that due to the cryoconcentration of HEC chains in NFLMP, the polymeric network of HEC MGs was formed from a solution with higher HEC concentration. As was mentioned before, the cryoconcentration of the gel precursors in NFLMP typically results in lowering the critical concentration of gelation (CCG). The lowering of CCG for MGs compared to the conventional gels prepared from the same feedstock is the common phenomenon in cryotropic gelation [Lozinsky, 2002].

The MGs are hydrophilic materials with inert surface when no active groups are presented on the cryogel surface. The pAAm-MGs were shown to not contain any non-reacted monomer (AAm) as was confirmed by gas liquid

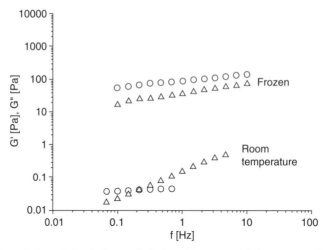

Figure 14.6. Variation of elastic (open circles) and loose moduli (open triangles) in the 0.1–10 Hz frequency range of 3wt% aqueous HEC solutions irradiated with UV-vis light at room temperature and in frozen state. Reproduced from [Petrov et al., 2006] with permission.

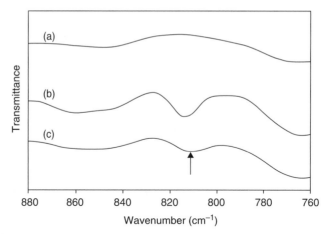

Figure 14.7. A fragment of FTIR spectra of dextran (a), glycidyl methacrylate derivatized dextran (dx-MA) (b) and polymerized at −20 °C dx-MA (c). Arrow indicates a peak at 813 cm^{-1} originating from the double bond of the methacrylate group. Reproduced from [Plieva et al., 2006c] with permission.

chromatography analysis [Plieva et al., 2004a]. When the MGs were prepared from macromer precursors (as dextran with grafted polymerizable double bonds, dextran-methacrylate, dextran-MA), the content of remaining non-reacted macromer (dextran-MA) was hardly detectable (Figure 14.7) as demonstrated by FTIR analysis [Plieva et al., 2006c].

The properties of MGs depend on degree and nature of cross-linkers used for the preparation of MGs. The highly cross-linked pAAm-MG monoliths (with

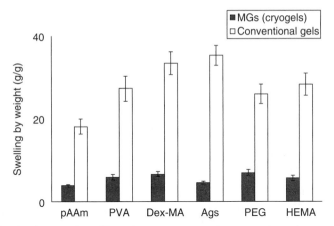

Figure 14.8. The degree of swelling of macroporous gels prepared at subzero temperatures (gray bar) and conventional gels prepared at room temperature of 20 °C (white bar) from the same initial reaction mixture. pAAm (polyacrylamide), PVA (polyvinyl alcohol), Dex-MA (dextran-methacrylate), Ags (agarose), PEG (polyethylene glycol) and HEMA (hydroxyethyl methacrylate). Reproduced from [Plieva et al., 2007a] with permission.

cross-linking ratio vinyl(monomers)/divinyl (cross-linker) of 5–10, mol/mol) had lower flow resistance compared to that of pAAm-MGs formed from the feedstock with low content of the cross-linker (MBAAm) in the reaction mixture (vinyl/divinyl ratio of 20–30, mol/mol). The swelling degree of highly cross-linked network of pAAm-MGs was much less compared to the swelling degree of the pAAm-MGs with low MBAAm content [Plieva et al., 2007a]. In general, the swelling degree for the MGs is much lower compared to that of conventional gels prepared from the same feedstock (Figure 14.8). The MGs prepared from both monomer or macromer gel precursors swell much less compared to the conventional gels (Figure 14.8). Lower swelling ability of MGs compared to conventional gels is one of the characteristic features of these macroporous materials.

For the MGs with "smart" properties (as poly-N-isopropylacrylamide MGs, pNIPAAm-MGs), faster stimuli response to the change of environmental conditions compared to that of conventional pNIPAAm gels was observed [Zhang and Chu, 2003; Galaev et al., 2007]. It is known that in aqueous solutions, pNIPAAm undergoes hydrophobic aggregation followed by the transition from soluble to insoluble state when the temperature is increased above a critical temperature of 32 °C [Schild, 1992]. The swelling degree of pNIPAAm-MGs prepared at subzero temperatures was much less compared to the conventional pNIPAAm gels prepared at 22 °C (Figure 14.9) [Zhang and Chu, 2003].

The swelling of pNIPAAm-MGs depended on the concentration of monomers in the initial reaction mixture and cross-linking degree [Galaev et al., 2007]. The sharp transition around 30 °C was observed for pNIPAAm-MGs in the temperature interval studied from 4 to 40 °C [Galaev et al., 2007]. The stimuli response

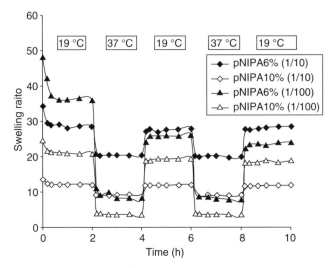

Figure 14.9. Swelling ratios of the pNIPAAm gels in distilled water at room temperature. Reproduced from [Galaev et al., 2007] with permission.

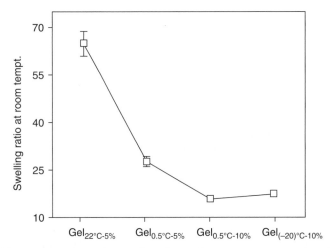

Figure 14.10. The time dependence of swelling of pNIPAAm-MGs produced under semi-frozen conditions from polymerization feeds with total monomer concentrations 6 and 10% and MBAAm(cross-linker)/NIPAAm ratios 1/10 and 1/100 mol/mol. Reproduced from [Zhang and Chu, 2003] with permission.

of pNIPAAm-MGs to a temperature change from 19 °C to 37 °C was very fast. The lower the total monomer concentration and the cross-linking degree of pNIPAAm-MGs, the higher was the change in swelling and the larger amplitude of mechanical deformation occurred when the temperature was changed from 19 °C to 37 °C and backwards (Figure 14.10).

14.4   PREPARATION OF MACROPOROUS GELS (MGs) FROM DIFFERENT GEL PRECURSORS

MGs with a broad range of porosities are produced at moderately low temperature, namely in a temperature range of −10 to −20 °C. The MGs prepared through the cryogelation technique can be divided in two main groups: thermo-reversible physically cross-linked MGs (where the MG network is formed through hydrogen-bond formation) and thermo-irreversible covalently cross-linked MGs (when the MG network is formed through covalent bond formation). Different macroporous cryogel systems were prepared through cryogelation approaches as potential materials for biomedical applications (Table 14.2). The porosity of such biomaterials can be varied to a large extent depending on the physical-chemical properties of the used gel precursors and particular application of MG.

14.4.1   Physically Cross-Linked MGs

The physically cross-linked MGs were prepared through physical gelation at subzero temperatures of both natural biocompatible polymers such as agarose [Plieva et al., 2007b] and collagen [Podorozhko et al., 2000] or synthetic polymer such as PVA [Bajpai and Saini, 2005a,b; Kokabi et al., 2007; Lozinsky, 1998; Lozinsky and Plieva, 1998; Nho and Park, 2001].

Among the physically cross-linked MG biomaterials, the MGs prepared from polyvinyl alcohol (PVA) are the most utilized (Table 14.2). PVA is known to be non-toxic [DeMerlis and Schoneker, 2003] and a readily available synthetic polymer widely used in biomedical [Hassan and Peppas, 2000; Hassan et al., 2000; Peppas and Mongia, 1997] and biotechnological [Lozinsky and Plieva, 1998] applications. PVA with high deacetylation degree (DH more than 97%) is a hydrophilic polymer that in concentrated aqueous solution can form weak gels during prolonged storage at room temperature because of the formation of hydrogen bonds between polymer molecules. The cryogelation technique facilitates the gelation process as a result of the increased concentration of the dissolved macromolecules in the unfrozen liquid microphase.

As a result of cryoconcentraton, PVA chains form ordered structures known as microcrystallinity zones which function as physical cross-links and are formed only when -OH groups are free to participate in such interactions [Hassan et al., 2000; Lozinsky, 1998].

Typically, the PVA with DH more than 97% is used for the preparation of physically cross-linked elastic cryogels with high mechanical strength and chemical stability. Two main approaches are used for the reinforcement of physically cross-linked PVA cryogels. First, the porosity and mechanical strength of PVA cryogels is regulated by the thawing rate; the lower the thawing rate, the higher the mechanical strength of the prepared PVA cryogels [Lozinsky, 1998]. The reason is that the slow thawing ensures the prolonged duration of the PVA sample at the temperature range of −5 to −1 °C. In this temperature region, the amount of unfrozen water is already sufficient to allow the movements of polymer chains

TABLE 14.2. The MGs Prepared Through Cryogelation Technique

Cryogels	Pore size, μm	Mechanism of gelation	Reference
Physically cross-linked			
PVA (DH > 97%)	Up to 1	Through hydrogen bond formation	[Bajpai and Saini 2005a,b; Kokabi et al., 2007; Lozinsky, 1998; Lozinsky et al., 1998; Nho et al., 2001]
Agarose cryogel	Up to 500	Through hydrogen bond formation	[Plieva et al., 2007b]
Chemically cross-linked			
Through cross-linking reaction using cross-linking agents			
PVA (DH < 90%)	Up to 80	Through chemical reaction at acidic pH using the glutaraldehyde (GA) as cross-linker	[Plieva et al., 2006b]
Chitosan	Up to 100	Through chemical reaction at pH 5–5.5 using the GA as cross-linker	[Noir et al., 2007]
Agarose	Up to 200	Through chemical reaction at pH 13 using the epichlorohydrin (ECH) as cross-linker	[Plieva et al., 2007b]
Alginate	Up to 100	Through reaction with metal ions	
Through free-radical polymerization reaction using APS/TEMED initiating system			
pAAm, pDMAAm, pHEMA, PEG, allyl-agarose, dextran-methacrylate	Up to 200		[Plieva et al., 2006a,c; Plieva et al., 2007a,b,c]
Through free-radical polymerization reaction using UV-vis light irradiation			
Gelatin-methacrylamide			[Dubruel et al., 2007; Vlierberghe et al., 2007]
Cellulose			[Petrov et al., 2006]

resulting in entanglement of macromolecular coils [Lozinsky, 1998; Lozinsky and Plieva, 1998]. Thus by simply controlling the thawing rate it is possible to prepare mechanically stable and highly-porous PVA cryogel during one cycle of freezing-thawing.

In another approach, the repetitive freezing-thawing technique during the preparation is used for the reinforcement of the PVA cryogels [Fray et al., 2007; Hassan et al., 2000; Peppas and Stauffer, 1991; Stauffer and Peppas, 1992; Watase and Nishinari, 1988]. Hassan and co-authors presented a novel group of PVA laminate cryogels that could be used for different pharmaceutical applications prepared through the additional freezing thawing technique [Hassan and Peppas, 2000; Hassan et al., 2000]. In that work, the fresh PVA solution was added to a previously formed gel and was then subjected to additional freeze-thawing cycles to create a layered structure. PVA-MGs found different applications in biomedicine due to the biocompatibility of PVA and excellent mechanical properties and elasticity which allow for withstanding extensive pressures [Jiang et al., 2004].

14.4.2 Covalently Cross-Linked MGs

Covalently cross-linked MGs are produced via two main approaches: through cross-linking reaction using an appropriate cross-linker; or through free radical cross-linking polymerization reaction using the respective initiators (Table 14.2). According to the first approach, the cross-linking reaction is performed in partially frozen media using the available cross-linkers such as, for example, glutaraldehyde (GA) and epichlorohydrin (ECH). Thus, agarose-based MGs were prepared through cross-linking of agarose chains with ECH at high pH value [Plieva et al., 2007b] and the chitosan- and PVA-based MGs were prepared through cross-linking reaction with GA in acidic medium [Noir et al., 2007; Plieva et al., 2006b] (Table 14.2).

According to the second approach, the covalently cross-linked MGs can be produced through free-radical cross-linking polymerization reaction using ammonium persulfate (APS) and N,N,N',N'-tetra-methyl-ethylenediamine (TEMED) initiating system [Dinu et al., 2007; Plieva et al., 2005, 2006; Yao et al., 2006a,b] or by UV irradiation of both aqueous solutions and moderately frozen aqueous systems [Petrov et al., 2006; Vlierberghe et al., 2007].

The APS/TEMED initiating system is one of the rare initiating systems that can be used to initiate the free-radical polymerization reaction of the vinyl monomers at subzero temperatures. In the free radical polymerization reactions, the concentrations of the initiator (APS) and activator (TEMED) have a great influence on the polymerization rate as well as on the molecular weight of the resulting polymers. The polymerization reaction starts with the reaction between APS and TEMED to form free radicals to initiate the polymerization reaction of the vinyl monomers/or macromonomers as well as the cross-linking of polymer chains with the cross-linking monomer (as MBAAm or polyethylene diacrylate, PEG-DA). Different MG systems were produced using the APS/TEMED initiating systems as pAAm-, pDMAAm-, pHEMA-, PEG-, pNIPAAm- dextran-MA- and allyl-agarose based MGs (Table 14.2). Among the chemically cross-linked monolithic MGs prepared through the free-radical polymerization reaction using the APS/TEMED initiating system, the pAAm based MGs are the most characterized [Dinu et al., 2007; He et al., 2007; Plieva et al., 2004a, 2006a, 2007c; Yao et al., 2006a,b].

The advantage of the UV irradiation is the cost efficiency and the very short time needed for an efficient gel formation. Cellulose based MGs were prepared through irradiation of the frozen aqueous solution of HEC with a Dymax 5000-EC UV curing equipment for one to five minutes [Petrov et al., 2006]. The frozen-thawed samples were opaque spongy materials, while all samples irradiated at room temperature were still liquid-like.

Porous gelatin materials with a gradient in pore-size were prepared by cryogenic treatment using temperature gradient between the top and the bottom phase of the sample [Dubruel et al., 2007; Vlierberghe et al., 2007]. For this purpose, gelatin was modified first with methacrylic anhydride to incorporate the polymerizable double bonds [Bulcke et al., 2000]. Then hydrogels were formed by gelation of an aqueous methacrylamide-modified gelatin solution, followed by radical cross-linking using a UV-active photoinitiator and chemically cross-linked hydrogels were subjected to a cryogenic treatment [Dubruel et al., 2007] (Table 14.2). By varying the conditions of the cryogenic treatment, gelatin MGs with different pore morphologies were prepared [Vlierberghe et al., 2007].

14.5   CHARACTERIZATION OF MGs

14.5.1   Pore Volume of MGs

The determination of absolute values of pore size in macroporous hydrophilic MGs presents a challenging problem. First, a significant amount of water is bound to the hydrophilic polymer backbone occupying some space in between polymer chains. This water is not exchanged freely with bulk water present in the macro-pores. Different methods were used for the determination of pore volume of pAAm-MGs [Plieva et al., 2005]. In the most typical case, more than 90% of pAAm-MGs (prepared from 6% monomer concentration) composed of large and highly interconnected pores, while the polymer bound water present less than 10% (Figure 14.11).

More than 70% of liquid can be squeezed from pAAm-MGs by mechanical compression. The total pore volume of pAAm-MGs was estimated using three different techniques (Table 14.3), namely: from water vapor adsorption experiments assuming that the pore volume is equal to the water volume inside the cryogel-minus volume of polymer-bound (adsorbed) water; from uptake of a good solvent, water and a poor solvent, cyclohexane. (As the hydrophilic polymer did not swell in cyclohexane, the uptake of cyclohexane reflected only the pore volume however, in the dry sample.); and from comparison of the densities of the dry and completely swollen cryogel samples.

All three methods gave consistent results with a clear tendency of decreasing total pore volume from ~90% for pAAm-MGs prepared from 6% monomer concentration to ~70% for pAAm-MGs prepared from 20% monomer concentration.

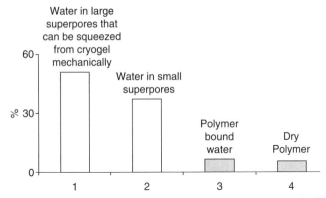

<u>Figure 14.11.</u> Composition of pAAm-MGs. Polymer bound water was quantified by the adsorption of water vapors by the dried cryogel sample. pAAm-MGs were dried in an oven at 60 °C to constant weight. The dried sample was incubated in a closed chamber saturated with water vapors but with no direct contact with water. The water in small pores was quantified as the difference between total water and mechanically squeezed + adsorbed water. Reproduced from [Plieva et al., 2004a] with permission.

TABLE 14.3. Pore Volume of pAAm-MGs Prepared at −12 °C from the Feedstock with Different Monomer Concentration

Monomer concentration in the feed, % w/v	Porosity, %		
	Water vapor adsorption	Cyclohexane uptake	Swelling
6	93	93	88.4
10	86.6	85	86.5
15	81.6	79.2	80.2
18	74.7	72.5	74
22	70.1	68	65.6

Reproduced from [Plieva et al., 2005] with permission.

The amount of bulk water in MG was determined using differential scanning calorimetric (DSC) analysis as the amount of freezable water that is not bound by hydrogen bonding [Kim et al., 2004; Plieva et al., 2005; Shibukawa et al., 1999]. The amount of freezable water decreased and the amount of bound water increased with increasing monomer concentration in the feed for the MGs prepared from PVA (Table 14.4). Pore volume estimated from DSC studies was in a good agreement with the values of pore volume obtained through water vapor adsorption studies as was shown for PVA-MGs [Plieva et al., 2006b].

Due to the presence of large (capillary-sized) and highly interconnected pores, a majority of MGs with pore volume in the range of 85–94% can be dried with no distortion of the porous structure. Dried MGs re-swell within seconds when contacted with water (Figure 14.12) [Plieva et al., 2007a]. This is one of the most important properties of these hydrophilic materials as drying simplifies storage of the MGs.

TABLE 14.4. Different States of Water in Monolithic PVA-MGs Prepared from Different PVA Concentration

PVA concentration in reaction mixture, % w/v	Total water[a], %	Free water[b], %		Bound water[c], %	
		DSC	Vapor ads.	DSC	Vapor ads.
3.5	95.6	91.8	90.7	3.8	4.9
5	94.7	89.6	88.0	5.1	6.7
8	94.4	88.0	84.9	6.4	9.5

Reproduced from [Plieva et al., 2006b] with permission.
[a]Total water content in cryoPVA was determined as difference between the swollen and dried cryogel.
[b]Free water was determined as freezable water using DSC or as difference between total and adsorbed water in water vapor adsorption experiments.
[c]Bound water was determined as the difference between total and free water when using DSC and as the amount of water adsorbed in water vapor adsorption experiments.

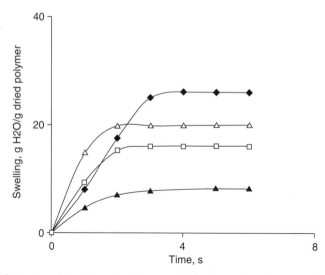

Figure 14.12. Swelling kinetics of different MGs: pAAm (closed diamonds), PEG (open triangles), dextran-MA (open squares) and PVA (closed triangles) after bringing dry samples in contact with water. Swelling kinetics was performed as described elsewhere [Plieva et al., 2005]. Reproduced from [Plieva et al., 2007a] with permission.

14.5.2 Characterization of Porous Structure Using Different Microscopy Techniques

There are no common techniques for the analysis of porous structures of hydrophilic materials. The most used technique for the analysis of pore size distribution in a porous material is mercury porosimetry, but it is not that well adaptable for the MGs, due to the soft and hydrophilic texture of these materials. Besides by the method described above, the porous structure of the MGs was studied using optical microscopy (OM) [Plieva et al., 2006b; Vlierberghe et al., 2007], scanning electron microscopy (SEM) [Dubruel et al., 2007; Plieva et al., 2004, 2006a; Vlierberghe et al., 2007], environmental scanning electron microscopy (ESEM) [Plieva et al., 2005, 2006b], confocal microscopy (CM) [Dubruel et al., 2007; Plieva et al., 2007a] and microcomputed tomography [Dubruel et al., 2007; Vlierberghe et al., 2007].

The cryogel backbone was colored with a dye or fluorescein-probe to be visible in OM and CM, respectively. The dye, Cibacrone Blue, was bound to the network of PVA to make the structure of PVA-MG visible in OM studies showing large interconnected pores surrounded by dense and microporous pore walls (Figure 14.13a). Gelatin cryogel scaffolds studied by optical microscopy showed the absence of "skin layer" which could be a problem for cell in-growth studies

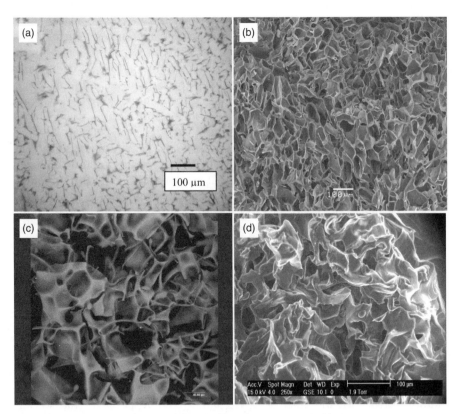

Figure 14.13. Porous structure of MGs visualized by different techniques: optical microscopy, OM (a), confocal microscopy, CM (b), scanning electron microscopy, SEM (c) and environmental scanning electron microscopy, ESEM (d). OM (a) is presented for PVA-MGs and reproduced from [Plieva et al., 2006b] with permission. CM (b) presented for pAAm-MGs and reproduced from [Plieva et al., 2006c] with permission. SEM (c) is presented for dextran-MA-MGs and reproduced from [Plieva et al., 2007a] with permission. The ESEM (d) is presented for PVA-MGs and reproduced from [Plieva et al., 2006b] with permission.

[Vlierberghe et al., 2007]. The absence of skin layer was shown also for agarose-based cryogels [Plieva et al., 2007b].

Scanning electron microscopy (SEM) technique, which is suitable to characterize the fine structures of porous materials only in the dried state, was shown to be the method of choice for the analysis of the porous structure of MGs [Plieva et al., 2006a,b]. The deformation of the porous structure of MGs due to the processing of the samples for SEM analysis was not that significant and fine porous structure was essentially preserved due to the mechanical stability of pore walls in MGs. The pore walls in elastic and spongy pAAm-MGs are formed from highly concentrated polymer network due to the pronounced concentration of the dissolved reagents. SEM images of dextran-MA-MGs showed the typical structure of the MG, consisting of μm-in-size interconnected pores surrounded by dense non-porous walls (Figure 14.13b).

On the other hand, confocal microscopy (CM) allows for the analysis of the shape and size of pores in the macroporous material and offers significant advantages over conventional microscopy in that it reduces "out-of-focus-blur" in images [Hanthamrongwit et al., 1996]. Sample preparation for CM is simple and less time consuming, simplifying the processes for fixation, dehydration, embedding, microtomy and staining required for optical microscopy. A CM image obtained for pAAm-MGs (with covalently bound fluoresceine-probe (fluoresceinamine, isomer I)) is presented in Figure 14.13c.

Other useful technique for characterizations of such materials has been environmental scanning electron microscopy (ESEM). The important advantage of the ESEM technology is the possibility of monitoring changes in the structure of the material whilst allowing the sample to dehydrate slowly [Rizzieri et al., 2003]. The ESEM images obtained for the PVA-MGs at high degrees of dehydration were similar to the SEM images showing the macroporous structure with interconnected pores of hundreds micrometers in size and thin and dense pore walls [Plieva et al., 2005] or microporous pore walls [Plieva et al., 2006b] (Figure 14.13d).

The microcomputed tomography was used for the analysis of porous structure of the gelatin macroporous gel, prepared through combination of cryogenic treatment of a chemically cross-linked gelatin gel, followed by removal of the ice crystals formed through lyophilization (freeze-drying technique) [Vlierberghe et al., 2007]. The 2D cross-sections of gelatin gel were used to segment the images and determine their 3D porosity and pore size distribution using the software (μCTanalySIS) [Vlierberghe et al., 2007]. For determination of the pore size distribution, each pore was filled with the largest sphere possible (the so-called "maximum opening"). The total volume filled by this maximum sphere was determined during the analysis. Subsequently, the software filled the total volume of each pore with a smaller sphere, while its total filling volume was determined. This process continued until the total volume of each pore was comprised with the smallest inscribed sphere, with a size of one voxel (Figure 14.14a). From this analysis, data for all pores were acquired. The microcomputed tomography (μ-CT) 3D images clearly showed that all pores in gelatin macroporous gels were interconnected [Vlierberghe et al., 2007]. All changes in porosity were possible to visualize using the 3D μ-CT images. For example, the 3D image of the rapidly cooled gelatin visualized very clearly a central region where the porosity was much lower compared to other parts of the macroporous gel (Figure 14.14b). This corresponded well with the zone where the two cooling surfaces (started from the top and bottom of the sample) coincided [Vlierberghe et al., 2007].

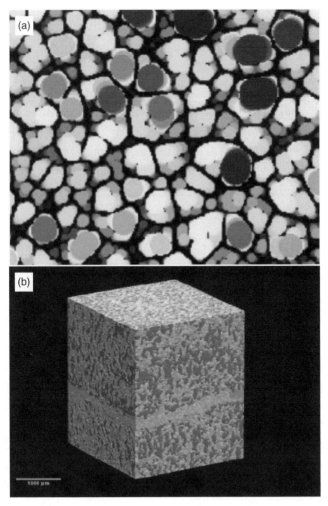

Figure 14.14. (a) Principle of the pore analysis performed by software (μCTanalysis) in microcomputed tomography analysis. Reproduced from [Vlierberghe et al., 2007] with permission. (b) Reconstruction of a section of the rapidly cooled gelatin (type IV), obtained using microcomputed tomography analysis. The pores are dark gray, and the scaffold material is light grey. The scale bar represents 1000 μm. Reproduced from [Vlierberghe et al., 2007] with permission.

14.6   BIOMEDICAL APPLICATION OF MGs

The main applications of MGs with different porosity are listed in Table 14.5 and are defined by their porosity, surface properties, elasticity and mechanical strength. Thus the highly elastic and mechanically stable MGs with pore size up to 100 μm (as physically cross-linked PVA-MGs) were shown as promising biocompatible porous materials for cartilage replacement [Covert et al., 2003; Jiang et al., 2004; Swieszowski et al., 2006].

The MGs with pore size up to 200 μm (which are characterized by high elasticity and sponge-like morphology) have an enormous potential as 3D porous scaffolds for cell culture applications. The highly elastic and sponge-like MGs meet most of the requirements to be suitable as 3D-scaffolds for cell cultivation. The MGs are highly porous, can be prepared from biocompatible precursors and can be produced in different formats. The MGs can be designed as non-degradable [Kumar et al., 2006a,b; Plieva et al., 2006a,b] or with controlled degree

TABLE 14.5. Biomedical Applications of MGs Prepared Through Cryogelation Technique and the Macroporous Materials Prepared from Similar Precursors Through Freeze-drying Technique

Polymer based	Approach used for the preparation of scaffolds	Pore size, μm	Application	References:
Poly(vinyl alcohol), PVA MGs	Cryogelation technique	Up to 1	Cartilage replacement	[Covert et al., 2003; Swieszowski et al., 2006; Jiang et al., 2004]
PVA cryogels with *Aloe Vera*	Cryogelation technique	Up to 1	Wound dressing	[Park and Nho, 2003]
	Freeze-drying	Up to 65	Wound healing	[You and Park, 2004]
Gelatin-based MGs	Freeze-drying	10–200	As 3D scaffold for cell culture	[Vlierberghe et al., 2007; Dubruel et al., 2007]
Gelatin-coated polyacrylamide and polydimethylacrylamide MGs	Cryogelation technique	10–200	As 3D scaffold for cell culture	[Kumar et al., 2006a,b; Nilsang et al., 2007a,b; Plieva et al., 2007c]
Dextran-based MGs	Cryogelation technique	10–100	As 3D scaffold for cell culture	[Bolgen et al., 2007a,b; Plieva et al., 2006c]

of degradation as was shown for the poly 2-hydroxyethyl methacrylate (pHEMA) based MGs [Bolgen et al., 2007a]. The incorporation of the degradable co-monomers (as 2-hydroxyehthylmethacrylate-L-Lactide HEMA-LLA) or macromers (as HEMA-LLA-dextran) into the polymeric backbone allows for developing MGs with open porous structure and controlled rate of degradation level [Bolgen et al., 2007b]. The dextran-MA based non-degradable MGs (pre-pared through the free radical polymerization of dextran-MA macromer at –20 °C) were stable for degradation under *in vitro* conditions (37 °C in PBS buffer, pH 7.2) for at least four months (Figure 14.15a) while incorporating HEMA-LLA and HEMA-LLA-dextran degradable grafts into the MGs network resulted in pronounced degradation (evaluated as loss of weight) of the MGs (Figure 14.15b).

Different MGs were tried as 3D-supports for cell culture applications. These MGs can be divided into two categories, one prepared from synthetic precursors and other MGs prepared from the natural biopolymers such as agarose, gelatin, chitosan and dextran. The pAAm MG, coated with gelatin (which is considered as one of the most common materials to facilitate the attachment of anchorage dependable cells [Bloch et al., 2005; Kumar et al., 2006a,b], were tested as poten-tial 3D-scaffolds for cell culturing. The human HT116 colon cancer cells were effectively attached and colonized onto the gelatin-coated pAAm MGs [Kumar et al., 2006a,b].

Another type of MG scaffolds was prepared on the basis of natural materials as agarose [Bloch et al., 2005], dextran [Bolgen et al., 2007a,b; Plieva et al., 2006c], gelatin [Dubruel et al., 2007] and chitosan (unpublished results). The agarose MG scaffolds, prepared at subzero temperature in the shape of small discs with thickness of two millimeters, had sponge-like morphology and interconnected pores (channels) with size up to 200–400 µm in diameter. The agarose scaffolds were coated with gelatin to facilitate the attachment of insulinoma cells (INS-1E). No toxic affect of the agarose cryogel sponge on cell viability and proliferation was found. However, the cells displayed low affinity to agarose per se. Insulinoma cells seeded on gelatin-coated sponges attached to the cryogel surface and proliferated. The cell monolayer covered 80% of the cryogel surface. Both cells attached to gelatin-coated agarose cryogels and cells attached to plastic dishes (used as control) demonstrated time-dependent increased insulin secretion and approximately equal insulin content [Bloch et al., 2005].

Mouse fibroblast 3T3-L1 cells were seeded into the dextran-MA based scaffolds to examine the cell attachment and proliferation [Plieva et al., 2006c]; 3T3-L1 fibroblasts demonstrated attachment to the gel surface and showed the spread and elongated shape characteristic for fibroblasts [Plieva et al., 2006c]. After eight days from the beginning of differentiation in the dex-MG scaffold, a change in cell morphology from elongated fibroblasts to regular, round adipo-cytes was observed. The biological function of the differentiated adipocytes in dex-MG scaffolds was confirmed by the lipolysis assay which showed more than 2.4 times increased glycerol release from the differentiated adipocytes in

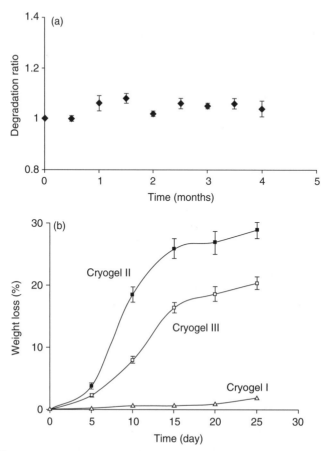

Figure 14.15. (a) Degradation ratio of Dextran-MA MG scaffold at incubation at 37 °C and pH 7.4. The dextran-MA MGs were prepared from 5% dextran-MA solution at −20 °C. Reproduced from [Plieva et al., 2006c] with permission. (b) Weight loss of non-degradable (cryogel I) and degradable (cryogel II and III) MGs. The MGs were dried in air to a constant weight and then placed in vials containing 5 ml saline PBS buffer (pH 7.4) at 37 °C. At selected time interval, the samples were removed from the medium, dried in the air overnight and weighted to determine weight loss. Cryogel I represents the MGs consisting of 90wt% HEMA and 10wt% HEMA-LLA. Cryogel II represents the degradable MGs consisting of 10wt% HEMA and 90wt% HEMA-LLA-dextran. Cryogel III represents the degradable MGs consisting of 10wt% HEMA-LLA and 90wt% HEMA-LLA-dextran. Reproduced from [Bolgen et al., 2007a] with permission.

comparison to the control, non-differentiated 3T3-L1 preadipocytes [Plieva et al., 2006c].

The tissue-like elasticity and open porous structure of the MG scaffolds are the unique properties of these materials. The size of pores, hydrophilic/hydrophobic balance and elasticity of pore walls can be varied to a large extent when preparing the MGs' scaffolds for cell culture application. By introducing special functionalities as ECM recognition elements or bioactive substances which induce tissue in-growth, it is possible to design the MG scaffolds with bioactive ligands. Besides, most of the MGs withstand sterilization by autoclaving [Plieva et al., 2004a,b] and can be dried and stored in dried state followed by fast re-swelling prior to use.

14.7 CONCLUSION AND OUTLOOK

Macroporous gels (MGs) with a broad variety of morphologies are prepared using cryotropic gelation technique meaning gelation at subzero temperatures. These highly elastic hydrophilic materials can be produced from practically any gel forming system with a broad range of porosities, from elastic and porous gels with pore size up to 1.0 µm till elastic and sponge-like gels with pore size up to 200 µm. The versatility of cryogelation technique is demonstrated by use of different routes of gel formation (hydrogen bonding, chemical cross-linking of polymers, free radical cross-linking polymerization reaction) mainly in an aqueous medium. Proper control over a solvent crystallization (formation of solvent crystals) and the rate of chemical reaction during the cryogelation allows for the reproducible preparation of cryogels with tailored properties. The gel surface chemistry can be designed depending on particular application. High mechanical strength of MGs combined with unique tissue-like elasticity and uniform porous structure with large interconnected pores will allow for numerous applications of MGs in tissue engineering field. The environmentally-friendly way of producing the MGs where no organic solvents are involved makes this approach favorable compared to the other mostly-used techniques for the production of macroporous biomaterials. Biodegradable as well as non-degradable MGs are produced depending on the chemistry of the gelation system.

ACKNOWLEDGMENTS

The authors acknowledge all authors whose works are cited in this chapter. The support from the Swedish Foundation for Strategic Research (area of Chemistry and Life sciences), Department of Biotechnology (DBT) and Department of Science and Technology (DST), Ministry of Science and Technology, India is also acknowledged.

REFERENCES

Akyurt M, Zaki G, Habeebullah B. 2002. Freezing phenomena in ice-water systems. Energ. Conv. Manag. 43: 1773–1789.

Bajpai A, Saini R. 2005a. Preparation and characterization of biocompatible spongy cryogels of poly(vinyl alcohol)-gelatin and study of water sorption behaviour. Polym. Int. 54: 1233–1242.

Bajpai A, Saini R. 2005b. Preparation and characterization of spongy cryogels of poly(vinyl alcohol)-casein system: water sorption and blood compatibility. Polymer Int. 54: 796–806.

Bennett DJ, Burford RP, Davis TP, Tilley HJ. 1995. Synthesis of porous hydrogel structure by polymerizing the continuous phase of a microemulsion. Polymer Int. 36: 219–226.

Bloch K, Lozinsky VI, Galaev IYu, Yavriyanz K, Vorobeychik M, Azarov D, Damashkaln LG, Mattiasson B, Vardi P. 2005. Functional activity of insulinoma cells (INS-1E) and pancreatic islets cultured in agarose cryogel sponges. J. Biomed. Mater. Res. 75A: 802–809.

Bolgen N, Plieva F, Galaev IYu, Mattiasson B, Piskin E. 2007a. A novel technique "cryogelation" for preparation of biodegradable tissue engineering scaffolds. J. Biomater. Sci. Polym. Ed. 18:1165–1179.

Bolgen N, Vargel I, Korkusuz P, Guzel E, Plieva F, Galaev IYu, Mattiasson B, Piskin E. 2007b. Tissue responses to novel tissue engineering biodegradable cryogel-scaffolds: an animal model. J. Biomed. Mater. Res. Part A, 2008, in press.

Bulcke AIVD, Bogdanov B, Rooze ND, Schacht EH, Cornelissen M, Berghmans H. 2000. Structural and rheological properties of methacrylamide modified gelatin hydrogels. Biomacromolecules 1: 31–38.

Burg KJL, Porter S, Kellam JF. 2000. Biomaterial developments for bone tissue engineering. Biomaterials 21: 2347–2359.

Cai Q, Yang J, Bei J, Wang S. 2002. A novel porous cells scaffold made of polylactide-dextran blend by combining phase-separation and particle-leaching techniques. Biomaterials 23: 4483–4492.

Chen J, Jo S, Park K. 1995. Polysaccharide hydrogels for protein drug delivery. Carbohyd. Polym. 28: 69–76.

Chen S-L, Lee T-S. 1998. A study of supercooling phenomenon and freezing probability of water inside horizontal cylinders. Intern. J. Heat Mas. Trans. 41: 769–783.

Chen S-L, Wang P-P, Lee T-S. 1999. An experimental investigation of nucleation probability of supercooled water inside cylindrical capsules. Exp. Therm. Fluid Sci. 18: 299–306.

Covert RJ, Ott RD, Ku DN. 2003. Friction characteristics of a potential articular cartilage biomaterial. Wear 255: 1064–1068.

Dainiak MB, Kumar A, Plieva F, Galaev IYu, Mattiasson B. 2004. Integrated isolation of antibody fragments from microbial cell culture fluids using supermacroporous cryogels. J. Chromatogr. A 1045: 93–98.

Dainiak MB, Kumar A, Galaev IYu, Mattiasson B. 2006. Detachment of affinity-captured bioparticles by elastic deformation of a macroporous hydrogel. Proc. Nat. Acad. Sci. USA 103: 849–854.

DeMerlis CC, Schoneker DR. 2003. Review of the oral toxicity of polyvinyl alcohol (PVA). Food Chem. Tech. 41: 319–326.

Dinu MV, Ozmen MM, Dragan ES, Okay O. 2007. Freezing as a path to build macroporous structures: superfast responsive polyacrylamide hydrogels. Polymer 48: 195–204.

Dubruel P, Unger R, Vlierberghe SV, Cnudde V, Jacobs PJS, Schacht E, Kirkpatrick CJ. 2007. Porous gelatin hydrogels: 2. *In vitro* cell interaction study. Biomacromolecules 8: 338–344.

Engström JA, Lindgren LJ, Helgee B. 2006. Synthesis of novel monomers and copolymers from 1-vinylpyrrolidin-2-one: attractive materials for drug delivery systems. Macromol. Chem. Phys. 207: 536–544.

Fray ME, Pilaszkiewicz A, Swieszkowski W, Kurzydlowski KJ. 2007. Morphology assessment of chemically modified and cryostructurated poly(vinyl alcohol) hydrogel. Eur. Polym. J. 43: 2035–2040.

Galaev IYu, Dainiak MB, Plieva F, Mattiasson B. 2007. Effect of matrix elasticity on affinity binding and release of bioparticles. Elution of bound cells by temperature-induced shrinkage of the smart macroporous hydrogel. Langmuir 23: 35–40.

Gunatillake PA, Adhikari R. 2003. Biodegradable synthetic polymers for tissue engineering. Eur. Cells Mater. 5: 1–16.

Hanthamrongwit M, Wilkinson R, Osborne C, Reid WH, Grant MH. 1996. Confocal laser-scanning microscopy for determining the structure of and keratinocyte infiltration through collagen sponges. J. Biomed. Mater. Res. 30: 331–339.

Hasirci V, Lewandowski K, Gresser JD, Wise DL, Trantolo DJ. 2001. Versatility of biodegradable biopolymers: degradability and *in vivo* applications. J. Biotechnol. 86: 135–150.

Hassan CM, Peppas NA. 2000. Structure and applications of poly(vinyl alcohol) hydrogels produced by convectional cross-linking or by freezing/thawing methods. Adv. Polym. Sci. 153: 37–65.

Hassan CM, Stewart JE, Peppas NA. 2000. Diffusional characteristics of freeze/thawed poly(vinyl alcohol) hydrogels: Applications to protein controlled release from multi-laminate devices. Eur. J. Pharm. Biopharm. 49: 161–165.

He X, Yao K, Shen S, Yun J. 2007. Freezing characteristics of acrylamide-based aqueous solution used for the preparation of supermacroporous cryogels via cryo-copolymerization. Chem. Eng. Sci. 62: 1334–1342.

Hennik WE, Nostrum CF. 2002. Novel crosslinking methods to design hydrogels. Adv. Drug Deliv. Rev. 54: 13–36.

Hentze H-P, Antonietti M. 2002. Porous polymers and resins for biotechnological and biomedical applications. Rev. Mol. Biotechnol. 90: 27–53.

Hollister SJ. 2005. Porous scaffold design for tissue engineering. Nature Mater. 4: 518–524.

Ito T, Yeo Y, Highley CB, Bellas E, Kohane DS. 2007. Dextran-based *in situ* cross-linked injectable hydrogels to prevent peritoneal adhesions. Biomaterials 28: 3418–3426.

Jiang H, Campbell G, Boughner D, Wan W-K, Quantz M. 2004. Design and manufacture of a polyvinyl alcohol (PVA) cryogel tri-leaflet heart valve prosthesis. Med. Engin. Phys. 26: 269–277.

Kabiri K, Omidian H, Zohuriaan-Mehr MJ. 2003. Novel approach to highly porous superabsorbent hydrogels: synergistic effect of porogens on porosity and swelling rate. Polymer Int. 52: 1158–1164.

Kaufman JD, Song J, Klapperich CM. 2006. Nanomechanical analysis of bone tissue engineering scaffolds. J Biomed Mater Res 81A: 611–623.

Kim SJ, Lee CK, Kim SI. 2004. Characterization of the water state of hyaluronic acid and poly(vinyl alcohol) interpenetrating polymer networks. J. Appl. Polym. Sci. 92: 1467–1472.

Kokabi M, Sirousazar M, Hassan ZM. 2007. PVA-clay nanocomposite hydrogels for wound dressing. Eur. Polym. J. 43: 773–781.

Kroupova J, Horak D, Pachernik J, Dvorak P, Slour M. 2006. Functional polymer hydrogels for embryonic stem cell support. J. Biomed. Mater. Res. Part B: Appl. Biomater. 76B: 315–325.

Kumar A, Plieva F, Galaev IYu, Mattiasson B. 2003. Affinity fractionation of lymphocytes using a monolithic cryogel. J. Immunol. Methods 283: 185–194.

Kumar A, Bansal V, Andersson J, Roychoudhury PK. Mattiasson B. 2006a. Supermacroporous cryogel matrix for integrated protein isolation: IMAC purification of urokinase from cell culture broth of a human kidney cell line. J. Chromatogr. A 1103: 35–42.

Kumar A, Bansal V, Nandakumar KS, Galaev IYu, Roychoudhury PK, Holmdahl R, Mattiasson B. 2006b. Integrated bioprocess for the production and isolation of urokinase from animal cell culture using supermacroporous cryogel matrices. Biotechnol. Bioeng. 93: 636–646.

Lai HL, Abu'khalil A, Craig DQM. 2003. The preparation and characterisation of drug-loaded alginate and chitosan sponges. Int. J. Pharm. 251: 175–181.

Levesque SG, Ryan RM, Shoichet MS. 2005. Macroporous interconnected dextran scaffolds of controlled porosity for tissue-engineering applications. Biomaterials 26: 7436–7446.

Levesque SG, Shoichet MS. 2006. Synthesis of cell-adhesive dextran hydrogels and macroporous scaffolds. Biomaterials 27: 5277–5285.

Liu J, Zhou Y-X. 2003. Freezing curve-based monitoring to quickly evaluate the viability of biological materials subject to freezing or thermal injury. Anal. Bioanal. Chem. 377: 173–181.

Liu Q, Hedberg EL, Liu Z, Bahulekar R, Meszlenyi RK, Mikos AG. 2000. Preparation of macroporous poly(2-hydroxyethyl methacrylate) hydrogels by enhanced phase separation. Biomaterials 21: 2163–2169.

Lozinsky VI. 1998. Cryotropic gelation of poly(vinyl alcohol) solutions. Russ. Chem. Rev. 67: 573–586.

Lozinsky VI. 2002. Cryogels on the basis of natural and synthetic polymers: preparation, properties and applications. Russ. Chem. Rev. 71: 489–511.

Lozinsky VI, Plieva FM. 1998. Poly(vinyl alcohol) cryogels employed as matrices for cell immobilization. 3.Overview of recent research and developments. Enzyme Microb. Technol. 23: 227–242.

Lozinsky VI, Plieva FM, Galaev IYu, Mattiasson B. 2002. The potential of polymeric cryogels in bioseparation. Bioseparation 10: 163–188.

Luyet BJ. 1966. An attempt at a systematic analysis of the notion of freezing rates and at an evaluation of the main contributory factors. Cryobiology 2: 198–205.

Mi F-L, Shyu S-S, Wu Y-B, Lee S-T, Shyong J-Y, Huang R-N. 2001. Fabrication and characterization of a sponge-like asymmetric chitosan membrane as a wound dressing. Biomaterials 22: 165–173.

Miralles G, Baudoin R, Dumas D, Baptiste D, Hubert P, Stoltz JF, Dellacherie E, Mainard D, Netter P, Payan E. 2001. Sodium alginate sponges with or without sodium hyaluronate: In vitro engineering of cartilage. J. Biomed. Mat. Res. 57: 268–278.

Nam YS, Park TG. 1999. Porous biodegradable polymeric scaffolds prepared by thermally induced phase separation. J. Biomed. Mater. Res. 47: 8–17.

Nho YC, Park KR. 2001. Preparation and properties of PVA/PVP hydrogels containing chitosan by radiation. J. Appl. Polym. Sci. 85: 1787–1794.

Nilsang S, Nandakumar KS, Galaev IYu, Rakshit SK, Holmdahl R, Mattiasson B, Kumar A. 2007a. Monoclonal Antibody Production Using a New Supermacroporous Cryogel Perfusion Reactor. Biotechnol. Prog. DOI: 10.1021/bp0700399.

Nilsang S, Nehru V, Plieva F, Nandakumar KS, Rakshit SK, Holdmahl R, Mattiasson B, Kumar A. 2007b. Three-dimensional culture for monoclonal antibody production by hybridoma cells Immobilized in macroporous gel particles/submitted/.

Noir ML, Plieva F, Hey T, Guiesse B, Mattiasson B. 2007. Macroporous molecularly imprinted polymer/cryogel composite systems for the removal of endocrine disrupting trace contaminants. J. Chromatogr. A 1154: 158–164.

O'Brien FJ, Harley BA, Yannas IV, Gibson L. 2004. Influence of freezing rate on pore structure in freeze-dried collagen-GAG scaffolds. Biomaterials 25: 1077–1086.

O'Brien FJ, Harley BA, Yannas IV, Gibson LJ. 2005. The effect of pore size on cell adhesion in collagen-GAG scaffolds. Biomaterials 26: 433–441.

Park KR, Nho YC. 2003. Preparation and characterization by radiation of hydrogels of PVA and PVP containing *Aloe Vera*. J. Appl. Polym. Sci. 91: 1612–1618.

Patel VR, Amiji MM. 1996. Preparation and characterization of freeze-dried chitosan-poly (ethylene oxide) hydrogels for site-specific antibiotic delivery in the stomach. Pharm. Res. 13: 588–593.

Peppas NA, Huang Y, Torres-Lugo M, Ward JH, Zhang J. 2000. Physicochemical foundations and structural design of hydrogels in medicine and biology. Annu. Rev. Biomed. Eng. 02: 9–29.

Peppas NA, Mongia NK. 1997. Ultrapure poly(vinyl alcohol)hydrogels with mucoadhesive drug delivery characteristics. Eur. J. Pharm. Biopharm. 43: 51–58.

Peppas NA, Stauffer SR. 1991. Reinforced uncross-linked poly(vinyl alcohol) gels produced by cyclic freezing-thawing processes: a short review. J. Contr. Release 16: 305–310.

Peters MC, Mooney DJ. 1997. Synthetic extracellular matrices for cell transplantation. Mater. Sci. Forum 250: 43–52.

Petrov P, Petrova E, Stamenova R, Tsvetanov CB, Riess G. 2006. Cryogels of cellulose derivatives prepared via UV irradiation of moderately frozen systems. Polymer 47: 6481–6484.

Plieva FM, Andersson J, Galaev IYu, Mattiasson B. 2004a. Characterization of polyacrylamide based monolithic columns. J. Sep. Sci. 27: 828–836.

Plieva F, Galaev IYu, Mattiasson B. 2007a. Macroporous gels prepared at subzero temperatures as novel materials for chromatography of particulate containing fluids and cell culture applications. J. Sep. Sci. 30: 1657–1671.

Plieva F, Huiting X, Galaev IYu, Bergenståhl B, Mattiasson B. 2006a. Macroporous elastic polyacrylamide gels prepared at subzero temperatures: control of porous structure. J. Mater. Chem. 16: 4065–4073.

Plieva F, Karlsson M, Aguilar M-R, Gomez D, Mikhalovsky S, Galaev IYu, Mattiasson B. 2007b. Porous structure of macroporous agarose gels prepared at subzero temperatures./manuscript/.

Plieva FM, Karlsson M, Aguilar M-R, Gomez D, Mikhalovsky S, Galaev IYu, Mattiasson B. 2006b. Pore structure of macroporous monolithic cryogels prepared from poly (vinyl alcohol). J. Appl. Polym. Sci. 100: 1057–1066.

Plieva FM, Karlsson M, Aguilar M-R, Gomez D, Mikhalovsky S, Galaev IYu. 2005. Pore structure in supermacroporous polyacrylamide based cryogels. Soft Matter 1: 303–309.

Plieva F, Oknianska A, Degerman E, Galaev IYu, Mattiasson B. 2006c. Novel supermacroporous dextran gels. J. Biomater. Sci. Polym. Edn 17: 1075–1092.

Plieva FM, Oknianska A, Mattiasson B. 2007c. Macroporous gel particles as robust matrices for cell immobilization. Biotechnol. J./in press/.

Plieva FM, Savina IN, Deraz S, Andersson J, Galaev IYu, Mattiasson B. 2004b. Characterization of supermacroporous monolithic polyacrylamide based matrices designed for chromatography of bioparticles. J. Chromatogr. B 807: 129–137.

Podorozhko EA, Kurskaya EA, Kulakova VK, Lozinsky VI. 2000. Cryotropic structuring of aqueous dispersions of fibrous collagen: influence of the initial pH values. Food Hydrocol. 14: 111–120.

Rizzieri R, Baker FS, Donald AM. 2003. A study of the large strain deformation and failure behaviour of mixed biopolymer gels via *in situ* ESEM. Polymer 44: 5927–5935.

Sannino A, Netti PA, Madaghiele M, Coccoli V, Luciani A, Maffezzoli A, Nicolais L. 2006. Synthesis and characterization of macroporous poly(ethylene glycol)-based hydrogels for tissue engineering application. J. Biomed. Mater. Res. 79A: 229–236.

Sawhney AS, Pathak CP, Hubbell JA. 1993. Bioerodible hydrogels based on photopolymerized poly(ethylene glycol)-co-poly(alpha-hydroxy acid) diacrylate macromers. Macromolecules 26: 581–587.

Schild HG. 1992. Poly(N-isopropylacrylamide): experiment, theory and application. Prog. Polym. Sci. 17: 163–249.

Shapiro L, Cohen S. 1997. Novel alginate sponges for cell culture and transplantation. Biomaterials 18: 583–590.

Shibukawa M, Aoyagi K, Sakamoto R, Oguma K. 1999. Liquid chromatography and differential scanning calorimetry studies on the states of water in hydrophilic polymer gel packing in relation to retention selectivity. J. Chromatogr. A 832: 17–27.

Srivastava A, Jain E, Kumar A. 2007. The physical characterization of supermacroporous poly(*N*-isopropylacrylamide) cryogel: mechanical strength and swelling/de-swelling kinetics. Mat. Sci. Eng. A 464: 93–100.

Stauffer SR, Peppas NA. 1992. Poly(vinyl alcohol) hydrogels prepared by freezing-thawing cyclic processing. Polymer 33: 3932–3936.

Swieszowski W, Ku DN, Bersee HEN, Kurzydlowski KJ. 2006. An elastic material for cartilage replacement in an arthritic shoulder joint. Biomaterials 27: 1534–1541.

Vijayasekaran S, Chirila T, Robertson TA, Lou X, Helenfitton J, Hicks CR, Constable IJ. 2000. Calcification of poly(2-hydroxyethyl methacrylate) hydrogel sponges implanted in the rabbit cornea: a 3-month study. J. Biomater. Sci. Polym. Ed. 11: 599–615.

Vlierberghe SV, Cnudde V, Dubruel P, Masschaele B, Cosijns A, Paepe ID, Jacobs PJS, Hoorebeke LV, Remon JP, Schacht E. 2007. Porous gelatin hydrogels: 1. Cryogenic formation and structure analysis. Biomacromolecules 8: 331–337.

Wan Y, Fang Y, Wu H, Cao X. 2007. Porous polylactide/chitosan scaffolds for tissue engineering. J. Biomed. Mater. Res. 80A: 776–789.

Watase M, Nishinari K. 1988. Thermal and reological properties of poly(vinyl alcohol) hydrogels prepared by repeated cycles of freezing and thawing. Macromol. Chem. 189: 871–880.

Wood CD, Cooper AI. 2001. Synthesis of macroporous polymer beads by suspension polymerization using supercritical carbon dioxide as a pressure-adjustable porogen. Macromolecules 34: 5–8.

Yao K, Shen S, Wang J, He X, Yu X. 2006a. Preparation of polyacrylamide-based super-macroporous monolithic cryogel beds under freezing-temperature variation conditions. Chem. Eng. Sci. 61: 6701–6708.

Yao K, Yun J, Shen S, Wang L, He X, Yu X. 2006b. Characterization of a novel continuous supermacroporous monolithic cryogel embedded with nanoparticles for protein chromatography. J. Chromatogr. A 1109: 103–110.

Yeong W-Y, Chua C-K, Leong K-F, Chandrasekaran M, Lee M-W. 2007. Comparison of drying methods in the fabrication of collagen scaffold via indirect rapid prototyping. J. Biomed. Mater. Res. Part B: Appl. Biomater. 82B: 260–266.

You Y, Park WH. 2004. Effect of PVA sponge containing chitooligosaccharide in the early stage of wound healing. J. Mater. Sci.: Materials in Medicine 15: 297–301.

Zhang X-Z, Chu C-C. 2003. Synthesis of temperature sensitive PNIPAAm cryogels in organic solvent with improved properties. J. Mater. Chem. 13: 2457–2464.

Section III

15

BIOMATERIAL APPLICATIONS

Ashok Kumar, Akshay Srivastava, and Era Jain

Department of Biological Sciences and Bioengineering, Indian Institute of Technology Kanpur, Kanpur, India

Contents

15.1	Overview	536
15.2	Introduction	536
15.3	Applications in Medicine, Biology, and Artificial Organs	537
	15.3.1 Cardiovascular Medical Devices	537
	15.3.2 Extracorporeal Artificial Organs	538
	15.3.3 Orthopedic Implants	538
	15.3.4 Dental Implantation	539
	15.3.5 Bioadhesive	541
	15.3.6 Opthalmologic Applications	541
	15.3.7 Cochlear Prosthesis	542
	15.3.8 Drug Delivery	544
	15.3.9 Tissue Engineering	545
	15.3.10 Array Technologies and Specific Medical Applications	546
15.4	Broad Overview of Biomaterial Applications Section	547
	Suggested Reading	550

Advanced Biomaterials: Fundamentals, Processing, and Applications, Edited by Bikramjit Basu, Dhirendra S. Katti, and Ashok Kumar
Copyright © 2009 The American Ceramic Society

535

15.1 OVERVIEW

The potential use of various types of advanced biomaterials for biomedical applications is ever-increasing and development of new types of biomaterials and their applications is becoming more and more important and challenging. A large number of biomaterials have received great success in their respective applications in human health; however, much needs to be done to improve the quality of these biomaterials and expand their applications for human healthcare. This introductory chapter on biomaterial applications provides a review of some of the successes and critical challenges of this field in health-related applications. A brief overview of some of the common biomaterial applications is also discussed.

15.2 INTRODUCTION

Biomaterials have shown potential to improve the quality of life for a large number of people every year. The range of applications is vast and includes important uses such as joint and limb replacements, artificial arteries and skin, contact lenses, and dental and orthopedic implants. While the implementation of some of these materials may be for medical reasons—such as the replacement of diseased tissues required to extend life expectancy—other reasons may include purely aesthetic ones such as breast implants or cosmetic surgeries. This increasing demand arises from an ageing population with higher quality-of-life expectations. The use of synthetic or natural materials to improve the health conditions of mankind is an established area of research. The range of available biomaterials is wide and ranges from hardest of metals like titanium to "tissue-like" soft polymeric hydrogels. The choice of biomaterial depends on the type of its application.

However, in early times the biomaterials that were used in their natural form without much processing often led to inflammation and non-biocompatibility. Modern biomaterial science is characterized by a growing emphasis on identification of specific design parameters that are critical to performance, and by a growing appreciation of the need to integrate biomaterial design with new insights emerging from studies of cell–matrix interactions, cellular signaling processes, and developmental and systems biology.

Several advances have been made in understanding disease mechanisms as well as human development and repair. These advances provide various clues that have improved the quality of biomaterials with better processing, specifically leading to improved biocompatibility. The advances in material science and other engineering fields have widened the scope of biomaterials by providing a clear understanding of the properties of materials and ways to improve them for specific applications. Biomaterials have an enormous impact on human health care. Applications include medical devices, diagnostics, sensors, drug delivery systems, and tissue engineering.

15.3   APPLICATIONS IN MEDICINE, BIOLOGY, AND ARTIFICIAL ORGANS

15.3.1   Cardiovascular Medical Devices

Cardiovascular medical devices (CMD) have been used for more than five decades for myriad applications that save, prolong, and enhance the quality of life. Still, complications are associated with available CMD devices that cause significant mortality rates, even years after implantation. Many different biomaterials are used in cardiovascular applications depending on the specific application and the design, for instance, carbon in heart valves and polyurethanes for pace maker leads (Figure 15.1). Heart valve prostheses are used to replace dysfunctional natural valves with substantial enhancement of both survival and quality of life. Metallic cylindrical mesh stents are inserted via catheters and without surgery during percutaneous transluminal coronary angioplasty (in which balloon is threaded into a diseased vessel and inflated, thereby deforming the atherosclerotic plaque and partially relieving the vessel). These inventions revolutionized the treatment of coronary artery disease and myocardial infarction. The synthetic

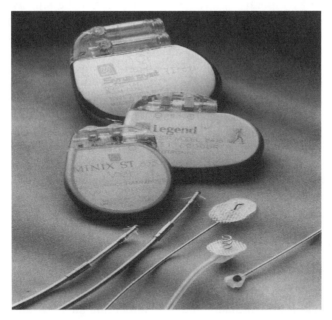

Figure 15.1. Various pacemaker component designs. Top: Three examples of titanium-encased pulse generators. Connector blocks, which serve to attach the pacemaker to the pacemaker lead, are shown at the top of each pulse generator. Bottom: Various types of insulated endocardial and myocardial leads. Note that the lead shown at the center of the figure has a silicone sewing pad and dacram mesh disk for implant fixation. *Adopted from chapter 1. overview of biomaterials and their use in medical devices, In: Handbook of materials for medical devices. Ed. J. R. Davis, ASM International (USA), 2003 pp. 1–11.*

vascular grafts are used to repair weakened vessels or bypass blockages, primarily in the abdomen and lower extremities. They are also used to obtain vascular access for hemodialysis treatment of patients with chronic renal failure. Devices to aid or replace the pumping function of the heart include intra-aortic balloon pumps, ventricular assist devices, and total implantable artificial hearts. Pacemakers and automatic internal cardiverter defibrillators are used widely to correct aberrant life-threatining cardiac arrhythmias (Figure 15.1).

Most of these devices either alleviate the health conditions for which they were implanted or provide otherwise enhanced function and serve well and for extended periods the patients who receive them. Nevertheless, device failure and/or other tissue-biomaterials interactions frequently cause clinically observable complications, reoperation or even death.

15.3.2   Extracorporeal Artificial Organs

The term "extracorporeal artificial organs" has been reserved for life support techniques requiring the online processing of blood outside the patient's body. The substitution, support, or replacement of organ functions is performed. When the need is only temporary or intermittent, support may be sufficient. The oldest and most widely employed extracorporeal artificial organs include kidney substitute, hemodialysis and hemofiltration for the treatment of chronic renal failure, fluid overload, and peritoneal dialysis. The blood treatment process of hemoperfusion and apheresis technologies, which include plasma exchange, plasma treatment, and cytapheresis, are used to treat metabolic and immunological diseases associated with blood. In addition, blood-gas exchangers are used for heart-lung bypass procedure, and bioartificial devices that employ living tissue in an extracorporeal circuit mainly involve artificial liver devices. Bioartificial liver (incorporated with hepatocyte) (BAL), constituted with extracorporeal blood circuit and bioreactor, is a developing novel medical technology, still in its pre-clinical stage. Currently nine bioartificial liver support devices are undergoing various stages of clinical trials, most of which utilize a hollow fiber technology. A much larger number of BAL systems in preclinical tests have been suggested to show an enhanced performance.

15.3.3   Orthopedic Implants

Metallic, ceramic and polymeric biomaterials are used in orthopedic applications. Metallic materials are normally used as load bearing implants such as pins and plates and femoral stems, and so on. Ceramics such as alumina and zirconia are used for wear applications in joint replacements, while hydroxyapatite is used for bone bonding applications to assist implant integration. Polymers such as ultra-high molecular weight polyethylene are used as articulating surfaces against ceramic components in joint replacements. Porous alumina has also been used as a bone spacer to replace large sections of bone that have had to be removed due to disease. A summary of prevalent orthopedic biomaterials and their primary

TABLE 15.1. Orthopedic Biomaterials and Their Primary Uses

Material	Primary use(s)
Metals	
Ti alloy (Ti-6%Al-4%V), Co-Cr-Mo alloy, Stainless steel	Bone plates, screws, TJA components, screws, cabling
Polymers	
Poly(methyl methacrylate) (PMMA), Ultrahigh-molecular weight polyethylene (UHMWPE), PLA, PLGA, HA/PLGA, PCL	Bone cement, low friction inserts for bearing surface in TJA, bone tissue engineering scaffolds, bone screws
Ceramics	
Alumina (Al_2O_3), Zirconia (ZrO_2)	Bearing surface TJA components, Hip joints (Figure 15.2), coating on bioimplants, bone filler, alveolar ridge augmentation
Composites	
HA/collagen, HA/gelatin, HA/PLGA, PLGA	Bone graft substitutes and tissue engineering scaffolds

uses are listed in Table 15.1. These materials are generally used for either fracture fixation or joint replacement. More specific orthopedic applications within these two categories are listed below.

- *Fracture fixation devices:* spinal fixation devices, fracture plates, wires, pins and screws, intramedullary devices and artificial ligaments.
- *Joint replacement:* hip, knee, ankle, shoulder and other joint arthroplasty.

15.3.4 Dental Implantation

A dental implant is an artificial tooth root replacement and is used in prosthetic dentistry to support restorations that resemble a tooth or group of teeth. There are several types of dental implants; the most widely accepted and successful is the osseointegrated implant, based on titanium that can be successfully fused into bone, when osteoblasts grow on and into the rough surface of the implanted titanium. This forms a structural and functional connection between the living bone and the implant. Variations on the implant procedure are the implant-supported bridge or implant-supported denture.

Three basic types of synthetic materials have been used for fabricating endosseous dental implants. These are metals and metal alloys, ceramics and carbons, and polymers. Metals and metal alloys, used for clinical and experimental implants, have included titanium and titanium alloys, tantalum, stainless steel, cobaltchromium alloys, gold alloys, and zirconium alloys, among others. These materials are selected based on their high corrosion resistance, strength, rigidity, ease of shaping and machining, and suitability for a wide range of sterilization techniques. Although the mechanisms that lead to osseointegration with titanium implants

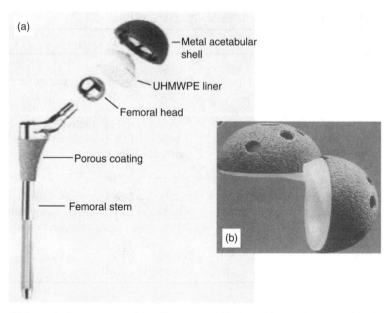

Figure 15.2. Typical components found in an assembled total hip replacement (THR) implant. It should be noted that this is one of many artificial joint designs used in THR arthroplasty. For example, implants secured by bone cements would not be porous coated. Similarly, the ultrahigh molecular weight polyethylene (UHMWPE) acetabular cup is sometimes not capped by a metal (cobalt- or titanium-base alloys or unalloyed tantalum) shell (a). Acetabular cup components, which are fitted over the femoral head, featuring plasma-sprayed shell with anatomic screw hole placement (b). *Adopted from chapter 1. overview of biomaterials and their use in medical devices, In: Handbook of materials for medical devices. Ed. J. R. Davis, ASM International (USA), 2003 pp. 1–11.*

are not fully known, metals in general do not form an interfacial bond with bone. The implant is typically connected to bone via a micro-mechanical interlock using a variety of surface designs and textures that are used to promote bony in-growth and improve the interfacial attachment. There are many implants available, each designed for a specific function. Most are made of titanium, an inert metal that has been proven to be effective at fusing with living bone, a process known as "osseointegration." The cylindrical or screw type implant, called "root form," is similar in shape to the root of a tooth with a surface area designed to promote good attachment to the bone. It is the most widely-used design and generally placed where there is plentiful width and depth of jawbone. Where the jawbone is too narrow or short for immediate placement of root form implants, the area may be enhanced with bone grafting to allow for their placement. When the jawbone is too narrow and not a good candidate for bone grafting, a special narrow implant, called "plate form," can be placed into the bone. In cases of advanced bone loss, the "subperiosteal" implant may be prescribed. It rests on top of the bone but under the gums. The actual implant procedure involves the surgical placement of the implant or implants, a healing period (osseointegration) and implant restoration to replace the missing tooth or teeth. The treatment may be a cooperative effort between a surgical dentist who actually places the implant and a restorative dentist who designs, prescribes, and inserts the final replacement teeth. Some dentists have advanced training and provide both of these services.

15.3.5 Bioadhesive

There are a number of adhesives and sealants that are suitable for short and/or long term biomedical applications. Typical adhesives used in medical products include silicones, epoxies, acrylics, and polyurethanes. But perhaps the most interesting materials are those that are aimed at surgical applications.

Today, most of these are based on cyanoacrylate materials. Two such commercial products are Dermabond—surgical glue that replaces suture and staples—and Liquid Band-Aid—a protective covering for cuts and scrapes that acts as a bandage. Both of these products have been developed by "Closure," a small start-up company located in Raleigh, North Carolina. Now Johnson & Johnson, one of the world's largest manufacturers of heath care products, has agreed to acquire the company. Biomaterials are not only used as adhesives for the human body, but are also being developed as sealants.

In addition to the two products mentioned above, Closure is developing several surgical sealants. Omnex, a vascular sealant is about to become available in Europe. This sealant can be used to glue blood vessels and will be the first surgical glue to be used inside the body. A sealant for use after lung cancer surgery is at least two years from commercialization, and an orthopedic sealant for tendon and muscle repair is at least three years from market. An especially useful fibrin glue composition comprises a biocompatible, bioabsorbable, hyaluronic acid derivative material, upon which are applied or chemically bonded fibrinogen and thrombin, along with other optional constituents, such as additional coagulation factors, anti-fibrinolytics, stabilizers, and biologically active substances. The fibrinogen, thrombin and other components can take the form of a dry preparation, an aqueous or nonaqueous preparation, or as a combination thereof. Such a fibrin glue composition can be placed directly on a wound site and is fully reabsorbed into the body.

Bioactive materials encourage specific reactions between the material and the surrounding tissue. One example of such a bioactive material is hydroxyapatite. This polymer is used as a porous coating on hip implants. The coating encourages growth of surrounding tissues that interlock into the pores to help stabilize the stem of the implant in the bone.

15.3.6 Opthalmologic Applications

The different types of eye medical devices such as Ophthalmic Tantalum Clip, Conformer Artificial Eye, Absorbable Implant, Eye Sphere, Extra Ocular Orbital Implant, Keratoprosthesis, Intraocular Lens, Scleral Shell, and Aqueous Shunt are all outcomes of biomaterial applications. The biomaterials for each of these devices are generally composed of PMMA, hydroxyapatite and silicon. Glass and artificial eyes have been made for thousands of years, the first ocular implants were developed about 100 years ago. These small spheres of glass or gold were later replaced by plastic or silicone spheres; but until recently, the basic design of these "first-generation" implants had changed little over the years. Artificial eyes are usually made of plastic (acrylic) or glass. Custom artificial eyes are hand-crafted by highly skilled ocularists (eye makers) to precisely match the natural eye. The first ocular implant made of hydroxyapatite was implanted in 1985, after several years of preliminary research. The eye muscles can be attached directly to this implant, allowing it to move within the orbit, just like the natural eye.

Bio-eye hydroxyapatite ocular implant has been described as "a dream come true" by eye care specialists, oculatists, and those familiar with the older, first-generation ocular implants. A keratoprosthesis made up of Silicone, hydroxyethyl methacrylate (PHEMA), divinyl glycol (DVG), and methyl methacrylate (MMA), is a device intended to restore vision to patients with severe bilateral corneal diseases for which corneal transplants are not an option. An extraocular orbital implant is a nonabsorbable device intended to be implanted during surgery, in which the eyeball or the contents of it are removed. The search for a well-tolerated orbital implant which gives an excellent appearance as well as good mobility has covered the gamut of autogenous and alloplastic materials and implant designs. Almost every conceivable material known to man has been used as an orbital implant, including magnets, gold, silver, glass, silicone, cartilage, bone, fat, cork, titanium mesh, acrylics, wool, rubber, catgut, peat, agar, asbestos, ivory, cellulose, paraffin, sponge, polyethylene, and hydroxyapatite.

In addition, a wide variety of implant shapes have been implanted in order to achieve an acceptable cosmetic result including: sphere; sphere with a truncated surface; sphere with a truncated surface and small knobs projecting from the surface; and so on. An ophthalmic tantalum clip is a malleable metallic device, intended to be permanently or temporarily implanted to bring together the edges of a wound to aid healing or prevent bleeding from small blood vessels in the eye. An intraocular lens, commonly called an IOL, is a tiny, lightweight, clear-plastic disk, which is placed in the eye during cataract surgery to replace the eye's natural lens. The biomaterial examples of IOL are described in Figure 15.3.

15.3.7 Cochlear Prosthesis

Cochlear prosthesis is being clinically used to restore functional hearing in patients suffering from profound sensorineural deafness. The device includes one or more electrodes implanted in or near cochlea to provide necessary electrical stimulation of the remaining auditory nerve fibers, thereby bypassing the defective sensory hair-cells. There are many different designs of these devices in various stages of testing, development, and availability. The therapeutic benefit of these devices depends upon the type of device and individual patients receiving a given device. Cochlear prostheses have evolved from laboratory experiment to a com-

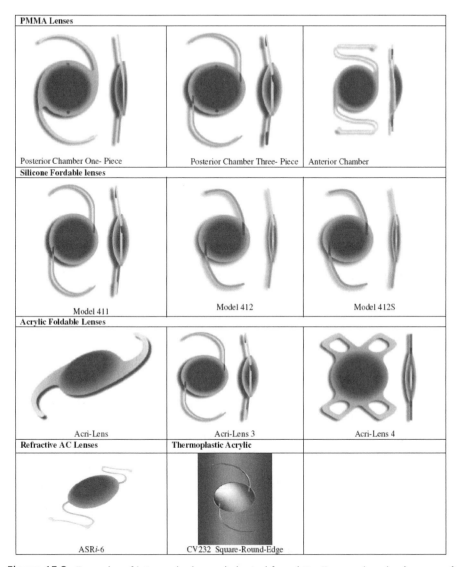

Figure 15.3. Examples of intraocular lenses (adopted from http://www.microviscphaco.com/) [I-Lens® Intraocular Lenses]

mercial technology that has benefited over 20,000 people. In the past 20 years, cochlear prostheses have become multi-channel systems. The first implants employed single electrodes, whereas present devices use up to 22 contacts inside the scala tympani. In most processing strategies, one electrode is driven at a time, although analog drives present currents to all electrodes simultaneously. A generic architecture of the cochlear prosthesis has been shown in Figure 15.4. There are currently three commercially available cochlear prosthesis, namely:

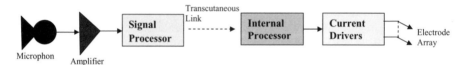

<u>Figure 15.4.</u> Schematic representation of cochlear prosthesis illustrating the generic architecture.

Nucleus Implant, The Clarion, and Med-EI implant. All are based on different strategies that process the incoming signals and send them to the electrodes, where they are finally converted into audio signals.

15.3.8 Drug Delivery

The most widespread use of biomaterials in the field of medicine is the area where the most-sought aim is to achieve targeted release of drug at predetermined rates. Drug-delivery systems can be synthesized with controlled composition, shape, size and morphology. Their surface properties can be manipulated to increase solubility, immunocompatibility, and cellular uptake. They can be used to deliver both small-molecule drugs and various classes of biomacromolecules, such as peptides, proteins, plasmid DNA and synthetic oligodeoxynucleotides. For this purpose, various synthetic, natural polymers have been employed in various forms such as implants, stealth particles, stimuli responsive hydrogels, and nanoparticles.

Recent examples are polymer-coated stents, which have recently been approved both in Europe and the United States. Another strategy that has been used in modifying a variety of natural and synthetic polymers has been the inclusion of polyethylene glycol (PEG) into the material to reduce non-specific effects of protein adsorption and colloidal aggregation. In addition, various controlled-release systems for proteins, such as human growth hormone, as well as molecules decorated with PEG, such as pegylated interferon, have recently been approved by regulatory authorities, and are showing how biomaterials can be used to positively affect the safety, pharmacokinetics and duration of release of important new drugs. Especially particulate drug delivery systems have found great attention in the research fields due to their various beneficial features over other systems. Some of the examples of particulate drug delivery systems are microcapsules and microspheres, liposomes which are being used for developing drug delivery systems mainly for cancer systems.

Apart from using modified polymers alone, polymer drug conjugates have also been used for formulation of these particulate devices. Some of the PLGA-based particulate drug delivery devices have reached commercialization, the most successful being the devices releasing luteinizing hormone for treatment of prostrate cancer. Various responsive polymers also find application in drug delivery, diagnostics and sensing. The most commonly used temperature responsive polymer for such applications is poly (N-isopropylacrylamide). The other responsive systems include pH-responsive polymers, and phase-separating polymer systems based on pluronics; pH-responsive polymer systems have been used as mucoadhesive, intracellular drug delivery, and enteric-coated drug delivery.

Another approach to creating a biomimetic-reversible system is the creation of an antigen-responsive hydrogel. Corresponding antibody pairs are used to form reversible non-covalent crosslinks in a polyacrylamide system. In the presence of excess-free antigen, the hydrogel swells, but in its absence, the gel collapses back to a crosslinked network. Swelling does not occur when foreign antigens are added, showing that the system is antigen specific. Release of a model protein such as haemoglobin has been demonstrated in response to specific antigens.

A more specialized case of drug delivery is delivery of DNA or genetic material to specific cells to modify the cellular behavior and treatment of various genetic disorders. Gene delivery requires appropriate molecular design, which is critical to achieving a successful outcome. Although viral vectors are highly effective, their use has raised serious safety concerns. To be effective, there are a number of attributes that the material must possess, including the ability to condense DNA to sizes of less than 150 nm, so that it can be taken up by receptor-mediated endocytosis, the ability to be taken up by endosomes in the cell and to allow DNA to be released in active form, and to enable it to travel to the cell's nucleus. Cationic polymers have been used mainly for this purpose along with modified poly(N-isopropylacrylamide). Another novel approach for gene therapy involves creating a triplex, where low-density lipoprotein is used for targeting and stearyl polylysine is used for DNA complexation. This approach has been used to deliver vascular endothelial cell growth factor to heart muscle to aid in treating blockage of blood vessels.

15.3.9 Tissue Engineering

The other major area where biomaterials find special applications is in tissue engineering. The research in this area is ever-expanding and encompasses tissue engineering of bone, blood vessel cartilage, cardiac tissue, peripheral nerve system, ligaments, liver and skin. By combining polymers with mammalian cells, it is now possible to make skin for patients who have burns or skin ulcers. Various other polymer/cell combinations are in clinical trials.

Traditional tissue engineering scaffolds were based on hydrolytically degradable macroporous materials; current approaches emphasize the control over cell behaviors and tissue formation by nano-scale topography that closely mimics the natural extracellular matrix (ECM). Materials composed of naturally occurring (biologically derived) building blocks, including extracellular matrix (ECM) components, are being studied for applications such as direct tissue replacement and tissue engineering. The ECM, a complex composite of proteins, glycoproteins and proteoglycans, provides an important model for biomaterials design. ECM-derived macromolecules (for example, collagen) have been used for many years in biomaterials applications. It is now possible to create artificial analogues of ECM proteins using recombinant DNA technology.

Through the design and expression of artificial genes, it is possible to prepare artificial ECM proteins with controlled mechanical properties and with domains chosen to modulate cellular behaviour. This approach avoids several important limitations encountered in the use of natural ECM proteins, including batch-to-batch (or source-to-source) variation in materials isolated from tissues, restricted flexibility in the range of accessible materials properties, and concerns about disease transmission associated with materials isolated from mammalian sources. Elastin-based systems have been of special interest in this regard. Urry and co-workers have shown over many years that simple repeating polypeptides related to elastin can be engineered to exhibit mechanical behaviour reminiscent of the intact protein.

The understanding that the natural ECM is a multifunctional nanocomposite motivated researchers to develop nanofibrous scaffolds through electrospinning or self-assembly. Nanocomposites containing nanocrystals have been shown to elicit active bone growth. Incorporation of cell adhesion ligands allows attachment and spreading of cultured cells, and in the specific case of materials for vascular grafts, retention of endothelial cell adhesion in the face of shear stresses is characteristic of the normal circulation.

Recent progress in the development of methods for incorporation of non-natural amino acids into recombinant proteins points the way to an alternative strategy for preparing artificial ECM proteins with diverse chemical, physical, and biological properties. Substantially more experience has been gained in evaluating the *in vivo* performance of engineered biomaterials based on polysaccharides. Alginate hydrogels bearing cell-adhesion ligands have been used as scaffolds for cell encapsulation and transplantation, and have yielded promising results in experiments directed towards the engineering of bone tissue capable of growth from small numbers of implanted cells. The prospect of growing tissues from small numbers of precursor cells is an attractive alternative to harvesting and encapsulating large cell masses before transplantation. Molecular self assembly of peptides or peptide-amphiphiles may also lead to unique biomaterials. A number of self assembled peptide systems have been developed, including systems that can potentially be used in tissue engineering and nanotechnology.

An alternative to synthesizing polymers composed of natural components is the synthesis of biomimetic polymers, which combine the information content and multifunctional character of natural materials (such as a particular amino acid sequence that might be desirable for cell attachment) with the tailorability of a synthetic polymer, such as control of molecular mass or polymer degradation, and the ability to impart appropriate mechanical properties. An example of this concept has been the synthesis of polymers composed of lactic acid and lysine.

15.3.10 Array Technologies and Specific Medical Applications

A related challenge arises in the engineering of materials for diagnostics and array technologies, in which large numbers (typically hundreds or thousands) of nucleic acids, "DNA chips," are characterized by high densities of biological information. Although these technologies are now highly developed and widely used, they are far from optimized. Additional challenges arise in the fabrication of protein arrays. Unlike nucleic acids, which share a common physical chemistry that is largely independent of sequence, proteins are highly diverse in terms of charge, hydrophobic character, and so on. There is as yet no consensus regarding the preferred method(s) of array fabrication, and further development will be required before protein arrays become widely available for use in research and clinical practice.

One area of increasing attention has been the development of shape-memory materials that have one shape at one temperature and another shape at a different temperature. Such materials might permit new medical procedures. For example, current approaches for implanting medical devices often require complex surgery followed by device implantation. Shape-memory materials might provide such an opportunity because they have the ability to memorize a permanent shape that can be substantially different from an initial temporary shape. Thus bulky devices could potentially be introduced into the body in a temporary shape, like a string, that could go through a small laproscopic hole, but then be expanded on demand into a permanent shape (for example, a stent, a sheet, and so on) at body temperature. New polymers have been synthesized with this concept in mind, including phase-segregated multiblock copolymers whose starting materials are known as biocompatible monomers, such as ε-caprolactone, p-dioxanone, and polydimethacarylate (Figure 15.5).

The development of high-throughput approaches to create novel biopolymers and screen them for various applications is garnering increased attention. For example, polymer libraries have been created and then screened for different applications. This type of high-throughput approach has also been used in the creation of gene therapy agents.

Microfabrication is a new approach that is gaining importance and may play a vital role in the development of new biomaterials and delivery systems. They have been used to make drug delivery silicon chips containing a combination of drugs in different wells and each drug can be released from the wells upon appropriate stimulation. Microfabrication has also been used in the creation of sensors for treatment of glaucoma as well as for needle-free drug delivery.

15.4 BROAD OVERVIEW OF BIOMATERIAL APPLICATIONS SECTION

In the application section of this book, various aspects of tissue engineering, synthetic heart valve and blood substitutes have been discussed. In particular some interesting aspects of neural tissue engineering have been included in the chapter contributed by Surya K. Mallapragada. Briefly, various aspect of differentiation and proliferation of neural progenitor cells (NPC) have been elaborated, including current state of the art research in this area. Different parameters affecting NPC differentiation and proliferation *in vitro*, especially the role of electric

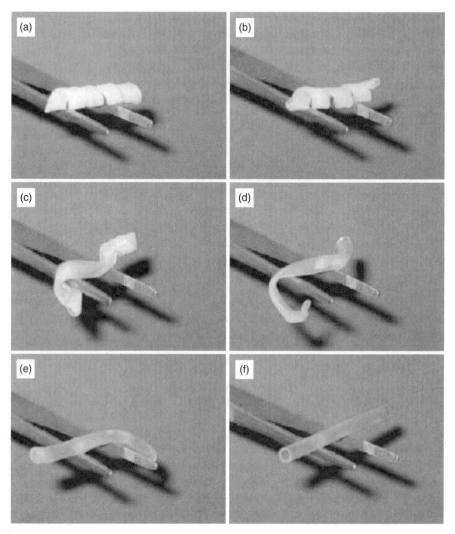

Figure 15.5. Time series of photographs showing recovery of a shape-memory tube. a–f, Start to finish of the process; total time, 10s at 50°C. The tube was made of a poly(ε-caprolactone) dimethacrylate polymer network (the M_n of the network's switching segments was 104) that had been programmed to form a flat helix. *Adopted from [3].*

stimulus in nervous system development and improving spinal cord injury, and the complexities involved in designing such studies have been emphasized.

The chapter by Chandra P. Sharma and K. Kaladhar demonstrates the upcoming importance of cell mimetic monolayer and their blood biocompatibility. The authors have included various approaches to design monolayer films on surface including the fundamentals involved in monolayer deposition on any surface. The effect of changing the composition of the lipid (mimicking the cell bilayer) monolayer, integration of various macromolecules (hydrophobic and hydrophilic) and variation of hydrophillicty balance by incorporating polyethylene glycol on the stability of monolayer deposition have been described. Thereafter various blood biocompatibility studies done on stable monolayers have been discussed.

Benefits of properly purified placental umbilical cord blood as an ideal and the true blood substitutes have been discussed in the chapter by Niranjan Bhattacharya. The author further supports this with the fact that placental cord is a rich mixture of fetal and adult hemoglobin, high platelet and WBC counts, and a plasma filled with cytokine and growth factors, as well as its hypo-antigenic nature and altered metabolic profile. All these potentialities make this blood a real and safe alternative to adult blood, especially in emergencies caused by any etiology of blood loss. Further, it may also be used to prevent ischemia and eventual hypoxic-triggered organ failure syndromes. The chapter also discusses some of the clinical experiences and safety studies of cord blood transfusion.

The coating of titanium nitride (TiN) and diamond like carbon (DLC) the two ceramic coating are discussed by Muraleedharan et al. for cardiovascular applications. Both DLC and TiN exhibit similar properties such as hardness, low frictional coefficient, high wear and corrosion resistance, chemical inertness, and very good processability. The substrate material can be chosen to provide the required strength for structural integrity, while coatings can be employed to enhance the blood compatibility. TiN and DLC coating exhibit very good tissue and blood compatibility and is well tolerated in biological environments. The chapter has given insight at the processing, characterization and applications of TiN and DLC coatings with a focus on cardiovascular applications.

The area of bone tissue engineering using cell-based nanocomposites and biomolecules are thoroughly discussed by S. Ramakrishna and cowokers. The authors have concluded that tissue-engineered constructs loaded with factors for cell proliferation and differentiation can revolutionize the clinical management of bone-related diseases and orthopedic applications. The functional nanofibrous composites made up of nano-hydroxyapatite and collagen meet the required property for a favorable cellular response. The mineralization is also more evident in nanofibrous scaffolds than in solid-walled scaffolds for bone constructs. The mesenchymal stem cells from bone marrow and the choice of growth factors and biomolecules to be incorporated are typically favored in bone repair. Such tissue-engineered nanomaterials will be the new-generation bone grafts, judging from the nascent state of regenerative medicine, fulfilling the desired characteristics of an ideal bone graft in terms of ostecconductivity, osteoinductivity, and osteogenecity.

The chapter by Lu et al. focuses on recently-emerged interface tissue engineering for achieving biological fixation of tissue-engineered grafts, in particular with its emphasis on regenerating the anatomic interface between soft tissues (such as ligaments, tendons, and cartilage) and bone. The area discussed can enable the development of integrated musculoskeletal tissue systems for total joint replacement. The anterior cruciate ligament-to-bone interface as a model system is reviewed as efforts in orthopedic interface tissue engineering.

The research focus on unique biocompatible injectable hydrogels for bio-medical applications is thoroughly elaborated upon by Nair et al. The chapter focuses on synthesis and application of photogelling polymer, thermogelling polymers, and hydrogels formed by fast chemical reaction/physical transitions. The chapter discusses recently-developed injectable hydrogel systems that can undergo sol-to-gel transformation in response to light irradiation, to temperature, and from chemical or physical reactions. The natural and synthetic polymers used for making injectable biomaterials are discussed and their potential applications introduced in this chapter.

SUGGESTED READING

1. Biomaterial Sciences. Editors: Buddy D. Ratner, Allan S. Hoffman, Frederick J. Schoen and Jck E. Lemons, (2004), Elsevier academic press (USA).
2. Handbook of materials for medical devices. Editor: J. R. Davis, (2003), ASM International, USA.
3. Robert Langer and David A. Tirrell. Designing materials for biology and medicine. Nature (2004) 428, 487–492.
4. Tissue Engineering: Fundamentals and Applications. Editor: Yoshito Ikada, (2006), Academic Press.

16

CELL-BASED NANOCOMPOSITES AND BIOMOLECULES FOR BONE TISSUE ENGINEERING

Michelle Ngiam[1], Susan Liao[2,3], Casey Chan[2,3], and S. Ramakrishna[2,4,5]

[1]*National University of Singapore (NUS) Graduate Program in Bioengineering NUS Graduate School (NGS) for Integrative Sciences and Engineering, Center for Life Sciences (CeLS), Singapore*
[2]*Division of Bioengineering, Faculty of Engineering, National University of Singapore, Singapore*
[3]*Department of Orthopedic Surgery, Yong Loo Lin School of Medicine, National University of Singapore, Singapore*
[4]*Department of Mechanical Engineering, Faculty of Engineering, National University of Singapore, Singapore*
[5]*National University of Singapore (NUS) Nanoscience & Nanotechnology Initiative, Singapore*

Contents

16.1 Introduction		552
16.2 Bone Grafts		553
16.2.1 Current Bone Grafts and Bone Graft Substitutes		553
16.2.2 Nanotechnology-Enabled Tissue Engineering		554
16.2.3 Factors for Bone Regeneration		554

Advanced Biomaterials: Fundamentals, Processing, and Applications, Edited by Bikramjit Basu, Dhirendra S. Katti, and Ashok Kumar
Copyright © 2009 The American Ceramic Society

16.3 Types of Materials for Bone Applications   559
    16.3.1 Bioceramics   559
    16.3.2 Polymers   560
            16.3.2.1 Natural Polymers   560
            16.3.2.2 Synthetic Polymers   560
    16.3.3 Nano-HA/Collagen-Based Composites   561
    16.3.4 Nanofibrous Composites   565
    16.3.5 Cell-Material Constructs (e.g., Stem Cell or Osteoblast/
            Material Constructs)   566
            16.3.5.1 Mesenchymal Stem Cells (MSCs)-Material Constructs   566
            16.3.5.2 Non-Mensenchymal Stem Cells (Non-MSCs)-Material
                      Constructs   569
    16.3.6 Peptide-Based Materials   570
    16.3.7 Gene-Based Materials   572
16.4 Sources of Stem Cells Used for Bone Tissue Engineering to Increase
      Osteogenic Differentiation   574
    16.4.1 Adipose-Derived Stem Cells   574
    16.4.2 Bone Marrow-Derived Stem Cells   575
    16.4.3 MSCs Derived from Other Sources   576
16.5 Current Perspective   577
16.6 Conclusion   578
      References   579

16.1 INTRODUCTION

In the twenty-first century, the world has evolved into a sophisticated society whereby affluence has a direct influence of increasing the average lifespan of an individual. The aging population is a worldwide phenomenon that brings a new set of problems as governments have to battle with the ever-increasing healthcare costs whilst delivering healthcare services which are accessible to the public. Degenerative bone disorders such as osteoporosis, osteoarthritis (OA) and Paget's disease are common in the elderly and often lead to fractures of the bone.

It is estimated that 40% of women over the age of 50 will experience an osteoporotic fracture. Consequently, joint diseases are prevalent in older patients, of which half of all chronic conditions will be associated with patients aged 65 years and above[1]. Paget's disease is a localized disorder of bone remodeling, affecting two to three percent of those over the age of 60 in the U.S.[2] Genetic bone disorders such as osteogenesis imperfecta (OI) or brittle-bone disease and fibrous dysplasia are some examples that also call for therapeutic treatments. The prevalence of OI was reported to range from one per 10,000, to one per 20,000 live births[3]. In such instances, bone grafts are employed to treat the ramifications of these diseases that is, to replace the loss of the natural bone.

Other cases that involve the use of bone grafts are trauma caused by either accidents or falls, and injuries due to sports. Conventional biomaterials that involve metals, ceramics, and non-degradable polymers are permanent implants, as these materials do not get resorb in the body. Yet, the risk of implant failure is prevalent and remnants of the failed implant will elicit an inflammatory response, hampering bone repair. This calls for a new generation of materials for bone applications, particularly tissue-engineered bone grafts, which will be dealt with in this chapter.

16.2 BONE GRAFTS

16.2.1 Current Bone Grafts and Bone Graft Substitutes

The gold standard for bone grafts is autologous bone grafts, also known as autografts, whereby healthy bone tissue is harvested from the patient and implanted in the diseased site. One of the major advantages of autografts is that there is no immunological response due to host compatibility and the presence of osteoprogenitor cells and bone morphogenetic proteins (BMPs) needed for bone regeneration. The main drawbacks are donor site immobility and risk of infection at the site of harvest. Allografts are grafts that are derived from another donor of the same species, often from cadavers that are freeze-dried. Some benefits of allografts include eliminating donor site morbidity caused by bone harvesting from the patient and a second operative procedure. One of the disadvantages of allografts is the possible immunological response in the patient as allografts are harvested from another donor. As such, there is a risk of disease transmission. Furthermore, donor shortage may also be an issue.

To circumvent some of the deficiencies associated with autografts and allografts, scientists have come up with bone graft substitutes, which consist of systems based on deminerialised bone matrix (DBM), bioceramics, BMPs, coral and composites. DBM is a processed product of allograft containing growth factors, collagen and proteins and it comes in various forms such as putty, injectable gel, granules or powder. Since DBM is further processed, the risk of disease transmission is reduced but it does not provide a strong framework for bone healing. Although bioceramics such as tricalcium phosphate (TCP) and hydroxyapatite (HA) do not carry the risk of disease transmission, due to the lack of bioactive molecules, bone regeneration may be impeded or the repair may occur at a slower rate.

Some researchers had attempted to combine autogenous bone grafts and DBM to treat tibial and femoral non-unions[4–6]. Out of thirty femoral non-unions cases, twenty-four were healed within six months after surgical intervention. Four patients needed a second plate before healing took place and the remaining two cases were lost to follow-up. Others have shown that demineralized bone matrix gel could be used as a supplement material to compensate for the lack of autograft volume without compromising the fusion rates as of those who used autografts alone[7]. Different manufacturers have their own procurement, demineralization, and sterilization procedures. Individual DBMs are often coupled with different carrier materials such as calcium sulfate, hyaluronic acid and glycerol. Donor variability is another concern in determining the osteoinductivity of the DBM material. It has been demonstrated that various commercially-available DBMs exhibited different biological properties for the induction of spinal fusion in an athymic rat model[8]. As such, there is a medical need to address these pertinent issues by developing a new class of tissue-engineered bone grafts for orthopedic applications.

16.2.2   Nanotechnology-Enabled Tissue Engineering

The principle of tissue engineering is to regenerate diseased/damaged tissue or organ by the use of biodegradable materials with or without biological factors. Through the extensive understanding of the structure and chemical composition of natural bone, bone grafts can be designed to mimic the native bone to achieve optimal performance.

The major components of natural bone are hydroxyapatite and Type I collagen. Two-third of bone by weight is nanophase hydroxyapatite which is the mineral constituent[9]. Type I collagen is the main structural protein, contributing up to 30% of the dry weight of bone and 90–95% of the non-mineral (organic) content[9,10]. Structurally, bone encompasses fiber bundles made up of collagenous nanofibrils. Besides collagen, non-collagenous proteins such as osteocalcin, osteopontin, osteonectin, bone sialoprotein, and so on, are part of the composition of bone. Other components also consist of calcium, phosphate, hydroxyl, carbonate, fluorine, sodium, magnesium, silicon, zinc and aluminum ions[9]. The hype of fabricating nano-scale materials or the like is due to the current advancement in nanotechnology, in areas such as electronics, filtration, catalysts, textiles, drug delivery, and so on.

In particular, tissue engineering is making waves in the research and development arena because of the seminal discoveries of enhanced absorption of biomolecules, such as vitronectin on the scaffold due to a high surface area-to-volume ratio[11], which is important for wound healing. The fibers or scaffolds being in nanometer scale (in diameter) are said to mimic the natural extracellular matrix (ECM), creating a more favorable environment for cellular interaction. Biodegradable materials are popular options for this new class of bone grafts. These materials can be either synthetic or natural polymers. Ultimately, researchers aim to develop bone grafts which surpass the status quo of existing bone grafts. A cocktail of growth factors and cells are usually integrated within the material as it is believed that the synergistic interactions between the material, cells, and growth factors will augment the effectiveness of such regenerative therapies in bone repair, as depicted in Figure 16.1.

16.2.3   Factors for Bone Regeneration

Besides diseases and trauma, several other factors affect osteogenesis. In cell culture experiments, dexamethosone, ascorbic acid, β-glycerophosphate, 1,25-Dihydroxyvitamin D3 are supplements to formulate an osteogenic media to

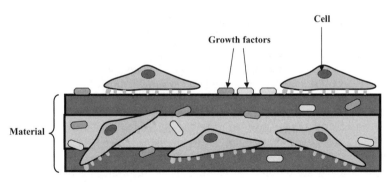

Figure 16.1. A typical tissue-engineered material construct, with the addition of cells and growth factors.

facilitate osteogenic differentiation of cells. For instance, dexamethasone stimulates proliferation and aids in the osteogenic lineage differentiation, ascorbic acid and 1,25-Dihydroxyvitamin D3 can be used for osteogenic induction, promotion of the deposition of matrix, increasing alkaline phosphatase (ALP) activity and osteocalcin production[12]. Ascorbic acid plays a role in the conversion of proline residues in collagen to hydroxyproline. β-glycerophosphate acts as a form of phosphate supply and plays a role in mineralization and osteoblastic processes. Free phosphates can induce the expression of osteoblastic markers such as osteopontin[13]. Other functions of phosphates include the production and nuclear export of an important osteogenic regulatory gene called core-binding factor α-1 (cbfa-1)[14]. Osteogenic supplements such as dexamethasone are often added in culture medium to direct osteogenic differentiation of either mesenchymal stem cells (MSCs), progenitor cells, or osteoblasts. Dexamethasone are bound to regulatory proteins and modulating the transcription of osteogenic genes[15–19]. Encapsulated human mesenchymal stem cells (hMSCs) exhibited an osteogenic effect when dexamethasone was released in a sustained manner over a month in a poly(ethylene glycol) (PEG) hydrogel due to the hydrolysis of the lactide ester bonds, where ALP and cbfa-1 were enhanced[16]. Table 16.1 shows an overview of the effects of various culture media supplements for osteogenesis *in vitro*[20–23]. Some of the benefits of using differentiation medium are expansion of cell number and cellular maturity, yet there may be an increased risk of cell contamination during culture, cell aging, time loss in terms of direct application of cells into patient, and so on.

BMPs are members of the transforming growth factor-β (TGF-β) family that are potent stimulators of bone regeneration. For instance, BMP-2, BMP-7, and so on, have been evaluated and shown that they have the capability to heal bone defects *in vitro* and *in vivo*. One particular study demonstrated that by using recombinant adenoviruses expressing BMPs, BMP-6 and BMP-9, in addition to BMP-2 showed the highest osteogenic activity (and to a lesser degree, BMP-4 and BMP-7) in both *in vitro* and *in vivo* settings. The osteogenic BMPs regulate a set of downstream target genes such as Ids, Dlx, and

TABLE 16.1. Effects of Culture Media Supplements on Osteogenic Markers *In Vitro*

Cells	Function	References
Human bone marrow-derived primary osteoblasts	1. Dexamethasone enhanced ALP activity but not BMP-2. 2. Dexamethasone caused the downregulation of Type I collagen. 3. Osteocalcin synthesis was dependent on Vitamin D. Dexamethasone or BMP-2 alone had no effects on the basal osteocalcin levels but in the presence of Vitamin D, BMP-2 increased osteocalcin synthesis, whilst dexamethasone suppressed the production of osteocalcin. 4. Parathyroid hormone-induced cyclic adenosine mono phosphate (cAMP) production was significantly increased with the treatment of dexamethasone. 5. Mineralization was enhanced in cultures containing BMP-2 and dexamethasone elicited mineralization to a lesser degree. 6. Dexamethasone significantly increased cell proliferation.	Ref[20]
Rat bone marrow stromal cells and osteoblastic MC3T3-E1 cells	**Bone marrow stromal cells** 1. Vitamin C was essential for doubling cell viability. 2. Dexamethasone and β-glycerophosphate reduced the cell proliferation rate. On the other hand, BMP, TGF-β, vitamin D sustained the growth rate given by Vitamin C. 3. Vitamin C in Dulbecco's modified Eagle (DME) medium was vital for the rapid proliferation. **MC3T3-E1 cells** 1. The incorporation of Vitamin C, Vitamin D, TGF-β and BMP did not give rise to a significant increase in cell proliferation. 2. Dexamethasone with Vitamin C and β-glycerophosphate increased the cell proliferation. 3. There was no increase of cells in the samples treated with Vitamin C in DME medium.	Ref[21]
Mouse embryo-derived NIH3T3 Fibroblasts	1. ALP activity was induced by 1α, 25-dihydroxyvitamin D3 in a dose-dependent manner and enhanced in the presence of dexamethasone. 2. Dexamethasone when used alone did not caused any detactable ALP expression. 3. Osteocalcin and osteopontin were produced in the presence of 1 α, 25-dihydroxyvitamin D3 and dexamethasone. 4. In the presence of β-glycerophosphate and L-ascorbic acid plus 1 α, 25-dihydroxyvitamin D3 and dexamethasone, extensive mineralization was observed.	Ref[22]

TABLE 16.1. *Continued*

Cells	Function	References
	5. The expression of Cbfa-1 was not significant in samples treated with 1 α, 25-dihydroxyvitamin D3 and dexamethasone at 3, 10 and 20 days as compared to the controls. No expression of type II or III Cbfa-1 was seen regardless of time point or treatment.	
Adipose-derived stem cells	1. Vitamin D3, β-glycerophosphate and ascorbic acid were required for mineralization.	Ref[23]
	2. Type I collagen secretion was upregulated by ascorbic acid and β-glycerophosphate.	
	3. Vitamin D3 induced osteonectin, osteopontin and osteocalcin expression.	
	4. Vitamin D3, β-glycerophosphate and ascorbic acid had a synergistic effect on sustained osteoblastic transcriptional gene expression such as runt-related transcription factor-2 (RUNX-2) and TAZ.	

CTGF during the early stages of osteogenic differentiation[24]. Specifically, BMP-2 and BMP-7 are some of the predominant BMPs used and are able to induce osteogenic differentiation and bone healing. In a study involving 450 patients with acute, diaphyseal, open tibial fractures, the risk of secondary intervention was greatly decreased in the rhBMP-2 group as compared to the control group (standard of care for long bone repair)[25]; rhBMP-2 seeded on resorbable collagen sponge can be used in spinal fusion and open fractures in patients as it is FDA-approved, while rhBMP-7 and bovine collagen or OP-1 is also FDA-approved and can be utilized as an alternative option to autografts in long bone non-unions and lumbar spinal fusion.

Despite the use of BMPs being potent inductors of osteogenic differentiation, the amounts of BMPs needed vary in humans and in animal studies. In humans, greater levels of BMPs are required for osteogenesis than in animals. It is evident that BMPs elicit a favorable response when added in culture medium or in material substrates. Yet there is a variability in terms of patient response to BMP treatment and minute amounts of BMPs in the nanogram range are sufficient to trigger bone formation *in vivo*[26–28]. On the other hand, at least a magnitude of six orders was reported to result in osteogenesis in human with a matrix substrate[29]. A controlled-delivery system of biomolecules or therapeutic agents can be achieved using tissue-engineered biomaterials.

Besides BMPs, other growth factors which are important for bone formation include insulin-like growth factor 1 (IGF-1), fibroblast growth factor (FGF-2) and vascular endothelial growth factor (VEGF). Table 16.2 shows the types of growth factors used in polymeric substrates for bone repair[30–38].

Smad, Smurf and Tob proteins are also part of the intricate network of the osteogenic pathway[39]. The administration of such growth factors can be utilized in

TABLE 16.2. Types of Growth Factors Used in Various Materials for Bone Regeneration

Materials	Form	Growth factors	Animal model	References
Collagen	Sponge	BMP-2	Goat, rat, rabbit	Refs[31,33]
Gelatin	Hydrogel	BMP-2	Rabbit	Ref[34]
		TGF-β1+IGF-1	Rat	Ref[36]
Alginate	Hydrogel	TGF-β3+BMP-2	Mouse	Ref[32]
PLGA	Scaffold	VEGF	Rat	Ref[38]
		VEGF+BMP-4	Mouse	Ref[30]
PLLA	Scaffold	TGF-β3	Sheep	Ref[37]
HA/TCP	Porous implant	TGF-β2	Dog	Ref[35]

tissue-engineered constructs to induce bony formation. Certain secreting proteins such as Wnts are known to be involved in cellular differentiation such as osteogenesis[40]. Notch signaling has been also said to have a non-promotive role in osteogenic differentiation of progenitor cells as ALP activity, osteocalcin, type I collagen and *in vitro* calcification were suppressive[41].

Heparan sulfate (HS) was assessed as a potential osteogenic agent in a rat model[42]. Five µg of HS was incorporated in the fibrin glue scaffolds and the release kinetics were analysed. More than 50% of HS was released with an initial burst phase in the first four hours, followed by a sustained release over four days during which 100% of HS was released. The released HS led to improved wound healing over a three-month period and increased ALP, RUNX-2 and osteopontin gene expression. In contrast, minimal healing was seen in the absence of HS after one and three months of implantation[42]. Growth factors such as FGF-2 and BMP-2 are susceptible to proteolytic degradation[43]. As such, HS comes in handy as it binds to several soluble proteins such as heparin-binding growth factors, providing a protective shield from extracellular proteases and aiding specific binding to their respective cell surface receptors[44].

Although researchers have established promising experimental data on different cells derived from various origins on a wide range of materials, much work is needed to be done in order for full scale production of these tissue-engineered bone grafts. The physiological mechanical properties and the remodeling of tissues for the restoration of physiological function are deemed to be one of the deciding factors for tissue engineering constructs to replace current bone grafts. Some have suggested that using additional tools such as "smart" scaffolds and bioreactors can accelerate the development of tissue engineered materials for various applications[45]. Bioreactors help create a "natural" environment for cell proliferation, growth and differentiation at optimal conditions such as 37 °C, 5% CO_2, and so on. Specialized bioreactors may also include features such as cyclic, rotational, or static loading to stress the cells to facilitate quicker extracellular matrix deposition or to increase mechanical strength of the material construct, and so on.

16.3 TYPES OF MATERIALS FOR BONE APPLICATIONS

It is of paramount importance that material selection should not be overlooked as the type of material selected plays a pivotal consideration of the success of bone tissue engineering as illustrated in this section of the chapter.

16.3.1 Bioceramics

Calcium phosphate materials have been used as bone substitutes because they possess excellent biocompatibility and osteoconduction characteristics. Materials such as Bioglass®, TCP and HA are some bioactive ceramics used in orthopedic applications. The bioceramic coatings on total joint replacement prostheses may also act as bonding agents between the implant and the native tissue. Some issues pertaining to these materials are inadequacies in bulk properties, lack of mechanical strength especially in load-bearing sites, problems in filling up large bony defects etc. Consequently, there is a medical need for a biomimetic material, which can solve the above-mentioned concerns, whilst improving bone formation *in vivo*.

Some researchers have successfully fabricated ceramic nanofibers such as HA and fluoro-hydroxyapatite (FHA) using an electrospinning technology[46]. The HA and FHA precursors were employed in sol-gel solutions and the solutions were subjected to aging and gelation processes. Subsequently, the sol-gel solutions were mixed with polyvinyl butyral (PVB) and used for electrospinning. By manipulating the sol concentration, the diameter of the fiber can range from micrometers to nanometers in size (1.55 μm to 240 nm). Other processing factors which affect the fiber diameter to a lesser extent are the injection rate and field strength of the electrospinning parameters. Apatite polycrystallines (approximately 30-to-40 nm) were observed. The FHA nanofibers exhibited greater chemical stability than HA nanofibers[46] and the release of fluorine ions was said to be beneficial in dental restoration applications because fluorine helped to prevent the dental caries formation and enhance mineralization and bone formation[47,48].

Biphasic calcium phosphate scaffolds comprising of β-tricalcium phosphate (β-TCP) matrix reinforced with HA nanofibers were produced by using a gel casting and polymer sponge techniques to improve material properties[49]. HA nanofibers were first synthesized via a biomimetic chemical precipitation method and incorporated with the β-TCP powder to make ceramic slurries. After polymerization of the monomers, a polyurethane foam with the desired shapes and sizes was then immersed into the ceramic slurries and subjected to sintering processes for the production of the nanocomposite scaffolds. The compressive strength and modulus increased as the HA nanofiber concentration increased. The HA nanofibers owing to their high surface energy can be easily diffused in the grain boundaries of the matrix during sintering. Scaffolds with 5wt% HA nanofibers had a compressive strength of 9.8 ± 0.3 MPa, comparable to the high end of the compressive strength of cancellous bone (2–10 MPa)[50].

In a separate study, bioactive glass nanofibers were electrospun with average diameters ranging from 85-to-400 nm[51]. The presence of polyvinyl pyrrolidone (PVP) and surfactant pluronic P123 (EO_{20}-PO_{70}-EO_{20}) resulted in the formation of smooth nanofibers and a reduction in diameter respectively. The nanofibers were subjected to simulated body fluid (SBF) whereby its ionic concentration was similar to human blood plasma and calcium phosphate nanoparticles were deposited on the nanofiber surfaces after six hours of SBF immersion. With increasing immersion periods, more apatite was seen and after twenty-four hours of immersion, the bioglass nanofibers were entirely covered with apatite layers. Unlike conventional bioglass fibers, the induction of apatite was accelerated on the bioglass nanofibers and this could be explained by virtue of the fact that the nanofibers had a large surface area that promoted apatite deposition.

16.3.2 Polymers

16.3.2.1 Natural Polymers. Natural polymers such as collagen, gelatin, chitosan, alginate, hyaluronan, fibrin and silk are frequently used in bone tissue engineering[52-61]. For instance, electrospun silk fibroin fibers were subjected to an alternate soaking method for nucleation and growth of apatite[61]. The fibers were first immersed in a calcium solution, followed by immersion in phosphate solution. Mineralization was achieved as apatite preferentially grew along the longitudinal direction of the fibers. The silk fibroin and acidic peptides allowed the controlled nucleation and growth of apatite minerals on the fibers[61]. In a separate study, porous hyaluronan-based materials coated with fibronectin that were implanted in osteochondral defects in rabbits exhibited improved bone repair as compared to those without the implantation of the hyaluronan-based materials[59]. One of the drawbacks of natural polymers is the lack of mechanical properties. Therefore, extensive investigations have been carried out in fine-tuning the material selection and design.

16.3.2.2 Synthetic Polymers. Synthetic materials are gaining popularity as alternative options because scaling up in production terms is not an issue and they are mechanically better than natural materials. The commonly used synthetic polymers encompass poly(lactic-co-glycolic) acid (PLGA), poly-l-lactide acid (PLLA) and polycaprolactone (PCL)[62-66]. Polyglycolic acid (PGA) is often used in medical applications (such as sutures) because it is a degradable product, since glycolic acid is a natural metabolite. Glycolic acid can also be excreted out of the body as urine. Polylactic acid (PLA) is also used and it is generally more hydrophobic than PGA. PLA has three isomeric forms, namely: d(−), l(+), and racimic (d, l). Poly(l)LA and poly(d)LA are semi-crystalline solids and have similar degradation rates as PGA. In general, the (l) isomer of lactic acid (LA) is preferred because it can be metabolized in the body. The degradation rate of PCL is slower than that of PLA and is a suitable material for long-term, drug delivery systems. One of the disadvantages of biodegrabable synthetic polymers is the release of acidic by-productions during degradation[67]. Typically, a combination of ceramic-based materials is incorporated into the synthetic materials to aid in bone integration of the graft material to the native host tissue.

16.3.3 Nano-HA/Collagen-Based Composites

Calcium phosphate (CaP) coatings are commonly deposited on orthopedic implants to improve on the biological properties, especially at the bone-implant interface. Plasma spraying, laser deposition and ion beam deposition are some of the methods used to coat CaP on implants[68]. Studies have shown that nanoscale topography of materials favor cellular response. As such, the fabrication of nano-phase HA has been evident in recent years. Electrostatic spray deposition, or electrospraying of nano-HA, is one such method, whereby nano-HA particles were first synthesized via a precipitation reaction using calcium hydroxide ($Ca(OH)_2$) and orthophosphoric acid (H_3PO_4) with a Ca/P ratio of 1.67, similar to natural bone. Subsequently, the nano-HA particles were suspended in ethanol to form a ceramic slurry for electrospraying[69].

As natural bone is a nanocomposite, investigators explore the possibilities of fabricating nanocomposite materials to marry the properties of at least two individual materials. In the author's previous work, the auhtors have successfully fabricated a composite that can act as a guided tissue regeneration (GTR) membrane for periodontal therapy. This three-layered graded membrane consists of one face of the material made of 8% nano-carbonated hydroxyapatite/collagen/polylactic-co-glycolic acid (nCHAC/PLGA) porous membrane, the non-porous opposite face made of pure PLGA and the middle layer made of 4% nCHAC/PLGA. The porous membrane allowed cellular penetration and the non-porous side of the membrane inhibited cellular adhesion. The composite was fabricated via a layer-by-layer casting method. As all three layers consisted of PLGA, the composite exhibited sufficient flexibility and mechanical strength. The nCHAC had the same constituent and had a nano crystal size that was similar to that of natural bone. As such, it can act as a template for mineralization to take place, attracting bone cells to the bone graft site during bone remodeling. PLGA was the choice of polymer because it is biodegrabable *in vivo*, and bone cells can deposit the osteoblastic components within the porous, degradable polymer over time, allowing it to be a suitable bone tissue engineered material, improving bone-biomaterial interface[70]. Composites that do not contain collagen can be produced via a hot temperature method such as hot pressing. Recently, a biomimetic self-assembly method that has been developed is said to be suitable for fabricating collagen-containing composites because collagen degrades rapidly in environments higher than the body temperature of 37 °C. In this method, illustrated in Figure 16.2[71], Type I collagen was first dissolved in acetic acid. Aqueous solutions of Ca^{2+} and PO_4^- were added into the mixture for the initial nucleation of apatite. To adjust the pH of the solution, drops of sodium hydroxide were carefully added until the pH was approximately eight. At this time, calcium phosphates begin to co-precipitate with the collagen. The precipitates were aged for two hours. Nano-HA can be retrieved via centrifugation[72,73].

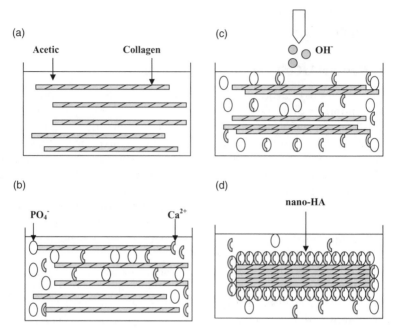

Figure 16.2. Biomimetic self-assembly method of producing nano-HA-collagen composite. (A): Type I collagen was dissolved in acetic acid. (B): Ca^{2+} and PO_4^- were added. (C) Drops of NaOH were incorporated into the solution for the co-precipitation of calcium phosphates with collagen. (D) Aging the precipitates for more than two hours. (E): Centrifugation of solution for the retrieval of nano-HA (not shown)[71] (Adapted from *Nanomedicine* (2006) 1(2), 177–188 with permission of Future Medicine Ltd.)

The nanoHA-collagen nanocomposite has nano-sized, bone-like apatite embedded in the collagen matrix. The three hierarchical levels—namely the calcified collagen fibrils, collagen molecules, and fibers—showcase an example of a self-assembly biomimetic material, where the crystallographic axes (*c*-axes) of the nano-HA crystals are intimately aligned with the longitudinal axes of the collagen fibrils. The nano-HA and collagen molecules co-precipitated into mineralized collagen fibrils are approximately 6 nm in diameter and 300 nm in length as shown in Figure 16.3[73]. The presence of this bone-like mineral is one of the prerequisites of good interfacial bonding with the orthopedic implants with the host's bone (i.e. osteoconductivity) and may trigger osteogenic differentiation of progenitor or bone cells (i.e. osteoinductivity). Table 16.3 summarizes the various types of nanocomposites and their respective cellular responses[70,72,74–86].

Although cell culture results were promising where osteoblasts adhered to the biomimetic nano-HA/collagen/PLA scaffold within two days of culture, subsequently proliferated within the pores of the materials and within a week, full confluence was achieved, the material was tested in an *in vivo* setting to evaluate its efficiency as a potential bone graft material[73]. A 15 mm segmental defect was

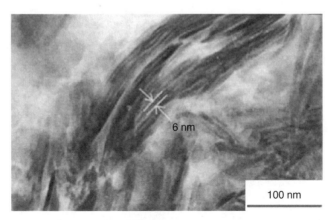

Figure 16.3. Transmission electron micrograph of a biomimetic self-assembly nano-HA/collagen composite.[73]

TABLE 16.3. Biomimetic Nano-HA/Collagen-based Composite for Bone Tissue Engineering

Nanocomposite	Cell/Growth factors	Tissue reactions	References
Nano-HA/Collagen	Osteogenic cells (*In vitro* and *in vivo*)	In a marrow cavity or bone fragment co-culture, interfacial bone formation at two weeks.	Refs[77,84,85]
Nano-HA/Collagen	Without/with BMP-2 (*In vivo*)	Resorbed by phagocytosis of osteoclast-like cells and form new bone in the surrounding area at 12 weeks.	Refs[75,76,81]
Nano-HA/Collagen	Chondroitin sulfate	No	Refs[74,80,83]
Nano-HA/Collagen/PLA	Osteoblasts (*In vitro*)	In-growth 400 μm depth of the porous scaffold.	Ref[79]
Nano-HA/Collagen/PLA	rhBMP-2 (*In vivo*)	8 weeks complete bone defect repair.	Refs[72,78]
Nano-carbonated HA/Collagen/PLGA	Osteoblasts (*In vitro*) (*In vivo*)	Enhance osteoblast and bone regeneration.	Refs[70,86]
Nano-HA/Collagen/Alginate	Fibroblasts/Osteoblasts (*In vitro*)	Positive affect on osteoblasts.	Ref[82]

made in the radius of 24 rabbits and the graft material was inserted into the defect with the incorporation of 0.5 mg of recombinant human bone morphogenetic protein-2 (rhBMP-2). Observations were made at 4, 8, 12 and 16 weeks, with six samples at each time point. Figure 16.4a shows the X-ray observation of the defect immediately after implantation. Figure 16.4b shows the X-ray result after 12 week of implantation where double cortical bone connection was formed. Histological

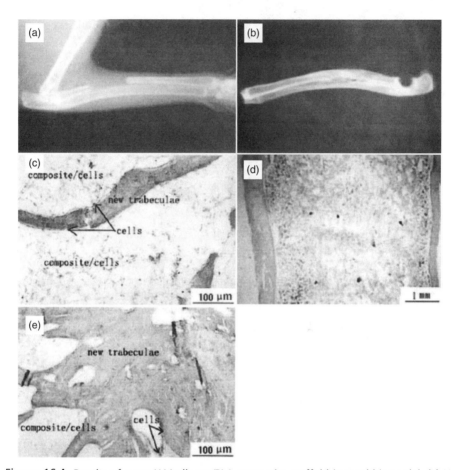

Figure 16.4. Results of nano-HA/collagen/PLA composite scaffold in a rabbit model. (a) X-ray result of defect immediately after implantation. (b) X-ray result after 12 weeks of post-implantation, where double cortical bone was connected. (c) Decalcified histology (Haematoxylin and Eosin or HE staining) at 8 weeks. (d) Histology (HE staining) at 12 weeks, with double cortical bone was connected completely, bone marrow and new trabeculae bone was formed in the vertex region. (e) Decalcified histology (HE staining) at 12 weeks, compare with (c) where more trabeculae bone was formed.[73] (See color insert.)

observation also indicated that within 12 weeks post-implantation, complete healing occurred and double cortical bone was connected to the defect (Figure 16.4d). Spherical cells adhered to the pores of the scaffold and appeared at the composite and new bone interface after eight weeks (Figure 16.4c). Trabeculae and bone marrow filled up the gaps left behind by the resorbed material. Figure 16.4e shows more trabeculae bone replacing the implant at 12 weeks than at eight weeks (Figure 16.4c).

The nano-HA/collagen/PLA composite did not give rise to any acidic by-products unlike pure PLA materials as the pH value of the culture media did not change, enabling cellular processes to take place. The authors postulated that the mineralized collagen may play a role in neutralizing the acidic PLA products[73]. The porous nature of the scaffold is a conducive environment for the deposition of bone matrix and mineralized collagen and may act as anchors for osteoblast adhesion. Further bone regeneration could be aided by the bone-cells in the scaffold[62,87,88]. Nutrient and waste transport are made possible via these pores as well. One study had reported that spinal fusion was achieved when rhBMP-2 in a collagen carrier was more homogeneous and underwent more remodeling than when rhBMP-2 was in an autograft regardless of the presence of a collagen carrier. In addition, the incorporation of rhBMP-2 led to a stiffer and stronger spinal fusion than those using autogenous grafts[89].

16.3.4 Nanofibrous Composites

Electrospun nanofibrous scaffolds were fabricated from a mixture of PCL, type I collagen and HA nanoparticles with an average fiber diameter of 180 ± 50 nm, characteristic of the collagen fiber bundle diameter of native bone. The presence of collagen in the nanofibers further improved the stiffness of the scaffold. In addition, the apatite particles were uniformly distributed on the fibers[90]. Electrospinning technology was also employed in producing hybrid membranes made of PLLA and HA. The presence of HA particles enhanced the tensile strength of the hybrid membranes and the increased elastic modulus and lower strain at failure were indicative of the fact that HA nanoparticles had made the nanofiber matrix stiffer and less plastic in deformation[91]. Table 16.4 shows some examples of various types of nanofibrous composites that have been successfully fabricated using electrospinning[92–96].

One of the advantages of nanofibrous scaffolds was that biomineralization was significantly enhanced on nanofibrous scaffolds than on solid-walled scaffolds[97]. Nanofibrous poly(L-lactic acid) (PLLA) scaffolds with interconnected pores were made using a phase separation method. Osteoblasts were seeded on the scaffolds and higher ALP activity and an earlier and enhanced expression of RUNX-2 protein and bone sialoprotein were observed on the nanofibrous scaffolds than on solid-walled scaffolds. In addition, the nanofibrous scaffolds seemed to promote the adsorption of proteins such as fibronectin and vitronectin as integrins associated with fibronectin ($\alpha v \beta 3$), vitronectin ($\alpha v \beta 3$) and collagen-binding ($\alpha 2 \beta 1$) were present at higher amounts than those grown on

TABLE 16.4. Electrospun Nanofibrous Composites with Calcium Salts

Calcium Salts (Nanoparticles)	Matrix	References
Hydroxyapatite	Polyhydroxybutyrate-co-valerate	Ref[92]
β-calcium phosphate	Polylactic acid	Ref[93]
Hydroxyapatite	Polycaprolactone	Ref[94]
Hydroxyapatite	Silk Fibroin	Ref[95]
Calcium carbonate	Polycaprolactone	Ref[96]

solid-walled scaffolds. These observations seemed to have an impact on osteo-blastic phenotype and cellular signaling, suggesting that nanofibrous materials were superior than solid-walled materials[97].

Improved mechanical properties and wettability were demonstrated on elec-trospun gelatin/PCL fibrous membranes than on pure gelatin or PCL membranes. Not only were bone marrow stromal cells favorably attached on the gelatin/PCL, but also the cells migrated into the scaffolds up to 114 µm after one week of culture[98].

16.3.5 Cell-Material Constructs (e.g. Stem Cell or Osteoblast/Material Constructs)

After material selection, factors such as the type of pre-treatment of the sub-strate, choice of cells to be seeded and culture environment (dynamic/static conditions, cyclic/static loading) have to be considered. To create a more favor-able environment for *in vivo* osteogenesis, many have attempted to pre-seed osteoblasts or MSCs on the bone-graft materials. Essentially, bone is made up of two main cell types, namely osteoblasts and osteoclasts. These bone cells, which are connected by gap junctions, allow cellular communications between the bone surface and the mineral matrix. Osteoblasts are involved in the production of Type I collagen and mineralization. The secretion of prostaglandin E_2 and inter-leukin-6 by osteoblasts stimulates osteoclasts, leading to bone resorption. In recent years, MSCs seem to be an attractive cell source because they are capable of differentiating into an osteoblastic lineage when induced in the appropriate conditions. The ECM secreted by MSCs can involved in several cellular processes such as the recruitment, proliferation, differentiation and maturation of progeni-tor cells. Physiologically, MSCs differentiates into mature matrix-secreting osteo-blasts, which progressively become osteocytes.

16.3.5.1 *Mesenchymal Stem Cells (MSCs)-Material Constructs.* For instance, coral, which has a natural architecture that resembles spongy bone, is said to be suitable as a bone graft material owing to its porosity (with an average pore size of 150 µm) because blood vessels and the deposition of the ECM and other cellular constituents can be intertwined within the graft, giving rise to an enhancement of material properties and stability. In this particular study, the authors have illustrated that the use of low level laser irradiation applied to a MSC/coral construct stimulated the proliferation and differentiation of MSC into an osteoblastic phenotype during the initial culture period and significantly induced *in vitro* osteogenesis over time. Higher levels of calcium deposition were seen in irradiated-treated samples at early (days three and six) and late culture periods (days 21 and 28).

On the other hand, phosphate deposition was enhanced in samples that were laser-treated in later culture periods (days 14, 21 and 28). The coral construct with MSC did not undergo laser irradiation. In addition, as an indicator of early osteo-blast differentiation, ALP activity was observed.

Laser-treated coral materials showed a significant level of ALP activity on day two of culture but at later culture stages (days 21 and 28), ALP activity was significantly reduced as compared to control samples. These results implied that low level laser irradiation quickens the differentiation of MSC into an osteoblastic phenotype during bone formation processes in early culture periods, whilst at later stages, cellular response and bone maintenance by osteocytes are predominant[99].

Mygind and co-workers studied the effect of different pore size of the coralline hydroxyapatite scaffolds and found out that scaffolds with an average pore size of 200 µm showed a greater rate of osteogenic differentiation based on increased ALP and enhanced expression of osteogenic markers such as osteocalcin, BMP-2, BSP-I (bone sialoprotein-I) and so on than a 500 µm pore-sized scaffold[100]. In this study, they had also showed that slightly fewer but more differentiated cells were found in the 200 µm pore-sized scaffold. These scaffolds reached full confluency more quickly than bigger pore-sized scaffolds, owing to a higher degree of cell-to-cell communication, resulting in a higher rate of osteoblastic differentiation.

On the other hand, a significant number of less-differentiated cells, that is, higher proliferation was associated with the bigger pore-sized scaffold, possibly due to its higher surface area to volume ratio, which could have facilitated cellular adhesion on day one of culture. Other probable reasons were that more cells are needed to fill up the voids in these bigger pore-sized scaffolds for 3D confluency, and that stimulated fluid flow aided in the proliferation process. By subjecting the constructs in a dynamic spinner flask as compared to a static cultivation, superior proliferation and differentiation of the cells within the scaffolds were observed, as seen in Figure 16.5. Osteoblast matrix production was more prominent in constructs that underwent dynamic cultivation[100].

Chastain et al. showed that MSCs isolated from adult bone marrow in 3D PLGA scaffolds expressed and maintained greater osteocalcin gene expression than in PCL over a period of five weeks. They hypothesized that the differential adsorption of certain ECM proteins in the serum-containing culture media and integrin-mediated attachment may be the reason of this difference. Type I collagen seemed to favor MSC adhesion to PLGA. However, vitronectin enhanced the attachment of MSC to PCL. Greater ALP activity was observed for the PLGA group after two weeks, suggesting osteogenesis was more predominant in the Type I collagen-mediated attachment of MSC to PLGA (more osteoconductive) than in vitronectin-mediated MSC attachment to PCL.

Chastain et al. acknowledged that the conformation and specific integrin-binding motifs in the ECM proteins and not just the identity of the ECM protein were some factors that modulated osteogenesis[101]. Other reasons for the preferential adsorption of the ECM proteins could be the wettability of the polymer, surface chemistry, nanotopography, and so on[102–105].

The MSCs fate to an osteogenic lineage was said to be dependent on certain cues, such as cell shape, which could be regulated by, for example, Rho A

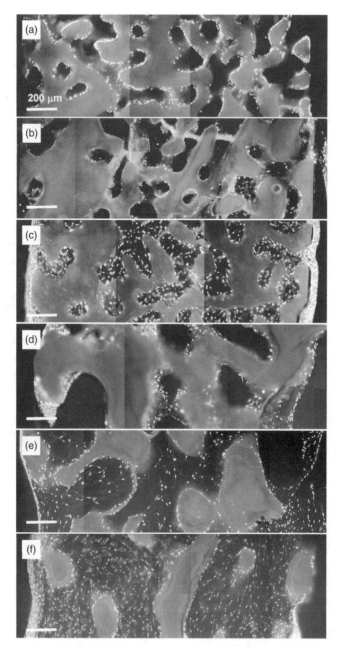

<u>Figure 16.5.</u> Hoechst-stained 20μm sections of the coral scaffold. Pictures taken from top to bottom of the scaffold at the central portion and merged using Photoshop software. (A) 200μm pore-sized scaffold at Day 1, (B) 200μm pore-sized scaffold at Day 21 with static cultivation, (C) 200μm pore-sized scaffold at Day 21 with dynamic cultivation, (D) 500μm pore-sized scaffold at Day 1, (E) 500μm pore-sized scaffold at Day 21 with static cultivation and (F) 500μm pore-sized scaffold at Day 21 with dynamic cultivation. Scale bar: 200μm.[100]

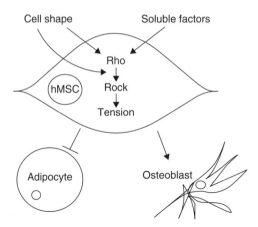

Figure 16.6. Cell shape, Rho A, Rock and cytoskeletal tension affects the fate of human MSCs (hMSCs) to an osteogenic or adipocytic lineage *in vitro*.[106]

modulation. Human MSCs (hMSCs) which were allowed to adhere and spread underwent osteogenesis. Local cues in the microenvironment and plating density were crucial for lineage-specific differentiation, as seen in the activation of the Rho A-Rock signaling pathway depicted in Figure 16.6[106].

16.3.5.2 Non-Mesenchymal Stem Cells (Non-MSCs)-Material Constructs.
Osteoblasts were seeded on hybrid membranes made of PLLA and HA. It was evident that the number of viable cells on PLLA/HA hybrid membranes was greater than that of those on pure PLLA membranes. This indicated that HA provided an osteoconductive environment for cell adhesion[91]. SaOS-2 osteoblast-like cells underwent biomineralization when cultured in the presence of multiphasic calcium phosphates that were synthesized via a self-propagating high temperature combustion synthesis (SHS) process, despite the fact that culture conditions favored cell quiescence[107]. Membrane vesicles with calcium phosphate and porous plate-like calcium phosphate structures were found to be adjacent to the cells. Pseudopodia and a flattened morphology of the cells were observed, suggesting that the cells had a normal metabolism and anchored to the heterogeneous calcium phosphates (mainly TCP and HA). The heterogeneous calcium phosphates had distinct crystalline regions as well as amorphous regions and the bulk porosity was spherical in nature. This heterogeneity and the hydrolysis of the amorphous phase resulted in the availability of calcium and phosphate that was said to have enhanced biomineralization[107].

Nanocrystalline silicon-substituted hydroxyapatite (SiHA) coatings on titanium (Ti) substrates were produced by magnetron co-sputtering and increased Si content resulted in decreased crystallite size[108]. There was a significant increase in osteoblast cell-growth density on coated SiHA Ti surfaces compared to uncoated Ti surfaces. It was observed that flattened cells were attached on the coated surfaces with enhanced ECM synthesis. Moreover, a distinct and well-defined cytoskeleton with actin stress fibers was present on coated surfaces, whereas on uncoated Ti surfaces, the actin filaments were not present in the cytoskeleton structure. Rapid bone mineralization was seen in those coatings with a high Si content (4.9 wt% Si) by Day 16 of culture. The draw-back of high Si content was that rapid dissolution of the coating was apparent because of the small HA crystal size; thus, the attachment of cells at very early stages may not be ideal. As such, it was found that 2.2 wt% Si was an ideal content for HA coatings[108].

16.3.6   Peptide-Based Materials

In tissue engineering, material design is of utmost importance. Attempts have been made to fabricate scaffolds to mimic the chemical composition and struc-tural properties of ECM because one would think that a tissue-engineered scaffold with these characteristics will have a better chance at enhancing tissue regeneration in the body. Structural proteins for example, collagen, are in the nanometer range and this nanotopography is said to affect cellular responses such as adhesion, proliferation, growth and differentiation. Since the native ECM is of a nanofibrous structure, several methods have been developed to make nanofibers or nanofibrous scaffolds, such as drawing, template synthesis, phase separation, self-assembly and electrospinning. Briefly, drawing involves a micropipette that is submersed in a droplet of solution and withdrawn to draw a fiber. In template synthesis, polymer is extruded through a porous mem-brane into a solidification solution for nanofiber formation. Phase separation is one method whereby separation of at least two different phases takes place, by the incorporation of polymer into a particular solvent; subsequently the freezing and freeze-drying processes give rise to a gel-like structure. For self-assembly method, smaller molecules act as building blocks to self-assemble fibers using specific bonds. Lastly, electrospinning uses a high voltage electric field to draw fibers out of a needle tip where the syringe is loaded with polymer solution[109–112].

In order to "coax" native cells to adhere to the biomaterials, so that the cells would not view the material as a "foreign" object, peptides design and develop-ment have been gaining much attention, because these peptides contain adhesion domains of the ECM, thereby they may have an impact on cell attachment, pro-liferation, and so on, and even inducing tissue formation.

Specifically, amphiphilic peptides with a carbon alkyl tail and other func-tional peptide motifs could be synthesized to form nanofibers via the self-assem-bly process[113,114]. Hosseinkhani et al. demonstrated that the incorporating MSC isolated from the femurs of rats into collagen sponge self-assembled peptide–amphiphile (PA) nanofiber hybrid scaffold in a bioreactor perfusion culture system had an impact on *in vitro* and *in vivo* osteogenic differentiation of the MSCs. The hybrid material that consists of a hydrogel (PA) and a sponge (collagen sponge reinforced with PGA fiber), when subjected in a perfusion culture or static culture, induced bone formation throughout the constructs, with

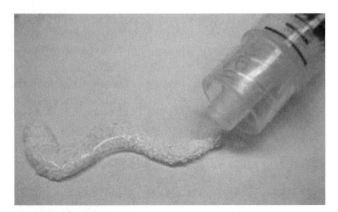

Figure 16.7. Anorganic bone mineral (ABM) embedded in hyaluronate hydrogel.[118]

those samples in the perfusion culture system exhibiting a greater and homogenous distribution of bone formation in a rat model. This was indicative that the flow velocity of the perfusion culture system accelerated the osteogenic differentiation of the MSCs[115].

A pivotal cell-binding domain of human Type I collagen located in the α-1 (I) chain sequence (P-15) has been studied[116,117]. The P-15 peptide was said to facilitate bone formation; therefore, this peptide had been used as a coating to mimic bone matrix components[118]. For instance, P-15 peptides were coated on anorganic bone mineral (ABM) particles and suspended in injectable hydrogels (such as hyaluronate (Hy) as seen in Figure 16.7, sodium alginate, carboxymethylcellulose) promoted cellular adhesion, osteoblastic activity, and mineral deposition. Preferential adhesion of osteoblast-like cells was observed on the hydrogels with P-15 peptide, with more cell coverage and scattering, suggestive that P-15 peptide also reinforced cellular migration. In the presence of P-15 peptide on ABM (with or without hydrogel), more actin and stress fibers were seen compared to ABM surfaces, which had little cell spreading and stress fibers, indicative of the adhesive properties of P-15 peptide. The upregulation of gene expression such as ALP, BMP-2 and BMP-7 after ten days of culture and mineralized matrix deposition after two weeks of culture in ABM/P-15/Hy were more prominent than those in ABM/Hy[118].

From the above-mentioned results, P-15 peptides seemed to stimulate bone repair and had a synergistic effect on osteogenic inductors such as BMPs. Studies have shown that BMPs and TGF-β interact with collagen to promote osteoblastic processes[119,120]. Instead of using reconstituted collagen, some advantages of P-15 peptide include minimal batch variations, possible large-scale production, ease of handling, greater stability, and so on[121,122]. One of the advantages of hydrogels is that they can be used in any bony defect, regardless of size and shape, although one must be cautious about cell viability, and the possibility of hampering cell migration may occur.

To improve the osteoinductive properties of bioceramics, grafting of RGD-containing (Arg-Gly-Asp) peptides on HA by silanization, cross-linking and thiol bonding were done to mediate cell attachment[123] via the ligand-receptor interactions with ECM proteins such as collagen, fibronectin, vitronectin, and laminin[124,125]. The argument of using smaller peptides was that these peptides were more resistant to proteolysis and possessed greater affinities to integrin receptors[123]. Biomolecules such as peptides, proteins, and other functional groups can be grafted onto the biomaterial's surface using plasma treatment without altering the construct's structural integrity and bulk properties, while improving the hydrophilicity of the material. Some have tried plasma-treatment as a form of surface modification on porous poly-l-lactic acid (PLLA) scaffolds to improve cell affinity[124]. A synthetic peptide derived from BMP-2 conjugated to a covalently cross-linked alginate gel was reported to show prolonged ectopic calcification, up to seven weeks in a rat model, inducing many osteoblast-like cells. Surprisingly, rhBMP-2 impregnated collagen gel showed maximum ectopic calcification after three weeks of implantation and the calcified products disappeared after five weeks. In addition, histological results showed that it induced several osteoclasts. Dense calcification was restricted in a particular region in the rhBMP-2 impregnated collagen gel, whereas the uniform calcification occurred in the BMP-2 peptide conjugated alginate gel. The results suggested that the peptide conjugated alginate gel had greater stability than the rhBMP-2 impregnated collagen gel[126]. It was postulated that MSCs from the muscle tissue (implant site in the rat model) could have migrated into the alginate gel and osteoblastic differentiation occurred after the stimulation of the BMP-2 derived synthetic peptide, subsequently osteoblasts released phosphorus ions and the carboxyl functional groups of the alginate gel stimulated apatite nucleation, with hydroxyapatite crystals being deposited on the gel[127]. Other synthetic peptides such as B2A2 which promoted rhBMP-2 bioactivity or B2A2-K-NS (an analog of B2A2) were said to augment osseous phenotypes in an osteoinductive environment[128,129].

16.3.7 Gene-Based Materials

Gene-based factor delivery systems can be designed in such a way that a gene encoding a target protein can be delivered. In this way, the upregulation and downregulation of a desired protein can be achieved. In bone repair, the upregulation of BMPs is generally favored.

One of the drawbacks of delivering osteoinductive growth factors from material constructs is that growth factors are easily degradable and material processing could potentially have destroyed them. Consequently, until now, there is no gold standard in terms of the optimal dose levels of growth factors to be added. By and large, the use of gene therapies in bone applications renders much attention as this facet of study provides an alternative option to bone repair. In essence, vectors are viral (such as retroviruses, adenoviruses, and so on) or non-viral (such as cationic lipid (CL) formulations and so on) tools that can be used for the delivery of recombinant proteins via the transfection, that is, transfer of DNA to the cell nucleus, applicable in both an *in vitro* or *in vivo* settings. For instance, the delivery of a gene encoding for an osteoinductive factor to target the cell-of-interest can galvanize the cells to produce the necessary factors at the location of bone pathology. The *in vivo* approach of gene therapy is to inject the genetically-modified vector or plasmid into the patient, although there might be interferences such as not being able to transfect the desired cell type or recombination with a wild-type vector. Alternatively, the patient's cells can be harvested and expanded *in vitro* prior to transfection before implantation. Nevertheless, this process is more cumbersome and time-consuming.

Bone marrow stromal cells that were isolated from rats were transfected with an adenovirus encoding cDNA for rhBMP-2 and seeded on PLGA/HA microspheres. In co-culture experiments (primary human MSCs and transfected cells), BMP-2 produced by the transfected cells promoted osteogenic differentiation and mineralization, with a significant increase in proliferation, ALP and calcium deposits than those MSCs which were co-cultured with non-transfected cells[130].

In another case, retrovirus encoding the CDNA for BMP-2 was used to transfect a murine stromal cell line and the transfected cells were cultured on the PLGA/HA material for a week. Results showed that the transfected cells attached onto the material and proliferation was seen. BMP-2 was continually expressed by the transfected cells. The material specimens were then implanted into the quadriceps muscle porch of severe combined immunedeficient (SCID) mice, with three sample groups namely PLGA/HA with $3\mu g$ of rhBMP-2 (positive control), PLGA/HA with BMP-2 producing W-20 cells, and PLGA/HA with non-transfected W-20 cells. No bone formation was observed in the PLGA/HA with non-transfected W-20 cells, whereas bone formation occurred in the PLGA/HA with the BMP-2 producing cells and PLGA/HA with rhBMP-2 groups, indicative of the potential application of retroviral gene transfer in concert with an appropriate material for bone regeneration[131].

Non-collagenous molecules in bone such as dentin matrix protein 1 (DMP1) has been reported to be involved in apatite nucleation[132,133]. Using genetically-engineered silk DMPI, combined with SBF treatment, calcium-deficient carbonated HA was formed. It was found that the carboxyl terminal domain of DMP1 induced HA nucleation. HA was absent in samples with no carboxyl terminal domains of the DMP1. Such studies showed that other macromolecules besides collagen were involved in HA nucleation and deposition[132].

Recombinant collagen technology has also been investigated extensively. It has been shown that recombinant human-like collagen synthesized from *Escherichia coli* (*E.coli*) underwent mineralization when the collagen was subjected to a series of chemical treatments involving $CaCl_2$ and NaH_2PO_4 solutions. Nano-HA crystals were deposited on the recombinant collagen fibrils, forming mineralized collagen fibers and the crystallographic *c*-axis alignment of the nano-HA crystals was parallel to the longitudinal axis of the collagen fibrils[134].

16.4 SOURCES OF STEM CELLS USED FOR BONE TISSUE ENGINEERING TO INCREASE OSTEOGENIC DIFFERENTIATION

In recent years, the rave on MSCs has been taking the scientific community by storm owing to its very nature of the cells. MSCs are non-hematopoetic stem cells which have the ability to become many tissues such as bone, adipose, cartilage, skin, muscle, tendon, and so on. MSCs can be derived from several sources and comprehensive studies have been done in hope of determining the ideal source of MSCs for bone applications as discussed in the subsequent sections of this chapter.

16.4.1 Adipose-Derived Stem Cells

Although for bone applications, bone marrow aspirates seem to be a "more" suitable choice for the extraction of stromal cells, the harvesting procedure for bone marrow is invasive and the number of stem cells from bone marrow varies from patient to patient, depending on medical condition and age. Bone marrow stromal cells can be as little as one in 10^7 to 10^8 cells[15]. The number of osteogenic progenitor cells found in bone marrow decreases from 66.2 ± 9.6 for every 10^6 cells in patients who are under 40 years of age. The number of these cells further decreases to 14.7 ± 2.6 per 10^6 cells in older patients[135]. In addition, the amount of bone marrow drawn from the patient is limited. To counter these issues, adipose tissue has been used as a source for stem cells as an enormous quantity of fatty tissue can be harvested. There are about 300 colonies per 100-mm dish for bone marrow samples and out of which one MSC per 33,000 nucleated cells are present[136]. In other studies, typically there are one MSC in every 50,000 or one MSC in every 100,000 nucleated cells, which constitute to about a few hundred MSCs for every milliliter of bone marrow[135,137]. The number of adherent bone marrow MSCs is about one in 10^5 nucleated cells[138]. For the confluency of bone marrow-derived stem cells plated between 20,000 to 400,000 cells/cm^2, it took about five to seven days[139,140]. Confluence was achieved within the same time period using the initial plating of 3,500 adipose derived stromal cells/cm^{2,141}.

Immortal adipose stromal cell lines (ATSCs) was developed by tranducing non-human primate-derived ATSCs with a retrovirus expressing TERT (catalytic protein subunit of the telomerase complex). The expression of TERT can be utilized for creating cell lines that can expand indefinitely while maintaining the multi-linage potential. The ATSC-TERT cells exhibited an increase level of telomerase activity and mean telomere length. These ATSC-TERT cells showed multi-lineage potential, on a lesser extent in untransduced cells *in vitro*. The duration of which calcium was produced by ATSC-TERT cells was greatly shortened (one week of culture), in comparison, calcium production occurred when native ATSCs was subjected to three to four weeks of culture in an osteogenic media. Enhanced expression of ostoblastic markers such as, osteoblast-specific factor 2, chondroitin sulfate proteoglycan etc. was associated with ATSC-TERT cells. These observations suggested that telomerase expression could open new avenues for bone repair[142]. The use of T-box (Tbx) factors—in particular, Tbx-3—was studied in human adipose tissue stromal cells (hADSCs) by using a lenti-virus si-RNA vector and it had proven that Tbx-3 played a role in proliferation and osteogenic differentiation of the stem cells[143].

16.4.2   Bone Marrow-Derived Stem Cells

Pittenger et al. indicated that by using stem cells from bone marrow aspirates from humans, the undifferentiated cells had the potential to differentiate into several lineages namely osteogenic, chodrogenic, adipocytic. When expanded to colonies, the multi-linage potential of the cells were maintained[17]. One study by Xin et al., showed that osteogenic and chondrogenic differentiation of human bone marrow derived stem cells when seeded on electrospun PLGA nanofiber scaffolds. The cells were treated with chondrogenic and osteogenic supplements. Figure 16.8 shows that in both 2D and 3D PLGA constructs, the cellular pheno-type *in vitro* after 14 days of cell seeding were retained[64].

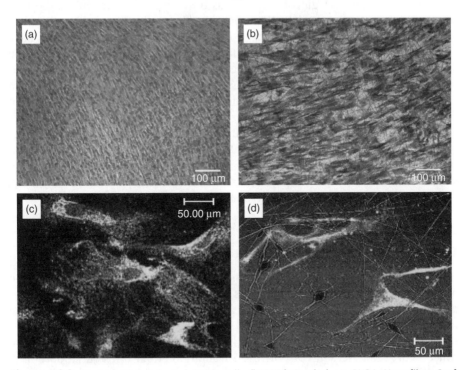

Figure 16.8. Human Mesenchymal Stem Cells (hMSCs) Seeded on PLGA Nanofiber Scaf-folds. (A) H&E staining showing hMSCs in 2D construct before trypsinization and cell seeding. (B) hMSCs on scaffold after Day 7. (C) hMSCs on 2D construct exhibited an elongated and spindle morphology at Day 14 as shown using a confocal microscope. (D) Attachment of hMSCs on 3D construct showed an elongated cellular morphology at Day 14 after cell seeding.[64]

hMSC from vertebral bodies cultured in serum-free conditions seemed to have preferential response to treatment with certain BMPs, with regards to osteo-induction. Amongst BMP-2, -4, -6 and -7, BMP-6 appeared to be a potent stimulus of osteoblastic differentiation and its gene expression was detected prior hMSC osteoblastic differentiation. The incorporation of BMP-6 to hMSC promoted the expression of osteoblastic genes such as Type I collagen, osteocalcin and bone sialoprotein. Furthermore, it stimulated key osteoblastic transcription factors such as cbfa-1/RUNX-2 and osterix. The synergistic effects led to an enhanced mineralization of extracellular matrix and hydroxyapatite deposition. It was shown that osteogenic growth factors such as IGF-1, β-fibroblast growth factor (β-FGF) and VEGF did not have direct osteoinductive effects on hMSC under serum-free media conditions. It was suggested that the above-mentioned growth factors, while essential in the function of osteoblasts or pre-osteoblasts and skeletal development, may not be sufficient in osteoblastic hMSC differentiation[144]. In a separate study, Boden and his colleagues showed that BMP-6 stimulates induced differentiation readily in rat calvarial cells, without glucocorticoid potentiation[145]. Similarly, the upregulation of BMP-6 production in rat calvarial cells in the presence of glucocorticoid was observed[144,146]. Conversely, the lack of sensitivity to BMP-2 and BMP-4 could be due to the expression of several families of secreted BMP antagonists, of which these antagonists could have a high affinity to BMP-2 and BMP-4, hindering their signaling, unlike BMP-6 and BMP-7 with a lower affinity to the antagonists[144]. Another explanation as to the lack of responsiveness of MSCs to certain BMPs could be due to a dose-dependant issue at which higher doses were essential for the induction of differentiation[147].

Surface chemistry was said to influence the MSC behavior with silane-modified surfaces as substrate materials in both basal and stimulated conditions[148], leading to the importance of studying the minute details of material science such as surface area, porosity, local acidification, degradation properties, and so on. This phenomenon also pertains to other cell types.

16.4.3   MSCs Derived from Other Sources

Umbilical cord blood (UCB), periosteum, synovium and muscle tissues are some of the alternate sources whereby MSCs can be derived[149–152]. Kern et al. delved the characteristics of three different tissues (UCB, bone marrow, and adipose tissue) as a human source of MSCs. There were no significant differences when morphology (fibroblastoid) and immune phenotype of the MSCs were concerned. All these sources portrayed a multipotential differentiation ability with the capability of formation of colony-forming unit-fibroblast (CFU-F) and expression of a set of surface proteins (e.g. CD44, CD73, CD29, CD90, HLA-1). The success rate of isolating MSCs was 100% for both the bone marrow and the adipose tissue samples. Conversely, the isolation rate for umbilical cord blood was 63%[149].

This observation could be attributed to the fact that the MSCs may be circulating in the prenatal organism and residing in tissues of the adult[153]. UCB showed the lowest colony frequency and contrary to adipose tissue with the highest colony frequency[149]. MSCs from UCB showed the longest culture period and the highest proliferation ability; MSCs from bone marrow had the shortest culture period and lowest proliferation ability. Another noteworthy point to be elaborated upon was that MSCs from UCB did not show adipogenic differentiation capacity, unlike those MSCs from bone marrow and adipose tissue, which showed osteogenic, chondrogenic, and adipogenic differentiation[149]. With regards to this, it is debated that a hierarchical or restricted differentiation capability of MSCs may be possible[17,154]. The proliferation rates of bone marrow, adipose and periosteum were similar after four, seven and eleven days of culture in a separate study. Osteogenic and chondrogenic differentiation were achieved in all the MSCs. Using a rabbit model, the authors demonstrated that bone-marrow and periosteum-derived MSCs had superior physeal arrest over adipose-derived MSCs[150].

For the comparative studies between bone marrow, adipose tissue, synovium, periosteum and skeletal muscle, bone marrow samples generated the greatest extent of calcification, followed by synovium, periosteum, adipose and muscle samples. For bone marrow samples, the colony number for every 10^3 nucleated cells was lower and cell number per colony was greater as compared to other tissue sources. The number of nucleated cells ($\times 10^3$) per volume or weight of tissue obtained was as follows: bone marrow (2045 ± 920), adipose tissue (22 ± 21), synovium (3 ± 4), periosteum (3 ± 6) and muscle (2 ± 1). Similarity in epitope profiles were found regardless of the tissue source[152]. A study also conducted on the immunological properties of bone marrow stromal cells and adipose tissue derived MSCs and concluded that their properties were maintained during pre- and post-osteogenic induction *in vitro* and seemed to be similar in both tissues[155].

16.5 CURRENT PERSPECTIVE

Advanced technologies are required in order to develop a hierarchical-assembled bone-like composite over several length scales for bone tissue applications. Room temperature fabrication techniques need further honing as biomimetic materials usually contain cells, proteins, growth factors and the like, and operating temperature is pivotal in their survival and integrity of the osteoblastic processes. The interplay between proteins, cells and materials renders further probing and understanding, so that these nuggets of knowledge can be translated into modulating biological pathways that are favorable for bone regeneration. Other critical issues involves maintaining sufficient material construct *in vivo* before osteogenesis can successfully take place, adequate material properties—especially in load-bearing sites—desirable material surface properties for the attraction of cells at the material-graft interface, amenability to contouring for implantation in different sizes and shapes of bony defects. Lastly, the graft has to support angiogenesis and vascularization for healing and bone remodeling.

Another noteworthy issue to address is that biological pathways are complex and the gene expression studies of certain bone markers may not project a holistic overview or analysis of the differentiation of progenitor or stem cells derived from various sources. As such, the choice of cells to be seeded on the graft materials based on preliminary gene expression results must always be tested in an *in vivo* setting, in order to fully evaluate the reliability of the cell-material construct. Current work on biological pathways is just a tip of the iceberg and still nebulous, as the portrayal of the evidence changes. Despite many studies that have shown promising results and have opened avenues for further evaluation, the intricate molecular interplay between growth factors, cells, proteins need to be extensively reviewed before synergistic cocktails can be formulated for effective bone formation.

Stem cell work needs to be investigated more thoroughly for the advancement of regenerative medicine in bone applications. The contributing factors that led to the conflicting results of the isolation, proliferative, and differentiation potential of MSCs derived from various sources can be elucidated by the fact that there are different tissue-harvesting techniques (which may be surgeon-dependent or donor-site dependent) as well as MSCs isolation methods that are employed. The amount of tissue harvested is another consideration when dealing with MCS numbers. Furthermore, patient variability such as age, gender and medical condition can impinge data consistency across the board[137,152]. Moreover, the scientific community needs to convince the general public of the notion of viral or gene delivery approaches in order for these options to be utilized clinically. Ideally, corroborative or contradictory evidence must be addressed, or, when necessary, reconciled to increase public confidence in these areas.

16.6 CONCLUSION

In conclusion, efficacious bone regeneration using tissue-engineered constructs loaded with factors that create a favorable environment *in vivo* can revolutionize the clinical management of bone-related diseases and orthopedic applications.

Suitable culture supplements such as dexamethasone, ascorbic acid, β-glycerophosphate, and so on, induced the proliferation and differentiation of several cell types. From the various studies, the functional property of nano-HA over conventional bioceramics such as TCP is favorable to cellular response. Material selection is also vital for the success of the tissue-engineered construct. One must weigh the pros and cons of both synthetic and natural polymers and decide which are deemed as the more important material properties needed to achieve the desired construct. Biomimetic mineralization of nanofibrous composites, especially those made of collagen and nano-HA, seemed to be promising because collagen and nano-HA are the main components of native bone. In addition, mineralization is more evident in nanofibrous scaffolds than in solid-walled scaffolds. Such nanofibrous scaffolds can be fabricated via an electrospinning technology. One of the disadvantages of electrospinning is the problem of scale-up production and much work is needed in this area in order to commercialize such scaffolds for bone repair.

MSCs from bone marrow are typically favored in bone repair, although results obtained from the use of MSCs from other sources have shown that these cells are in no way inferior to that of bone-marrow derived MSCs. The cascade of the orchestrated processes of gene expression in biological pathways renders further investigation so that the interplay between the various biomolecules and proteins can be understood. This would greatly facilitate the material selection and the choice of growth factors and biomolecules to be incorporated into the material constructs.

It is conceivable that such tissue-engineered nano-materials will be the new generation of bone grafts, judging from the nascent state of regenerative medicine, fulfilling the desired characteristics (for example, material chemistry, surface area, mechanical integrity, angiogensis, optimal concentration of cells residing in the material, potential for possible drug delivery, and so on) of an ideal bone graft in terms of osteoconductivity, osteoinductivity and osteogenicity. Due to the complexity of bone regeneration, the ideal delivery system needs to address several issues such as the controlled release of biomolecules from the carrier material and structural similarity as natural bone.

REFERENCES

1. Woolf AD. The Bone and Joint Decade 2000–2010. Ann Rheum Dis 59, 81–82. 2000.
2. Siris ES. Paget's Disease of Bone. J Bone Miner Res 13(7), 1061–1065. 1998.
3. Engelbert RH, Pruijs HE, Beemer FA, Helders PJ. Osteogenesis Imperfecta in Childhood: Treatment Strategies. Arch Phys Med Rehabil 79, 1590–1594. 1998.
4. Johnson EE, Urist MR. Human bone morphogenetic protein allografting for reconstruction of femoral nonunion. Clin Orthop 371, 61–74. 2000.
5. Johnson EE, Urist MR, Finerman GA. Repair of segmental defects of the tibia with cancellous bone grafts augmented with human bone morphogenetic protein. A preliminary report. Clin Orthop 236, 249–257. 1998.
6. Johnson EE, Urist MR, Finerman GA. Bone morphogenetic protein augmentation grafting of resistant femoral nonunions. A preliminary report. Clin Orthop 230, 257–265. 1998.
7. Morone MA, Boden SD. Experimental posterolateral lumbar spinal fusion with a demineralized bone matrix gel. Spine 23, 159–167. 1998.
8. Peterson B, Whang PG, Iglesias R, Wang, JC, Lieberman JR. Osteoinductivity of Commercially Available Demineralized Bone Matrix. Preparations in a Spine Fusion Model. J Bone Joint Surg Am 86, 2243–2250. 2004.
9. Vallet-Regi M. Ceramics for medical applications. J Chem Soc Dalton Trans 100, 97–108. 2001.
10. Landis WJ, Song MJ, Leith A. Mineral and organic matrix interaction in normally calcifying tendon visualized in three dimensions by high-voltage electron microscopic tomography and graphic image reconstruction. J Struct Biol 110, 39–54. 1993.

11. Woo KM, Chen VJ, Ma PX. Nano-fibrous scaffolding architecture selectively enhances protein adsorption contributing to cell attachment. J Biomed Mater Res 67(A), 531–537. 2003.

12. Liu P, Oyajobi BO, Russell RG, Scutt A. Regulation of osteogenic differentiation of human bone marrow stromal cells: interaction between transforming growth factor-beta and 1,25(OH)(2) vitamin D(3) *In vitro*. Calcif Tissue Int 65(2), 173–180. 1999.

13. Beck GR Jr., Zerler B, Moran E. Phosphate is a specific signal for induction of osteopontin gene expression. Proc Natl Acad Sci U S A 97(15), 8352–8357. 2000.

14. Fujita T, Izumo N, Fukuyama R, Meguro T, Nakamuta H, Kohno T, Koida M. Phosphate provides an extracellular signal that drives nuclear export of Runx2/Cbfa1 in bone cells. Biochem Biophys Res Commun 280(1), 348–352. 2001.

15. Reyes M, Verfaillie CM. Characterization of multipotent adult progenitor cells, a subpopulation of mesenchymal stem cells. Ann N Y Acad Sci 938, 231. 2001.

16. Nuttelman CR, Tripodi MC, Anseth KS. Dexamethasone-functionalized gels induce osteogenic differentiation of encapsulated hMSCs. J Biomed Mater Res A 76(1), 183–195. 2006.

17. Pittenger MF, Mackay AM, Beck SC, Jaiswal RK, Douglas R, Mosca JD, Moorman MA, Simonetti DW, Craig S, Marshak DR. Multilineage Potential of Adult Human Mesenchymal Stem Cells. Science 284, 143. 1999.

18. Peter SJ, Liang CR, Kim DJ, Widmer MS, Mikos AG. Osteoblastic phenotype of rat marrow stromal cells cultured in the presence of dexamethasone, beta-glycerolphosphate, and Lascorbicacid. J Cell Biochem 71, 55–62. 1998.

19. Atmani H, Audrain C, Mercier L, Chappard D, Basle MF. Phenotypic effects of continuous or discontinuous treatment with dexamethasone and/or calcitriol on osteoblasts differentiatedfrom rat bone marrow stromal cells. J Cell Biochem 85, 640–650. 2002.

20. Jørgensen NR, Henriksen Z, Sørensen OH, Civitelli R. Dexamethasone, BMP-2, and 1,25-dihydroxyvitamin D enhance a more differentiated osteoblast phenotype: validation of an *in vitro* model for human bone marrow-derived primary osteoblasts. Steroids 69, 219–226. 2004.

21. Taira M, Nakao H, Takahashi J, Araki Y. Effects of two vitamins, two growth factors and dexamethasone on the proliferation of rat bone marrow stromal cells and osteoblastic MC3T3-E1 cells. J Oral Rehabil 30, 697–701. 2003.

22. Shui C, Scutt AM. Mouse Embryo-Derived NIH3T3 Fibroblasts Adopt an Osteoblast-Like Phenotype When Treated With 1a,25-Dihydroxyvitamin D3 and Dexamethasone In-vitro. J Cell Physiol 193, 164–172. 2002.

23. Gupta A, Leong DT, Bai HF, Singh SB, Lim TC, Hutmacher DW. Osteo-maturation of adipose-derived stem cells required the combined action of vitamin D3, β-glycerophosphate, and ascorbic acid. Biochem Biophys Res Commun 362, 17–24. 2007.

24. Luu HH, Song WX, Luo X, Manning D, Luo J, Deng ZL, Sharff KA, Montag AG, Haydon RC, He TC. Distinct Roles of Bone Morphogenetic Proteins in Osteogenic Differentiation of Mesenchymal Stem Cells. J Orthop Res 25(5), 665–677. 2007.

25. Nordsletten L. Recent developments in the use of bone morphogenetic protein in orthopaedic trauma surgery. Curr Med Res Opin S13–S17: S23. 2006.

26. Groeneveld EH, Burger EH. Bone morphogenetic proteins in human bone regeneration. Eur J Endocrinol 142, 9–21. 2000.

27. Diefenderfer DL, Osyczka AM, Reilly GC, Leboy PS. BMP responsiveness in human mesenchymal stem cells. Connect Tissue Res 44 (Suppl 1), 305–311. 2003.

28. Lane JM. BMPs: why are they not in everyday use? J Bone Joint Surg Am 83A (Suppl 1), S161–S163. 2001.

29. Service RF. Tissue engineers build new bone. Science 289, 1498–1500. 2000.

30. Huang YC, Kaigler DK, Rice KG, Krebsbach PH, Mooney DJ. Combined angiogenic and osteogenic factor delivery enhances bone marrow stromal cell-driven bone regeneration. J Bone Miner Res 20, 848–857. 2005.

31. Hsu HP, Zanella JM, Peckham SM, Spector M. Comparing ectopic bone growth induced by rhBMP-2 on an absorbable collagen sponge in rat and rabbit models. J Orthop Res 24, 1660–1669. 2006.

32. Simmons CA, Alsberg E, Hsiong S, Kim WJ, Mooney DJ. Dual growth factor delivery and controlled scaffold degradation enhance *in vivo* bone formation by transplanted bone marrow stromal cells. Bone 35, 562–569. 2004.

33. Welch RD, Jones AL, Bucholz RW, Reinert CM, Tjia JS, Pierce WA, Wozney JM, Li XJ. Effect of recombinant human bone morphogenetic protein-2 on fracture healing in a goat tibial fracture model. J Bone Miner Res 13, 1483–1490. 1998.

34. Yamamoto M, Takahashi Y, Tabata Y. Enhanced bone regeneration at a segmental bone defect by controlled release of bone morphogenetic protein-2 from a biodegradable hydrogel. Tissue Eng 12, 1305–1311. 2006.

35. Sumner DR, Turner TM, Urban RM, Leven RM, Hawkins M, Nichols EH, McPherson JM, Galante JO. Locally delivered rhTGF-beta2 enhances bone ingrowth and bone regeneration at local and remote sites of skeletal injury. J Orthop Res 19, 85–94. 2001.

36. Srouji S, Rachmiel A, Blumenfeld I, Livne E. Mandibular defect repairby TGF-beta and IGF-1 released from a biodegradable osteoconductive hydrogel. J Craniomaxillofac Surg 33, 79–84. 2005.

37. Maissen O, Eckhardt C, Gogolewski S, Glatt M, Arvinte T, Steiner A, Rahn B, Schlegel U. Mechanical and radiological assessment of the influence of rhTGFbeta-3 on bone regeneration in a segmental defect in the ovine tibia: pilot study. J Orthop Res 24, 1670–1678. 2006.

38. Kaigler D, Wang Z, Horger K, Mooney DJ, Krebsbach PH. VEGF scaffolds enhance angiogenesis and bone regeneration in irradiated osseous defects. J Bone Miner Res 21, 735–744. 2006.

39. Yoshida Y, von Bubnoff A, Ikematsu N, Blitz IL, Tsuzuku JK, Yoshida EH, Umemori H, Miyazono K, Yamamoto T, Cho KWY. Tob proteins enhance inhibitory Smad-receptor interactions to repress BMP signaling. Mech Dev 120, 629–637. 2003.

40. Gaur T, Lengner CJ, Hovhannisyan H, Bhat RA, Bodine PVN, Komm BS, Javed A, van Wijnen AJ, Stein JL, Stein GS, Lian JB, Canonical WNT. Signaling Promotes Osteogenesis by Directly Stimulating Runx2 Gene Expression. J Biol Chem 280(39), 33132–33140. 2005.

41. Shindo K, Kawashima N, Sakamoto K, Yamaguchi A, Umezawa A, Takagi M, Katsube K, Suda H. Osteogenic differentiation of the mesenchymal progenitor cells, Kusa is suppressed by Notch signaling. Exp Cell Res 290, 370–380. 2003.

42. Woodruff MA, Rath SN, Susanto E, Haupt LM, Hutmacher DW, Nurcombe V, Cool SM. Sustained release and osteogenic potential of heparansulfate-doped fibrin glue scaffolds within a rat cranial model. J Mol Hist 38(5), 425–433. 2007.

43. Babensee JE, McIntyre LV, Mikos AG. Growth factor delivery for tissue engineering. Pharm Res 17, 497–504. 2000.

44. Zhang X, Sobue T, Hurley MM. FGF-2 increases colonyformation, PTH receptor, and IGF-1 mRNA in mouse marrow stromal cells. Biochem Biophys Res Commun 290, 526–531. 2002.

45. Freed LE, Guilak F, Guo EX, Gray ML, Tranquillo R, Holmes JW, Radisic M, Sefton MV, Kaplan D, Vunjak-Novakovic V. Advanced Tools for Tissue Engineering: Scaffolds, Bioreactors, and Signaling. Tissue Eng 12, 3285–3305. 2006.

46. Kim HW, Kim HE. Nanofiber generation of hydroxyapatite and fluro-hydroxyapatite bioceramics. J Biomed Mater Res (B): App Biomater 77B, 323–328. 2006.

47. Marie PJ, De Vernejoul MC, Lomri A. Stimulation of bone formation in osteoporosis patients treated with fluoride associated with increased DNA synthesis by osteoblastic cells *in vitro*. J Bone Miner Res 7, 103–113. 1992.

48. de Leeuw NH. Resisting the onset of hydroxy-apatite dissolution through the incorporation of fluoride. J Phys Chem B 108, 1809–1811. 2004.

49. Ramay HRR, Zhang M. Biphasic calcium phosphate nanocomposite porous scaffolds for load-bearing bone tissue engineering. Biomaterials 25, 5171–5180. 2004.

50. Gibson LJ. The mechanical behaviour of cancellous bone. Biomechanics 18, 317–328. 1985.

51. Xia W, Zhang D, Chang J. Fabrication and in vitro biomineralization of bioactive glass (BG) nanofibres. Nanotechnology 18, 1–7. 2007.

52. Zhang W, Liao SS, Cui FZ. Hierarchical Self-Assembly of Nano-Fibrils in Mineralized Collagen. Chem Mater 15, 3221–3226. 2003.

53. Zhang W, Huang ZL, Su-San L, Cui FZ. Nucleation Sites of Calcium Phosphate Crystals during Collagen Mineralization. J Am Ceram Soc 86(6), 1052–1054. 2003.

54. Malafaya PB, Pedro AJ, Peterbauer A, Gabriel C, Redl H, Reis RL. Chitosan particles agglomerated scaffolds for cartilage and osteochondral tissue engineering approaches with adipose tissue derived stem cells. J Mater Sci Mater Med 16, 1077–1085. 2005.

55. Awad HA, Wickham MQ, Leddy HA, Gimble JM, Guilaka F. Chondrogenic differentiation of adipose-derived adult stem cells in agarose, alginate, and gelatin scaffolds. Biomaterials 25, 3211–3222. 2004.

56. Shih YRV, Chen CN, Tsai SW, Wang YJ, Lee OK. Growth of Mesenchymal Stem Cells on Electrospun Type I Collagen Nanofibers. Stem Cells 24, 2391–2397. 2006.

57. Oliveira JM, Rodrigues MT, Silva SS, Malafaya PB, Gomes ME, Viegas CA, Dias IR, Azevedo JT, Mano JF, Reis RL. Novel hydroxyapatite/chitosan bilayered scaffold for osteochondral tissue-engineering applications: Scaffold design and its performance when seeded with goat bone marrow stromal cells. Biomaterials 27 27, 6123–6137. 2006.

58. Karp JM, Sarraf F, Shoichet MS, Davies JE. Fibrin-filled scaffolds for bone-tissue engineering: An *in vivo* study. J Biomed Mater Res 71A (1), 162–171. 2004.

59. Solchaga LA, Yoo JU, Lundberg M, Dennis JE, Huibregtse BA, Goldberg VM, Caplan AI. Hyaluronan-based Polymers in the Treatment of Osteochondral Defects. J Orthop Res 18(5), 773–780. 2000.

60. Marolt D, Augst A, Freed LE, Vepari C, Fajardo R, Patel N, Gray M, Farley M, Kaplan D, Vunjak-Novakovic G. Bone and cartilage tissue constructs grown using human bone marrow stromal cells, silk scaffolds and rotating bioreactors. Biomaterials 27, 6138–6149. 2006.

61. Li C, Jin HJ, Botsaris GD, Kaplan DL. Silk apatite composites from electrospun fibers. J Mater Res 20(12), 3374–3384. 2005.

62. Ishaug SL, Crane GM, Miller MJ. Bone formation by three dimensional stromal osteoblast culture in biodegrable polymer scaffolds. J Biomed Mater Res 36, 17–28. 1997.

63. Williams JM, Adewunmi A, Schek RM, Flanagan CL, Krebsbach PH, Feinberg SE, Hollister SJ, Das S. Bone tissue engineering using polycaprolactone scaffolds fabricated via selective laser sintering. Biomaterials 26(23), 4817–4827. 2005.

64. Xin X, Hussain M, Mao JJ. Continuing differentiation of human mesenchymal stem cells and induced chondrogenic and osteogenic lineages in electrospun PLGA nanofiber scaffold. Biomaterials 28, 316–325. 2007.

65. Ciapetti G, Ambrosio L, Marletta G, Baldini N, Giunti A. Human bone marrow stromal cells: *In vitro* expansion and differentiation for bone engineering. Biomaterials 27, 6150–6160. 2006.

66. Liao SS, Cui FZ. *In Vitro* and *in Vivo* Degradation of Mineralized Collagen-Based Composite Scaffold: Nanohydroxyapatite/Collagen/Poly(L-lactide). Tissue Eng 10, 73–80. 2004.

67. Gunatillake PA, Adhikari R. Biodegradable synthetic polymers for tissue engineering. Euro Cell Mat 5, 1–16. 2003.

68. Christenson EM, Anseth KS, van den Beucken JJJP, Chan CK, Ercan B, Jansen JA, Laurencin CT, Li WJ, Murugan R, Nair LS, Ramakrishna S, Tuan RS, Webster TJ, Mikos AG. Nanobiomaterial Applications In Orthopaedics. J Orthop Res 25, 11–22. 2007.

69. Huang J, Jayasinghe SN, Best SM, Edirisinghe MJ, Brooks RA, Bonfield W. Electrospraying of a nano-hydroxyapatite suspension. Journal of Materials Science M 39, 1029–1032. 2004.

70. Liao S, Wang W, Uo M, Ohkawa S, Akasaka T, Tamura K, Cui FZ, Watari F. A three-layered nano-carbonated hydroxyapatite/collagen/PLGA composite membrane for guided tissue regeneration. Biomaterials 26, 7564–7571. 2005.

71. Chan CK, Sampath Kumar TS, Liao S, Murugan R, Ngiam M, Ramakrishna S. Biomimetic Nanocomposites for Bone Graft Applications. Nanomedicine 1(2), 177–188. 2006.

72. Liao S, Watari F, Uo M, Ohkawa S, Tamura K, Wang W, Cui FZ. The Preparation and Characteristics of a Carbonated Hydroxyapatite/Collagen Composite at Room Temperature. J Biomed Mater Res B Appl Biomater 74(2), 817–821. 2005.

73. Liao SS, Cui FZ, Zhang W, Feng QL. Hierarchically Biomimetic Bone Scaffold Materials: Nano-HA/Collagen/PLA Composite. J Biomed Mater Res B Appl Biomater 69(2), 158–165. 2004.

74. Rhee SH, Suetsugu Y, Tanaka J. Biomimetic configurational arrays of hydroxyapatite nanocrystals on bio-organics. Biomaterials 22, 2843–2847. 2001.

75. Kikuchi M, Ikoma T, Itoh S, Matsumoto HN, Koyama Y, Takakuda K, Shinomiya K, Tanaka J. Biomimetic synthesis of bone-like nanocomposites using the

self-organization mechanism of hydroxyapatite and collagen. Comp Sci Technol 64(6), 819–825. 2004.

76. Itoh S, Kikuchi M, Koyama Y, Takakuda K, Shinomiya K, Tanaka J. Development of a hydroxyapatite/collagen nanocomposite as a medical device. J Cell Transplant 13(4), 451–461. 2004.

77. Du C, Cui FZ, Zhang W, Feng QL, Zhu XD, de Groot K. Formation of calcium phosphate/collagen composites through mineralization of collagen matrix. J Biomed Mater Res 50, 518–527. 2000.

78. Liao SS, Guan K, Cui FZ, Shi SS, Sun TS. Lumbar Spinal Fusion With a Mineralized Collagen Matrix and rhBMP-2 in a Rabbit Model. Spine 28(17), 1954–1960. 2003.

79. Liao SS, Cui FZ, Zhu Y. Osteoblasts Adherence and Migration through Three-dimensional Porous Mineralized Collagen Based Composite: nHAC/PLA. J Bioact Comp Pol 19, 117. 2004.

80. Rhee SH, Tanaka J. Self-assembly phenomenon of hydroxyapatite nanocrystals on chondroitin sulfate. J Mater Sci Mater Med 13, 597–600. 2002.

81. Kikuchi M, Itoh S, Ichinose S, Shinomiya K, Tanaka J. Self organization mechanism in a bone-like hydroxyapatite/collagen nanocomposite synthesized *in vitro* and its biological reaction *in vivo*. Biomaterials 22, 1705–1711. 2001.

82. Zhang SM, Cui FZ, Liao SS, Zhu Y, Han L. Synthesis and biocompatibility of porous nano-hydroxyapatite/collagen/alginate composite. J Mater Sci: Mater Med 14, 1–5. 2003.

83. Rhee SH, Tanaka J. Synthesis of a hydroxyapatite/collagen/chondroitin sulphate nanocomposite by a novel precipitation method. J Am Ceram Soc 84(2), 459–461. 2001.

84. Du C, Cui FZ, Zhu XD, de Groot K. Three-dimensional nano-HAp/collagen matrix Loading with osteogenic cells In organ culture. J Biomed Mater Res 44, 407–415. 1999.

85. Du C, Cui FZ, Feng QL, Zhu XD, de Groot K. Tissue response to nano-hydroxyapatite/collagen composite implants in marrow cavity. J Biomed Mater Res 42, 540–548. 1998.

86. Liao S, Yokoyama A, Wang W, Zhu Y, Watari F, Ramakrishna S, Chan C. In-vitro and In-vivo behaviors of the Three Layered Nano-carbonated Hydroxyapatite/Collagen/ PLGA Composite Membrane. J Bioactive Compat Polym in Press. 2006.

87. Jones SJ, Boyde A. The migration of osteoblasts. Cell Tissue Res 184, 197–182. 1977.

88. Du C, Su XW, Cui FZ, Zhu XD. Morphological behaviour of osteoblasts on diamond-like carbon coating and amorphous C-N film in organ culture. Biomaterials 19, 651–658. 1998.

89. Schimandle JH, Boden SD, Hutton WC. Experimental spinal fusion with recombinant human bone morphogenetic protein-2. Spine 20, 1326–1337. 1995.

90. Catledge SA, Clem WC, Shrikishen N, Chowdhury S, Stanishevsky AV, Koopman M, Vohra YK. An electrospun triphasic nanofibrous scaffold for bone tissue engineering. Biomed Mater 2, 142–150. 2007.

91. Sui G, Yang X, Mei F, Hu X, Chen G, Deng X, Ryu S. Poly-L-lactic acid/hydroxyapatite hybrid membrane for bone tissue regeneration. J Biomed Mater Res 82A, 445–454. 2007.

92. Ito Y, Hasuda H, Kamitakahara M, Ohtsuki C, Tanihara M, Kang IK, Kwon OH. A composite of hydroxyapatite with electrospun biodegradable nanofibers as a tissue engineering material. J Biosci Bioeng 100(1), 43–49. 2005.

93. Fan HS, Wen XT, Tan YF, Wang R, Cao HD, Zhang XD. Compare of electrospinning PLA and PLA/â-TCP scaffold in vitro. PRICM 5: the Fifth Pacific Rim International Conference on Advanced Materials and Processing, PTS 1–5 Mater Sci Forum Part 1, 475–479, 2379–2382. 2005.

94. Thomas V, Jagani S, Johnson K, Jose MV, Dean DR, Vohra YK, Nyairo E. Electrospun bioactive nanocomposite scaffolds of polycaprolactone and nanohydroxyapatite for bone tissue engineering. J Nanosci Nanotechnol 6(2), 487–493. 2006.

95. Li C, Vepari C, Jin HJ, Kim HJ, Kaplan DL. Electrospun silk-BMP-2 scaffolds for bone tissue engineering. Biomaterials 27, 3115–3124. 2006.

96. Fujihara K, Kotaki M, Ramakrishna S. Guided bone regeneration membrane made of polycaprolactone/calcium carbonate composite nano-fibers. Biomaterials 26, 4139–4147. 2005.

97. Woo KM, Jun JH, Chen VJ, Seo J, Baek JH, Ryoo HM, Kim GS, Somerman MJ, Ma PX. Nano-fibrous scaffolding promotes osteoblast differentiation and biomineralization. Biomaterials 28, 335–343. 2007.

98. Zhang Y, Ouyang H, Lim CT, Ramakrishna S, Huang ZM. Electrospinning of Gelatin Fibers and Gelatin/PCL Composite Fibrous Scaffolds. J Biomed Mater Res Part B: Appl Biomater 72B, 156–165. 2005.

99. Abramovitch-Gottlib L, Naveh TGD, Geresh S, Rosenwaks S, Bar I, Vago R. Low level laser irradiation stimulates osteogenic phenotype of mesenchymal stem cells seeded on a three-dimensional biomatrix. Las Med Sci 20, 138–146. 2005.

100. Mygind T, Stiehler M, Baatrup A, Li H, Zou X, Flyvbjerg A, Kassem M, Bunger C. Mesenchymal stem cell ingrowth and differentiation on coralline hydroxyapatite scaffolds. Biomaterials 28, 1036–1047. 2007.

101. Chastain SR, Kundu AK, Dhar S, Calvert JW, Putnam AJ. Adhesion of mesenchymal stem cells to polymer scaffolds occurs via distinct ECM ligands and controls their osteogenic differentiation. J Biomed Mater Res A 78(1), 73–85. 2006.

102. Calvert JW, Marra KG, Cook L, Kumta PN, DiMilla PA, Weiss LE. Characterization of osteoblast-like behavior of cultured bone marrow stromal cells on various polymer surfaces. J Biomed Mater Res 52, 279–284. 2000.

103. Keselowsky BG, Collard DM, Garcia AJ. Integrin binding specificity regulates biomaterial surface chemistry effects on cell differentiation. Proc Natl Acad Sci USA 102(17), 5953–5957. 2005.

104. Miller DC, Haberstroh KM, Webster TJ. Mechanism(s) of increased vascular cell adhesion on nanostructured poly(lacticco-glycolic acid) films. J Biomed Mater Res A 73(4), 476–484. 2005.

105. Webster TJ, Schadler LS, Siegel RW, Bizios R. Mechanisms of enhanced osteoblast adhesion on nanophase alumina involve vitronectin. Tissue Eng 7(3), 291–301. 2001.

106. McBeath R, Pirone DM, Nelson CM, Bhadriraju K, Chen CS. Cell Shape, Cytoskeletal Tension, and RhoA Regulate Stem Cell Lineage Commitment. Dev Cell 6, 483–495. 2004.

107. Ayers R, Nielsen-Preiss S, Ferguson V, Gotolli G, Moore JJ, Kleebe HJ. Osteoblast-like cell mineralization induced by multiphasic calcium phosphate ceramic. Mat Sci Eng C 26, 1333–1337. 2006.

108. Thian ES, Huang J, Best SM, Barber ZH, Brooks RA, Rushton N, Bonfield W. The response of osteoblasts to nanocrystalline silicon-substituted hydroxyapatite thin films. Biomaterials 27, 2692–2698. 2006.

109. Ramakrishna S, Fujihara K, Teo WE, Lim TC, Ma Z. An introduction to electrospinning and nanofibers. Singapore: World Scientific Publishing, 7–16. 2005.

110. Ma Z, Kotaki M, Inai R, Ramakrishna S. Potential of nanofiber matrix as tissue-engineering scaffolds. Tissue Eng 11(1/2), 101–109. 2005.

111. Subbiah T, Bhat GS, Tock RW, Parameswaran S, Ramkumar SS. Electrospinning of nanofibers. J of Appl Polym Sci 96, 557–569. 2005.

112. Teo WE, Ramakrishna S. A review on electrospinning design and nanofiber assemblies. Nanotechnology 17, R89–R106. 2006.

113. Hartgerink JD, Beniash E, Stupp SI. Self-assembly and mineralization of peptide-amphiphile nanofibers. Science 294, 1684–1688. 2001.

114. Silva GA, Czeisler C, Niece KL, Beniash E, Harrington DA, Kessler JA, Stupp SI. Selective differentiation of neural progenitor cells by high epitope density nanofibers. Science 303, 1352–1355. 2001.

115. Hosseinkhani H, Hosseinkhani M, Tian F, Kobayashi H, Tabata Y. Ectopic bone formation in collagen sponge self-assembled peptide–amphiphile nanofibers hybrid scaffold in a perfusion culture bioreactor. Biomaterials 27, 5089–5098. 2006.

116. Bhatnagar RS, Qian JJ, Gough CA. The role in cell binding of a b-bend within the triple helical region in collagen α1 (I) chain: structural and biological evidence for conformational tautomerism on fiber surface. J Biomol Struct Dyn 14, 547–560. 1997.

117. Bhatnagar RS, Qian JJ, Wedrychowska A, Sadeghi M, Wu YM, Smith N. Design of biomimetic habitats for tissue engineering with P-15, a synthetic peptide analogue of collagen. Tissue Eng 5, 53–65. 1999.

118. Nguyen H, Qian JJ, Bhatnagar RS, Li S. Enhanced cell attachment and osteoblastic activity by P-15 peptide-coated matrix in hydrogels. Biochem Biophys Res Commun 311, 179–186. 2003.

119. Mizuno M, Kuboki Y. TGF-β accelerated the osteogenic differentiation of bone marrow cells induced by collagen matrix. Biochem Biophys Res Commun 211, 1091–1098. 1995.

120. Jikko A, Harris SE, Chen D, Mendrick DL, Damsky CH. Collagen integrin receptors regulate early osteoblast differentiation induced by BMP-2. J Bone Miner Res 14, 1075–1083. 1999.

121. DeLustro F, Condell RA, Nguyen MA, McPherson JM. A comparative study of the biologic and immunologic response to medical devices derived from dermal collagen. J Biomed Mater Res 20, 109–120. 1986.

122. Meade KR, Silver FH. Immunogenicity of collagenous implants. Biomaterials 11, 176–180. 1990.

123. Durrieu MC, Pallu S, Guillemot F, Bareille R, Amedee J, Baquey CH. Grafting RGD containing peptides onto hydroxyapatite to promote osteoblastic cells adhesion. J Mater Sci: Mater Med 15, 779–786. 2004.

124. Ho MH, Hou LT, Tu CY, Hsieh HJ, Lai JY, Chen WJ, Wang DM. Promotion of Cell Affinity of Porous PLLA Scaffolds by Immobilization of RGD Peptides via Plasma Treatment. Macromol BioSci 6, 90–98. 2006.

125. Ruoslahti E, Pierschbacher MD. New perspectives in cell adhesion: RGD and integrins. Science 238, 491–497. 1987.

126. Saito A, Suzuki Y, Ogata SI, Ohtsuki C, Tanihara M. Prolonged ectopic calcification induced by BMP-2–derived synthetic peptide. J Biomed Mater Res A 2004 70(1), 115–121. 2004.

127. Tanahashi M, Matsuda T. Surface functional group dependence on apatite formation on self-assembled monolayers in a simulated body fluid. J Biomed Mater Res 34, 305–315. 1997.

128. Lin X, Elliot JJ, Carnes DL, Fox WC, Pena LA, Campion SL, Takahashi K, Atkinson BL, Zamora PO. Augmentation of Osseous Phenotypes *In vivo* with a Synthetic Peptide. J Orthop Res 25, 531–539. 2007.

129. Lin X, Zamora PO, Albright S, Glass JD, Pena LA. Multi domain synthetic peptide B2A2 synergistically enhances BMP-2 in-vitro. J Bone Miner Res 20, 693–703. 2005.

130. Kofron MD, Zhang J, Lieberman JR, Laurencin CT. Genetically modified mesodermal-derived cells for bone tissue engineering. IEEE Eng Med Biol Mag 22, 57–64. 2003.

131. Laurencin CT, Attawia MA, Lu LQ, Borden MD, Lu HH, Gorum WJ, Lieberman JR. Poly(lactide-co-glycolide)/hydroxyapatite delivery of BMP-2-producing cells: a regional gene therapy approach to bone regeneration. Biomterials 22, 1271–1277. 2001.

132. Huang J, Wong C, George A, Kaplan DL. The effect of genetically engineered spider silk-dentin matrix protein 1 chimeric protein on hydroxyapatite nucleation. Biomaterials 28, 2358–2367. 2007.

133. He G, Tom Dahl T, Veis A, George A. Nucleation of apatite crystals in vitro by self-assembled dentin matrix protein 1. Nat Mat 2, 552–558. 2003.

134. Zhai Y, Cui FZ. Recombinant human-like collagen directed growth of hydroxyapatite nanocrystals. J Crystal Growth 291, 202–206. 2006.

135. D'Ippolito G, Schiller PC, Ricordi C, Roos BA, Howard GA. Age-related osteogenic potential of mesenchymal stromal stem cells from human vertebral bone marrow. J Bone Miner Res 14(7), 1115–1122. 1999.

136. Lennon DP, Caplan AI. Isolation of human marrow-derived mesenchymal stem cells. Exp Hema 34, 1604–1605. 2006.

137. Muschler GF, Nitto H, Boehm CA, Easley KA. Age- and gender-related changes in the cellularity of human bone marrow and the prevalence of osteoblastic progenitors. J Orthop Res 19, 117–125. 2001.

138. Bruder SP, Jaiswal N, Haynesworth SE. Growth Kinetics, Self-Renewal, and the Osteogenic Potential of Purified Human Mesenchymal Stem Cells During Extensive Subcultivation and Following Cryopreservation. J Cell Biochem 64, 278–294. 1997.

139. Wexler SA, Donaldson C, Denning-Kendall P, Rice C, Bradley B, Hows JM. Adult bone marrow is a rich source of human mesenchymal stem cells but umbilical cord and mobilized adult blood are not. Br J Haematol 121, 368–374. 2003.

140. Jaiswal N, Haynesworth SE, Caplan AI, Bruder SP. Osteogenic differentiation of purified, culture expanded human mesenchymal stem cells *in vitro*. J Cell Biochem 64, 295–312. 1997.

141. Gronthos S, Franklin DM, Leddy HA, Robey PG, Storms RW, Gimble JM. Surface Protein Characterization of Human Adipose Tissue-Derived Stromal Cells. J Cell Physiol 189, 54–63. 2001.

142. Kang SK, Putnam L, Dufour J, Ylostalo J, Jung JS, Bunnell BA. Expression of Telomerase Extends the Lifespan and Enhances Osteogenic Differentiation of Adipose Tissue–Derived Stromal Cells. Stem Cells 22, 1356–1372. 2004.

143. Lee HS, Cho HH, Kim HK, Bae YC, Baik HS, Jung JS. Tbx3, a transcriptional factor, involves in proliferation and osteogenic differentiation of human adipose stromal cells. Mol Cell Biochem 296, 129–136. 2007.

144. Friedman MS, Long MW, Hankenson KD. Osteogenic Differentiation of Human Mesenchymal Stem Cells Is Regulated by Bone Morphogenetic Protein-6. J Cell Biochem 98, 538–554. 2006.

145. Boden SD, McCuaig K, Hair G, Racine M, Titus L, Wozney JM, Nanes MS. Differential effects and glucocorticoid potentiation of bone morphogenetic protein actionduring rat osteoblast differentiation *in vitro*. J Endocrinology 137, 3401–3407. 1996.

146. Boden SD, Hair G, Titus L, Racine M, McCuaig K, Wozney JM, Nanes MS. Glucocorticoid-induced differentiationof fetal rat calvarial osteoblasts is mediated by bonemorphogenetic protein-6. J Endocrinology 138, 2820–2828. 1997.

147. Diefenderfer DL, Osyczka AM, Reilly GC, Leboy PS. BMP responsiveness in human mesenchymal stem cells. Connect Tissue Res 44(Suppl 1), 305–311. 2003.

148. Curran JM, Chen R, Hunt JA. The guidance of human mesenchymal stem cell differentiation *in vitro* by controlled modifications to the cell substrate. Biomaterials 27, 4783–4793. 2006.

149. Kern S, Eichler H, Stoeve J, Klüter H, Bieback K. Comparative Analysis of Mesenchymal Stem Cells from Bone Marrow, Umbilical Cord Blood, or Adipose Tissue. Stem Cells 24, 1294–1301. 2006.

150. Hui JHP, Li L, Teo YH, Ouyang HW, Lee EH. Comparative Study of the Ability of Mesenchymal Stem Cells Derived from Bone Marrow, Periosteum, and Adipose Tissue in Treatment of Partial Growth Arrest in Rabbit. Tissue Eng 11, 904–912. 2005.

151. Yoshimura H, Muneta T, Nimura A, Yokoyama A, Koga H, Sekiya I. Comparison of rat mesenchymal stem cells derived from bone marrow, synovium, periosteum, adipose tissue, and muscle. Cell Tissue Res 327(3), 449–462. 2007.

152. Sakaguchi Y, Sekiya I, Yagishita K, Muneta T. Comparison of Human Stem Cells Derived From Various Mesenchymal Tissues: Superiority of Synovium as a Cell Source. Arthritis Rheum 52(8), 2521–2529. 2005.

153. Erices A, Conget P, Minguell JJ. Mesenchymal progenitor cells in human umbilical cord blood. Br J Hematol 109, 235–242. 2000.

154. Muraglia A, Cancedda R, Quarto R. Clonal mesenchymal progenitors from human bone marrow differentiate *in vitro* according to a hierarchical model. J Cell Sci 113, 1161–1166. 2000.

155. Niemeyer P, Kornacker M, Mehlhorn A, Seckinger A, Vohrer J, Schmal H, Kasten P, Eckstein V, Sudkamp NP, Krause U. Comparison of Immunological Properties of Bone Marrow Stromal Cells and Adipose Tissue–Derived Stem Cells Before and After Osteogenic Differentiation *In Vitro*. Tissue Eng 13(1), 111–121. 2007.

17

ORTHOPEDIC INTERFACE TISSUE ENGINEERING: BUILDING THE BRIDGE TO INTEGRATED MUSCULOSKELETAL TISSUE SYSTEMS

Helen H. Lu, Kristen L. Moffat, and Jeffrey P. Spalazzi

Biomaterials and Interface Tissue Engineering Laboratory, Department of Biomedical Engineering, Columbia University, New York, New York

Contents

17.1 Overview 589
17.2 Design Considerations in Interface Tissue Engineering 590
17.3 Mechanism of Interface Regeneration: Role of Heterotypic
     Cellular Interactions 593
17.4 Structure-Function Relationship at the Interface 596
17.5 Multi-Phased Scaffold Design for Interface Tissue Engineering 599
17.6 Summary and Challenges in Interface Tissue Engineering 603
     Acknowledgments 603
     References 604

17.1 OVERVIEW

Over the past two decades, the field of tissue engineering has focused on formulating and validating a consistent experimental methodology for *ex vivo* tissue

Advanced Biomaterials: Fundamentals, Processing, and Applications, Edited by Bikramjit Basu, Dhirendra S. Katti, and Ashok Kumar

regeneration. Application of these tissue-engineering methods (Langer and Vacanti 1993; Skalak 1988) to musculoskeletal tissue regeneration has yielded significant advances whereby bone—(Agrawal and Ray 2001; Byers and Garcia 2004; El Ghannam, Ducheyne, and Shapiro 1995; Laurencin C.T. et al. 1999; Lu et al. 2003; Mikos et al. 1993; Richardson et al. 2001; Shea et al. 2000; Yaszemski et al. 1996; Zhang and Ma 1999), cartilage—(Almarza and Athanasiou 2004; Caterson et al. 2002; Freed et al. 1993; Hung et al. 2003; Kim et al. 2003; Klein et al. 2003; Li et al. 2005; Lu et al. 2001; Mauck et al. 2000; Riley et al. 2001; Vunjak-Novakovic et al. 1996), ligament—(Altman et al. 2002; Cooper et al. 2005; Dunn et al. 1995; Jackson, Heinrich, and Simon 1994; Lu et al. 2005; Musahl et al. 2004; Whitesides et al. 2001; Woo et al. 1999) and tendon-like—(Carpenter, Thomopoulos, and Soslowsky 1999; Derwin et al. 2004; Garvin et al. 2003; Goh et al. 2003; Juncosa et al. 2003; Zhang and Chang 2003) tissues have been engineered *in vitro* and *in vivo*.

Building upon these successes, the emphasis in the field of orthopedic tissue engineering has recently shifted from tissue *formation* to tissue *function* (Butler, Goldstein, and Guilak 2000). A critical area in the current functional tissue engineering effort focuses on the integration of tissue engineered grafts with the host environment as well as with each other. To this end, interface tissue engineering has emerged as a promising strategy for achieving biological fixation of tissue-engineered soft tissue grafts, in particular with its emphasis on regenerating the anatomic interface between soft tissues (that is, ligaments, tendons, cartilage) and bone. Furthermore, this newly-engineered interface will serve as the bridge between soft tissue and bone, and thereby enabling the development of integrated musculoskeletal tissue systems for total joint replacement.

This chapter will discuss tissue engineering-based strategies for the regeneration of the native interface between soft tissue and subchondral bone. It will begin with a discussion of design considerations in interface tissue engineering. Subsequently, using the anterior cruciate ligament-to-bone interface as a model system, current efforts in orthopedic interface tissue engineering will be reviewed. Existing challenges and future directions in this emerging area will also be presented.

17.2 DESIGN CONSIDERATIONS IN INTERFACE TISSUE ENGINEERING

In the musculoskeletal system, soft tissues such as ligaments—which connect bone to bone—or tendons—which join muscle to bone—must integrate seamlessly with subchondral bone in order to function in unison to facilitate physiologic joint motion. The insertion of ligaments or tendons into subchondral bone is often achieved through a characteristic fibrocartilage interface with well-defined spatial variations in cell type and matrix composition (Benjamin et al. 1991; Benjamin, Evans, and Copp 1986; Cooper and Misol 1970; Messner 1997; Niyibizi et al. 1995; Niyibizi et al. 1996; Petersen and Tillmann 1999; Sagarriga et al. 1996; Thomopoulos et al. 2003; Wang et al. 2006; Wei and Messner 1996). By design, this controlled matrix heterogeneity minimizes the formation of stress concentrations, enabling the transfer of complex loads between two distinct types of tissue (Benjamin, Evans, and Copp 1986; Woo et al. 1983). Current soft tissue reconstruction methods utilizing autologous or allogeneic grafts unfortunately fail to preserve or reform the native soft tissue-to-bone insertion, and the absence of this critical interface compromises graft function and long-term clinical outcome. Moreover, tissue engineered grafts for soft tissue repair or regeneration also face similar challenges in graft-to-bone integration.

For interface tissue engineering, it is essential to devise rational strategies aimed at regenerating the soft tissue-to-bone interface, and subsequently applying these tissue engineering strategies to design *integrative* fixation devices capable of promoting the biological fixation of soft tissue grafts to bone. Using the anterior cruciate ligament (ACL) as a model system, strategies for the regeneration of a biomimetic interface between ACL reconstruction grafts and subchondral bone have been formulated (Lu and Jiang 2006). The ACL is the primary knee joint stabilizer and inserts into bone through a characteristic fibrocartilage interface, with controlled spatial variations in cell type and matrix composition (Benjamin, Evans, Rao, Findlay, and Pemberton 1991; Benjamin, Evans, and Copp 1986; Cooper and Misol 1970; Messner 1997; Niyibizi, Visconti, Kavalkovich, and Woo 1995; Niyibizi, Sagarrigo, Gibson, and Kavalkovich 1996; Petersen and Tillmann 1999; Sagarriga, Kavalkovich, Wu, and Niyibizi 1996; Thomopoulos, Williams, Gimbel J.A., Favata, and Soslowsky 2003; Wang, Mitroo, Chen, Lu, and Doty 2006; Wei and Messner 1996). The ACL-to-bone junction consists of three distinct tissue regions: ligament, fibrocartilage, and bone (Figure 17.1).

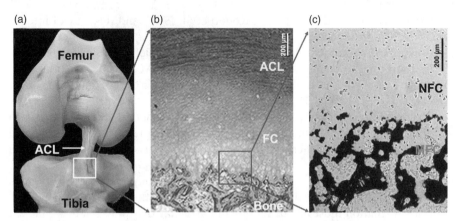

Figure 17.1. Multi-tissue Matrix Organization at the Ligament-to-Bone Insertion. A) The anterior cruciate ligament (ACL) connects the femur and tibia through two insertion sites (anterior view). B) The multi-tissue organization of the ACL-to-bone insertion, transiting from the ACL to the fibrocartilage (FC) region, and then to the bone region (Modified Goldner's Masson Trichrome). C) The fibrocartilage interface is further divided into the non-mineralized fibrocartilage (NFC) and mineralized fibrocartilage (MFC) zones (von Kossa).

The fibrocartilage region is further divided into non-mineralized and mineralized fibrocartilage zones (Figure 17.1C). The ligament proper contains fibroblasts embedded in a collagen I and III matrix. The non-mineralized fibrocartilage matrix consists of ovoid fibrochondrocytes, and collagen types I and II are distributed within a proteoglycan-rich matrix. In the mineralized fibrocartilage zone, hypertrophic fibrochondrocytes are surrounded by a calcified matrix containing collagen X (Niyibizi, Sagarrigo, Gibson, and Kavalkovich 1996; Petersen and Tillmann 1999). The fibrochondrocyte phenotype at the ACL-bone interface has been found to be similar to that of articular chondrocytes (Sun, Moffat, and Lu 2007). The last region is the subchondral bone, within which osteoblasts, osteocytes and osteoclasts reside in a mineralized type I collagen matrix. The specific organization and controlled matrix heterogeneity found at the ACL insertion are believed to minimize the formation of stress concentrations and, in turn, facilitate the transfer of complex loads between soft and hard tissues (Benjamin, Evans, and Copp 1986; Woo and Buckwalter 1988).

The ACL is the most frequently injured knee ligament (Johnson 1982), with over 100,000 ACL reconstruction procedures performed annually in the United States alone (American Academy of Orthopedic Surgeons 1997; Gotlin and Huie 2000). Autologous soft tissue or hamstring tendon-based grafts are increasingly utilized for ACL reconstruction due to donor site morbidity associated with bone-patellar tendon-bone grafts (Barrett et al. 2002; Beynnon et al. 2002). While these reconstruction grafts may restore the physiological range of motion and joint function through mechanical fixation, graft integration is not achieved as disorganized scar tissue forms within the bone tunnels and the native insertion site is lost during reconstruction. Without an anatomical interface, the graft-bone junction has limited mechanical stability (Kurosaka, Yoshiya, and Andrish 1987; Robertson, Daniel, and Biden 1986; Rodeo et al. 1999), and this lack of integration is the primary cause of graft failure (Friedman et al. 1985; Jackson et al. 1987; Kurosaka, Yoshiya, and Andrish 1987; Robertson, Daniel, and Biden 1986; Yahia 1997). Therefore, to enable the biological fixation of ACL reconstruction grafts, the regeneration of the multi-tissue interface between soft tissue and bone is critical.

Based on the complex multi-tissue organization inherent at the soft tissue-to-bone junction, it is likely that interface formation will require *multiple types* of cells, a *scaffold* system which supports interactions between these different cell types, and the development of distinct yet continuous *multi-tissue regions* mimicking the structure of the native insertion through physical and biochemical stimuli. For functional soft tissue-to-bone integration, the mechanism governing interface formation must be elucidated, in particular the role of heterotypic cellular interactions in fibrocartilage formation and multi-tissue regeneration. These interactions may be examined using multi-scale co-culture models that can determine the relevance of homotypic and heterotypic cellular communications for interface regeneration and homeostasis. In addition, the success of any interface tissue engineering effort will require an in-depth understanding of the structure-function relationship at the native insertion in order to identify interface-relevant design parameters. These understandings will collectively enable the design of stratified scaffolds optimized for supporting heterotypic cellular interactions as well as the development of controlled matrix heterogeneity and multi-tissue stratification mimicking those found at the soft tissue-to-bone junction. Recent advances in each of these three critical areas in interface tissue engineering will be discussed in the following sections.

17.3 MECHANISM OF INTERFACE REGENERATION: ROLE OF HETEROTYPIC CELLULAR INTERACTIONS

An understanding of the basic mechanisms governing interface regeneration is required for any successful interface tissue engineering effort. One of the fundamental questions to be addressed is how distinct boundaries between different types of connective tissues are re-established post injury. As described above and shown in Figure 17.1, the native ACL-bone insertion consists of a linear progression of three distinct matrix regions: ligament, fibrocartilage, and bone, each exhibiting a characteristic cellular phenotype and extracellular matrix composition. Currently, the mechanisms of interface regeneration and homeostasis of these multi-tissue boundaries are not known. It is likely that communication among the cell types residing within these three distinct tissue regions—namely fibroblasts, fibrochondrocytes and osteoblasts—plays an important role in interface homeostasis and regeneration post injury.

While tendon-to-bone healing following ACL reconstruction does not lead to the re-establishment of the native insertion, it has been well documented that a fibrovascular tissue is formed within the bone tunnel (Anderson et al. 2001; Batra et al. 2002; Blickenstaff, Grana, and Egle 1997; Chen et al. 2003; Chen et al. 1997; Eriksson, Kindblom, and Wredmark 2000; Grana et al. 1994; Liu et al. 1997; Panni et al. 1997; Rodeo et al. 1993; Song et al. 2004; Thomopoulos et al. 2002; Yoshiya et al. 2000). This layer later matures and reorganizes into fibrocartilage-like or fibrovascular tissue during the healing process. While this neo-fibrocartilage tissue is non-anatomical, these observations demonstrate that a fibrocartilage-like tissue can be regenerated *in vivo* between soft tissue and bone. Specifically, fibrocartilage formation is usually localized to areas where the tendon graft *directly contacts* the bone. When damage to the interface region during injury results in the non-physiologic exposure of normally segregated tissue types (that is, bone and ligament), heterotypic cellular interactions (osteoblast-fibroblast) are likely critical for initiating and directing the repair response that results in the regeneration of a fibrocartilage interface between these two types of tissue. Moreover, *in vivo* cell-tracking studies have revealed that the tendon graft is populated by host cells within one week of implantation (Kobayashi et al. 2005).

Since the source and nature of these host cells are not known, cell types other than osteoblasts and fibroblasts may be involved in fibrocartilage formation. When Fujioka et al. sutured the Achilles tendon to its original attachment site, both cellular organization resembling that of the native insertion and the deposition of collagen type X were observed (Fujioka et al. 1998). Based on these observations, Lu and Jiang (Lu and Jiang 2006) proposed a working hypothesis for interface regeneration, which stated that heterotypic interactions between osteoblasts and fibroblasts can lead to phenotypic changes or trans-differentiation of osteoblasts and/or fibroblasts that will result in interface regeneration. In addition, these interactions can promote the recruitment of progenitor or stem cells to the tendon-bone interface. Influenced by these heterotypic cellular communications, stem cells can differentiate into fibrochondrocytes and are responsible for fibrocartilage formation.

To test this hypothesis, several *in vitro* studies evaluating the role of osteoblast-fibroblast interactions on interface regeneration have been reported (Jiang, Nicoll, and Lu 2005; Tsai et al. 2005; Wang et al. 2007; Wang and Lu 2005). Both co-culture and tri-culture models of interface-relevant cell types have been used to determine the effects of cell communication on the development of fibro-cartilage-specific markers *in vitro*. Wang et al. conducted the first reported study to examine interactions between ligament fibroblasts and osteoblasts (Wang et al. 2007), where a 2D co-culture model permitting both physical contact and cellular interactions was designed to emulate the *in vivo* condition in which the tendon is in direct contact with bone tissue following ACL reconstruction. In this model, osteoblasts and fibroblasts were first seeded on opposite sides of a tissue culture well. The cells were separated by a hydrogel divider preformed in the center of the well. Once the cells reached confluence, the divider was removed, allowing the osteoblasts and fibroblasts to migrate and interact within the interface region (Figure 17.2A).

It was found that osteoblast-fibroblast interaction led to a decrease in cell proliferation (Figure 17.2B), a reduction in osteoblast-mediated mineralization, accompanied by an increase in the mineralization potential of fibroblasts.

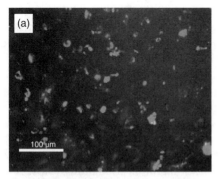 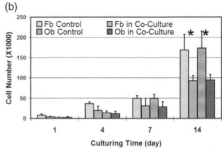

<u>Figure 17.2.</u> Effects of Heterotypic Cellular Interactions on Cellular Phenotypes. A) Co-culture of fibroblasts (green, CFDA-SE) and osteoblasts (red, CM-Dil) at the Interface region (bar = 100 μm). B) Effects of co-culture on cell growth (Wang, Shan, Choi, Oh, Kepler, Chen, and Lu 2007). The co-culture of fibroblasts and osteoblasts led to decreased proliferation of each cell type when compared controls (*p < 0.05). (See color insert.)

Subsequent conditioned media studies have revealed that both autocrine and paracrine factors were responsible for the changes in phenotype observed during osteoblast-fibroblast co-culture (Shan, Wang, and Lu 2007). In addition to fibroblasts and osteoblasts, chondrocytes are also present at the interface.

Recently, Jiang et al. evaluated osteoblast and chondrocyte interactions using a monolayer-micromass model (Jiang, Nicoll, and Lu 2005). This co-culture model permits direct physical contact between these two cell types, while maintaining the required 3D chondrocyte culture using the micromass culture. Similar to the findings of Wang et al. (Wang et al. 2007), osteoblast mineralization potential was significantly reduced due to heterotypic cellular interactions. These results collectively suggest that osteoblast-fibroblast interactions modulate cell phenotypes and may lead to trans-differentiation. It is likely that osteoblast-fibroblast and osteoblast-chondrocyte interactions are key modulators of cell phenotypes at the graft-to-bone junction. It is not known, however, which or if any of these cells are directly responsible for interface regeneration. Fibroblast trans-differentiation was anticipated as the ACL-bone insertion site fibrocartilage may be derived from ligamentous tissue during development (Nawata et al. 2002). The heterotypic cellular interactions most likely also have a down-stream effect, either in terms of cell trans-differentiation into fibrochondrocytes or in the recruitment and differentiation of pluripotent cells for fibrocartilage formation.

While osteoblast-fibroblast interactions resulted in phenotypic changes and the expression of interface-relevant markers, a fibrocartilage-like interface was not formed *in vitro* in the above osteoblast–fibroblast co-culture study. Thus, chondrogenic cells such as fibrochondrocyte precursors, chondrocytes, or stimulated stem cells may be involved in interface regeneration. When Lim et al. (Lim et al. 2004) coated tendon grafts with mesenchymal stem cells embedded in a fibrin gel, the formation of a zone of cartilaginous tissue between graft and bone was observed, suggesting a potential role for stem cells in fibrocartilage formation. Expanding upon their co-culture model, Wang et al. (Wang and Lu 2005) later evaluated the effects of cellular interactions on stem cell differentiation by tri-culturing fibroblasts, osteoblasts and bone marrow-derived mesenchymal stem cells (MSCs). In the tri-culture model, fibroblasts and osteoblasts were seeded on cover-slips on the left and right sides of a culture well, and the MSCs were loaded into the hydrogel insert and maintained in 3D culture.

Under the influence of osteoblast-fibroblast interactions, MSC proliferation remained unchanged, and these cells exhibited a similar level of alkaline phosphatase activity and proteoglycan synthesis as that of the insertion fibrochondrocytes. Moreover, under stimulation by osteoblast-fibroblast interactions, MSCs produced a type II collagen-containing matrix. These observations suggest that osteoblast-fibroblast interactions may indeed promote the differentiation of MSCs into insertion fibrochondrocytes and facilitate the eventual repair of the ligament-to-bone junction.

Findings from these *in vitro* examinations of heterotypic cellular interactions utilizing novel cellular interaction models provide preliminary validation of the hypothesis that osteoblast-fibroblast interactions promote the induction of interface-specific markers in progenitor or stem cells, and demonstrate the effects of heterotypic cellular interactions in regulating the maintenance of specific cellular phenotypes at multi-tissue junctions. While the nature of the regulatory molecules and the mechanism behind these interactions remains elusive, cell communication is likely to be significant for interface regeneration as well as homeostasis (Jiang et al. 2007; Lu and Jiang 2006).

17.4 STRUCTURE-FUNCTION RELATIONSHIP AT THE INTERFACE

In addition to elucidating the mechanism of interface regeneration, understanding the interface structure-function relationship will also be important for functional scaffold design for interface tissue engineering. Butler et al. (Butler, Goldstein, and Guilak 2000) proposed that, for functional tissue engineering, it is critical to determine the material properties of the tissue to be replaced, as well as to quantify the *in vivo* strains and stresses experienced by the native tissue. Therefore, the structural and material properties of the insertion site must be characterized in order to re-engineer the functional interface between soft tissue and bone. Moreover, the biomimetic design parameters can serve as outcome criteria for determining the success of the tissue engineered interfaces.

The inherent multi-tissue organization and heterogeneity in matrix composition at the interface are likely related to the nature and distribution of the mechanical stress experienced at the region. Knowledge of mechanical properties of the insertion site has been largely derived from theoretical predictions (Matyas et al. 1995; Thomopoulos et al. 2003). Thomopoulos et al. examined the variation in biomechanical properties of the supraspinatus tendon-to-bone insertion in a rodent model (Thomopoulos et al. 2003). Using the Quasi-Linear Viscoelastic model (Fung 1972), the viscoelastic behavior of the tendon-to-bone insertion was predicted to vary along the length of the tendon, with superior elastic and viscoelastic properties predicted for the tendon-to-fibrocartilage transition compared to the fibrocartilage-to-bone transition (Thomopoulos et al. 2003). These reports strongly suggest that the matrix organization at the tendon-to-bone transition is optimized to sustain both tensile and compressive stresses.

The direct measurement of interface mechanical properties has been difficult due to the complexity and the relative small scale of the interface, in general ranging from 100 µm to 1 mm in length (Cooper and Misol 1970; Gao and Messner 1996; Wang, Mitroo, Chen, Lu, and Doty 2006; Woo and Buckwalter 1988). Recently, using the novel functional imaging method of ultrasound elastography (Konofagou and Ophir 2000), Spalazzi et al. conducted the first experimental determination of the strain distribution at the ACL-to-bone interface (Spalazzi, Gallina, Fung-Kee-Fung, Konofagou, and Lu 2006). In this study, the tibiofemoral joint was mounted on a material testing system and loaded in tension in the tibial orientation while radiofrequency (RF) data were collected over time. Axial elastograms between successive RF frames were then generated using cross-correlation and recorrelation techniques. Elastography analyses revealed that the displacement under applied tension across the insertion is region-dependent (Figure 17.3A), with the highest displacement found at the ACL, then decreasing in magnitude from the interface to bone.

These regional differences suggest an increase in tissue stiffness from ligament to bone. In addition, both tensile and compressive strain components were detected at the insertion while the knee was loaded in tension. These findings are in agreement with finite-element model analyses of the medial collateral ligament (MCL) performed by Matyas et al., which predicted that the maximum principal tensile stresses are located in the MCL mid-substance, while the maximum principal compressive stresses occurred near the distal edge of the MCL-to-bone insertion (Matyas, Anton, Shrive, and Frank 1995).

Fibrocartilage is often localized in the anatomical regions subjected to compressive loading (Vogel 1995; Vogel and Koob 1989). It is thus likely that the insertion fibrocartilage will also bear the compressive strain detected in the elastography analysis (Spalazzi, Gallina, Fung-Kee-Fung, Konofagou, and Lu 2006). Recently, Moffat et al. performed the first experimental determination of the compressive mechanical properties of the ACL–bone interface (Moffat et al. 2005). Combining microscopic mechanical testing with optimized digital image correlation methods (Wang et al. 2003), the region-dependent changes in interface mechanical properties were quantified. In this method, the cells residing in the interface were first stained with Hoechst nuclear dye in order to enhance texture correlation following the methods of Wang et al. (Wang et al. 2002).

The samples were subsequently loaded in a custom unconfined compression microscopy device. Displacement under the applied load was then imaged using epifluorescence microscopy and digital image analysis was performed to determine the mechanical properties. As shown in Figure 17.3B, the incremental displacement decreased gradually from the non-mineralized to mineralized fibrocartilage to bone, indicating an increase in tissue stiffness across these regions. The interface also exhibited a region-dependent decrease in strain and a significantly higher elastic modulus for the mineralized fibrocartilage when compared to the non-mineralized fibrocartilage zone (Moffat, Chahine, Hung, Ateshian, and Lu 2005). These regional mechanical responses enable a gradual transition rather than an abrupt increase in tissue strain across the insertion, and are likely intrinsic to the multi-tissue ACL-to-bone interface, as they were evident under both the applied tension and compression. These observations collectively demonstrate the functional importance of the fibrocartilage interface in mediating load transfer between soft and hard tissue.

Given the structure-function dependence inherent in the biological system, the region-dependent changes in mechanical properties reported by Moffat et al. (Moffat, Chahine, Hung, Ateshian, and Lu 2005) are likely correlated to changes in matrix organization and composition across the interface. Characterization of the insertion site using Fourier Transform Infrared Imaging (FTIR-I) (Spalazzi, Boskey, and Lu 2007) and X-ray analysis (Moffat, Chahine, Hung, Ateshian, and Lu 2005) revealed an abrupt change in calcium and phosphorous content progressing from ligament, to interface, then to bone (Moffat et al. 2006; Spalazzi

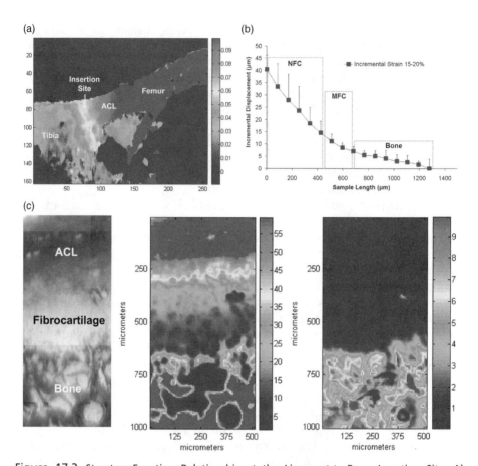

Figure 17.3. Structure-Function Relationship at the Ligament-to-Bone Insertion Site. A) Elastographic analysis of the ACL-to-Bone insertion under uniaxial tension (Spalazzi, Gallina, Fung-Kee-Fung, Konofagou, and Lu 2006). Displacement map calculated from ultrasound radiofrequency data (increase in magnitude in mm: *blue to red*, bar = 5 mm). A region-dependent decrease in displacement resulted from increasing tissue stiffness from the ligament to fibrocartilage interface and then to bone. B) Microcompression testing of the ACL-to-Bone insertion revealed region-specific increase in tissue stiffness from the non-mineralized (NFC) to mineralized (MFC) and to bone (Moffat, Chahine, Hung, Ateshian, and Lu 2005). In the displacement curve, the slope of the curve in each region represents the strain, with lower strain measured in the MFC compared to the NFC zone. C) Matrix composition and distribution at the ACL-to-Bone insertion site as determined by FTIR-I analysis (Spalazzi, Boskey, and Lu 2007). i) Light images of tissue regions from which IR spectra were collected. ii) Amide I peak integration area maps indicating regional variations in collagen content. iii) Maps of mineral-to-matrix ratio showing mineral presence is only detectable in the mineralized fibrocartilage and bone regions. (See color insert.)

et al. 2004; Sun, Moffat, and Lu 2007). Specifically, FTIR-I analysis of the interface found that calcium phosphate presence was only detected at the mineralized fibrocartilage and bone regions (Figure 17.3C). It is likely that the measured increase in elastic modulus is directly related to the presence of calcium phosphate within the mineralized fibrocartilage region of the interface. It has been suggested that the quantity of calcified tissue at the insertion may be positively correlated to the force transmitted across the calcified zone (Benjamin, Evans, Rao, Findlay, and Pemberton 1991), and warrants further evaluation. In addition to the mineral phase, large extracellular matrix molecules such as collagen or proteoglycans are also expected to play a role in maintaining the structure-function profiles at the soft tissue-to-bone interface, and should be further investigated.

In summary, theoretical and experimental evaluations of the interface suggest that a structure-function relationship exists at the ligament-to-bone insertion. As such, more in-depth determination of the chemical and mechanical properties of the insertion at the nano-, micro-, and macro-scale levels are needed for providing key design parameters for interface tissue engineering. The development and application of novel characterization methods with the requisite resolution to quantify both structural and functional variations across multi-tissue regions will be essential for augmenting the current understanding of this complex interface.

17.5 MULTI-PHASED SCAFFOLD DESIGN FOR INTERFACE TISSUE ENGINEERING

Investigations of the role of heterotypic cellular interactions in interface regeneration, as well as interface structure-function relationships, are invaluable for biomimetic scaffold design in orthopedic interface tissue engineering. It is likely that interface formation will require *multiple types* of cells, a *scaffold* system which supports interactions between different cell types, and the development of distinct yet continuous *multi-tissue regions* through physical and biochemical stimuli. Therefore, the design of biomimetic, multi-phased scaffolds able to promote heterotypic cellular interactions and multi-tissue formation will be critical for interface tissue engineering.

Stratified scaffold design has been researched for orthopedic tissue engineering, and in particular for osteochondral applications (Gao et al. 2001; Hollister, Maddox, and Taboas 2002; Lu et al. 2005; Niederauer et al. 2000; Schaefer et al. 2000; Yu, Grynpas, and Kandel 1997). The first generation of the stratified scaffolds were formed by joining together two different scaffold phases by sutures or sealants. Schaefer et al. (Schaefer, Martin, Shastri, Padera, Langer, Freed, and Vunjak-Novakovic 2000) seeded bovine articular chondrocytes on PGA meshes and periosteal cells on PLGA/polyethylene glycol foams, and subsequently sutured these separate constructs together at one or four weeks after seeding. Integration between the two scaffolds was observed to be superior when brought together at week one instead of four, suggesting the importance of cellular interactions immediately post-seeding. Similarly, Gao et al. (Gao, Dennis, Solchaga, Awadallah, Goldberg, and Caplan 2001) seeded mesenchymal stem cell (MSC)-differentiated chondrogenic cells in a hyaluronan sponge and MSC-differentiated osteogenic cells in a porous calcium phosphate scaffold. These scaffolds were then joined by fibrin sealant and implanted subcutaneously in syngeneic rats, with continuous collagen fibers observed between the two scaffolds six weeks following implantation. Shortly after, Sherwood et al. designed a *continuous* biphasic scaffold using the TheriForm™ 3D printing process and evaluated chondrocyte response on this scaffold (Sherwood et al. 2002). Using a sequential polymerization technique, Alhadlaq and Mao fabricated bi-layered human mandibular condyle-shaped osteochondral constructs with MSC-derived chondrocytes and osteoblasts encapsulated in distinct layers of polyethylene glycol-diacrylate hydrogel (Alhadlaq and Mao 2005). Distinct cartilaginous and osseous regions were observed post-implantation in a subcutaneous model, with integration between the two layers. These studies demonstrate the importance of multi-phased scaffold design for multi-tissue formation.

Due to the complexity inherent at the soft tissue-to-bone interface and the need to replace more than one type of tissue, stratified scaffold design is critical for interface tissue engineering. The aforementioned biphasic construct studies represent a significant advancement over strategies which have focused on regenerating only a single type of tissue on a construct with homogenous properties. In addition, advanced scaffold design must take into consideration the regeneration of the interface region between distinct tissue types. A biomimetic substrate is essential for maintaining the mechanical strength and structural support, as well as for providing the optimal growth environment for fibrocartilage formation (Lu and Jiang 2006).

The multi-tissue transition from ligament to fibrocartilage and to bone at the insertion site poses significant challenges for interface tissue engineering as more than three distinct types of tissue are present. In addition to supporting the growth and differentiation of relevant cell types, the *ideal scaffold* for interface tissue engineering must direct heterotypic and homotypic cellular interactions while promoting the formation and maintenance of controlled matrix heterogeneity. Consequently, the scaffold should exhibit a gradient of structural and material properties mimicking those of the native insertion zone.

Compared to a homogenous structure, a scaffold with pre-designed inhomogeneity may better sustain and transmit the distribution of complex loads inherent at the ACL-to-bone interface. The interface scaffold must also be biodegradable and exhibit mechanical properties comparable to those of the ligament insertion site. Finally, the tissue engineered graft must be easily adaptable with current ACL reconstruction grafts, or pre-incorporated into the design of ligament replacement grafts, in order to enable *in vivo* graft integration. Modeled after the native ACL-to-bone interface and inspired by the structure-function relationship inherent at the ACL-to-bone interface, Spalazzi et al. were the first to report on the design of a multi-phased scaffold for interface tissue engineering (Spalazzi

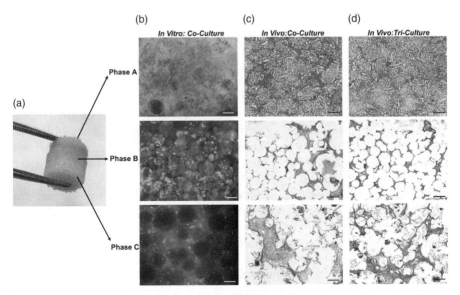

Figure 17.4. Biomimetic Multiphasic Scaffold for Interface Tissue Engineering: Design, *In Vitro* and *In Vivo* Testing. A) Multi-phased scaffold modeled after the three regions of the interface: *Phase A* for soft tissue, *Phase B* for the fibrocartilage region and *Phase C* for Bone (Spalazzi, Doty, Moffat, Levine, and Lu 2006). B) *In vitro* co-culture of fibroblasts and osteoblasts on the triphasic scaffold resulted in phase-specific cell distribution and controlled matrix heterogeneity (Spalazzi, Doty, Moffat, Levine, and Lu 2006). Fibroblasts (Calcein AM, *green*) localized in Phase A and osteoblasts (CM-Dil, *red*) in Phase C at day 1 and day 28. Both cell types migrated into Phase B by day 28 (bar = 200 μm). C) *In vivo* evalution of the multi-phased scaffold co-cutlured with fibroblasts and osteoblasts revealed abundant tissue infiltration and matrix production at four weeks (Spalazzi, Dagher, Doty, Guo, Rodeo, and Lu 2006). (Modified Goldner's MassonTrichrome, bar = 200 μm). D) *In vivo* evalution of the multi-phased scaffold tri-cutlured with fibroblasts, chondrocytes, and osteoblasts revealed abundant tissue infiltration and matrix production at four weeks (Spalazzi, Dagher, Doty, Guo, Rodeo, and Lu 2006). (Modified Goldner's MassonTrichrome, bar = 200 μm). (See color insert.)

et al. 2006). Specifically, the scaffold consisted of three distinct yet continuous phases (Figure 17.4A), with each designed for a particular cell type and tissue region found at the interface: Phase A for fibroblasts and soft tissue formation, Phase B as an interface region intended for fibrochondrocytes and fibrocartilage formation, and Phase C (Lu, El Amin, Scott, and Laurencin 2003) for osteoblasts and bone tissue.

Both co-culture and tri-culture of the interface relevant cell types on the triphasic scaffold have been reported, and the feasibility of using this model system for interface tissue engineering has been evaluated (Spalazzi, Doty, Moffat,

Levine, and Lu 2006; Spalazzi, Dagher, Doty, Guo, Rodeo, and Lu 2006). Spalazzi et al. (Spalazzi, Doty, Moffat, Levine, and Lu 2006) seeded fibroblasts and osteoblasts onto Phase A and Phase C, respectively. Phase B was left unseeded. After four weeks, the fibroblasts and osteoblasts each proliferated within their respective phases and both cell types migrated into the interface phase (Figure 17.4B). The stratified scaffold design enabled spatial control of cell distribution, with both osteoblasts and fibroblasts localized in their respective regions, while restricting their interaction to the interface region. This controlled cell distribution also resulted in the formation of cell type-specific matrix on each phase, with a mineralized matrix detected only in Phase C, and an extensive type I collagen matrix found on both Phases A and B. When the tri-phasic scaffold co-cultured with osteoblasts and fibroblasts was evaluated in a subcutaneous athymic rat model, abundant tissue formation was observed on both Phase A and Phase C. As shown in Figure 17.4C, extensive tissue infiltration and vascularization was observed in all three phases. Cells migrated into Phase B, and increased matrix production was evident in this interface region. Extracellular matrix production compensated for the temporal decrease in scaffold mechanical properties, and more importantly, controlled matrix heterogeneity was maintained *in vivo*.

Similar to the findings of the 2D co-culture model, while both anatomic ligament- and bone-like regions were found on the tri-phasic scaffold *in vitro* and *in vivo*, no fibrocartilage-like tissue was formed in the interface region. Recently, Spalazzi et al. extended their *in vivo* evaluation by tri-culturing osteoblasts, chondrocytes and fibroblasts on the multi-phasic scaffold (Spalazzi, Dagher, Doty, Guo, Rodeo, and Lu 2006). Specifically, articular chondrocytes were encapsulated in a hydrogel matrix and loaded into Phase B of the scaffold, while ligament fibroblasts and osteoblasts were pre-seeded onto Phase A and Phase C, respectively. After two months *in vivo*, an extensive collagen-rich matrix was prevalent in all three phases of the tri-cultured scaffolds, and the mineralized matrix was again confined to the bone region (Phase C). In addition, a fibrocartilage-like region of chondrocyte-like cells embedded in a matrix of collagen types I and II as well as glycosaminoglycans was observed in the tri-cultured group.

These promising *in vitro* and *in vivo* results suggest that a fibrocartilage region can indeed be formed in tri-culture, and demonstrate the potential of the multi-phased scaffold for interface regeneration. Moreover, this scaffold can be used as a model system to elucidate the mechanism for multi-tissue regeneration, determining the role of heterotypic cellular interactions as well as the effects of biochemical and biomechanical stimulation for interface tissue engineering. Heterotypic cellular interactions are likely facilitated by physiological loading, which can mediate cytokine transport between different cell types and tissue regions. Additionally, nutrient transport (Botchwey et al. 2003; Botchwey et al. 2004; Cartmell et al. 2003; Mauck et al. 2003; Mauck, Hung, and Ateshian 2003; Porter et al. 2005) through the scaffold and bioreactor cultures (Altman et al. 2002; Botchwey et al. 2001; Darling and Athanasiou 2003; Freed, Martin, and Vunjak-Novakovic 1999; Freed, Vunjak-Novakovic, and Langer 1993; Yu et al.

2004) will be critical for optimizing the stratified scaffolds designed for interface regeneration.

17.6 SUMMARY AND CHALLENGES IN INTERFACE TISSUE ENGINEERING

Interface tissue engineering is an emerging research area that focuses on the integration of soft tissue to bone by regenerating the functional transition between these distinct tissue types. Building upon previous advances in tissue engineering, interface tissue engineering aims to develop innovative technologies for multi-tissue regeneration, with the extended goal of addressing the challenges of *biological* fixation of tissue-engineered grafts with each other and with the host environment. Current efforts in interface tissue engineering are guided by the working hypothesis that tissue-to-tissue interfaces may be regenerated by controlling the interaction between relevant cell types using a stratified scaffold with a pre-designed biomimetic gradient of structural and functional properties.

The success of any interface tissue engineering effort will require a systematic characterization of the structure-function relationship existing at the native insertion site, as well as the elucidation of the mechanisms governing interface regeneration. While the majority of research in this field has focused on interface formation, the engineering of multiple tissue types must also address the problem of maintaining the stability of pre-formed tissue regions. Moreover, the effects of biological, physical and chemical stimulation on interface regeneration are not known and must be investigated. These understandings will be instrumental for formulating the optimal tissue engineering strategies for interface regeneration and the formation of complex musculoskeletal tissue systems.

In summary, interface tissue engineering via the regeneration of an anatomical soft tissue-to-bone interface will enable long term graft function and biological fixation. The multi-phasic scaffold design principles and co-culturing methodologies optimized through interface tissue engineering can lead to the realization of integrative fixation devices for orthopedic repair. Moreover, by bridging distinct tissue types, interface tissue engineering will be instrumental for the *ex vivo* development and *in vivo* translation of integrated musculoskeletal tissues with biomimetic complexity and functionality.

ACKNOWLEDGMENTS

The authors would like to gratefully acknowledge all collaborators and members of the Biomaterials and Interface Tissue Engineering Laboratory at Columbia University who have contributed to our interface tissue engineering research program. We would also like to thank Columbia University Science and Technology Ventures, the Whitaker Foundation, the Wallace H. Coulter Foundation, and the National Institutes of Health (NIAMS), and National Science Foundation GK-12 Graduate Fellowship (KLM, JPS) for supporting our studies.

REFERENCES

Agrawal, C. M. and R. B. Ray. 2001. Biodegradable polymeric scaffolds for musculoskeletal tissue engineering. *Journal of Biomedical Materials Research* 55, no. 2:141–150.

Alhadlaq, A. and J. J. Mao. 2005. Tissue-engineered osteochondral constructs in the shape of an articular condyle. *J Bone Joint Surg Am* 87, no. 5:936–944.

Almarza, A. J. and K. A. Athanasiou. 2004. Design characteristics for the tissue engineering of cartilaginous tissues. *Ann Biomed Eng* 32, no. 1:2–17.

Altman, G. H., R. L. Horan, H. H. Lu, J. Moreau, I. Martin, J. C. Richmond, and D. L. Kaplan. 2002. Silk matrix for tissue engineered anterior cruciate ligaments. *Biomaterials* 23, no. 20:4131–4141.

Altman, G. H., H. H. Lu, R. L. Horan, T. Calabro, D. Ryder, D. L. Kaplan, P. Stark et al. 2002. Advanced bioreactor with controlled application of multi-dimensional strain for tissue engineering. *J Biomed Eng* 124, no. 6:742–749.

American Academy of Orthopedic Surgeons. 1997. Arthoplasty and Total Joint Replacement Procedures: United States 1990 to 1997. United States.

Anderson, K., A. M. Seneviratne, K. Izawa, B. L. Atkinson, H. G. Potter, and S. A. Rodeo. 2001. Augmentation of tendon healing in an intraarticular bone tunnel with use of a bone growth factor. *Am J Sports Med* 29, no. 6:689–698.

Barrett, G. R., F. K. Noojin, C. W. Hartzog, and C. R. Nash. 2002. Reconstruction of the anterior cruciate ligament in females: A comparison of hamstring versus patellar tendon autograft. *Arthroscopy* 18, no. 1:46–54.

Batra, G. S., J. W. Harrison, T. M. Clough, and A. S. Paul. 2002. Failure of anterior cruciate ligament reconstruction following calcification of the graft. *Knee* 9, no. 3:245–247.

Benjamin, M., E. J. Evans, and L. Copp. 1986. The histology of tendon attachments to bone in man. *J Anat* 149:89–100.

Benjamin, M., E. J. Evans, R. D. Rao, J. A. Findlay, and D. J. Pemberton. 1991. Quantitative differences in the histology of the attachment zones of the meniscal horns in the knee joint of man. *J Anat* 177:127–134.

Beynnon, B. D., R. J. Johnson, B. C. Fleming, P. Kannus, M. Kaplan, J. Samani, and P. Renstrom. 2002. Anterior cruciate ligament replacement: comparison of bone-patellar tendon-bone grafts with two-strand hamstring grafts. A prospective, randomized study. *J Bone Joint Surg Am* 84-A, no. 9:1503–1513.

Blickenstaff, K. R., W. A. Grana, and D. Egle. 1997. Analysis of a semitendinosus autograft in a rabbit model. *Am J Sports Med* 25, no. 4:554–559.

Botchwey, E. A., M. A. Dupree, S. R. Pollack, E. M. Levine, and C. T. Laurencin. 2003. Tissue engineered bone: measurement of nutrient transport in three-dimensional matrices. *J Biomed Mater Res A* Oct 1;67, no. 1:357–367.

Botchwey, E. A., S. R. Pollack, E. M. Levine, E. D. Johnston, and C. T. Laurencin. 2004. Quantitative analysis of three-dimensional fluid flow in rotating bioreactors for tissue engineering. *J Biomed Mater Res A* 69, no. 2:205–215.

Botchwey, E. A., S. R. Pollack, E. M. Levine, and C. T. Laurencin. 2001. Bone tissue engineering in a rotating bioreactor using a microcarrier matrix system. *J Biomed Mater Res* 55, no. 2:242–253.

Butler, D. L., S. A. Goldstein, and F. Guilak. 2000. Functional tissue engineering: the role of biomechanics. *J Biomech Eng* 122, no. 6:570–575.

Byers, B. A. and A. J. Garcia. 2004. Exogenous Runx2 expression enhances *in vitro* osteoblastic differentiation and mineralization in primary bone marrow stromal cells. *Tissue Eng* 10, no. 11–12:1623–1632.

Carpenter, J. E., S. Thomopoulos, and L. J. Soslowsky. 1999. Animal models of tendon and ligament injuries for tissue engineering applications. *Clin Orthop Relat Res* no. 367 Suppl:S296–S311.

Cartmell, S. H., B. D. Porter, A. J. Garcia, and R. E. Guldberg. 2003. Effects of medium perfusion rate on cell-seeded three-dimensional bone constructs *in vitro*. *Tissue Eng* 9, no. 6:1197–1203.

Caterson, E. J., W. J. Li, L. J. Nesti, T. Albert, K. Danielson, and R. S. Tuan. 2002. Polymer/alginate amalgam for cartilage-tissue engineering. *Ann NY Acad Sci* 961:134–138.

Chen, C. H., W. J. Chen, C. H. Shih, C. Y. Yang, S. J. Liu, and P. Y. Lin. 2003. Enveloping the tendon graft with periosteum to enhance tendon-bone healing in a bone tunnel: A biomechanical and histologic study in rabbits. *Arthroscopy* 19, no. 3:290–296.

Chen, C. S., M. Mrksich, S. Huang, G. M. Whitesides, and D. E. Ingber. 1997. Geometric control of cell life and death. *Science* 276, no. 5317:1425–1428.

Cooper, J. A., H. H. Lu, F. K. Ko, J. W. Freeman, and C. T. Laurencin. 2005. Fiber-based tissue-engineered scaffold for ligament replacement: design considerations and *in vitro* evaluation. *Biomaterials* 26, no. 13:1523–1532.

Cooper, R. R. and S. Misol. 1970. Tendon and ligament insertion. A light and electron microscopic study. *J Bone Joint Surg Am* 52, no. 1:1–20.

Darling, E. M. and K. A. Athanasiou. 2003. Articular cartilage bioreactors and bioprocesses. *Tissue Eng* 9, no. 1:9–26.

Derwin, K., C. Androjna, E. Spencer, O. Safran, T. W. Bauer, T. Hunt, A. Caplan, and J. Iannotti. 2004. Porcine small intestine submucosa as a flexor tendon graft. *Clin Orthop Relat Res* no. 423:245–252.

Dunn, M. G., J. B. Liesch, M. L. Tiku, and J. P. Zawadsky. 1995. Development of fibroblast-seeded ligament analogs for ACL reconstruction. *J Biomed Mater Res* 29, no. 11:1363–1371.

El Ghannam, A. R., P. Ducheyne, and I. M. Shapiro. 1995. Bioactive material template for *in vitro* synthesis of bone. *J Biomed Mater Res* 29, no. 3:359–370.

Eriksson, K., L. G. Kindblom, and T. Wredmark. 2000. Semitendinosus tendon graft ingrowth in tibial tunnel following ACL reconstruction: a histological study of 2 patients with different types of early graft failure. *Acta Orthop Scand* 71, no. 3:275–279.

Freed, L. E., J. C. Marquis, A. Nohria, J. Emmanual, A. G. Mikos, and R. Langer. 1993. Neocartilage formation *in vitro* and *in vivo* using cells cultured on synthetic biodegradable polymers. *J Biomed Mater Res* 27, no. 1:11–23.

Freed, L. E., I. Martin, and G. Vunjak-Novakovic. 1999. Frontiers in tissue engineering. *In vitro* modulation of chondrogenesis. *Clin Orthop* no. 367 Suppl:S46–S58.

Freed, L. E., G. Vunjak-Novakovic, and R. Langer. 1993. Cultivation of cell-polymer cartilage implants in bioreactors. *J Cell Biochem* 51, no. 3:257–264.

Friedman, M. J., O. H. Sherman, J. M. Fox, W. Del Pizzo, S. J. Snyder, and R. J. Ferkel. 1985. Autogeneic anterior cruciate ligament (ACL) anterior reconstruction of the knee. A review. *Clin Orthop* no. 196:9–14.

Fujioka, H., R. Thakur, G. J. Wang, K. Mizuno, G. Balian, and S. R. Hurwitz. 1998. Comparison of surgically attached and non-attached repair of the rat Achilles tendon-bone interface. Cellular organization and type X collagen expression. *Connect Tissue Res* 37, no. 3–4:205–218.

Fung, Y. C. 1972. Stress-strain-history relations of soft tissues in simple elongation. In *Biomechanics: Its Foundations and Objectives*, eds. Fung, Y. C., N. Perrone, and M. Anliker, 181–208 (San Diego: Prentice-Hall).

Gao, J., J. E. Dennis, L. A. Solchaga, A. S. Awadallah, V. M. Goldberg, and A. I. Caplan. 2001. Tissue-engineered fabrication of an osteochondral composite graft using rat bone marrow-derived mesenchymal stem cells. *Tissue Eng* 7, no. 4:363–371.

Gao, J. and K. Messner. 1996. Quantitative comparison of soft tissue-bone interface at chondral ligament insertions in the rabbit knee joint. *J Anat* 188, no. Pt 2:367–373.

Garvin, J., J. Qi, M. Maloney, and A. J. Banes. 2003. Novel system for engineering bioartificial tendons and application of mechanical load. *Tissue Eng* 9, no. 5:967–979.

Goh, J. C., H. W. Ouyang, S. H. Teoh, C. K. Chan, and E. H. Lee. 2003. Tissue-engineering approach to the repair and regeneration of tendons and ligaments. *Tissue Eng* 9 Suppl 1:S31–S44.

Gotlin, R. S. and G. Huie. 2000. Anterior cruciate ligament injuries. Operative and rehabilitative options. *Phys Med Rehabil Clin N Am* 11, no. 4:895–928.

Grana, W. A., D. M. Egle, R. Mahnken, and C. W. Goodhart. 1994. An analysis of autograft fixation after anterior cruciate ligament reconstruction in a rabbit model. *Am J Sports Med* 22, no. 3:344–351.

Hollister, S. J., R. D. Maddox, and J. M. Taboas. 2002. Optimal design and fabrication of scaffolds to mimic tissue properties and satisfy biological constraints. *Biomaterials* 23, no. 20:4095–4103.

Hung, C. T., E. G. Lima, R. L. Mauck, E. Taki, M. A. LeRoux, H. H. Lu, R. G. Stark, X. E. Guo, and G. A. Ateshian. 2003. Anatomically shaped osteochondral constructs for articular cartilage repair. *J Biomech* 36, no. 12:1853–1864.

Jackson, D. W., E. S. Grood, S. P. Arnoczky, D. L. Butler, and T. M. Simon. 1987. Cruciate reconstruction using freeze dried anterior cruciate ligament allograft and a ligament augmentation device (LAD). An experimental study in a goat model. *Am J Sports Med* 15, no. 6:528–538.

Jackson, D. W., J. T. Heinrich, and T. M. Simon. 1994. Biologic and synthetic implants to replace the anterior cruciate ligament. *Arthroscopy* 10, no. 4:442–452.

Jiang, J., N. L. Leong, J. C. Mung, C. Hidaka, and H. H. Lu. 2007. Interaction between zonal populations of articular chondrocytes suppresses chondrocyte mineralization and this process is mediated by PTHrP. *Osteoarthritis Cartilage*, In press.

Jiang, J., S. B. Nicoll, and H. H. Lu. 2005. Co-culture of osteoblasts and chondrocytes modulates cellular differentiation *in vitro*. *Biochem Biophys Res Commun* 338, no. 2:762–770.

Johnson, R. J. 1982. The anterior cruciate: a dilemma in sports medicine. *Int J Sports Med* 3, no. 2:71–79.

Juncosa, N., J. R. West, M. T. Galloway, G. P. Boivin, and D. L. Butler. 2003. *In vivo* forces used to develop design parameters for tissue engineered implants for rabbit patellar tendon repair. *J Biomech* 36, no. 4:483–488.

Kim, T. K., B. Sharma, C. G. Williams, M. A. Ruffner, A. Malik, E. G. McFarland, and J. H. Elisseeff. 2003. Experimental model for cartilage tissue engineering to regenerate the zonal organization of articular cartilage. *Osteoarthritis Cartilage* 11, no. 9:653–664.

Klein, T. J., B. L. Schumacher, T. A. Schmidt, K. W. Li, M. S. Voegtline, K. Masuda, E. J. Thonar, and R. L. Sah. 2003. Tissue engineering of stratified articular cartilage from chondrocyte subpopulations. *Osteoarthritis Cartilage* 11, no. 8:595–602.

Kobayashi, M., N. Watanabe, Y. Oshima, Y. Kajikawa, M. Kawata, and T. Kubo. 2005. The fate of host and graft cells in early healing of bone tunnel after tendon graft. *Am J Sports Med* 33, no. 12:1892–1897.

Konofagou, E. E. and J. Ophir. 2000. Precision estimation and imaging of normal and shear components of the 3D strain tensor in elastography. *Phys Med Biol* 45, no. 6:1553–1563.

Kurosaka, M., S. Yoshiya, and J. T. Andrish. 1987. A biomechanical comparison of different surgical techniques of graft fixation in anterior cruciate ligament reconstruction. *Am J Sports Med* 15, no. 3:225–229.

Langer, R. and J. P. Vacanti. 1993. Tissue Engineering. *Science* 260, no. 5110:920–926.

Laurencin C. T., A. A. Ambrosio, M. Borden, and J. A. Cooper. 1999. Tissue Engineering: Orthopedic Applications. In *Annual Review of Biomedical Engineering*, eds. Yarmush, M. L., K. R. Diller, and M. Toner, 19–46.

Li, W. J., R. Tuli, C. Okafor, A. Derfoul, K. G. Danielson, D. J. Hall, and R. S. Tuan. 2005. A three-dimensional nanofibrous scaffold for cartilage tissue engineering using human mesenchymal stem cells. *Biomaterials* 26, no. 6:599–609.

Lim, J. K., J. Hui, L. Li, A. Thambyah, J. Goh, and E. H. Lee. 2004. Enhancement of tendon graft osteointegration using mesenchymal stem cells in a rabbit model of anterior cruciate ligament reconstruction. *Arthroscopy* 20, no. 9:899–910.

Liu, S. H., V. Panossian, R. al Shaikh, E. Tomin, E. Shepherd, G. A. Finerman, and J. M. Lane. 1997. Morphology and matrix composition during early tendon to bone healing. *Clin Orthop Relat Res*, no. 339:253–260.

Lu, H. H., J. A. Cooper, Jr., S. Manuel, J. W. Freeman, M. A. Attawia, F. K. Ko, and C. T. Laurencin. 2005. Anterior cruciate ligament regeneration using braided biodegradable scaffolds: *in vitro* optimization studies. *Biomaterials* 26, no. 23:4805–4816.

Lu, H. H., S. F. El Amin, K. D. Scott, and C. T. Laurencin. 2003. Three-dimensional, bioactive, biodegradable, polymer-bioactive glass composite scaffolds with improved mechanical properties support collagen synthesis and mineralization of human osteoblast-like cells *in vitro*. *J Biomed Mater Res* 64A, no. 3:465–474.

Lu, H. H. and J. Jiang. 2006. Interface tissue engineering and the formulation of multiple-tissue systems. *Adv Biochem Eng Biotechnol* 102:91–111.

Lu, H. H., J. Jiang, A. Tang, C. T. Hung, and X. E. Guo. 2005. Development of controlled heterogeneity on a polymer-ceramic hydrogel scaffold for osteochondral repair. *Bioceramics 17 Key Engineering Materials* 284–286:607–610.

Lu, L., X. Zhu, R. G. Valenzuela, B. L. Currier, and M. J. Yaszemski. 2001. Biodegradable polymer scaffolds for cartilage tissue engineering. *Clin Orthop* no. 391 Suppl:S251–S270.

Matyas, J. R., M. G. Anton, N. G. Shrive, and C. B. Frank. 1995. Stress governs tissue phenotype at the femoral insertion of the rabbit MCL. *J Biomech* 28, no. 2:147–157.

Mauck, R. L., C. T. Hung, and G. A. Ateshian. 2003. Modeling of neutral solute transport in a dynamically loaded porous permeable gel: implications for articular cartilage biosynthesis and tissue engineering. *J Biomed Eng* 125, no. 5:602–614.

Mauck, R. L., M. A. Soltz, C. C. Wang, D. D. Wong, P. H. Chao, W. B. Valhmu, C. T. Hung, and G. A. Ateshian. 2000. Functional tissue engineering of articular cartilage through dynamic loading of chondrocyte-seeded agarose gels. *J Biomech Eng* 122, no. 3:252–260.

Mauck, R. L., C. C. Wang, E. S. Oswald, G. A. Ateshian, and C. T. Hung. 2003. The role of cell seeding density and nutrient supply for articular cartilage tissue engineering with deformational loading. *Osteoarthritis Cartilage* 11, no. 12:879–890.

Messner, K. 1997. Postnatal development of the cruciate ligament insertions in the rat knee. morphological evaluation and immunohistochemical study of collagens types I and II. *Acta Anatomica* 160, no. 4:261–268.

Mikos, A. G., G. Sarakinos, S. M. Leite, J. P. Vacanti, and R. Langer. 1993. Laminated three-dimensional biodegradable foams for use in tissue engineering. *Biomaterials* 14:323–330.

Moffat, K. L., N. O. Chahine, C. T. Hung, G. A. Ateshian, and H. H. Lu. 2005. Characterization of the mechanical properties of the ACL-Bone insertion. *Proceedings of the ASME Summer Bioengineering Conference*, I-67.

Moffat, K. L., W. S. Sun, N. O. Chahine, P. E. Pena, S. S. Doty, C. T. Hung, G. A. Ateshian, and H. H. Lu. 2006. Characterization of the Mechanical Properties and Mineral Distribution of hte Anterior Cruciate Ligament-to-Bone Insertion Site. *Proceedings of the IEEE Engineering in Medicine and Biology Society*, 2366–2369.

Musahl, V., S. D. Abramowitch, T. W. Gilbert, E. Tsuda, J. H. Wang, S. F. Badylak, and S. L. Woo. 2004. The use of porcine small intestinal submucosa to enhance the healing of the medial collateral ligament—a functional tissue engineering study in rabbits. *J Orthop Res* 22, no. 1:214–220.

Nawata, K., T. Minamizaki, Y. Yamashita, and R. Teshima. 2002. Development of the attachment zones in the rat anterior cruciate ligament: changes in the distributions of proliferating cells and fibrillar collagens during postnatal growth. *J Orthop Res* 20, no. 6:1339–1344.

Niederauer, G. G., M. A. Slivka, N. C. Leatherbury, D. L. Korvick, H. H. Harroff, W. C. Ehler, C. J. Dunn, and K. Kieswetter. 2000. Evaluation of multiphase implants for repair of focal osteochondral defects in goats. *Biomaterials* 21, no. 24:2561–2574.

Niyibizi, C., Visconti C. Sagarrigo, G. Gibson, and K. Kavalkovich. 1996. Identification and immunolocalization of type X collagen at the ligament-bone interface. *Biochem Biophys Res Commun* 222, no. 2:584–589.

Niyibizi, C., C. S. Visconti, K. Kavalkovich, and S. L. Woo. 1995. Collagens in an adult bovine medial collateral ligament: immunofluorescence localization by confocal microscopy reveals that type XIV collagen predominates at the ligament-bone junction. *Matrix Biol* 14, no. 9:743–751.

Panni, A. S., G. Milano, L. Lucania, and C. Fabbriciani. 1997. Graft healing after anterior cruciate ligament reconstruction in rabbits. *Clin Orthop* no. 343:203–212.

Petersen, W. and B. Tillmann. 1999. Structure and vascularization of the cruciate ligaments of the human knee joint. *Anat Embryol (Berl)* 200, no. 3:325–334.

Porter, B., R. Zauel, H. Stockman, R. Guldberg, and D. Fyhrie. 2005. 3-D computational modeling of media flow through scaffolds in a perfusion bioreactor. *J Biomech* Mar;38, no. 3:543–549.

Richardson, T. P., M. C. Peters, A. B. Ennett, and D. J. Mooney. 2001. Polymeric system for dual growth factor delivery. *Nat Biotechnol* 19, no. 11:1029–1034.

Riley, S. L., S. Dutt, Torre R. De La, A. C. Chen, R. L. Sah, and A. Ratcliffe. 2001. Formulation of PEG-based hydrogels affects tissue-engineered cartilage construct characteristics. *J Mater Sci Mater Med* 12, no. 10–12:983–990.

Robertson, D. B., D. M. Daniel, and E. Biden. 1986. Soft tissue fixation to bone. *Am J Sports Med* 14, no. 5:398–403.

Rodeo, S. A., S. P. Arnoczky, P. A. Torzilli, C. Hidaka, and R. F. Warren. 1993. Tendon-healing in a bone tunnel. A biomechanical and histological study in the dog. *J Bone Joint Surg Am* 75, no. 12:1795–1803.

Rodeo, S. A., K. Suzuki, X. H. Deng, J. Wozney, and R. F. Warren. 1999. Use of recombinant human bone morphogenetic protein-2 to enhance tendon healing in a bone tunnel. *Am J Sports Med* 27, no. 4:476–488.

Sagarriga, Visconti C., K. Kavalkovich, J. Wu, and C. Niyibizi. 1996. Biochemical analysis of collagens at the ligament-bone interface reveals presence of cartilage-specific collagens. *Arch Biochem Biophys* 328, no. 1:135–142.

Schaefer, D., I. Martin, P. Shastri, R. F. Padera, R. Langer, L. E. Freed, and G. Vunjak-Novakovic. 2000. *In vitro* generation of osteochondral composites. *Biomaterials* 21, no. 24:2599–2606.

Shan, J. M., I. E. Wang, and H. H. Lu. 2007. Osteoblast-Fibroblast Interactions Modulate Cell Phenotypes Through Paracrine and Autocrine Regulations. *Trans Orthop Res Soc* 32:30.

Shea, L. D., D. Wang, R. T. Franceschi, and D. J. Mooney. 2000. Engineered bone development from a pre-osteoblast cell line on three-dimensional scaffolds. *Tissue Engineering* 6, no. 6:605–617.

Sherwood, J. K., S. L. Riley, R. Palazzolo, S. C. Brown, D. C. Monkhouse, M. Coates, L. G. Griffith, L. K. Landeen, and A. Ratcliffe. 2002. A three-dimensional osteochondral composite scaffold for articular cartilage repair. *Biomaterials* 23, no. 24:4739–4751.

Skalak, R. 1988. Tissue engineering: proceedings of a workshop, held at Granlibakken, Lake Tahoe, California, February 26–29, 1988. New York, NY: Liss.

Song, E. K., S. M. Rowe, J. Y. Chung, E. S. Moon, and K. B. Lee. 2004. Failure of osteointegration of hamstring tendon autograft after anterior cruciate ligament reconstruction. *Arthroscopy* 20, no. 4:424–428.

Spalazzi, J. P, A. L. Boskey, and H. H. Lu. 2007. Region-dependent variations in matrix collagen and mineral distribution across the femoral and tibial anterior cruciate ligament-to-bone insertion sites. *Trans Orthop Res Soc* 32:891.

Spalazzi, J. P., K. D. Costa, S. B. Doty, and H. H. Lu. 2004. Characterization of the mechanical properties, structure, and composition of the anterior cruciate ligament-bone insertion site. *Trans Orthop Res Soc* 29:1271.

Spalazzi, J. P., E. Dagher, S. B. Doty, X. E. Guo, S. A. Rodeo, and H. H. Lu. 2006. *In vivo* evaluation of a tri-phasic composite scaffold for anterior cruciate ligament-to-bone integration. *Proceedings of the IEEE Engineering in Medicine and Biology Society*, 525–528.

Spalazzi, J. P., S. B. Doty, K. L. Moffat, W. N. Levine, and H. H. Lu. 2006. Development of Controlled Matrix Heterogeneity on a Triphasic Scaffold Orthopedic Interface Tissue Engineering. *Tissue Engineering* 12, no. 12:3497–3508.

Spalazzi, J. P., J. Gallina, S. D. Fung-Kee-Fung, E. E. Konofagou, and H. H. Lu. 2006. Elastographic imaging of strain distribution in the anterior cruciate ligament and at the ligament-bone insertions. *J Orthop Res* 24, no. 10:2001–2010.

Sun, W. S., K. L. Moffat, and H. H. Lu. 2007. Characterization of Fibrochondrocytes Derived from the Ligament-Bone Insertion. *Trans Orthop Res Soc* 32:200.

Thomopoulos, S., G. Hattersley, V. Rosen, M. Mertens, L. Galatz, G. R. Williams, and L. J. Soslowsky. 2002. The localized expression of extracellular matrix components in healing tendon insertion sites: an *in situ* hybridization study. *J Orthop Res* 20, no. 3:454–463.

Thomopoulos, S., G. R. Williams, J. A. Gimbel, M. Favata, and L. J. Soslowsky. 2003. Variations of biomechanical, structural, and compositional properties along the tendon to bone insertion site. *J Orthop Res* 21, no. 3:413–419.

Tsai, J., I. E. Wang, L. C. Kam, and H. H. Lu. 2005. Novel micropatterned fluidic system for osteoblast and fibroblast co-culture. *Transactions of the International Symposium on Ligaments and Tendons* 5:33.

Vogel, K. G. 1995. Fibrocartilage in tendon: a response to compressive load. In *Repetitive Motion Disorders of the Upper Extermity*, eds. Gordon, S. L., S. L. Blair, and L. J. Fine, 205–215 (Rosemont, Illinois: American Academy of Orthopedic Surgeons).

Vogel, K. G. and T. J. Koob. 1989. Structural specialization in tendons under compression. *Int Rev Cytol* 115:267–293.

Vunjak-Novakovic, G., L. E. Freed, R. J. Biron, and R. Langer. 1996. Effects of mixing on the composition and morphology of tissue- engineered cartilage. *Aiche Journal* 42, no. 3:850–860.

Wang, C. C., N. O. Chahine, C. T. Hung, and G. A. Ateshian. 2003. Optical determination of anisotropic material properties of bovine articular cartilage in compression. *J Biomech* 36, no. 3:339–353.

Wang, C. C., J. M. Deng, G. A. Ateshian, and C. T. Hung. 2002. An automated approach for direct measurement of two-dimensional strain distributions within articular cartilage under unconfined compression. *J Biomech Eng* 124, no. 5:557–567.

Wang, I. E. and H. H. Lu. 2005. Tri-culture of bovine anterior cruciate ligament fibroblasts, osteoblasts and chondrocytes with application in interface tissue engineering. *Trans Orthop Res Soc* 30:1522.

Wang, I. E., J. M. Shan, R. Y. Choi, S. Oh, C. K. Kepler, F. H. Chen, and H. H. Lu. 2007. Role of Fibroblast-Osteoblast Interactions on the Formation of the Ligament-to-Bone Interface. *J Orthop Res* In press.

Wang, I. N., S. Mitroo, F. H. Chen, H. H. Lu, and S. B. Doty. 2006. Age-dependent changes in matrix composition and organization at the ligament-to-bone insertion. *J Orthop Res* 24, no. 8:1745–1755.

Wei, X. and K. Messner. 1996. The postnatal development of the insertions of the medial collateral ligament in the rat knee. *Anat Embryol (Berl)* 193, no. 1:53–59.

Whitesides, G. M., E. Ostuni, S. Takayama, X. Jiang, and D. E. Ingber. 2001. Soft lithography in biology and biochemistry. *Annu Rev Biomed Eng* 3:335–373.

Woo, S. L. and J. A. Buckwalter. 1988. AAOS/NIH/ORS workshop. Injury and repair of the musculoskeletal soft tissues. Savannah, Georgia, June 18–20, 1987. *J Orthop Res* 6, no. 6:907–931.

Woo, S. L., M. A. Gomez, Y. Seguchi, C. M. Endo, and W. H. Akeson. 1983. Measurement of mechanical properties of ligament substance from a bone-ligament-bone preparation. *J Orthop Res* 1, no. 1:22–29.

Woo, S. L., K. Hildebrand, N. Watanabe, J. A. Fenwick, C. D. Papageorgiou, and J. H. Wang. 1999. Tissue engineering of ligament and tendon healing. *Clin Orthop Relat Res* no. 367 Suppl:S312–S323.

Yahia, L. 1997. *Ligaments and Ligamentoplasties*. Berlin Heidelberg: Springer Verlag.

Yaszemski, M. J., R. G. Payne, W. C. Hayes, R. Langer, and A. G. Mikos. 1996. Evolution of bone transplantation: molecular, cellular and tissue strategies to engineer human bone. *Biomaterials* 17, no. 2:175–185.

Yoshiya, S., M. Nagano, M. Kurosaka, H. Muratsu, and K. Mizuno. 2000. Graft healing in the bone tunnel in anterior cruciate ligament reconstruction. *Clin Orthop* no. 376:278–286.

Yu, H., M. Grynpas, and R. A. Kandel. 1997. Composition of cartilagenous tissue with mineralized and non-mineralized zones formed *in vitro*. *Biomaterials* 18, no. 21:1425–1431.

Yu, X., E. A. Botchwey, E. M. Levine, S. R. Pollack, and C. T. Laurencin. 2004. Bioreactor-based bone tissue engineering: the influence of dynamic flow on osteoblast phenotypic expression and matrix mineralization. *Proc Natl Acad Sci USA* 101, no. 31:11203–11208.

Zhang, A. Y. and J. Chang. 2003. Tissue engineering of flexor tendons. *Clin Plast Surg* 30, no. 4:565–572.

Zhang, R. and P. X. Ma. 1999. Poly(alpha-hydroxyl acids)/hydroxyapatite porous composites for bone-tissue engineering. I. Preparation and morphology. *J Biomed Mater Res* 44, no. 4:446–455.

18

CELLS OF THE NERVOUS SYSTEM AND ELECTRICAL STIMULATION

Carlos Atico Ariza and Surya K. Mallapragada

Chemical and Biological Engineering, Iowa State University, Ames, Iowa

Contents

18.1 Overview   614
18.2 Cells in the Nervous System   614
18.3 Neural Progenitor Cells   616
    18.3.1 History of Postnatal Neurogenesis   616
    18.3.2 NPCs in the Brain   617
    18.3.3 NPC Fate Identification   618
    18.3.4 Possible NPC Applications   619
18.4 Central Nervous System Damage and Repair   620
    18.4.1 Repair Strategies   621
18.5 Electrical Stimulation   621
    18.5.1 Physiological Endogenous Electric Fields   622
    18.5.2 Electrical Stimulation of the Nervous System   623
    18.5.3 DC Electric Fields *In Vivo*   623
    18.5.4 Electromagnetic Stimulation *In Vivo*   624
    18.5.5 Therapeutic Electrical Stimulation in the CNS   624
    18.5.6 Extracellular Electrical Stimulation *In Vitro*   625

Advanced Biomaterials: Fundamentals, Processing, and Applications, Edited by Bikramjit Basu,
Dhirendra S. Katti, and Ashok Kumar

        18.5.6.1 Stimulation Methodology   626
        18.5.6.2 Signal Selection   626
        18.5.6.3 Electrode Material   627
        18.5.6.4 Changes in Hydrogen Concentration   627
     18.5.7 Cellular Response to Electric Field *In Vitro*   628
18.6 Neurons in Electric Fields   629
     18.6.1 Axon Guidance   629
     18.6.2 Cellular Level Changes Due to EFs   630
     18.6.3 Receptor Accumulation and Autoregulation   631
     18.6.4 Calcium   633
18.7 Neural Progenitor Cells and Electric Fields   633
18.8 Conclusions   634
     Acknowledgments   634
     Dedication   634
     References   635

18.1   OVERVIEW

A potential cell-based therapy for Alzheimer's disease, spinal cord injury and other non-treatable damage to the central nervous system (CNS) is the use of neural progenitor cells (NPCs). To exploit the therapeutic potential of NPCs, scientists must first learn how to control the differentiation and proliferation of NPCs. NPC characterization *in vivo* can be cumbersome due to the myriad of stimulants found in the neurogenic niche. Thus, the identification of stimulants that affect NPC differentiation and proliferation is best performed *in vitro*. Examples of such cues are soluble and insoluble proteins secreted by other cells, membrane-bound signaling proteins, and topography. One additional consideration is the electric gradient that is present in the developing and adult nervous system. In the developing nervous system, a rostral to caudal electric field guides growth and development of the nervous system. At this time there are also neural progenitor cells present, which are differentiating into the cells that make up the nervous system. Yet, the effect of electrical stimulation on neural progenitor cells is yet to be studied. So this chapter focuses on recent studies that may give an inkling of the relationship between electrical stimulation and the proliferation, growth and differentiation of neural progenitor cells. Briefly, the main subjects covered in this text are the effect of electric fields on neurons, the use of electrical stimulation to improve spinal cord injury, and the complexity of investigating electrical stimulation of cells *in vitro*.

18.2   CELLS IN THE NERVOUS SYSTEM

The central nervous system (CNS) is comprised of two types of cells, neurons and glia. There exist 10 to 50 times more glial cells than neurons in the CNS of vertebrates. Glial cells provide support and structure to the CNS; insulate axons with myelin; perform housekeeping duties regularly and during injury; guide migrating neurons and direct the outgrowth of axons in development; regulate presynaptic terminals at the nerve-muscle junction; and more. Not forgetting that neurons have subcategories, the glial cells within the nervous system are further categorized into microglia and macroglia. Macroglia are further subcategorized in the CNS and the peripheral nervous system (PNS) into oligodendrocytes, astrocytes, and Schwann cells, respectively.

First, consider microglia. As the name implies, microglia are typically much smaller than the cells found in the CNS and are the smallest of the glial cells. Microglia are phagocytes produced outside the nervous system and are unrelated physiologically and developmentally to the other cells of the CNS. Microglia are not phagocytotic until they are mobilized or become activated because of injury, disease, or infection of the nervous system. The brain owes its limited immunological response to microglia, because microglia remove apoptotic cells and are activated during injury.

Second, oligodendrocytes in the CNS and Schwann cells in the PNS are responsible for making the transmission of neuronal signals more efficient. They do this by insulating axons with sheaths of a lipid-based substance called myelin. The sheaths are created by oligodendrocytes/Schwann cells densely wrapping their membranous processes around the axon repeatedly. A single oligodendrocyte can myelinate an average of 15 internodes/axons. Schwann cells, by comparison, only envelop one internode/axon. The myelin produced by Schwann cells is not chemically the same as that produced by oligodendrocytes, but are very similar.

Lastly, astrocytes derive their name from the Greek word *astron*, which means of the stars. The reason for this name is easily understood when observing astrocytes *in vitro*, since their cell bodies resemble stars. Astrocytes are the most numerous cells in the CNS and were once consider solely supportive cells. One thought is that astrocytes filter nutrients to neurons, since astrocytes have end-feet at both capillaries and neurons. These end-feet encircle capillaries in the brain, helping make an impermeable blood barrier know as the blood-brain barrier. Neurotoxic substances and high concentrations of neurotransmitters such as norepinephrine and glutamate are prevented from entering or accumulation in damaging concentrations in the brain, respectively, by the blood-brain barrier.

The functions that astrocytes perform are indispensable for the survival of neurons *in vivo*. Astroglial functions were once considered to be purely supportive. What is known about glia and how they are viewed is partly due to precedence given to neurons over other cells when studying the nervous system. Previous attention was mainly given to neurons because of their intriguing capabilities such as the transmission of signals via the action potential. Therefore, astrocytes were studied for their relevance to neurons. Recently, however, astrocytes and other cells in the CNS are shown to serve a more profound role due to the discovery of neurogenesis (Ma et al. 2005). This adds to the problem of clearly categorizing or defining what astrocytes are (Kimelberg 2004). In other words, the neurogenic niche is influenced by astrocytes, making astrocytes more than mere support cells for neurons.

18.3   NEURAL PROGENITOR CELLS

Neural Progenitor Cells (NPCs) are present in the adult nervous system through-out life, can self-renew but not indefinitely, and give rise to (differentiate into) cells of the nervous system (neurons and glial cells) (Gage 2000; Turner et al. 1990; Turner and Cepko 1987; Baizabal et al. 2003). (See Figure 18.1). However, in the adult CNS, differentiation occurs in specific niches. Some of the locations where NPCs are found within the adult nervous system are the olfactory bulb (Fisher 1997; Baizabal et al. 2003), hippocampus (Gage et al. 1995), sub-ventricular zone (Palmer et al. 1997) and spinal cord (Weiss et al. 1996; Kehl et al. 1997; Shihabuddin et al. 1997). The following section will provide additional detail about these cells. The research performed in the author's group characterizes the behavior of NPCs from the hippocampus of rats and humans under different environmental conditions.

18.3.1   History of Postnatal Neurogenesis

Originally, it was thought that neurogenesis[1] in mammals only occurred in the early developmental stages (Cajal 1913). In 1913, Santiago Ramon y Cajal deter-mined that neurons were generated only before birth (Ramon y Cajal 1913).

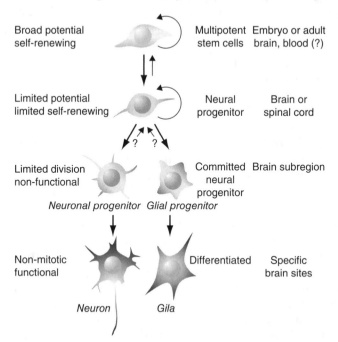

Broad potential self-renewing	Multipotent stem cells	Embryo or adult brain, blood (?)
Limited potential limited self-renewing	Neural progenitor	Brain or spinal cord
Limited division non-functional	Committed neural progenitor	Brain subregion

Neuronal progenitor   Glial progenitor

| Non-mitotic functional | Differentiated | Specific brain sites |

Neuron   Gila

Figure 18.1. Neural Progenitor Cells (Gage 2000), reprinted with permission from AAAS.

1. Neurogenesis: a process of generating functional neurons from progenitor cells. This process in-cludes proliferation and neuronal fate specification of neural progenitors, and maturation and func-tional integration of neuronal progeny into neuronal circuits.

Limited laboratory techniques prevented successful investigations into specula-
tions of dividing cells in the postnatal CNS. Thus, Ramon y Cajal's work became
a dogma for about 90 years, despite evidence that began to prove otherwise
starting in 1961. For a detailed historical timeline see (Ming and Song 2005) and
(Gross 2000).

In 1982, Bromodeoxyuridine (5-bromo-2-deoxyuridine, BrdU) was successfully used to detect neurogenesis in mice (Gratzner 1982) and later in humans
(Eriksson et al. 1998). BrdU labeling is still used to identify adult neurogenesis
and isolate NPCs from the brain. Once NPCs were cultured successfully *in vitro*,
the functionality of differentiated neurons was electrophysiological tested to
established that NPCs were indeed capable of producing neurons.

Then, a very important study of the telencephalon (brain region) in song birds
related neurogenesis with learning (Alvarez-Borda et al. 2004). Furthermore,
synaptic activity and integration of new neurons into preexisting neural networks
has been shown in the CNS, specifically in the olfactory bulb (Saghatelyan et al.
2003; Belluzzi et al. 2003). Still, much is unknown. Future challenges lie in understanding why neurogenesis occurs only in certain areas of the brain; what functions neurogenesis serves; and how neurogenesis is endogenously directed.

18.3.2 NPCs in the Brain

Within the brain, there are two zones that are most proliferative or neurogenic:
the sub ventricular zone (SVZ) of the lateral ventricles, and the subgranular zone
(SGZ) of the dentate gyrus in the hippocampus (Gage 2002; Ming and Song
2005). These two areas are being extensively investigated because of their ability
to maintain neurogenesis or neural progenitor cells throughout adult life (Doetsch
2003). It should also be noted that outside these areas, there are proliferating
progenitor cells that give rise to glial cells but not to neurons (Horner et al. 2000;
Gage 2000; Rakic 2002; Magavi et al. 2000).

Yet, purified proliferating cells, dissected out of many regions in the adult
brain (Palmer et al. 1999), even non-neurogenic regions, such as the spinal cord
(Shihabuddin et al. 2000; Shihabuddin et al. 1997; Palmer et al. 1999), can produce
neurons *in vitro*, when cultured in the presence of FGF (Palmer et al. 1999), and
after grafting into neurogenic regions *in vivo* (Kondo and Raff 2000), such as the
dentate gyrus (Shihabuddin et al. 2000).

The exact phenotype or identity of the most primitive cells that are truly
adult stem cells (least differentiated with indefinite self-renewal) in the adult
CNS, which terminally differentiate into glia and neurons, has not been clearly
established. Some evidence indicates that a subpopulation of ependymal cells in
the lining of the third ventricle are stem cells (Johansson et al. 1999). Yet other,
more convincing evidence points to a subset of cells in the SVZ that are astrocyte-
like (GFAP expressing) as being adult stem cells (Doetsch et al. 1999), as described
in a recent review by Alvarez-Buylla (Alvarez-Buylla et al. 2002). The resolution
of this issue is crucial in understanding neurogenesis and the development of cell-
based therapies for the nervous system (Alvarez-Buylla et al. 2002; Lindvall et al.

2004). In either case, more evidence is needed to identify the location of stem cells in the adult brain.

The way scientists think of the CNS and CNS therapies continues to change, as evidence accumulates for the use of NPCs in CNS injury. Studies are indicating that the CNS has greater self-repair potential than was once believed, in part due to investigations into NPC behavior. For example, degeneration of motor neurons seems to trigger a response in NPC proliferation, migration and neurogenesis in the lumbar region of the adult spinal cord (Chi et al. 2006).

The SVZ and SGZ, as well as other areas with NPC activity, serve as models for the study of neurogenesis *in vivo* because of migration, differentiation, and maturation of NPCs. These areas are interesting because the mature daughter progenitor cells that arise from asymmetric cell divisions[2], in both the SVZ and dentate gyrus of the hippocampus, migrate to distinct targeted areas as they mature. At the targets, the progenitor cells may completely differentiate or become quiescent (Watts et al. 2005). Cellular signaling occurs throughout this process. Thus, within these niches lie guidance, fate-specific, and proliferative cues that control NPC behavior. Suspected cues are being studied to discern the complex task of controlling NPCs.

Cues or signals can be proteins that make up the extracellular matrix or proteins that come from surrounding cells, such as secreted soluble proteins and membrane-bound proteins that come in contact with progenitor cells. Proteins used for interaction or communication between NPCs and astrocytes, oligodendrocytes or neurons are of interest because these CNS cells are involved in every phase of neurogenesis in the adult brain. Astrocytic cues are of particular interest because astrocytes are the most abundant cell type in the brain and are found in neurogenic niches.

18.3.3   NPC Fate Identification

To determine the fate of differentiated NPCs and to distinguish other cell types when co-cultured with NPCs, immunocytochemistry and fluorescence microscopy are used. Most often NPCs are derived from transgenic (genetically modified) mice that express green fluorescent protein (GFP). The GFP in NPCs is ubiquitous, making NPCs easily distinguished from other cells when co-cultured with non-GFP cells using a fluorescent microscope.

In ICC, antibodies with specific antigenic targets are used to identify proteins that are unique to certain cell types. These antibodies are tagged with fluorescent probes that when exposed to a specific excitation wavelength(s) emit light allowing the probes to be visualized. So if the cell is fluorescent, it contains the cell-type-specific protein identified by the antibody. This does not conclusively prove that the cells identified are of a specific type, unless their functionality is tested.

---

2. Asymmetric cell division refers to daughter cells that differ in fate produced from the same cell. For example, a stem cell can asymmetrically divide to produce one daughter cell like itself, able to continue as a stem cell, and one daughter unlike itself, able to differentiate.

TABLE 18.1. Antibodies Used to Identify Neural Cell Types

Cell Type	Marker	Description
Progenitor	Nestin	Intermediate filament protein expressed in both neuronal and glial progenitors
Neuron	TUJ1	Epitope of type III β-tubulin
	MAP2ab	Microtubule associated protein 2ab
Astrocyte	GFAP	Glial Fibrilary Acidic Protein, an astrocyte specific intermediate filament
Oligodendrocytes	RIP	

However, this method is used by almost all researchers to determine what cells types stem cells have differentiated into.

The proteins (antigens) or antibodies commonly used to identify cells that differentiate from NPCs are listed in Table 18.1.

18.3.4 Possible NPC Applications

Currently, NPCs are one of the most investigated progenitor cells because of their ability to produce neurons and the demand for a bioengineered solution to neurodegenerative diseases and nervous system injury (Fisher 1997; Baizabal et al. 2003; Goh et al. 2003; McDonald et al. 2004). For example, neurons lost due to Parkinson's or Alzheimer's diseases may be potentially replaced using NPCs. First, however, stem or progenitor cells must be completely understood to be used as an effective therapy, in any tissue.

One aspect of stem cell behavior that must be carefully characterized is the adoption of a final cell fate. At first, it was believed that stem cell fate was genetically programmed or intrinsically controlled (Rakic 1981). Later, evidence demonstrated that cell fate is dependent on environmental cues or extrinsic signals that trigger changes in behavior (O'Neill and Schaffer 2004). The dependence of NPCs on the surrounding environment has been shown in many *in vivo* transplantations. For example, transplanted NPCs in the developing eye of a rat can migrate, integrate, and adopt similar morphology of adjoined but distinct cell layers in the retina (fluorescent in Figure 18.2) (Sakaguchi et al. 2003). The signals that lead NPCs to migrate into a specific layer and adopt the surrounding layer's morphology are unknown.

Determining the cues that allow or prevent stem cells to integrate into tissues is crucial for the advancement of cell-mediated therapies and cellular biology. If stem cells cannot be controlled *in vivo*, adverse effects, such as the formation of teratomas, can arise when applied therapeutically, especially in the case of pluripotent stem cells. In clinical trials, fetal neural tissue implanted into patients with Parkinson's disease alleviated the symptoms of some patients (Fillmore et al. 2005); yet, the inability to control stem cell behavior exacerbated the symptoms of others (O'Neill and Schaffer 2004; Barinaga 2000). Thus, if scientists are to overcome today's limited ability to treat major damage to the CNS using

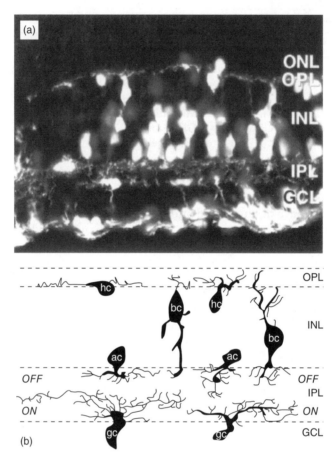

<u>Figure 18.2.</u> NPCs implanted into the developing retina (Sakaguchi et al. 2003). Used with permission from Blackwell Publishing Ltd.

stem cells, then scientists must first completely learn to control stem cells (Lindvall et al. 2004; Marshall et al. 2006). Additionally, understanding the processes that occur in the diseased or injured CNS is necessary for cell-based therapies to overcome limited therapeutic capability.

18.4   CENTRAL NERVOUS SYSTEM DAMAGE AND REPAIR

Generally, when injury occurs in the body, the immune system's macrophages remove damaged cells and debris while releasing substances that promote healing or growth. However, the blood-spine barrier slows and limits macrophage entry only to the site of trauma where the blood-spine barrier is weak (Lazarov-Spiegler et al. 1996; Schmidt and Leach 2003). When the spinal cord is injured, neurons and neural connections are destroyed and debris is created. Many glycoproteins found in the debris inhibit axonal[3] growth (Caroni and Schwab 1988; Cadelli and Schwab 1991). Since the immune system's intervention is slow in the CNS—compared to the peripheral nervous system (PNS)—and restricted, the injury is not properly "cleaned" and healing substances are not delivered. Furthermore, astrocyte proliferation is activated (Kakulas and Taylor 1992) producing a physical and chemical (astrocyte secrete soluble factors) barrier, known as the "glial scar," through which surviving neurons cannot extend their axons (Geller and Fawcett 2002). Simply stated, an inhospitable environment which prevents axonal growth (Houle and Tessler 2003; McKerracher 2001) emerges and remains after CNS injury.

18.4.1   Repair Strategies

Since the PNS can regenerate when damaged, early attempts to repair the CNS involved PNS tissue transplants (Horner et al. 2002). In 1980, PNS tissue grafted into damaged regions of the brain and spinal cord promoted axonal re-growth of CNS axons (Richardson et al. 1980; Benfey and Aguayo 1982). Grafts composed of similar tissues, such as fetal spinal cord tissue (Reier et al. 1986), also showed beneficial results. Further research made nerve grafts the main approach when repairing transections of the PNS. However, additional surgery is necessary to remove donor tissue, and after grafting, total nerve function is not restored. Therefore, a bioengineered solution that does not depend on donor tissue and will restore total nerve function is needed in both the CNS and PNS.

Recent approaches to nerve repair investigate chemical, biological, physical, and electrical stimuli to improve regenerative conditions. Chemical approaches use pharmacological agents that mimic the action of neurotransmitters and prevent cell death or interfere with inhibitors of axonal growth (Chierzi and Fawcett 2001; Rutkowski et al. 2004; McKerracher 2001). Biological strategies utilize cells that secrete recuperative substances or replace damaged cells altogether (for example, stem cells) (Baizabal et al. 2003; Okano 2002; McDonald et al. 2004). Physical techniques employ bridges or conduits that link together a transected nerve (Vroemen et al. 2003; Miller et al. 2002), and/or patterned surfaces that guide cells in the proper direction (Recknor et al. 2005). Lastly, electrical, magnetic or electromagnetic stimulation can be applied to injured nerves, which has been shown to stimulate axonal growth and improve recovery time (Pfeifer et al. 2004; Mohapel et al. 2004; Sisken 1992; Shapiro et al. 2005).

18.5   ELECTRICAL STIMULATION

The use of electrical stimulation as an investigative or therapeutic tool was not taken very seriously 100 or so years ago. Most electro-therapeutic treatments were considered quackery, providing no beneficial outcome. Shown in Figure 18.3 is an apparatus designed to immerse a patient in an electric field (EF) or

---

3. Axons are fibrolytic projections that extend from neurons and form connections or synapses with target cells for communication.

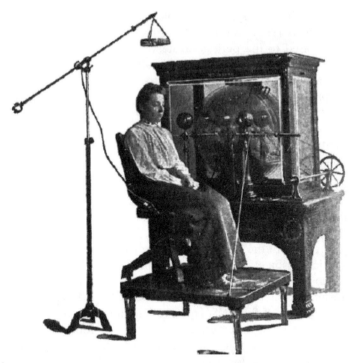

Figure 18.3. Nineteenth century "Electric Air Treatment" (Borgens 1989; McCaig et al. 2005). Used with permission from The American Physiological Society.

"negative breeze" meant to cure a broad range of ailments, even baldness. A metal receptor above the patient's head and a metal plate placed beneath the patient acted as the cathode and anode, respectively. The metal plate was connected to a static-electricity generator (inside a wooden cabinet in Figure 18.3). A patient might be occasionally shocked due to faulty or incorrectly grounded wires, but no therapeutic benefit came from such a device (Borgens 1989).

Such treatments were stopped by the next century, thanks to knowledge gained in human electrophysiology. However, the elimination of bogus treatments did not bring demise to electrotherapeutic treatment. Instead, the field advanced as evidence began to show correlations between electricity and anatomy. The role of electric fields (EFs) in tissues is still being investigated, but now the field of bioelectricity or electrical therapy is held with higher scientific regard.

18.5.1 Physiological Endogenous Electric Fields

The well-known action potential, one of the most significant discoveries in electrophysiology, is a momentary reversal in the potential difference across a plasma membrane (as in a nerve cell or muscle fiber) that occurs when a cell has been activated by a stimulus. The action potential is, in part, what makes neurons so unique from most other cells in the body. However, there is another electrical phenomenon discovered before the action potential, which is not usually mentioned in regular curriculum. That phenomenon is known as the injury potential and occurs when a nerve or other tissue is damaged. The injury potential is a voltage gradient established within the extracellular and intracellular space due to current flowing out of a wound.

In intact epithelium, a uniform potential is maintained perpendicular to the plane of the epithelium. Due to asymmetrically distributed membrane-bound ion channels and pumps on epithelial cells, dissimilar concentrations of ionic species are separated by the epithelium. Na^+ channels are more numerous at the apical side of the epithelium, while K^+ channels and Na^+/K^+-ATPase (pump) are localized at the basolateral membrane of epithelial cells. This causes the concentration of K^+ and Na^+ at the basolateral side of the epithelium to be larger than the apical side, establishing a potential difference across the epithelium. Thus, a concentration gradient drives ions to the apical side where possible, such as between the cells. Gap junctions unite epithelial cells, creating a resistance to the flow of ionic species from the basolateral to the apical side of the epithelium (Nuccitelli 2003).

A break occurs across multiple cell layers, as occurs in injury, creates a low resistance pathway for ionic current to flow between the basolateral and apical sides of the epithelium. Therefore, a potential gradient (or EF) with a positive vector pointing toward the wound is created. The EF that arises due to a wound is found in the subepithelium or at the basolateral side of the epithelium and runs parallel to the plane of the epithelium. The EF or injury potential guides wound healing by making cells migrate in the direction of the wound. Furthermore, the rate of mitosis increases, the mitotic spindle aligns perpendicularly to the EF, and neurite outgrowth is directed in the direction of the EF vector (Nuccitelli 2003).

For most cell types that respond to EFs or the injury potential, there seems to be a minimum EF strength that will elicit a cellular response and an EF strength that maximizes the response. In the case of the human corneal endothelial cells, alignment of their mitotic spindles perpendicularly to the vector of a DC EF is most prominent at 200 mV/mm (Zhao et al. 1999). There are two recent, illustrated, thorough and well-written articles about the injury potential related to wound healing and the history of the injury potential (McCaig et al. 2005; Nuccitelli 2003).

18.5.2 Electrical Stimulation of the Nervous System

Electrical stimulus has been applied therapeutically to improve the regeneration of nerve cells in the PNS. The type of EFs used can be direct (DC), alternating current (AC), and electromagnetic. The sciatic nerve of rats is a common model used to study the regeneration of the PNS. The two types of trauma commonly studied are crush lesions and transections. After the animal is injured, the electrical stimulation is applied and the results are evaluated.

18.5.3 DC Electric Fields *In Vivo*

The use of DC EFs to treat nervous system injury is effective at stimulating regrowth of axons as long as the cathode is present distally, otherwise no benefits are observed (Pomeranz et al. 1984). When an EF is created in air, electrons flows form the anode to the cathode. However, when an EF is applied through tissue or culture media, ions carry the charge from the anode to the cathode. The movement of ions from anode to cathode is the reason that DC EFs are generally effective only when the cathode is placed past the injury in the direction of desired growth. Conversely, if the cathode is placed proximally to the injury, the EF vector will be against the direction of desired growth, which seems to hinder regeneration (Winter et al. 1981).

DC EFs show similar types of improvements in the regeneration of nerves. For example, electrodes placed intraluminally in transected rat sciatic nerves were used to apply a weak-DC EF. After treatment, the regenerated-axonal distance in the rats sciatic nerve was 69% longer than that of untreated rats (Sisken 1992). However, the age of the treated rat has an effect on the improved rate of recovery due to DC EF treatment. The application of a DC EF in ten-month-old rats showed an increase in recovery rate (measured by a behavioral test) of 21% compared to controls (Pomeranz and Campbell 1993). However, younger rats (three-months-old) did not have significant improvement in recovery. The unaltered recovery rate in younger rates is thought to be due to younger rats having a better healing ability than older rats: two- to three-months-old rats heal 24% faster than nine to ten-months-old rats (Campbell and Pomeranz 1993).

18.5.4   Electromagnetic Stimulation *In Vivo*

P. Jagadeesh and D. Wilson (Wilson and Jagadeesh 1976) were one of the first teams to explore the effects of electromagnetic fields on nerve regeneration by stimulating the median-unlar nerves with a radio frequency signal (5–120 mV/cm^2) (Wilson and Jagadeesh 1976). Transected median-ulnar nerves were stimulated for 15 minutes each day for up to 60 days. From observations seen 30 days from the start of treatment, the animals treated with the pulsed electromagnetic field (PEMF) showed significant restoration of nerve conduction activity and larger diameter nerve fibers, compared to untreated rats (Wilson and Jagadeesh 1976). Similarly, rats with transected sciatic nerves were completely subjected to PEMF. Treated rats regained motor function in four weeks instead of untreated rats, which regained motor function in eight weeks (Ito and Bassett 1983). Additionally, sinusoidal electromagnetic fields were applied to a crushed sciatic nerve model with similar results. However, regeneration was attributed to earlier stages in re-growth of the transected nerve (Sisken 1992).

18.5.5   Therapeutic Electrical Stimulation in the CNS

Jagadeesh and Wilson extended their studies of electrical stimulation from the PNS to the CNS using cats. Cats were treated with PEMF stimulation after transversely cutting half-way into the spinal cord (hemicordotomy). The PEMF treatment consisted of 50 mW/cm^2 at 400 pulses/second applied 30 minutes each day for one month. After three months, the spinal cord was dissected, sectioned, and histologically analyzed. In treated cats, extent of scarring was reduced and neurons traversed the region of the hemicordotomy (Wilson and Jagadeesh 1976). Therefore, electrical stimulation has shown potential in achieving axonal growth across the glial scar, which is one of the greatest challenges in spinal cord repair.

More recent use of electrical stimulation to repair spinal cord injury (SCI) has also been researched in guinea pigs and dogs. The research of Borgens et al. in guinea pigs, first demonstrated that axons could grow into the glial scar and in some cases around the glial scar (Borgens, Blight, and Murphy 1986; Borgens, Blight, Murphy et al. 1986). However, axons were not shown to grow through the glial scar. Despite this, functional recovery occurred in guinea pigs with SCI treated with a 200 µV/mm voltage gradient was demonstrated (Borgens et al. 1987). Behavioral recovery was studied using the cutaneous trunci muscle reflex, a useful reflex when studying SCI recovery (Blight et al. 1990). This led to trials in dogs (Borgens et al. 1999) using implantable electrical stimulators. The trials in dogs used an oscillating electrical field switching polarity every 15 minutes as opposed to the previous studies in guinea pigs where the field did not oscillate. The use of an oscillating EF on dogs with SCI showed improvement in every category of functional evaluation at six weeks and six months, with no reverse trend. The stimulators used in dogs were designed for future use in human clinical trials in humans. Recently, human phase 1 clinical trials of SCI with oscillating electric field stimulation were shown to be safe and neurologically beneficial to patients. No severe adverse effects were observed after one year of treatment in ten patients and there was an improvement in somatosensory tests (Shapiro et al. 2005). These trials are evidence that electrical stimulation may achieve significant therapeutic use. However, these trials have failed to show benefits if implemented after the initial recovery period post SCI. Yet, other studies that use functional electrical stimulation in combination with locomotive training to treat chronic SCI have shown to help rehabilitate walking (Barbeau et al. 2002). In either case, electrical stimulation was shown to have a promising future in the regeneration of the spinal cord, and possibly in the entire nervous system.

18.5.6   Extracellular Electrical Stimulation *In Vitro*

When undertaking extracellular stimulation, one encounters the complexity of merging into one, three fields of study: electrical engineering, electrochemistry, and cellular biology. There are many possible choices to make when designing a system to stimulate cells. The electrical stimulation apparatuses and the characteristics of the stimuli that may be applied gives researchers a myriad of conditions or stimuli to choose from. This can be frustrating when determining the appropriate variable combination that will produce a desired result. The probability of discerning those values can require many repetitions and thorough statistical analysis. Since experiments are done on live cells/tissue, one must consider possible electrochemical reactions that occur when placing electrodes in cell culture media/tissue. Electrode and stimulation device material must be chosen wisely as not to affect the health of the cells or render the electrodes useless. Most cells are sensitive to minute changes in the media and thus any change in the media will usually negatively affect the cells. Finally, the assays used to determine the effect of electrical/electromagnetic/magnetic stimulation have to be carefully thought of and incorporated into the design. For example, when analyzing changes in stem-cell differentiation, a set-up must be created that allows one to stimulate many cells at once yet have separable sets of cells that can be analyzed immunocytochemically. So, when designing such an apparatus, many stipulations must be considered.

18.5.6.1 Stimulation Methodology. First, there are many ways to stimulate cells with a form of electricity. One characteristic that most devices have in common is the way in which stimulation is applied to the cells. Usually an EF is created around growing or proliferating cells. Ironically, this is essentially a scaled down version of the electric air bath that served no therapeutic purpose (Figure 18.3). This EF can be applied in two fashions, with electrodes submerged in the media and electrodes that surround the chamber where the cell are grown. There are numerous electrodes or ways to apply a direct stimulus to the media these include: micro-wires placed on or near the cells slated for stimulation (Salimi and Martin 2004), semiconductor-based multi-electrode arrays (Jimbo and Kawana 1992; Sisken et al. 1993; Kawana 1996; Borkholder 1998; Grumet et al. 2000; van Bergen et al. 2003; Bieberich and Anthony 2004; Nam et al. 2004), electrically-conducting polymers (Schmidt et al. 1997; Kotwal and Schmidt 2001), agar saline bridges (Zhao et al. 1996), and graphite rods (Berger et al. 1994).

Furthermore, cells can be grown on a surface that is electrically conductive and serves as one of the electrodes (working electrode). For this, most groups use a potentiostat: an instrument that holds a constant voltage across the growth media, by varying the current in response to changes in resistance. Two electrodes are placed in the media, one for the potentiostat to measure the voltage change (reference electrode) and the other to deliver the electrical stimulus (counter electrode) to the cells via the media. The counter electrode acting as the opposing terminal that completes the circuit with the electrically conductive surface or reference electrode (Kimura et al. 1998). Of course, the working electrode must allow the cells to grow without any abnormality.

Others have stimulated cells without direct electrodes to media contact, greatly reducing changes in pH, the possibility of contamination, and electrode by-products due to electrochemical reactions, the caveat being that more power is needed to supply a field of similar strength compared to electrodes placed directly in the growth media where the cells are maintained. One of the simplest ways to achieve this is to use parallel metal plates (that is, stainless steal) to create a capacitive EF that surrounds petri dishes (Hartig et al. 2000). Similarly, electromagnetic stimulation through a large solenoid (Grassi et al. 2004) or with other arrangements (Walker et al. 1994; Longo et al. 1999; Lohmann et al. 2000; McFarlane et al. 2000; Tattersall et al. 2001), and magnetic fields (Blackman et al. 1993; Trabulsi et al. 1996; Arias-Carrion et al. 2004) have been used.

18.5.6.2 Signal Selection. Second, the electrical signal that is chosen for stimulation has many variables. The stimulus can be direct current (DC—

constant voltage) (Bawin et al. 1986; Bikson et al. 2004), alternating current (Bawin et al. 1984; Bawin et al. 1986), biphasic, or monophasic (pulses with only either positive or negative components) (Zeck and Fromherz 2001; Fromherz 2003). Furthermore, the signal can be modified in terms of frequency, amplitude, impulse duration, impulse delay, and waveform. Typical waveforms used are square or rectangular (Zeck and Fromherz 2001; Fromherz 2003; Mitchell et al. 1992), triangular and sinusoidal (Grumet 1994; Grumet et al. 2000). Most function generators now allow unique waveforms to be created so the signal possibilities are endless. The biggest constraints when applying electrical stimulation to live cells or tissue is that the current should not cause cell death.

18.5.6.3 Electrode Material. When considering the material to be used as electrodes, one must consider cost, reusability, reversibility, and how the material may affect the cells. Some common electrode materials used in electrophysiology are Ag/AgCl, Pt, graphite and gold. These electrodes are used to establish an EF directly in the media, converting the flow of electrons into the flow of ions and vice versa, allowing current to be passed in a consistent manner.

Ag/AgCl electrodes are economical and reversible, yet they are exhaustible and brittle. They can also become imbalanced when using two half-cells to drive create an EF. In other words, differences in the concentration of AgCl can build up on the electrodes. This decreases or increases the amount of current that is being applied (depending on direction of applied current) from one electrode to the other. To equilibrate, electrodes can be connected and placed in the same saline solution (typically that used for experiments). To increase the lifetime of the electrodes, when using a DC current, electrodes should alternated as cathode and anode, so that the AgCl that is removed (anode) can then be regenerated (cathode) and vice versa. In other words, the amount of current and time that passes through the electrode as a cathode should be approximately the same when using that same electrode as an anode to limit electrode exhaustion and keep electrodes balanced.

Graphite electrodes are not easily exhaustible and do not accumulate ionic species. Graphite is a good electrode material because of high electrical conductivity; acceptable corrosion resistance; high purity; inertness with ionic species; low cost; and ease of fabrication into composite structures. However, graphite is brittle and will easily crumble when handled.

Platinum is inexhaustible and does not accumulate ionic species, but is expensive. Pt does not produce material byproducts; however, H_2 and O_2 gas are produced by electrolysis of water. To minimize water electrolysis, it is best to maintain a low current, no larger than 1 mA (Katzberg 1974). If electrolysis of water occurs, the pH of the media will change, harming cells residing in the media.

18.5.6.4 Changes in Hydrogen Concentration. With the complexity of choosing a signal, it is logical to attempt a constant DC signal that eliminates variables (for example, frequency, waveform, and so on) and allows any effect to be correlated with the strength and time of stimulation. The caveat is that the pH of the media will be changed when using a constant current, so one must design a system that prevents cells from experiencing change in pH to use DC. Solving this problem can often be difficult. Most often media perfusion is a good solution, but this increases the risk of contamination.

One other solution is the use of agar or agarose salt bridges to prevent electrochemical byproducts and changes in pH caused by the electrodes to enter the media. However, the saline in the salt bridges will diffuse out and media will diffuse into the salt bridge when stimulating cells for an extended period and temperatures close to the agar gelation temperature. The concentration difference between the media and agar-saline bridge drives the diffusion of salt into the media and of media into the salt bridge. Diffusion will be slower at room temperature than at incubator temperature which is 37 °C. At temperatures close to 37 °C agar is close or at its gelation temperature allowing diffusion in and out of the agar. Additionally, agar has been shown to cause changes in the genetic material of cells when an electromagnetic field is applied. This may not be related to DC stimulation but should be taken as a precaution (Cohen et al. 1988). Therefore, using agar salt bridges is an appropriate solution for experiments on cold-blooded animal cells, but for mammalian cells, agarose gel bridges and media perfusion is better.

18.5.7   Cellular Response to Electric Field *In Vitro*

The effect of any electrical stimulation is not predictable or the same for all cell types. There is no individual signal that results in the same cellular response in all cell types, although a strong electric signal that passes high enough current through the cell will cause cell death. A thorough review, written by Nuccitelli et al., where the effects of *in vitro* electrical stimulation on several cells types are listed (Nuccitelli 2003), shows that no single response to an identical stimulus is the same for all cell types. The cells mentioned in the list by Nuccitelli et al. were stimulated with DC EFs. Cells types that have been stimulated with other methodologies are: PC12 cells (Kimura et al. 1998; Schmidt et al. 1997), astroglial cells (Koyama et al. 1997), HeLa cancer cells (Manabe et al. 2004), and epithelial cells (Zhao et al. 1996), again, with no identical response to a particular stimulus.

The focus of this chapter is on electrical stimulation related to the nervous system; therefore, studies with PC12 and astroglial cells are considered here in greater detail. PC12 cells were stimulated with rectangular impulses of 200 mV and 400 mV, peak-to-peak, with frequencies of 50 Hz, 100 Hz, 500 Hz and 1 kHz for 96 hours. The result was that PC12 cells matured and extended neurites without the use of NGF. In other words, electrical stimulation caused the cells to differentiate into more mature neurons, which normally only occurs by incorporating NGF into the media (Kimura et al. 1998).

In the latter study, astroglial cells were shown to secrete NGF when an electrical stimulation was applied. A 10 Hz, sine wave with a potential difference of +0.3 V was shown to maximize the amount of NGF secreted into the media. These two studies are related since they both show that electrical stimulation affects the dependency on or the quantity of secreted NGF. These relationships help determine the mechanisms or pathways through which electrical stimulation alters cell behavior.

18.6 NEURONS IN ELECTRIC FIELDS

Despite the different cell types investigated using electrical stimulation, neurons are probably the most thoroughly researched in this context, with myocardial cells following the lead. The relationship between neurons and EFs has been investigated, mostly using neurons derived from cold-blooded animals, which eliminates the need for equipment such as temperature and CO_2 controlled incubators.

The work of McCaig et al. on spinal cord neurons from embryonic frogs (*Xenopus laevis*) using an agar bridge setup (McCaig et al. 2005) is a great example. McCaig et al. investigated the effects of EFs on axon guidance or turning, axonal growth rate, growth cone receptors, secondary messengers and cytoskeletal proteins.

18.6.1 Axon Guidance

Galvanotropism occurs at different thresholds for different cells types (Nuccitelli 2003). The same can be said about the different types of neurons and the strength of the EF needed to initiate neurites turning. Thresholds as low as 7 mV/mm have been reported to initiate neurite growth cone turning (Nuccitelli 2003). If neurite turning were dependent only on EF strength, then determining an underlying mechanism would not be such a daunting task.

Surface adhesion molecules or extracellular matrix components effect the influence an EF has on cells (Rajnicek et al. 1998). Laminin is often applied after another surface adhesion protein such as poly L-lysine (PLL) or poly L-ornithine. Neurons examined by Rajnicek et al. turned cathodally in the presence of an EF on culture plastic (control). Neurite on laminin or on PLL with laminin remained cathodal, although not as prominent as on culture plastic. However, on PLL, neurite growth under an EF changed direction (compared to control) toward the anode (Rajnicek et al. 1998). PLL is strongly cationic demonstrating neurite galvanotropism (guidance due to an EF) to be dependent on surface charge, but surface charge alone was not sufficient to cause a complete change in growth.

A misconception can be that neurites turn towards the cathode because most experiments were carried out using embryonic *Xenopus* neurons to demonstrate neurites are directed towards the cathode in an EF (McCaig et al. 1994) (Figure 18.4). Yet, cathodal turning has been shown mainly for motor neurons (Hinkle et al. 1981) and for cold blooded animals such as *Xenopus*. However, the direction towards which neurites extend varies for other neuronal cell types. For example, processes from sensory neurons do not turn (Jaffe and Poo 1979), and neurites

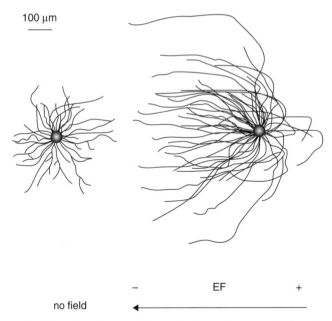

100 µm

–   EF   +

no field

Figure 18.4. Cathodal turning of axons from embryonic *Xenopus* spinal cord neurons, modified from (McCaig et al. 2005). Used with permission of The American Physiological Society.

from PC12 turn towards the anode (Cork et al. 1994). Therefore, neuronal cell type, EF strength and extracellular matrix proteins influence the behavior of neurons when grown in an EF. Furthermore, evidence shows that hippocampal neurons and astrocytes align perpendicularly to electric fields *in vitro* (Rajnicek el al. 1992; Alexander et al. 2006).

Thus, the influence an EF can have on neurites is dependent on EF strength, time of exposure, nerve cell type, the charge on the substratum (on which the cells are cultured), and for axonal turning, if the neuronal projection is axonal or dendritic (McCaig et al. 2005). These variables create a complicated puzzle when determining the cellular mechanics that produce responses to EFs.

18.6.2   Cellular Level Changes Due to EFs

It has been proposed that neural growth cone guidance or galvanotaxis in an EF is due to an accumulation or concentration of receptor and voltage gated channels in the membrane facing the direction of movement or turning (Figure 18.5A). The receptors and channels involved are similar to those involved in chemotropic guidance. For example, in neurons, poly-saccharide-binging plant lectins receptors, such as, concanavalin A receptor (Patel and Poo 1982) and acetylcholine receptors (AChRs) (Poo 1981; Stollberg and Fraser 1988) are asymmetrically distributed due to an EF. Similarly, in corneal epithelial cells and fibroblasts, epidermal growth factor rector (EGFR) becomes unequally distributed (McCaig et al. 2005). These receptors were shown to accumulate, in an EF, on areas of the cell membrane facing the cathode.

Since more than one type of AChR exists, the dependency of neurite guidance on nicotinic and muscarinic AChR in an EF was tested. When nicotinic AChRs were blocked with D-tubocurare cathodal turning did not occur, but when muscarinic AChRs were blocked with the antagonist atropine and/or suramin, cathodal turning was enhanced (Erskine and McCaig 1995). Atropine and suramin are also P2-purinoceptor and bFGF receptor antagonists. Therefore, the interaction of P2-purinoceptors and bFGF receptors with an EF cannot be ruled out.

The release of ACh can be enhanced using neurotrophins NT-3 and brain derived neurotorphic factor (BDNF) as demonstrated in embryonic *Xenopus* neuromuscular synapses. The addition of either NT-3 or BDNF to media of cells grown in an EF enhanced growth cone attraction three-fold at 150 mV/mm, and also reduced the threshold required for cathodal guidance. This effect was shown to be dependent on trkB and trkC receptors by blocking NT-3-trk receptor interaction using antagonist K252a. Not all growth factors tested enhanced growth cone turning, for example, nerve growth factor (NGF) and ciliary neuronotrophic factor (CNTF) had no affect on growth cone guidance (McCaig et al. 2000).

These results implicate three receptors in the regulation of EF induced growth cone turning or nuerite guidance: P2-purinoceptor, bFGF receptor and AChR. Therefore, there does not seem to be a single receptor responsible for galvanotaxis or growth cone guidance by an EF. Instead, combinations of signals dictate whether cells are guided by an EF.

18.6.3 Receptor Accumulation and Autoregulation

The accumulation of membrane receptors in an EF is not precisely understood. However, electrophoresis and electroosmosis have been experimentally and theoretically shown to be driving forces in the migration of membrane bound proteins due to an EF. Briefly, most membrane receptors are proteins with an overall negative charge, which electrophoretic force dictates should accumulate towards the anode (+) facing side of the membrane (Jaffe 1977). Yet, water molecules are polar and surround negatively-charged proteins. The surrounding positively charged water molecules cause the proteins to migrate toward the cathode (−). This is known as electroosmosis. Thus, electroosmosis counteracts the electrophoretic effect when proteins are negatively charged, which is usually the case. More on this theory can be explored in an interesting article on macromolecular movement on the membranes of cells by McLaughlin and Poo (McLaughlin and Poo 1981).

When receptors bind their ligands, a conformational change usually occurs, which can change how the receptor migrates in an EF (possibly due to changes in the proteins overall charge). Therefore, cells sometimes do not respond to an applied EF if ligands are bound to their receptors. This was demonstrated using concanavalin A (Con A), which recognizes a commonly occurring sugar structure, (α-linked mannose, found in many membrane bound glycoproteins. The use of

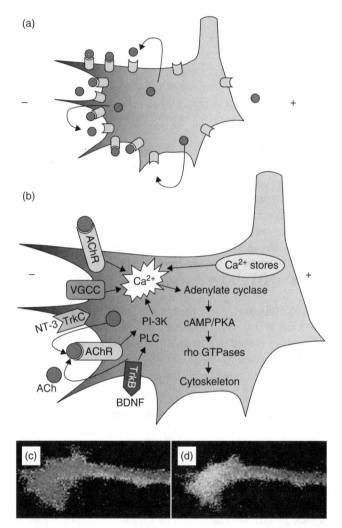

Figure 18.5. Growth cone changes due to an EF (McCaig et al. 2005). Used with permission from The American Physiological Society. (See color insert.)

Con A prevented 88% of neurites from responding to a small EF; where without Con A, 75% of neurites turned towards the cathode (McCaig 1989).

Receptor migration and accumulation can affect the behavior of a cell partly because of autoregulation. A good example of this is the AChR (yellow in Figure 18.5). As mentioned previously, AChRs accumulate at the cathode-facing side of the growth cone. Also at the growth cone, acetylcholine (ACh; green in Figure 18.5) is spontaneously released, regulating cone growth by activating nearby AChR. Since AChRs accumulate on the cathode facing side of the growth cone in an EF, AChR signaling cascades initiate inside the growth cone closer to the cathode promoting preferential growth toward the cathode (Figure 18.5A).

18.6.4 Calcium

Calcium seems to play a very important role in the mechanism of growth cone turning; substantial research by McCaig et al. has led to such a hypothesis: "Cathodal turning requires influx of Ca^{2+} via voltage-gated Ca^{2+} channels (VGCC) and Ca^{2+} release from ryanodine and thapsigargin-sensitive intracellular stores. Activation of AChRs (yellow) by spontaneous release of Ach (green) induces cytoplasmic Ca^{2+} elevation further, since the receptors are 'leaky'" to Ca^{2+}. Activation of the trkC and trkB receptors is also required for cathodal turning. Addition of NT-3, the ligand for the trkC receptor (blue) or brain-derived neurotrophic factor (BDNF), the ligand for the trkB receptor (magenta) to the culture medium enhances the cathodal response. This implicates the AChR further because NT-3 and BDNF stimulate release of ACh from the growth cone, therefore enhancing the asymmetric signaling via AChRs at the cathodal side of the growth cone. trkB receptors and AChRs activate the phospholipase C (PLC), phosphatidylinositol 3-kinase (PI-3K) pathway, elevating intracellular Ca^{2+} even further. Ca^{2+} elevation stimulates cAMP production via adenylate cyclase. cAMP activates the protein kinase C-dependent kinase (PKA), which affects signaling by the rho family of small GTPases (rac1, rhoA, and cdc42).

Activation of rac1 and cdc42 by PKA stimulate lamellipodial and filopodial formation, respectively. This is hypothesized to underlie the EF-stimulated orientation of filopodia and lamellipodia on the cathode-facing sides of growth cones, which are essential for cathodal orientation. Inhibition of rhoA by PKA activation cathodally prevents cathodal growth cone collapse, but relatively low levels of PKA signaling anodally permit rhomediated growth cone collapse, further enhancing growth cone asymmetry. This leads to asymmetric tension within the growth cone and turning toward the cathode. (McCaig et al. 2005) (Figure 18.5B) Support for this theory can be visualized using fluorescent Ca^{2+} labeling within growth cones (Figure 18.5C and D). When exposed to an EF of 120 mV/mm, the Ca^{2+} present in the growth cone increases (Figure 18.5D), compared to the little Ca^{2+} prior to EF exposure (Figure 18.5C).

18.7 NEURAL PROGENITOR CELLS AND ELECTRIC FIELDS

NPCs share some characteristics with neurons; some of the same receptors and ion channels may be affected by an EF. One example is the TrkB signaling cascade, which is known for promoting differentiation of neural progenitor cells (Sieber-Blum 1991). Changes in these or other membrane bound proteins may influence the TrkB cascade or other signaling cascades, causing changes in differentiation, such as the preferential adoption or increase in a specific cell fate over another when NPCs are exposed to an EF. Another example is bFGF, which is known to control the proliferation of NPCs, and as mentioned above, seems to be involved in growth-cone guidance. Furthermore, migration of corneal epithelial cells in an EF was not possible at low EF strength unless growth factors such as EGF, bFGF and TGF-β1 were used (Zhao et al. 1996). Finally, calcium channels also seem to be involved in the differentiation of NPCs into neurons. When L-type Ca^{2+} channels are blocked the rate of differentiation into neurons ($TUJ1^+/MAP2ab^+$) decreases (D'Ascenzo et al. 2006). Speculation provides possible routes for EF to influence NPC differentiation. Once these routes are investigated, a mechanism for the differentiation of NPCs in an EF will be even more rigorous to establish than that of mature neurons, because differentiation is also complex and not well understood.

18.8 CONCLUSIONS

If the differentiation of NPCs were completely controllable and the use of electrical stimulation to treat CNS damage continues to improve, then cell-based and electrical-stimulatory therapies should be developed in the near future. The use of electrical stimulation as a therapeutic tool is already showing promising results in clinical trials by improving recovery in SCI patients (Shapiro et al. 2005). NPC-based therapies are also being investigated, but more progress is needed before clinical trials can be undertaken. Once NPC proliferation, growth and differentiation are completely understood, cell-based clinical trials can begin. The use of NPCs as a cell-based therapy has enormous potential to treat cases where neural cell damage occurs. Despite the complexity in understanding how electrical stimulation affects the CNS cells, understanding how NPCs may be used in combination with electrical stimulation is worthwhile. Combing these two fields of research could produce techniques that treat injury or disease in the CNS.

ACKNOWLEDGMENTS

Authors would like to thank NSF-AGEP and NIH (RO1GM072005) for financial support.

DEDICATION (by Carlos Atico Ariza)

I dedicate this work to my family, especially … my father, Atico Ariza, who despite a short life full of hardship and turmoil, provided our family with everything we needed. My mother, widowed seven years after my birth, has taught me exceptional lessons that have lasted throughout my life. Finally, to the only grandmother I have known, Amalia Mercader Arrien, who has changed the lives of many, including my father, by being a compassionate and benevolent person.

REFERENCES

Alexander, J., B. Fuss, and R.J. Colello. 2006. Electric field-induced astrocyte alignment directs neurite outgrowth. *Neuron Glia Biol.* 2 (2):93–103.

Alvarez-Borda, B., B. Haripal, and F. Nottebohm. 2004. Timing of brain-derived neurotrophic factor exposure affects life expectancy of new neurons. *Proc Natl Acad Sci U S A* 101 (11):3957–61.

Alvarez-Buylla, A., B. Seri, and F. Doetsch. 2002. Identification of neural stem cells in the adult vertebrate brain. *Brain Res Bull* 57 (6):751–8.

Arias-Carrion, O., L. Verdugo-Diaz, A. Feria-Velasco, D. Millan-Aldaco, A. A. Gutierrez, A. Hernandez-Cruz, and R. Drucker-Colin. 2004. Neurogenesis in the subventricular zone following transcranial magnetic field stimulation and nigrostriatal lesions. *J Neurosci Res* 78 (1):16–28.

Baizabal, J. M., M. Furlan-Magaril, J. Santa-Olalla, and L. Covarrubias. 2003. Neural stem cells in development and regenerative medicine. *Arch Med Res* 34 (6):572–88.

Barbeau, H., M. Ladouceur, M. M. Mirbagheri, and R. E. Kearney. 2002. The effect of locomotor training combined with functional electrical stimulation in chronic spinal cord injured subjects: walking and reflex studies. *Brain Res Brain Res Rev* 40 (1–3):274–91.

Barinaga, M. 2000. Fetal neuron grafts pave the way for stem cell therapies. *Science* 287 (5457):1421–2.

Bawin, S. M., A. R. Sheppard, M. D. Mahoney, M. Abu-Assal, and W. R. Adey. 1986. Comparison between the effects of extracellular direct and sinusoidal currents on excitability in hippocampal slices. *Brain Res* 362 (2):350–4.

Bawin, S. M., A. R. Sheppard, M. D. Mahoney, and W. R. Adey. 1984. Influences of sinusoidal electric fields on excitability in the rat hippocampal slice. *Brain Res* 323 (2):227–37.

Belluzzi, O., M. Benedusi, J. Ackman, and J. J. LoTurco. 2003. Electrophysiological differentiation of new neurons in the olfactory bulb. *J Neurosci* 23 (32):10411–8.

Benfey, M., and A. J. Aguayo. 1982. Extensive elongation of axons from rat brain into peripheral nerve grafts. *Nature* 296 (5853):150–2.

Berger, H. J., S. K. Prasad, A. J. Davidoff, D. Pimental, O. Ellingsen, J. D. Marsh, T. W. Smith, and R. A. Kelly. 1994. Continual electric field stimulation preserves contractile function of adult ventricular myocytes in primary culture. *Am J Physiol* 266 (1 Pt 2):H341–9.

Bieberich, E., and G. E. Anthony. 2004. Neuronal differentiation and synapse formation of PC12 and embryonic stem cells on interdigitated microelectrode arrays: contact structures for neuron-to-electrode signal transmission (NEST). *Biosens Bioelectron* 19 (8):923–31.

Bikson, M., M. Inoue, H. Akiyama, J. K. Deans, J. E. Fox, H. Miyakawa, and J. G. Jefferys. 2004. Effects of uniform extracellular DC electric fields on excitability in rat hippocampal slices *in vitro. J Physiol* 557 (Pt 1):175–90.

Blackman, C. F., S. G. Benane, and D. E. House. 1993. Evidence for direct effect of magnetic fields on neurite outgrowth. *Faseb J* 7 (9):801–6.

Blight, A. R., M. E. McGinnis, and R. B. Borgens. 1990. Cutaneus trunci muscle reflex of the guinea pig. *J Comp Neurol* 296 (4):614–33.

Borgens, R. B., A. R. Blight, and M. E. McGinnis. 1987. Behavioral recovery induced by applied electric fields after spinal cord hemisection in guinea pig. *Science* 238 (4825):366–9.

Borgens, R. B., A. R. Blight, and D. J. Murphy. 1986. Axonal regeneration in spinal cord injury: a perspective and new technique. *J Comp Neurol* 250 (2):157–67.

Borgens, R. B., A. R. Blight, D. J. Murphy, and L. Stewart. 1986. Transected dorsal column axons within the guinea pig spinal cord regenerate in the presence of an applied electric field. *J Comp Neurol* 250 (2):168–80.

Borgens, R. B., J. P. Toombs, G. Breur, W. R. Widmer, D. Waters, A. M. Harbath, P. March, and L. G. Adams. 1999. An imposed oscillating electrical field improves the recovery of function in neurologically complete paraplegic dogs. *J Neurotrauma* 16 (7):639–57.

Borgens, R. B. 1989. *Electric fields in vertebrate repair: natural and applied voltages in vertebrate regeneration and healing.* New York: A.R. Liss.

Borkholder, D. A. 1998. Cell Based Biosensors Using Microelectrodes. PhD, Department of Electrical Engineering, Stanford University, San Francisco.

Cadelli, D. S., and M. E. Schwab. 1991. Myelin-associated inhibitors of neurite outgrowth and their role in CNS regeneration. *Ann N Y Acad Sci* 633:234–40.

Cajal, S. R. Y. 1913. Degeneration and Regeneration of the Nervous System. London: Oxford University Press. Original edition, 1913.

Campbell, J. J., and B. Pomeranz. 1993. A new method to study motoneuron regeneration using electromyograms shows that regeneration slows with age in rat sciatic nerve. *Brain Res* 603 (2):264–70.

Caroni, P., and M. E. Schwab. 1988. Two membrane protein fractions from rat central myelin with inhibitory properties for neurite growth and fibroblast spreading. *J Cell Biol* 106 (4):1281–8.

Chi, L., Y. Ke, C. Luo, B. Li, D. Gozal, B. Kalyanaraman, and R. Liu. 2006. Motor neuron degeneration promotes neural progenitor cell proliferation, migration, and neurogenesis in the spinal cords of amyotrophic lateral sclerosis mice. *Stem Cells* 24 (1):34–43.

Chierzi, S., and J. W. Fawcett. 2001. Regeneration in the mammalian optic nerve. *Restor Neurol Neurosci* 19 (1–2):109–18.

Cohen, M. M., S. Schwartz, A. Kunska, J. Satish, and A. Hamburger. 1988. The effect of tissue culture agar on chromosome breakage, sister-chromatid exchanges and clonogenicity in human cells. *Mutat Res* 208 (3–4):201–5.

Cork, R. J., M. E. McGinnis, J. Tsai, and K. R. Robinson. 1994. The growth of PC12 neurites is biased towards the anode of an applied electrical field. *J Neurobiol* 25 (12):1509–16.

D'Ascenzo, M., R. Piacentini, P. Casalbore, M. Budoni, R. Pallini, G. B. Azzena, and C. Grassi. 2006. Role of L-type Ca2+ channels in neural stem/progenitor cell differentiation. *Eur J Neurosci* 23 (4):935–44.

Doetsch, F. 2003. A niche for adult neural stem cells. *Curr Opin Genet Dev* 13 (5):543–50.

Doetsch, F., I. Caille, D. A. Lim, J. M. Garcia-Verdugo, and A. Alvarez-Buylla. 1999. Subventricular zone astrocytes are neural stem cells in the adult mammalian brain. *Cell* 97 (6):703–16.

Eriksson, P. S., E. Perfilieva, T. Bjork-Eriksson, A. M. Alborn, C. Nordborg, D. A. Peterson, and F. H. Gage. 1998. Neurogenesis in the adult human hippocampus. *Nat Med* 4 (11):1313–7.

Erskine, L., and C. D. McCaig. 1995. Growth cone neurotransmitter receptor activation modulates electric field-guided nerve growth. *Dev Biol* 171 (2):330–9.

Fillmore, H. L., K. L. Holloway, and G. T. Gillies. 2005. Cell replacement efforts to repair neuronal injury: a potential paradigm for the treatment of Parkinson's disease. *Neuro-Rehabilitation* 20 (3):233–42.

Fisher, L. 1997. Neural Precursor Cells: Applications for the Study and Repair of the Central Nervous System. *Neurobiology of Disease* 4:1–22.

Fromherz, P. 2003. Neuroelectronic Interfacing: Semiconductor Chips with Ion Channels, Nerve Cells, and Brain. In *Nanoelectronics and Information Technology: Advanced Electronic Materials and Novel Devices*, edited by R. Waser. Berlin: Wiley-VCH.

Gage, F. H. 2000. Mammalian neural stem cells. *Science* 287 (5457):1433–8.

———. 2002. Neurogenesis in the adult brain. *J Neurosci* 22 (3):612–3.

Gage, F. H., P. W. Coates, T. D. Palmer, H. G. Kuhn, L. J. Fisher, J. O. Suhonen, D. A. Peterson, S. T. Suhr, and J. Ray. 1995. Survival and differentiation of adult neuronal progenitor cells transplanted to the adult brain. *Proc Natl Acad Sci U S A* 92 (25):11879–83.

Geller, H. M., and J. W. Fawcett. 2002. Building a bridge: engineering spinal cord repair. *Exp Neurol* 174 (2):125–36.

Goh, E. L., D. Ma, G. L. Ming, and H. Song. 2003. Adult neural stem cells and repair of the adult central nervous system. *J Hematother Stem Cell Res* 12 (6):671–9.

Grassi, C., M. D'Ascenzo, A. Torsello, G. Martinotti, F. Wolf, A. Cittadini, and G. B. Az-zena. 2004. Effects of 50 Hz electromagnetic fields on voltage-gated Ca2+ channels and their role in modulation of neuroendocrine cell proliferation and death. *Cell Calcium* 35 (4):307–15.

Gratzner, H. G. 1982. Monoclonal antibody to 5-bromo- and 5-iododeoxyuridine: A new reagent for detection of DNA replication. *Science* 218 (4571):474–5.

Gross, C. G. 2000. Neurogenesis in the adult brain: death of a dogma. *Nat Rev Neurosci* 1 (1):67–73.

Grumet, A. E., J. L. Wyatt, Jr., and J. F. Rizzo, 3rd. 2000. Multi-electrode stimulation and recording in the isolated retina. *J Neurosci Methods* 101 (1):31–42.

Grumet, A. E. 1994. Extracellular electrical stimulation of retinal ganglion cells. Thesis M.S.—Massachusetts Institute of Technology Dept. of Electrical Engineering and Computer Science 1994.

Hartig, M., U. Joos, and H. P. Wiesmann. 2000. Capacitively coupled electric fields accelerate proliferation of osteoblast-like primary cells and increase bone extracellular matrix formation *in vitro*. *Eur Biophys J* 29 (7):499–506.

Hinkle, L., C. D. McCaig, and K. R. Robinson. 1981. The direction of growth of differentiating neurones and myoblasts from frog embryos in an applied electric field. *J Physiol* 314:121–35.

Horner, P. J., A. E. Power, G. Kempermann, H. G. Kuhn, T. D. Palmer, J. Winkler, L. J. Thal, and F. H. Gage. 2000. Proliferation and differentiation of progenitor cells throughout the intact adult rat spinal cord. *J Neurosci* 20 (6):2218–28.

Horner, P. J., M. Thallmair, and F. H. Gage. 2002. Defining the NG2-expressing cell of the adult CNS. *J Neurocytol* 31 (6–7):469–80.

Houle, J. D., and A. Tessler. 2003. Repair of chronic spinal cord injury. *Exp Neurol* 182 (2):247–60.

Ito, H., and C. A. Bassett. 1983. Effect of weak, pulsing electromagnetic fields on neural regeneration in the rat. *Clin Orthop Relat Res* (181):283–90.

Jaffe, L. F. 1977. Electrophoresis along cell membranes. *Nature* 265 (5595):600–2.

Jaffe, L. F., and M. M. Poo. 1979. Neurites grow faster towards the cathode than the anode in a steady field. *J Exp Zool* 209 (1):115–28.

Jimbo, Y., and A. Kawana. 1992. Electrical stimulation and recording from cultured neurons using a planar electrode array. *Bioelectrochemistry and Bioenergetics* 29:193–204.

Johansson, C. B., S. Momma, D. L. Clarke, M. Risling, U. Lendahl, and J. Frisen. 1999. Identification of a neural stem cell in the adult mammalian central nervous system. *Cell* 96 (1):25–34.

Kakulas, B. A., and J. R. Taylor. 1992. Pathology of injuries of the vertebral column and spinal cord. In *Handbook of Clinical Neurology*, edited by P. J. Vinken, P. J. Bruyn, H. L. Klauwens, and H. L. Frankel. Amsterdam: Elsevier.

Katzberg, A. A. 1974. The induction of cellular orientation by low-level electrical currents. *Ann N Y Acad Sci* 238:445–50.

Kawana, A. 1996. Formation of a simple model brain on microfabricated electrode arrays. In *Nanofabrication and Biosystems: Integrating materials science, engineering, and biology*, edited by J. L. Hoch HC, and Craighead HG. New York: Cambridge University Press.

Kehl, L. J., C. A. Fairbanks, T. M. Laughlin, and G. L. Wilcox. 1997. Neurogenesis in post-natal rat spinal cord: a study in primary culture. *Science* 276 (5312):586–9.

Kimelberg, H. K. 2004. The problem of astrocyte identity. *Neurochem Int* 45 (2–3):191–202.

Kimura, K., Y. Yanagida, T. Haruyama, E. Kobatake, and M. Aizawa. 1998. Electrically induced neurite outgrowth of PC12 cells on the electrode surface. *Med Biol Eng Comput* 36 (4):493–8.

Kondo, T., and M. Raff. 2000. Oligodendrocyte precursor cells reprogrammed to become multipotential CNS stem cells. *Science* 289 (5485):1754–7.

Kotwal, A., and C. E. Schmidt. 2001. Electrical stimulation alters protein adsorption and nerve cell interactions with electrically conducting biomaterials. *Biomaterials* 22 (10):1055–64.

Koyama, S., T. Haruyama, E. Kobatake, and M. Aizawa. 1997. Electrically induced NGF production by astroglial cells. *Nat Biotechnol* 15 (2):164–6.

Lazarov-Spiegler, O., A. S. Solomon, A. B. Zeev-Brann, D. L. Hirschberg, V. Lavie, and M. Schwartz. 1996. Transplantation of activated macrophages overcomes central nervous system regrowth failure. *Faseb J* 10 (11):1296–302.

Lindvall, O., Z. Kokaia, and A. Martinez-Serrano. 2004. Stem cell therapy for human neurodegenerative disorders-how to make it work. *Nat Med* 10 Suppl:S42–50.

Lohmann, C. H., Z. Schwartz, Y. Liu, H. Guerkov, D. D. Dean, B. Simon, and B. D. Boyan. 2000. Pulsed electromagnetic field stimulation of MG63 osteoblast-like cells affects differentiation and local factor production. *J Orthop Res* 18 (4):637–46.

Longo, F. M., T. Yang, S. Hamilton, J. F. Hyde, J. Walker, L. Jennes, R. Stach, and B. F. Sisken. 1999. Electromagnetic fields influence NGF activity and levels following sciatic nerve transection. *J Neurosci Res* 55 (2):230–7.

Ma, D. K., G. L. Ming, and H. Song. 2005. Glial influences on neural stem cell development: cellular niches for adult neurogenesis. *Curr Opin Neurobiol* 15 (5):514–20.

Magavi, S. S., B. R. Leavitt, and J. D. Macklis. 2000. Induction of neurogenesis in the neocortex of adult mice. *Nature* 405 (6789):951–5.

Manabe, M., M. Mie, Y. Yanagida, M. Aizawa, and E. Kobatake. 2004. Combined effect of electrical stimulation and cisplatin in HeLa cell death. *Biotechnol Bioeng* 86 (6): 661–6.

Marshall, C. T., C. Lu, W. Winstead, X. Zhang, M. Xiao, G. Harding, K. M. Klueber, and F. J. Roisen. 2006. The therapeutic potential of human olfactory-derived stem cells. *Histol Histopathol* 21 (6):633–43.

McCaig, C. D. 1989. Studies on the mechanism of embryonic frog nerve orientation in a small applied electric field. *J Cell Sci* 93 (Pt 4):723–30.

McCaig, C. D., A. M. Rajnicek, B. Song, and M. Zhao. 2005. Controlling cell behavior electrically: current views and future potential. *Physiological reviews* 85 (3):943–78.

McCaig, C. D., L. Sangster, and R. Stewart. 2000. Neurotrophins enhance electric field-directed growth cone guidance and directed nerve branching. *Dev Dyn* 217 (3):299–308.

McCaig, D., D. W. Allan, L. Erskine, A. M. Rajnicek, and R. Stewart. 1994. Growing Nerves in an Electric Field. *Neuroprotocols: A Companion to Methods In Neurosciences* 4:134–141.

McDonald, J. W., D. Becker, T. F. Holekamp, M. Howard, S. Liu, A. Lu, J. Lu, M. M. Platik, Y. Qu, T. Stewart, and S. Vadivelu. 2004. Repair of the injured spinal cord and the potential of embryonic stem cell transplantation. *J Neurotrauma* 21 (4):383–93.

McFarlane, E. H., G. S. Dawe, M. Marks, and I. C. Campbell. 2000. Changes in neurite outgrowth but not in cell division induced by low EMF exposure: influence of field strength and culture conditions on responses in rat PC12 pheochromocytoma cells. *Bioelectrochemistry* 52 (1):23–8.

McKerracher, L. 2001. Spinal cord repair: strategies to promote axon regeneration. *Neurobiol Dis* 8 (1):11–8.

McLaughlin, S., and M. M. Poo. 1981. The role of electro-osmosis in the electric-field-induced movement of charged macromolecules on the surfaces of cells. *Biophys J* 34 (1):85–93.

Miller, C., S. Jeftinija, and S. Mallapragada. 2002. Synergistic effects of physical and chemical guidance cues on neurite alignment and outgrowth on biodegradable polymer substrates. *Tissue Eng* 8 (3):367–78.

Ming, G. L., and H. Song. 2005. Adult neurogenesis in the mammalian central nervous system. *Annu Rev Neurosci* 28:223–50.

Mitchell, R. H., A. H. Bailey, J. M. Anderson, and W. S. Gilmore. 1992. Electrical stimulation of cultured myocardial cells. *J Biomed Eng* 14 (1):52–6.

Mohapel, P., C. T. Ekdahl, and O. Lindvall. 2004. Status epilepticus severity influences the long-term outcome of neurogenesis in the adult dentate gyrus. *Neurobiol Dis* 15 (2):196–205.

Nam, Y., J. C. Chang, B. C. Wheeler, and G. J. Brewer. 2004. Gold-coated microelectrode array with thiol linked self-assembled monolayers for engineering neuronal cultures. *IEEE Trans Biomed Eng* 51 (1):158–65.

Nuccitelli, R. 2003. A role for endogenous electric fields in wound healing. *Curr Top Dev Biol* 58:1–26.

O'Neill, A., and D. V. Schaffer. 2004. The biology and engineering of stem-cell control. *Biotechnol Appl Biochem* 40 (Pt 1):5–16.

Okano, H. 2002. Stem cell biology of the central nervous system. *J Neurosci Res* 69 (6):698–707.

Palmer, T. D., E. A. Markakis, A. R. Willhoite, F. Safar, and F. H. Gage. 1999. Fibroblast growth factor-2 activates a latent neurogenic program in neural stem cells from diverse regions of the adult CNS. *J Neurosci* 19 (19):8487–97.

Palmer, T. D., J. Takahashi, and F. H. Gage. 1997. The adult rat hippocampus contains primordial neural stem cells. *Mol Cell Neurosci* 8 (6):389–404.

Patel, N., and M. M. Poo. 1982. Orientation of neurite growth by extracellular electric fields. *J Neurosci* 2 (4):483–96.

Pfeifer, K., M. Vroemen, A. Blesch, and N. Weidner. 2004. Adult neural progenitor cells provide a permissive guiding substrate for corticospinal axon growth following spinal cord injury. *Eur J Neurosci* 20 (7):1695–704.

Pomeranz, B., and J. J. Campbell. 1993. Weak electric current accelerates motoneuron regeneration in the sciatic nerve of ten-month-old rats. *Brain Res* 603 (2):271–8.

Pomeranz, B., M. Mullen, and H. Markus. 1984. Effect of applied electrical fields on sprouting of intact saphenous nerve in adult rat. *Brain Res* 303 (2):331–6.

Poo, M. 1981. *In situ* electrophoresis of membrane components. *Annu Rev Biophys Bioeng* 10:245–76.

Rajnicek, A. M., K. R. Robinson, and C. D. McCaig. 1998. The direction of neurite growth in a weak DC electric field depends on the substratum: contributions of adhesivity and net surface charge. *Dev Biol* 203 (2):412–23.

Rajnicek, A.M., N.A. Gow, and C.D. McCaig. 1992. Electric field-induced orientation of rat hippocampal neurons *in vitro*. *Exp. Physiol.* 77 (1):229–32.

Rakic, P. 1981. Neuronal-glial interaction during brain development. *Trends in Neurosciences* 4:184–187.

Rakic, P. 2002. Adult neurogenesis in mammals: an identity crisis. *J Neurosci* 22 (3): 614–8.

Ramon y Cajal, S. 1913. *Degeneration and Regeneration of the Nervous System*. London: Oxford: Univ. Press.

Recknor, J. B., D. S. Sakaguchi, and S. K. Mallapragada. 2005. Growth and differentiation of astrocytes and neural progenitor cells on micropatterned polymer films. *Ann N Y Acad Sci* 1049:24–7.

Reier, P. J., B. S. Bregman, and J. R. Wujek. 1986. Intraspinal transplantation of embryonic spinal cord tissue in neonatal and adult rats. *J Comp Neurol* 247 (3):275–96.

Richardson, P. M., U. M. McGuinness, and A. J. Aguayo. 1980. Axons from CNS neurons regenerate into PNS grafts. *Nature* 284 (5753):264–5.

Rutkowski, G. E., C. A. Miller, S. Jeftinija, and S. K. Mallapragada. 2004. Synergistic effects of micropatterned biodegradable conduits and Schwann cells on sciatic nerve regeneration. *Journal of Neural Engineering* 1 (3):151.

Saghatelyan, A., A. Carleton, S. Lagier, A. de Chevigny, and P. M. Lledo. 2003. Local neurons play key roles in the mammalian olfactory bulb. *J Physiol Paris* 97 (4–6): 517–28.

Sakaguchi, D. S., S. J. Van Hoffelen, and M. J. Young. 2003. Differentiation and morphological integration of neural progenitor cells transplanted into the developing mammalian eye. *Ann N Y Acad Sci* 995:127–39.

Salimi, I., and J. H. Martin. 2004. Rescuing transient corticospinal terminations and promoting growth with corticospinal stimulation in kittens. *J Neurosci* 24 (21): 4952–61.

Schmidt, C. E., and J. B. Leach. 2003. Neural tissue engineering: strategies for repair and regeneration. *Annu Rev Biomed Eng* 5:293–347.

Schmidt, C. E., V. R. Shastri, J. P. Vacanti, and R. Langer. 1997. Stimulation of neurite outgrowth using an electrically conducting polymer. *Proc Natl Acad Sci U S A* 94 (17):8948–53.

Shapiro, S., R. Borgens, R. Pascuzzi, K. Roos, M. Groff, S. Purvines, R. B. Rodgers, S. Hagy, and P. Nelson. 2005. Oscillating field stimulation for complete spinal cord injury in humans: a phase 1 trial. *J Neurosurg Spine* 2 (1):3–10.

Shihabuddin, L. S., P. J. Horner, J. Ray, and F. H. Gage. 2000. Adult spinal cord stem cells generate neurons after transplantation in the adult dentate gyrus. *J Neurosci* 20 (23):8727–35.

Shihabuddin, L. S., J. Ray, and F. H. Gage. 1997. FGF-2 is sufficient to isolate progenitors found in the adult mammalian spinal cord. *Exp Neurol* 148 (2):577–86.

Sieber-Blum, M. 1991. Role of the neurotrophic factors BDNF and NGF in the commitment of pluripotent neural crest cells. *Neuron* 6 (6):949–55.

Sisken, B. F., J. Walker, and M. Orgel. 1993. Prospects on clinical applications of electrical stimulation for nerve regeneration. *J Cell Biochem* 51 (4):404–9.

Sisken, B. F. 1992. Electrical stimulation of nerves and their regeneration. *Bioelectrochemistry and Bioenergetics* 29 (1):121–126.

Stollberg, J., and S. E. Fraser. 1988. Acetylcholine receptors and concanavalin A-binding sites on cultured Xenopus muscle cells: electrophoresis, diffusion, and aggregation. *J Cell Biol* 107 (4):1397–408.

Tattersall, J. E., I. R. Scott, S. J. Wood, J. J. Nettell, M. K. Bevir, Z. Wang, N. P. Somasiri, and X. Chen. 2001. Effects of low intensity radiofrequency electromagnetic fields on electrical activity in rat hippocampal slices. *Brain Res* 904 (1):43–53.

Trabulsi, R., B. Pawlowski, and A. Wieraszko. 1996. The influence of steady magnetic fields on the mouse hippocampal evoked potentials *in vitro*. *Brain Res* 728 (1):135–9.

Turner, D. L., and C. L. Cepko. 1987. A common progenitor for neurons and glia persists in rat retina late in development. *Nature* 328 (6126):131–6.

Turner, D. L., E. Y. Snyder, and C. L. Cepko. 1990. Lineage-independent determination of cell type in the embryonic mouse retina. *Neuron* 4 (6):833–45.

van Bergen, A., T. Papanikolaou, A. Schuker, A. Moller, and B. Schlosshauer. 2003. Long-term stimulation of mouse hippocampal slice culture on microelectrode array. *Brain Res Brain Res Protoc* 11 (2):123–33.

Vroemen, M., L. Aigner, J. Winkler, and N. Weidner. 2003. Adult neural progenitor cell grafts survive after acute spinal cord injury and integrate along axonal pathways. *Eur J Neurosci* 18 (4):743–51.

Walker, J. L., J. M. Evans, P. Resig, S. Guarnieri, P. Meade, and B. S. Sisken. 1994. Enhancement of functional recovery following a crush lesion to the rat sciatic nerve by exposure to pulsed electromagnetic fields. *Exp Neurol* 125 (2):302–5.

Watts, C., H. McConkey, L. Anderson, and M. Caldwell. 2005. Anatomical perspectives on adult neural stem cells. *J Anat* 207 (3):197–208.

Weiss, S., C. Dunne, J. Hewson, C. Wohl, M. Wheatley, A. C. Peterson, and B. A. Reynolds. 1996. Multipotent CNS stem cells are present in the adult mammalian spinal cord and ventricular neuroaxis. *J Neurosci* 16 (23):7599–609.

Wilson, D. H., and P. Jagadeesh. 1976. Experimental regeneration in peripheral nerves and the spinal cord in laboratory animals exposed to a pulsed electromagnetic field. *Paraplegia* 14 (1):12–20.

Winter, W. G., R. C. Schutt, B. F. Sisken, and S. D. Smith. 1981. Effects of low levels of direct current on peripheral nerve regeneration. Paper read at 27th Annual Orthopedic Research Society, February 24–26, at Las Vegas, Nevada.

Zeck, G., and P. Fromherz. 2001. Noninvasive neuroelectronic interfacing with synaptically connected snail neurons immobilized on a semiconductor chip. *Proc Natl Acad Sci U S A* 98 (18):10457–62.

Zhao, M., A. Agius-Fernandez, J. V. Forrester, and C. D. McCaig. 1996. Orientation and directed migration of cultured corneal epithelial cells in small electric fields are serum dependent. *J Cell Sci* 109 (Pt 6):1405–14.

Zhao, M., J. V. Forrester, and C. D. McCaig. 1999. A small, physiological electric field orients cell division. *Proc Natl Acad Sci U S A* 96 (9):4942–6.

19

PLACENTAL UMBILICAL CORD BLOOD: A TRUE BLOOD SUBSTITUTE

Niranjan Bhattacharya

Advisor, Biomedical Research and Consultant, Advanced Medical Research Institute (AMRI) Hospitals, Gol Park, B.P.Poddar Hospitals, Alipore, Apollo Gleneagle Hospital, and Vidyasagore Hospital, Calcutta, India

Contents

19.1 Overview   644
19.2 The Problem of Safe Blood Transfusion and the Global Scenario   644
19.3 The Search for a True Blood Substitute and Its Problems   645
19.4 Wastage of the Placenta and Its Content   648
19.5 Rationality for the Use of Cord Blood as a True Blood Substitute   649
19.6 Cord Blood Stability in Room Temperature and Time   650
19.7 Contemporary Clinical Experience and Safety Studies of Cord Blood Transfusion   652
19.8 Special Properties of Cord Blood Transfusion   656
19.9 Conclusion   658
    Acknowledgment   659
    References   659

Advanced Biomaterials: Fundamentals, Processing, and Applications, Edited by Bikramjit Basu, Dhirendra S. Katti, and Ashok Kumar
Copyright © 2009 The American Ceramic Society

643

19.1　OVERVIEW

The current generation of blood substitutes are actually poor RBC substitutes, which primarily carry out only the oxygen-carrying function of hemoglobin. Ideally such agents should replicate the functions of platelets, plasma coagulation factors, and their various activation processes, a true volume expansion, carrying and activating immune cells (WBC), and so forth, as well as oxygen carrying functions.

Properly screened placental umbilical cord blood, freshly collected after the birth of a healthy baby, is an ideal and true blood substitute with enormous clinical potential. This blood has a rich mix of fetal and adult hemoglobin, in addition to a high platelet count and coagulation factors, and contains WBCs and plasma filled with cytokine and growth factors. The constituents of this precious blood are developmentally hypo-antigenic and also maintain an altered metabolic profile. All these factors make it a real and safe alternative to adult blood, especially in emergencies caused by any etiology of blood loss. It may also have the potential to prevent ischemia and eventual hypoxic-triggered organ failure syndromes.

19.2　THE PROBLEM OF SAFE BLOOD TRANSFUSION AND THE GLOBAL SCENARIO

The need to develop a blood substitute is now urgent, not only because of increasing concern over the worldwide HIV/AIDS epidemic, but also because of sudden terrorist attacks and other disaster scenarios, which appear to have become endemic and which compel a requirement for safe blood or blood substitutes to save lives. The storage of frozen blood to combat such emergencies is often a complex, cumbersome and costly task.

It is a well-known fact that a large number of war casualties die as a result of hemorrhagic shock. Bellamy projected in 1984 that the percentage of wounded soldiers who die in battlefields would increase from 20% to 26% unless the soldiers are evacuated within two hours, and 32% if not evacuated within 24 hours (1). The majority of soldiers and civilians killed in action, crossfire, or bombings die due to blood loss from compressible wounds. These deaths could be prevented if there was a timely transfusion of blood or a blood substitute. The real problem, however, is the availability of safe, screened blood for immediate use emergencies.

The imperative of having a steady supply of blood for transfusion is also highlighted in a report of the World Health Organization (WHO) in 2000. This revealed that there are about 500,000 pregnancy-related deaths globally, and at least 25% of the maternal deaths are due to a loss of blood (2).

So far as the safety of blood meant for transfusion is concerned, Sloand et al. reported in 1995 that an estimated 13 million units of blood worldwide are not tested against human immunodeficiency viruses (HIV) or hepatitis viruses. Moreover, in some developing countries, 80% of the blood supply comes from paid donors or replacement donors (family, friends or acquaintances), even when the percentage of infection in the population is high (3).

19.3   THE SEARCH FOR A TRUE BLOOD SUBSTITUTE AND ITS PROBLEMS

Blood is made of a fluid called plasma in which are suspended many tiny living cells. These are mostly red blood cells (RBCs), with some white blood cells (WBCs), which are also called leukocytes, and smaller cells called platelets. The cellular components make up 45% of the blood volume. Through a complex process, which incorporates the oxygen-carrying pigment, the hemoglobin, inside the RBC (instead of carrying oxygen in the plasma itself), the evolutionary process increased by about 100 times the oxygen carrying capacity of blood and its metabolic process in higher vertebrates. If hemoglobin is extra-cellular and intra-vascular, it exerts more osmotic pressure than plasma protein. As a result, water will be drawn from the tissue space and will load the intra-vascular compartment. By the inclusion of the hemoglobin component inside the cell (RBC), the viscosity of the blood remains low, water is not drawn from the tissue space and the flow of blood with its large protein content is made possible.

In addition, RBC membranes contain enzymes that protect the hemoglobin from degradation and allow it to work for three months at a stretch. If there is a lack of enzymes in the membrane, free hemoglobin leaves it at risk of oxidative damage by the haem molecule.

Furthermore, membrane-free hemoglobin is always subject to oxidative denaturation and it also acts as a trigger for hypertensive episodes. Through evolution, the oxygen-free carrying pigment in invertebrates became intracellular for better tissue perfusion in response to growth and metabolic demands, in lower vertebrates to higher vertebrates.

It is the pigment, hemoglobin, which gives red blood cells its color. Hemoglobin is a complex protein containing iron, which is found in no other cell. It has an affinity for oxygen, which varies with the pH (acidity) of the tissues. The red blood cells carry oxygen from air in the lungs to all the cells of the body. The waste product (carbon dioxide) is carried by cells from various tissues to the lungs, where it is once more exchanged for oxygen. The usual range of hemoglobin in a normal adult is between 12 and 15 gms/dl.

The search for an oxygen-carrying substitute for blood began in 1940, during the great wars as reported by Amberson (4). It was during World War II that the military realized the difficulties in transporting whole blood and began a search to find an alternative. However, technology at that time did not support the development or large-scale production of highly purified products.

It was during the 1980s that the need for oxygen-based blood substitutes became even more critical with the growing incidence of HIV/AIDS. The risk of infection from HIV and hepatitis B and C viruses caused international concern.

The resultant search for a true blood substitute has led to the selection and isolation of a group of hemoglobin-based oxygen carriers from human as well as bovine sources of hemoglobin, which can provide the respiratory functions of hemoglobin alone. It should be noted that none of these have passed through the Phase III clinical trials of the United States. Other problems related to these carriers are prohibitory costs and an unacceptable level of complications.

However, experimentation has continued in this area, using human RBC to bovine RBC, particularly its chemically or genetically modified forms. A report in *Nature* in 2003 also noted that there has been extraction from sea creatures (*Arenicola Marina*), that is, the sea worm, for potential human use (5). But animal hemoglobin, it should be mentioned, can trigger allergic reactions and even damage the kidneys.

Any blood substitute must be safe and efficacious before it can be used clinically. However, safety and efficacy may have many interpretations. Thus, the ideal blood substitute continues to be elusive, particularly because its function must include the properties of an oxygen-carrying volume expander which is free of any risk of infection or adverse effects; there must also be a lack of antigenicity so that it can be administered unmatched without any fear of immune reactions. The substitute must also have a stable shelf life and an intravascular half-life of several weeks to months. It must be easy to produce in mass quantities, and its cost should not be prohibitive for wide-scale use. If the advances in the field are briefly examined, it can be seen that hemoglobin-based blood substitutes include human blood, bovine blood, and recombinant technology. Human blood comes from outdated red blood cells, and the main disadvantage of this source may be its lack of availability. Bovine blood is widely available in slaughterhouses, but initial studies suggest some antigenicity. Bovine hemoglobin has a P-50 that is closer to human hemoglobin when in red blood cells than human stroma-free hemoglobin.

Recombinant hemoglobin has an advantage over bovine and human hemoglobin in that the genetic code can be modified to produce hemoglobin with the most desirable properties and the fewest adverse effects, as reported by Cohn (6, 7), Creteur et al. in (8), Frietsch et al. (9), Goodnough et al. (10), and Gould et al. (11).

Stroma-free hemoglobin has been investigated as an oxygen carrier since the 1940s, when researchers realized that native hemoglobin is not antigenic. These stroma-free hemoglobin solutions have many advantages over red blood cells, including a shelf life of approximately two years at room temperature for some products and the ability to withstand sterilization. Solutions of acellular hemoglobin are not as effective at oxygenation as packed red blood cells because of their high affinity for oxygen. Therefore, modifications are made to the hemoglobin to decrease oxygen affinity and to attenuate the adverse effects of stroma-free hemoglobin. Unfortunately, the initial attempts of transfusing stroma-free hemoglobin produced renal dysfunction, coagulopathy, and hypertension [Rochan et al. (12), Messmer et al. (13), Luterman et al. (14)].

There have been several attempts to produce an effective blood substitute. Hungerer et al. reported that Diaspirin–cross-linked hemoglobin (DCLHb) (15) or Hemassist, from Baxter Healthcare, is a DCLHb tetramer made from outdated human blood. This product underwent Phase III clinical trials for coronary artery bypass grafting procedures and was determined to decrease the need for transfused packed red blood cells. The adverse effects include hypertension and gastrointestinal distress.

The first recombinant hemoglobin product, rHb 1.1 or Optro, is a genetically-engineered variant of human hemoglobin and the product could be genetically altered to produce more favorable characteristics [Sakai (16)]. Its current intravascular half-life is two to nineteen hours and is dose-dependent. It has similar adverse effects when compared to DCLHb, including vasoconstriction, gastrointestinal distress, fevers, chills, and backache.

There are other promising products like Poly-SFH, or PolyHeme, which is made from pyridoxylated, polymerized, outdated human blood or Polyethylene glycol (PEG) hemoglobin. This product is currently being evaluated for use in cancer therapy to increase tumor oxygenation and enhance the efficacy of radiation and chemotherapy.

There is another interesting product with potentialities known as Hemolink, which is human hemoglobin polymerized with a ring-opened raffinose structure creating intratetrameric and intertetrameric cross-linking. Hemolink, too, is derived from outdated human red cells, which makes future availability a concern. This product can be stored at 4 °C for at least one year.

Apart from these, HbOC-201, or Hemopure, is a promising product. This is a polymerized form of bovine hemoglobin. Bovine hemoglobin has a P-50 of 30 mm Hg, which is closer to human hemoglobin than stroma-free hemoglobin. The advantages of this product include its availability and its ability to be stored at room temperature. Its intravascular half-life is 8 to 23 hours and is dose-dependent. Hemopure has a shelf life of 36 months at room temperature. It has been used in patients undergoing elective abdominal aortic surgery; this product also increased mean arterial pressure and systemic vascular resistance.

However, as mentioned, none of these products passed the FDA Phase III trial, and as such they are unavailable for unrestricted global use [Henkel-Honke and Oleck (17)].

From 1970 onwards, perfluorocarbons (PFCs), too, have been investigated as blood substitutes [Jin (18)]. Replacing the hydrogen atoms of hydrocarbons with fluorine atoms creates these products. PFCs have a high affinity for oxygen, approximately ten to twenty times higher than plasma or water. The oxygen content of PFCs is directly proportional to oxygen partial pressure; therefore, patients require supplemental oxygen. The first product to be marketed was a mixture of perfluorodecalin and perfluorotripropylamine emulsified with Pluronic F-68 called Fluosol-DA. Ultimately, this product was ineffective at significantly improving oxygen delivery in case of acute hemorrhage. Other shortfalls of Fluosol-DA included a short effective intravascular half-life, temperature instability, low oxygen-carrying capacity, and a poor shelf life. Its major adverse effects included acute complement activation, uptake by the reticuloendothelial system, and disruption of normal pulmonary surfactant.

Liposome-encapsulated hemoglobin (LEH) has also been found to be an effective oxygen carrier, without the adverse effects of vasoconstriction [Kawaguchi et al. (19)]. Liposome encapsulation appears to increase plasma retention time; however, adverse immune interactions occur with liposome. This product has an advantage because it can be freeze-dried and stored at room temperature.

In actuality, the most commonly-used volume replacement solution is the Ringer-Lactate solution. If modified hemoglobin or fluorochemicals are added to Ringers solution so that it can act as an oxygen carrier, and to also increase the colloid osmotic pressure, even then the functions of clotting and antioxidants will not be performed.

It has been observed by many sources that treatment with so-called blood substitutes is not too effective in combating a potential injury in life-threatening conditions, which have latent possibilities for ischemia-reperfusion injuries, for instance, sustained ischemia in stroke, severe hemorrhagic shock with intestinal ischemia, prolonged cerebral ischemia, and so on.

Since these substitutes do not contain any red blood cell antioxidant enzymes such as catalase and superoxide dismutase, the hemoglobin in the blood substitutes can break down more easily to release heme and iron in the presence of oxidants in ischemia-reperfusion and thus intensify injuries.

Therefore, newer generation blood substitutes are being tried which may contain antioxidants as in the case of polyhemogloin-catalase-superoxide dismutase. In fact, artificial oxygen carriers are not real blood substitutes. They serve to carry oxygen to tissues and are either hemoglobin-based or perfluorocarbon-based. No artificial oxygen carriers are currently approved for clinical use in the United States.

19.4 WASTAGE OF THE PLACENTA AND ITS CONTENT

In the animal kingdom, swallowing the afterbirth by the mother is a general norm. Even herbivorous animals, such as the cow, swallow the placenta after the birth of their babies. Humans, so far, had not seemed to realize the potential of the afterbirth.

However, recent research suggests that the placenta may prove to be a non-controversial source of hematopoietic and mesenchymal stem cells as well as endothelial progenitor cells. There is now widespread successful utilization of cord blood collected from the placenta after the birth of healthy babies as a stem cell source in the treatment of pediatric hematological malignancies after myeloablative conditioning. Since matching requirements for this type of transplant are not as strict as for hematopoietic stem cell sources, cord blood began gaining acceptance in adult patients lacking bone marrow donors [Cornetta et al. (20)]. Apart from oncology, the efficacy of the clinical use of cord blood has been noted in Hurler's syndrome, difficult spinal injuries, Burger's disease, refractory anemia and many more intractable and congenital diseases, apart from stroke [Newcomb et al. (21)], myocardial ischaemia [Leor et al. (22)], and also in inducing angiogenesis, only to name a few common clinical conditions.

The most important advantage is the less-strict HLA matching requirement. This is because cord blood is a much more developmentally immature source of stem cells as opposed to stem cells derived from adult sources. It has the additional advantage of easy availability. A source of hematopoietic cells, cord blood contains potent angiogenesis-stimulating cells. Several phenotypes have been ascribed to cord blood angiogenic-stimulating cells. In one report, the $CD34^+$, $CD11b^+$ fraction, which is approximately less than half of the $CD34^+$ fraction of cord blood, was demonstrated to possess the ability to differentiate into functional endothelial cells *in vitro* and *in vivo* [Hildbrand et al. (23)]. Mesenchymal stem cells are another important constituent of cord blood. These are classically defined as adhering to plastic and expressing a non-hematopoietic cell surface phenotype, consisting of $CD34^-$, $CD45^-$, HLA-DR$^-$, while possessing markers such as STRO-1, VCAM, CD13, CD29, CD44, CD90, CD105, SH-3, and STRO-1 [De Ugarte et al. (24)]. To date, mesenchymal stem cells have been purified from the placenta, scalp tissue, bone marrow, adipose tissue and cord blood [Kadivar et al. (25)]. The transdifferential properties of mesenchymal stem cells into hepatocytes, cardiomyocyte, and neuronal cell line, to name a few, have now been scientifically proven. Cord blood mesenchymal stem cells are capable of expansion to approximately 20 times, whereas adipose derived cells expand to an average of eight times, and bone marrow derived cells expand five times, [Kern et al. (26)]. Cells with markers and activities resembling embryonic stem cells have also been found in cord blood. Zhao et al. (27) identified a population of $CD34^-$ cells expressing OCT-4, Nanog, SSEA-3 and SSEA-4, which could differentiate into cells of the mesoderm, ectoderm and endoderm lineage.

A "cocktail" of these three elements may perhaps be used in the future to treat one of the more than 80 diseases that have responded to stem cell transplantation. Thus, it may have the potential to treat degenerative diseases such as heart disease, endocrine disorders such as diabetes, and neurodegenerative diseases such as stroke, Alzheimer's disease, Parkinson's disease and spinal cord injuries, and so on. However, stem cells constitute only .01% of the nucleated cells (hematopoietic stem cells, which is similar to that found in bone marrow: approximately 0.1–0.8 $CD34^+$ cells per 100 nucleated cells) of placental blood. The rest, that is, 99.99% of the placental blood, is discarded as trash. The global wastage of placental blood with all its potentials amounts to approximately ten billion milliliters per annum (at the current birth rate of 100 million per year). It should also be remembered that the so-called placental barrier, which is one of nature's finest biological sieves, screens this blood.

19.5 RATIONALITY FOR THE USE OF CORD BLOOD AS A TRUE BLOOD SUBSTITUTE

Cord blood is the blood collected aseptically from the placenta after the birth of a healthy baby. The blood volume of a term fetus is approximately 80–85 ml/kg.

The placental vessel at term contains approximately 150 ml of blood. Cord blood contains three types of hemoglobin, HbF, HbA, HbA2, of which HbF constitutes the major fraction (50–85 percent). HbA accounts for 15% to 40% of hemoglobin, and HbA2 is present only in trace amounts at birth. HbF has a greater oxygen affinity than HbA. The oxygen tension at which the hemoglobin of the cord blood is 50% saturated is 19 to 20 millimeters of Hg, six to eight millimeters Hg lower than that of normal adult blood. This shift to the left of the hemoglobin oxygen dissolution curve results from poor binding of the two to three diphosphoglycerate of the HbF.

Cord blood is the richest source of fetal hemoglobin. Fetal hemoglobin is a natural stress response to hemoglobin synthesis. An attempt is made to preserve and augment this in case of thalassemia by providing hydoxyurea or other similar drug support. Other conditions such as pregnancy, diabetes, thyroid disease, or anti-epileptic drug therapy, can also increase the fetal hemoglobin concentration. Fetal hemoglobin has an abundant source, that is, the placenta. In India alone, there are more than 20 million placentas produced as afterbirth every year.

Cord blood has some other advantages. It is common knowledge that blood viscosity is a major determinant of blood flow. Whole blood is a non-Newtonian fluid, that is, its viscosity increases with decreasing shear rate (flow rate). Blood viscosity is determined by hematocrit, plasma viscosity, red cell aggregation and red cell deformability. The overall viscosity of the cord blood is less than that of adult blood and has the potential to improve tissue perfusion and oxygen transfer.

19.6   CORD BLOOD STABILITY IN ROOM TEMPERATURE AND TIME

Moreover, the stability of cord blood at room temperature has also been proven. Osmotic fragility studies of the cord blood were conducted with .45% NaCl (N = 40) at 4 °C, 35 °C and 40 °C, with a time gap of 24 hours, 48 hours, 7 days and 14 days, along with oxyhemoglobin (mmole/ml) and plasma hemoglobin (mg/ml) assessment in identical schedule. The studies proved that the cord blood was reasonably stable at room temperature, as shown in Table 19.1.

This blood has been successfully transfused, after meeting the ethical and scientific formalities for safe transfusion, by a medical research team in Calcutta, India, as an alternative emergency source of blood transfusion in the background of anemia and emaciation of any etiology from surgery to medicine, that is, from HIV or thalassemia to leprosy, or from advanced cancer to patients with a crippling polyarthritis condition, and so on.

Before transfusion, aseptically collected umbilical cord blood was routinely screened for HIV 1 and 2, Hepatitis B and C, Malaria, Syphilis, blood grouping, and so on. Red cell serology and other biosafety precautions and quality assurances were strictly adhered to. The potential complications of the blood transfusion therapy can be grossly divided under two categories, that is, immunological

TABLE 19.1. Early Study Results on the Stability of Cord Blood at Temperature and Time

Temp	Time			
	24 hr	48 hr	7 days	14 days
4°C	12.5 + 3.5	32.7 + 4.2	45.5 + 2.8	82.7 + 4.5
35°C	16.5 + 2.8	20.4 + 4.4	53.6 + 3.8	100
40°C	45.4 + 6.7	77.9 + 3.6	92.3 + 4.9	100

Mean Fragility (% hemolysis in 0.45% NaCl) with Standard deviation (N = 40)

Temp	Time			
	24 hr	48 hr	7 days	14 days
4°C	0.33 + .18	0.32 + .18	0.27 + .08	0.28 + .17
35°C	0.32 + .06	0.29 + .08	0.24 + .04	—
40°C	0.16 + .02	0.09 + .01	—	—

Mean Oxyhemoglobin (mmole/ml) with Standard deviation (N = 34)

Temp	Time			
	24 hr	48 hr	7 days	14 days
4°C	6.06 + .86	6.33 + .73	7.09 + .79	9.64 + 1.9
35°C	4.59 + .57	7.63 + .84	10.3 + 2.6	—
40°C	10.5 + 1.3	13.7 + 2.5	—	—

Mean Plasma hemoglobin (mg/ml) with Standard Deviation (N = 36)

and non-immunological reactions. The findings of the research showed that there was not a single case of immunological or non-immunological reaction noted from 1999 [Bhattacharya et al. (28)], when this blood was first transfused, to 2006, when this phase of the study ended. This indicated the safety potential of cord blood.

Following the publication of the first report of this study in 2001, there was a subsequent report on the safe use of cord blood to combat pediatric anemia in Africa [Hassall et al. (29)]. However, it must be pointed out that the use of cord blood was actually reported much earlier [Halbrecht (30)], in fact, before the invention of the RH system and the introduction of modern screening procedures. There were no blood bank services at that time and practically no screening for infection and its transmission. Moreover, the study occurred before the invention of acid citrate dextrose (ACD) solution in 1943, which reduces the volume of anticoagulant, permits transfusion of greater volumes of blood, and allows longer-term storage. But in spite of these drawbacks, the study reported that cord blood could be safely used as a substitute for peripheral blood for performing transfusions.

19.7   CONTEMPORARY CLINICAL EXPERIENCE AND SAFETY STUDIES OF CORD BLOOD TRANSFUSION

Millions of people are saved every year as a result of blood transfusions. At the same time, particularly in developing countries, many still die because of an inadequate supply of safe blood and blood products. A reliable supply of safe blood is essential to improve health standards at several levels, especially for women and children, and particularly in the poorer sections of society anywhere in the world. Half-a-million women still die of complications related to pregnancy and childbirth, and 99% of these are in developing countries. Hemorrhage accounts for 25% of the complications and is the most common cause of maternal death. In children, other than complicated diseases, malnutrition, thalassaemia and severe anemia are prevalent diseases that require blood transfusion. Over 80 million units of blood are collected every year, but the tragedy is that only 39% of this is collected in the developing world which contains 82% of the global population.

The authors' clinical research over the past ten years has shown that cord blood can be used safely as a blood substitute. Moreover, this blood has higher hemoglobin content and growth factors, which have the potential to benefit patients in varying diseases.

A brief survey of the work done by the present research group will illustrate this point. In one instance, seventy-eight units of placental umbilical cord whole blood (from 1 April 1999 to 30 April 2005), collected after lower uterine cesarean section (LUCS) from consenting mothers (56 ml–138 ml mean 82 ml +/– 5.6 ml SD, median 84 ml, mean packed cell volume 49.7 +/– 4.2 SD, mean percent hemoglobin concentration 16.6 g/dl +/– 1.5 g/dl SD) was transfused to diabetes patients with microalbuminuria and severe anemia, necessitating transfusion.

After collection, the blood was transfused, in most cases immediately after completion of the essential norms of transfusion. In rare cases, it was kept in the refrigerator and transfused within 72 hours of collection to a suitable recipient. For inclusion in this study, the patient's percent plasma hemoglobin had to be 8 g/dl or less (the pretransfusion hemoglobin in this series varied from 5.2 g/dl to 7.8 g/dl) in the background of Type II diabetes (fasting sugar 200 mg or more), along with features of microalbuminuria (albumin excretion 30–299 mg/g creatinine). There were 39 informed consenting patients. The patients were randomized into two groups: Group A (control cases N = 15), and Group B (study group N = 24). In Group A, the rise of hemoglobin (Hbg) after two units of adult blood transfusion was 1.5 to 1.8 g/dl, as seen after a 72-hour blood sample assessment. The rise of Hbg in Group B as noted after 72 hours of two units of freshly collected cord blood transfusion was .6 g/dl to 1.5 g/dl.

Each patient received two of four units of freshly-collected cord blood transfusion (two units at a time), depending on availability and compatibility. Microalbuminuria was assessed in both groups after one month of treatment with transfusion and other identical support. The mean result for Group A was 152 +/– 18 mg SD of albumin per gram of creatinine excreted through 24-hour urine (pre-transfusion mean excretion was 189 +/– 16 mg in this group) and

103 +/– 16 mg SD of albumin excretion per gram of creatinine in 24-hour excretion of urine in Group B (pretransfusion mean excretion was 193 +/– 21 mg). Univariate analysis using Fisher's exact test was performed for the results of Groups A and B. The difference between Group A and B values and its comparison with the pre-transfusion microalbuminuria appeared to be statistically significant (p < .003). No clinical, immunological or non-immunological reaction has been detected so far in either group [Bhattacharya (31)].

In another study, cord blood transfusions were tested in 39 patients with severe anemia of which 22 patients were infected with Plasmodium falciparum and 17 patients with Plasmodium vivax. For inclusion in this study, too, the patient's plasma hemoglobin had to be 8 gm% or less. The pre-transfusion haemoglobin in the malaria infected patients in this study varied from 5.4 gm/dl to 7.9 gm/dl for falciparum infection and 6.3 gm/dl–7.8 gm/dl in vivax-infected patients. The rise of haemoglobin as estimated after 72 hours of the transfusion of two units of cord blood was 0.5 gm/dl to 1.6 gm/dl (Figure 19.1). What is interesting is the fact that there was a slow but sustained rise of haemoglobin on the seventh day after transfusion (series 3).

A univariate analysis using Fisher's exact test was performed for the results of Series 2 (rise of haemoglobin after 72 hours from pre-transfusion value) and Series 3 (rise of haemoglobin after seven days from pre-transfusion value). The difference between Series 2 and Series 3 values and its comparison with the pre-transfusion haemoglobin appeared to be statistically significant (p < .003). This effect could be due to the bone marrow stimulating effect of the different cytokine systems of the placental blood (Figure 19.2). No immunological or non-immunological reaction or adverse metabolic impact on the recipient has been encountered so far. There was no detected change of serum creatinine

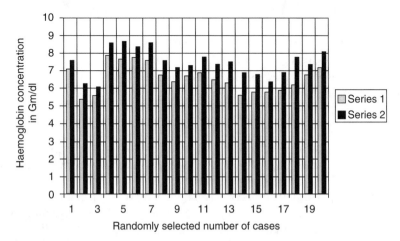

Figure 19.1. Graphical impact of 2 units of cord blood transfusion on the host after 72 hours. Series 1: pre-transfusion haemoglobin in gm/dl. Series 2: post-transfusion haemoglobin in gm/dl (after 72 hours).

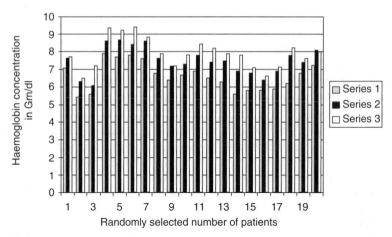

Figure 19.2. Graphical impact of 2 units of cord blood transfusion on the host after 72 hours and 7 days. Series 1: pre-transfusion haemoglobin in gm/dl. Series 2: post-transfusion haemoglobin in gm/dl after 72 hours. Series 3: post-transfusion haemoglobin in Gm/dl after 7 days.

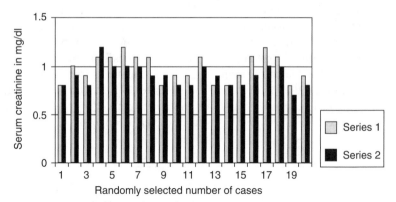

Figure 19.3. Graphical impact of 2 units of cord blood transfusion on the host's creatinine level as seen after 72 hours. Series 1: pre-transfusion Creatinine in mg/dl. Series 2: post-transfusion Creatinine in mg/dl after 72 hours.

(Figure 19.3), urea (Figure 19.4), glucose (Figure 19.5), bilirubin (Figure 19.6), on the recipients of two units of cord blood, when compared to the pre-transfusion level. There was also an improvement of appetite and a sense of well being in all the recipients of cord blood transfusion [Bhattacharya (32)].

In yet another study, 92 units of ABO matched HLA mismatched cord blood transfusion were made to combat severe anemia in the background of beta thalassemia (hemoglobin concentration varying from 3.5 to 5.9 g/dl with mean hemoglobin 4.6 g/dl). This transfusion was extremely effective in 14 patients as an emergency substitute of adult conc. RBC transfusion (male:female ratio 1:1, age varying from six months to 38 years). In this series, the collection of the blood

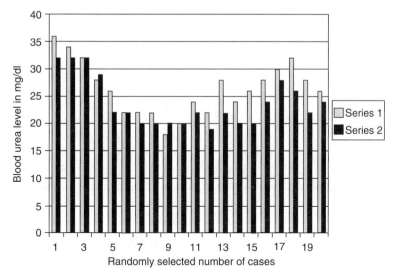

Figure 19.4. Graphical impact of 2 units of cord blood transfusion on the host's urea level as seen after 72 hours. Series 1: pre-transfusion Urea level in mg/dl. Series 2: post-transfusion Urea level in mg/dl after 72 hours.

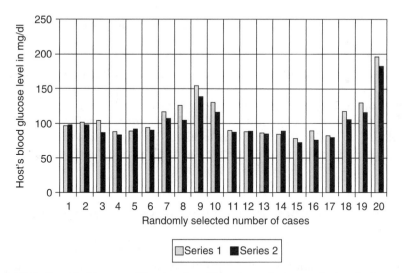

Figure 19.5. Graphical impact of 2 units of cord blood transfusion on the host's glucose level as seen after 72 hours. Series 1: pre-transfusion glucose in mg/dl. Series 2: post-transfusion glucose in mg/dl (after 72 hours).

varied from 57 ml–136 ml mean 84 ml +/– 7.2 ml SD, median 87 ml, mean packed cell volume 45 +/– 3.1 SD, mean hemoglobin concentration 16.4 g/dl +/– 1.6 g/dl SD. After collection, the blood was immediately preserved in the refrigerator and transfused within 72 hours of collection from the consenting mother under-

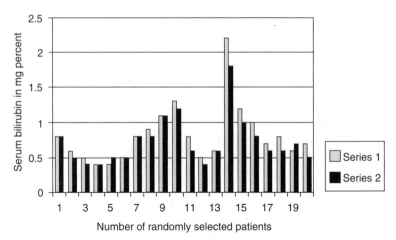

Figure 19.6. Graphical impact of 2 units of cord blood transfusion on the host's bilirubin level as seen after 72 hours. Source: Malar J. 2006; 5: 20.

going lower uterine cesarean section. Here, too, no case of immunological or non-immunological reaction was encountered [Bhattacharya (33)].

In another extensive study conducted between April 1, 1999 and 2005, the investigator transfused cord blood in 129 informed consenting patients (54 men and 75 women). Patient ages varied from two years to 86 years. Seventy-three patients (56.58%) suffered from advanced cancer and 56 (43.42%) patients had other diseases like ankylosing spondylitis, lupus erythematosus, rheumatoid arthritis, aplastic anemia, and thalassemia major. There was no transfusion related problem in this series as well [Bhattacharya (34)].

In a recent article published in *Med Hypotheses* in 2007, the authors, Chaudhuri A, Hollands P, and Bhattacharya N, have discussed the immense potentialities of cord blood use in acute ischaemic stroke to prevent neurological damages [Chaudhuri, Hollands, and Bhattacharya, (35)].

19.8   SPECIAL PROPERTIES OF CORD BLOOD TRANSFUSION

Cord blood use and its effect on the host system have several dimensions. One significant observation from the studies mentioned is that transfusion of hypoantigenic cord blood in a non-myloablated recipient has a transplant impact on the host system, which raises a serious question regarding the necessity of myeloablation and/or immunosupression on donor recipient HLA mismatch.

The author noted this impact in several cases. In a recently published article, the author reported the experience of transfusion of 123 units of placental umbilical cord whole blood (62 ml–154 ml mean 85 ml +/– 8.4 ml SD, median 82 ml, mean packed cell volume 48.8 +/– 4.2 SD, mean percent hemoglobin concentration 16.3 g/dl +/– 1.6 g/dl SD; after collection the blood was immediately preserved in a refrigerator and transfused within 72 hours of collection), which was collected after lower uterine cesarean section (LUCS), and transfused to 16 consenting HIV-positive patients (12 cases had full-blown AIDS) with anemia and emaciation. Apart from the correction of anemia, there was also definite improvement in the energy and fatigue levels in individuals with HIV, that is, physical functioning, a sense of well-being and weight gain from two to five pounds, within three to ten months of the commencement of transfusion. There was also an immediate rise in CD34 levels of peripheral blood in the HLA-randomized host after transfusion, without any clinical graft versus host reaction [Bhattacharya (36)].

Another study was conducted, comprising 106 units (48 ml–148 ml mean 81 ml +/– 6.6 ml SD, median 82 ml, mean packed cell volume 49.4 +/– 3.1 SD, mean percent hemoglobin concentration 16.3 g/dl +/– 1.7 g/dl SD) of ABO matched, HLA randomized placental umbilical cord whole blood transfusion (taken from consenting mothers after LUCS) to 21 informed consenting patients with tuberculosis and anemia (from 1 April 1999 to August 2005) who had plasma hemoglobin of 8 g/dl percent or less. The patients received two to twenty-one units of freshly collected blood without encountering any clinical, immunological or nonimmunological reactions. Three days after completion of the placental umbilical cord blood transfusion, the peripheral blood hematopoietic stem cell (CD34) estimation revealed a rise from the pretransfusion base level (.09%), varying from 2.99% to 33%, which returned to base level in 66.66% at the three-month CD34 re-estimation, without provoking any clinical graft vs. host reaction in any of the patients [Bhattacharya (37)].

In another report on the experience of combating anemia in the background of autoimmune diseases like rheumatoid arthritis, 78 units (42 ml–136 ml mean 80.6 ml +/– 3.6 ml SD, median 82.4 ml, mean packed cell volume 48.2 +/– 2.1 SD, mean percent hemoglobin concentration 16.4 g/dl +/– 1.5 g/dl SD) of placental umbilical cord whole blood was transfused (from 1 April 1999 to 31 March 2005) to 28 informed, consenting patients with advanced rheumatoid arthritis who had plasma hemoglobin of 8 g/dl or less. Three days after completion of the transfusion of placental umbilical cord blood, the peripheral blood hematopoietic stem cell (CD34) estimation revealed a rise from the pretransfusion base level (.09%), varying from 2.03 to 23% [Bhattacharya (38)].

The author has also reported the experience of 74 units (50 ml–146 ml mean, 86 ml +/– 7.6 ml SD, median 80 ml, mean packed cell volume 48 +/– 4.1 SD, mean percent hemoglobin concentration 16.2 g/dl +/– 1.8 g/dl) of placental umbilical cord whole blood collection (from 1 April 1999 to 31 August 2006) transfused to 16 informed, consenting patients suffering from leprosy with plasma hemoglobin 8 g/dl or less. Fifteen males and one female, aged 12 to 72 years (mean 48.4 years) participated in this trial, of which five cases were having pausibacillary-type (PB) infection and 11 cases were suffering from multibacillary-type (MB) infection. Seven days after completion of the placental umbilical cord blood transfusion, the peripheral blood hematopoietic stem cell (CD34) estimation revealed a rise from the pretransfusion base level (.09%), varying from 3.6% to 16.2%, in 75% of the cases, without provoking any clinical graft versus host reaction in any of the leprosy victims. This value returned to normal within three months in most cases (80%) [Bhattacharya (39)].

Another study attempted to ascertain the fate of hematopoietic stem cells (CD34) after placental umbilical cord whole blood transfusion, as assessed from the peripheral blood CD34 level 72 hours after cord blood transfusion in sex- and HLA-randomized patients and its prognostic implications.

In a small study of six cases of cancer patients, a patient with breast sarcoma received the lowest amount of cord blood (six units), while another patient with breast cancer received the largest amount (32 units). The youngest patient, a 16-year-old boy suffering from non-Hodgkin's lymphoma, received eight units of cord blood to combat anemia. Other patients received amounts varying from 7–15 units: a patient with metachronous lymph node metastasis received 15 units, another patient suffering from breast cancer received 14 units, and one with lung cancer received seven units. There was no transfusion-related clinical immunological or nonimmunological reaction. Studies of CD34 levels showed an initial rise followed by a fall in two cases, two cases registered very little effect on the CD34 level, that is, no change from the baseline, and one case demonstrated a very slow rise from the baseline. However, one case showed a frequent steep rise up to 99% and a sustained high CD34 level. This patient is alive with clinical remission of the disease [Bhattacharya (40)]. These reports of ABO matched HLA randomized transfusion with varying degrees of transplant impact on the host raises serious questions about the requirement of myeloablation [Riordan et al. (41)].

19.9   CONCLUSION

There are about 100 million births per year globally. In India alone there are more than 20 million births, which implies production of that many placentas. These are normally thrown away. However, one of the products of the placenta is cord blood, which has immense potential.

Hematopietic stem cells from cord blood are now harvested in many laboratories all over the world and stored in cord blood banks, but they constitute only .01% of the nucleated cells of the cord blood. The rest, that is 99.99% of the blood, which is wasted, is rich in fetal hemoglobin, growth factors and cytokine-filled plasma. Moreover, in the womb, the fetus benefits from the mother's in-built defenses against diseases and the placental environment is basically infection free in the case of a healthy newborn.

To combat the emergency requirement of blood in natural or man-made disaster management, both civil and military, these precious hypo-immune fetal cells with an altered metabolic profile are a gift of nature, entrapped inside the placenta. Moreover, placental cord blood itself could be a readily available source of blood not only in the under-resourced countries of the world, but also in case of any genuine requirement for a blood substitute anywhere in the world, especially at times of crisis.

The term "blood substitute" is actually a misnomer, because only a part of the total functions of blood, that is, oxygen delivery and volume expansion only, are replaced by any available so-called substitute. Cord blood, because of its rich mix of fetal and adult hemoglobin, high platelet and WBC counts, and a plasma filled with cytokine and growth factors, as well as its hypo-antigenic nature and altered metabolic profile, has all the potentialities of a real and safe alternative to adult blood during emergencies due to any etiology of blood loss. The viscosity of cord blood is less than that of adult blood and this may help tissue perfusion and oxygen transfer better. No clinical, immunological, or non-immunological reactions have been encountered so far in this type of transfusion. The observed transient rise of CD34 after transfusion has immense potential for immunotherapy and for its bone marrow replenishing impact, the possibilities of which are currently under intense scientific scrutiny. It has, in addition, all the qualities to prevent ischemia and eventual hypoxic-triggered organ failure syndromes. Therefore, placental umbilical cord whole blood may actually prove to be a better blood substitute, with additional therapeutic use, than any substitute currently in the market.

ACKNOWLEDGMENT

The author acknowledges with gratitude the patients who volunteered for the work. The Dept. of Science and Technology, Government of West Bengal, supported the work with a grant to the investigator (Dr Niranjan Bhattachaya) from 1999–2002. Without its support, the work presented in this chapter could not have been done.

Dr. Niranjan Bhattacharya worked on the problem since 1999 and drafted this chapter in its present format.

REFERENCES

1. Bellamy RF. "The Causes of Death in Conventional Land Warfare-Implications for Combat Casualty Care Research," MilMed 1984;149:55–62.
2. World Health Organization. International Federation of Red Cross and Red Crescent Societies, "Safe blood starts with me," Geneva, World Health Organization 2000:12.
3. Sloand EM, Pitt E, Klein HG. "Safety of blood supply," JAMA 1995;274:1368–1373.
4. Amberson WR, Mulder AG, Steggerda FR, et al. Mammalian life without red blood corpuscles. Science 1933;78:106–107.
5. Hannah Hoag. "Blood substitute from worm show promise-hemoglobin from sea creature could replace red cells," 4 June 2003 http://www.nature.com/nsu/030602/030602-7html.
6. Cohn SM. Is blood obsolete? J Trauma 1997 Apr;42(4):730–732.
7. Cohn SM. Blood substitutes in surgery. Surgery 2000 Jun;127(6):599–602.

8. Creteur J, Sibbald W, Vincent JL. Hemoglobin solutions—not just red blood cell substitutes. Crit Care Med 2000 Aug;28(8):3025–3034.

9. Frietsch T, Lenz C, Waschke KF. Artificial oxygen carriers. Eur J Anaesthesiol 1998 Sep;15(5):571–584.

10. Goodnough LT, Scott MG, Monk TG. Oxygen carriers as blood substitutes. Past, present, and future. Clin Orthop 1998 Dec;(357):89–100.

11. Gould SA, Moore EE, Hoyt DB, et al. The first randomized trial of human polymerized hemoglobin as a blood substitute in acute trauma and emergent surgery. J Am Coll Surg 1998 Aug;187(2):113–120; discussion 120–122.

12. Rochon G, Caron A, Toussaint-Hacquard M, Alayash AI, Gentils M, Labrude P, Stoltz JF, Menu P. Hemodilution with stroma-free [correction of stoma-free] hemoglobin at physiologically maintained viscosity delays the onset of vasoconstriction. Hypertension 2004 May;43(5):1110–1115. Epub 2004 Mar 29.

13. Messmer K, Jesch F, Endrich B, Hobbhahn J, Peters W, Schoenberg M. Tissue PO2 during reanimation with hemoglobin solutions. Eur Surg Res 1979;11(3):161–171.

14. Luterman A, Canizaro PC, Carrico CJ, Horovitz JH, Glover W. Improvement of oxygen—carrying properties of stoma-free hemoglobin solution with acetrizoate sodium. Surg Forum 1976;27(62): 62–64.

15. Hungerer S, Nolte D, Botzlar A, Messmer K. Effects of Diaspirin Crosslinked Hemoglobin (DCLHb) on microcirculation and local tissue pO2 of striated skin muscle following resuscitation from hemorrhagic shock. Artif Cells Blood Substit Immobil Biotechnol 2006;34(5):455–471.

16. Sakai H, Yuasa M, Onuma H, Takeoka S, Tsuchida E. Synthesis and physicochemical characterization of a series of hemoglobin-based oxygen carriers: objective comparison between cellular and acellular types. Bioconjug Chem 2000 Jan–Feb;11(1):56–64.

17. Henkel-Honke T, Oleck M. Artificial oxygen carriers: a current review. AANA J 2007 Jun;75(3):205–211.

18. Jin Y, Saito N, Harada KH, Inoue K, Koizumi A. Historical trends in human serum levels of perfluorooctanoate and perfluorooctane sulfonate in Shenyang, China. Tohoku J Exp Med 2007 May;212(1):63–70.

19. Kawaguchi AT, Fukumoto D, Haida M, Ogata Y, Yamano M, Tsukada H. Liposome-encapsulated hemoglobin reduces the size of cerebral infarction in the rat: evaluation with photo chemically induced thrombosis of the middle cerebral artery. Stroke 2007 May;38(5):1626–1632. Epub 2007 Mar 29.

20. Cornetta K, Laughlin M, Carter S, Wall D, Weinthal J, Delaney C, Wagner J, Sweetman R, McCarthy P, Chao N. Umbilical cord blood transplantation in adults: results of the prospective Cord Blood Transplantation (COBLT). Biol Blood Marrow Transplant 2005;11:149–160.

21. Newcomb JD, Ajmo CT Jr., Sanberg CD, Sanberg PR, Pennypacker KR, Willing AE. Timing of cord blood treatment after experimental stroke determines therapeutic efficacy. Cell Transplant 2006;15:213–223.

22. Leor J, Guetta E, Feinberg MS, Galski H, Bar I, Holbova R, Miller L, Zarin P, Castel D, Barbash IM, Nagler A. Human umbilical cord blood-derived CD133+ cells enhance function and repair of the infarcted myocardium. Stem Cells 2006;24:772–780.

23. Hildbrand P, Cirulli V, Prinsen RC, Smith KA, Torbett BE, Salomon DR, Crisa L. The role of angiopoietins in the development of endothelial cells from cord blood CD34+ progenitors. Blood 2004;104:2010–2019.

24. De Ugarte DA, Alfonso Z, Zuk PA, Elbarbary A, Zhu M, Ashjian P, Benhaim P, Hedrick MH, Fraser JK. Differential expression of stem cell mobilization-associated molecules on multi-lineage cells from adipose tissue and bone marrow. Immunol Lett 2003;89:267–270.

25. Kadivar M, Khatami S, Mortazavi Y, Shokrgozar MA, Taghikhani M, Soleimani M. In vitro cardiomyogenic potential of human umbilical vein-derived mesenchymal stem cells. Biochem Biophys Res Commun 2006;340:639–647.

26. Kern S, Eichler H, Stoeve J, Kluter H, Bieback K. Comparative Analysis of Mesenchymal Stem Cells from Bone Marrow, Umbilical Cord Blood or Adipose Tissue. Stem Cells 2006.

27. Zhao Y, Wang H, Mazzone T. Identification of stem cells from human umbilical cord blood with embryonic and hematopoietic characteristics. Exp Cell Res 2006;312:2454–2464.

28. Bhattacharya N, Mukherijee K, Chettri MK, Banerjee T, Mani U, Bhattacharya S. A study report of 174 units of placental umbilical cord whole blood transfusion in 62 patients as a rich source of fetal hemoglobin supply in different indications of blood transfusion. Clin Exp Obstet Gynecol 2001;28(1):47–52.

29. Hassall O, Bedu-Addo G, Adarkwa M, Danso K, Bates I. Umbilical-cord blood for transfusion in children with severe anaemia in under-resourced countries. Lancet 2003;361:678–679.

30. Halbrecht J. Fresh and stored placental blood. Lancet 1939;2:1263.

31. Bhattacharya N. Placental umbilical cord blood transfusion: a new method of treatment of patients with diabetes and microalbuminuria in the background of anemia. Clin Exp Obstet Gynecol 2006;33(3):164–168.

32. Bhattacharya N. A preliminary study of placental umbilical cord whole blood transfusion in under resourced patients with malaria in the background of anaemia. Malar J 2006 Mar 23;5:20.

33. Bhattacharya N. Placental umbilical cord blood transfusion in transfusion-dependent beta thalassemic patients: a preliminary communication. Clin Exp Obstet Gynecol 2005;32(2):102–106.

34. Bhattachary N. Placental umbilical cord whole blood transfusion: a safe and genuine blood substitute for patients of the under-resourced world at emergency. J Am Coll Surg 2005 Apr;200(4):557–563.

35. Chaudhuri A, Hollands P, Bhattacharya N. Placental umbilical cord blood transfusion in acute ischaemic stroke. Med Hypotheses. 2007 Jun 1; [Epub ahead of print].

36. Bhattacharya N. A preliminary report of 123 units of placental umbilical cord whole blood transfusion in HIV-positive patients with anemia and emaciation. Clin Exp Obstet Gynecol 2006;33(2):117–121.

37. Bhattacharya N. Placental umbilical cord whole blood transfusion to combat anemia in the background of tuberculosis and emaciation and its potential role as an immuno-adjuvant therapy for the under-resourced people of the world. Clin Exp Obstet Gynecol 2006;33(2):99–104.

38. Bhattacharya N. Placental umbilical cord whole blood transfusion to combat anemia in the background of advanced rheumatoid arthritis and emaciation and its potential role as immunoadjuvant therapy. Clin Exp Obstet Gynecol 2006;33(1):28–33.

39. Bhattacharya N. Transient spontaneous engraftment of CD34 hematopoietic cord blood stem cells as seen in peripheral blood: treatment of leprosy patients with anemia by placental umbilical cord whole blood transfusion. Clin Exp Obstet Gynecol 2006;33(3):159–163.

40. Bhattacharya N. Spontaneous transient rise of CD34 cells in peripheral blood after 72 hours in patients suffering from advanced malignancy with anemia: effect and prognostic implications of treatment with placental umbilical cord whole blood transfusion. Eur J Gynaecol Oncol 2006;27(3):286–290.

41. Riordan NH, Chan K, Marleau AM, Ichim TE. Cord blood in regenerative medicine: do we need immune suppression? J Transl Med 2007;5:8.

20

SUPPORTED CELL MIMETIC MONOLAYERS AND THEIR BLOOD COMPATIBILITY

K. Kaladhar and Chandra P. Sharma

Biosurface Technology Division, BMT Wing, Sree Chithra Tirunal Institute for Medical Science and Technology, Thiruvananthapuram, Kerala, India

Contents

20.1 Overview	664
20.2 Dense Thin Solid Films	664
20.3 Biomimetic Approaches in Surface Modification	664
20.3.1 Air/Water and Air/Solid Properties of Thin Solid Films of Lipids	665
20.3.2 Optimization of Heterogeneous Phospholipids/Glycolipid/ Cholesterol Ternary Lipid Composition, Lateral Stability Improvement, and Preliminary Blood Compatibility Studies	667
20.3.3 Air/Water Interfacial Properties of TSF	668
20.3.4 Macromolecule Incorporation into Lipid Thin Solid Films	668
20.3.5 Optimization of Deposition Parameters	670
20.3.6 Surface Properties of Supported Thin Solid Films	671
20.3.7 Biological Interactions onto These Surfaces	672
20.4 Calcification Studies	673
20.5 Protein Interaction Studies	673
20.6 Blood Cell Adhesion Studies	674
20.7 Platelet Adhesion and Activation Studies	674

Advanced Biomaterials: Fundamentals, Processing, and Applications, Edited by Bikramjit Basu, Dhirendra S. Katti, and Ashok Kumar

20.8 Conclusions   675
     Acknowledgments   675
     References   675

20.1 OVERVIEW

This chapter reviews the biological interactions to material surface with a perspective of developing miniaturized biomedical devices. These interactions are surface initiated, and the various surface modification strategies are reviewed. Particularly, the opportunities of exploring Thin Solid Films (TSF) for this purpose are reviewed. Biomimicry of cell membrane components for the development of TSF for biomaterial application are reviewed with an emphasis for its development and a study of various physical, chemical and biological properties of the TSF at air/water or air/solid interface are reviewed.

20.2 DENSE THIN SOLID FILMS

Dense thin solid films (TSF) of few nanometers (a monolayer) with desired functional properties have been extensively explored for electronic[1] and computing[2] applications. There is immense opportunity of these TSF, for bioactive post synthetic surface modification of biomaterials and devices, such as bio-sensors, detectors, displays, electronic circuit components, and so on.[3] The self-assembly of the amphiphilic molecules such as surfactants, lipids, and amphiphilic polymeric brushes to form two dimensional (2D) TSF could be laterally stabilized on various kinds of materials. Such composite systems (developed in nano to macro scale) can do controlled ligand supplementation by avoiding biofouling for an optimum performance under diverse biological conditions.

20.3 BIOMIMETIC APPROACHES IN SURFACE MODIFICATION

Biomimetic approaches were found to be successful in various disciplines. Biological membrane biomimicry could be explored for the post-synthetic surface modification of nanodevices and materials using TSF. Cell membranes form the cell boundaries are fluid and dynamic as well as effectively participating in the biological communication processes. This is attributed to the properties of the membrane components, which govern the fluidity, packing, and orientation of the surface groups[4]. The lipids form the major class of the structural elements, and are heterogeneous across the membrane. The trans membrane lipid heterogenecity is closely controlled in living systems and is disrupted under pathological conditions. Surfaces modified with the heterogeneous lipid compositions and lipid protein as well as lipid-macromolecular interactions could be explored for tissue[5] and blood-compatible surface modification[6] applications such as drug and gene delivery.

20.3.1 Air/Water and Air/Solid Properties of Thin Solid Films of Lipids

Amphiphiles can self-assemble at an air/water or air/ solid interface. Based on the nature of thin film formed from different amphiphiles, they can be deposited onto a polymer substrate by various techniques, such as thermal evaporation, sputtering, electro deposition, molecular beam epitaxy, and adsorption from solution, Langmuir-Blodgett Technique, and Self-assembly[7]. Langmuir-Blodgett trough facility is versatile for studies at air/solid and air/water interface. Irwing Langmuir was the first to perform systematic studies on floating surfactant monolayers[8]. However, the first detailed description of sequential monolayer transfer was given several years later by Katherine Blodgett[9]. These built up thin solid films are therefore known as Langmuir-Blodgett films.

The most important indicator of the monolayer properties of an amphiphilic molecule (depending upon the properties) is given by measuring the surface pressure as a function of the area of water surface available for each molecule. This is carried out at constant temperature and is known as surface pressure-area isotherm. Figure 20.1 shows the typical pattern of surface pressure-area isotherm.

A number of distinct regions are immediately apparent on examining the isotherm. These regions are called phases. A simple terminology used to classify different monolayer phases of fatty acids has been proposed by W. D. Harkins[10]. This is applicable to different kinds of molecules at the air/water interface. At large, the monolayers exist in the gaseous state (G); on compression, they undergo a phase transition to the liquid expanded state (L_1). Upon further compression

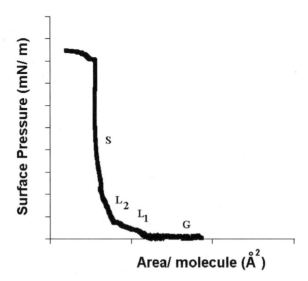

Figure 20.1. π-A isotherm. Gaseous state (G), liquid expanded (L_1), Liquid Condensed (L_2), Solid (S) state.

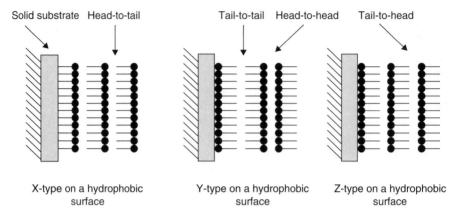

Figure 20.2. Mono and multi layer of thin solid films transferred from the air/water interface to the solid supports.

the L_1 phase undergoes a transition to the Liquid Condensed state (L_2) and even at higher concentrations the monolayer reaches the Solid (S) state. If the monolayer is further compressed after reaching the S state, it will collapse into three-dimensional structures.

Apart from these interfacial studies, LB apparatus could also be used for transferring the mono- and multi-layers into solid substrates. The deposition process is schematically illustrated in Figure 20.2. The LB deposition is traditionally carried out in the solid phase. However, amphiphiles can seldom be successfully deposited at surface pressures lower than 10 mN/m and surface pressures above 40 mN/m, due to lower film rigidity-related problems. When the solid substrate is hydrophilic, the first layer is deposited by raising the solid substrate from the subphase through the monolayer, whereas if the solid substrate is hydrophobic the first layer is deposited by lowering the substrate into the subphase through the monolayer. The deposited (supported) monolayers can be characterized by various techniques including Transfer ratio. This is defined as the ratio between the decrease in monolayer area during a deposition stroke and the area of the substrate. A transfer ratio of one and above has been considered as a complete wetting of the polymer surface by the monolayer[11].

An alternative strategy to deposit the monolayer is Langmuir-Shaffer technique. This technique differs from the vertical technique described above only in the sense that the solid substrate is horizontally lowered in contact with the monolayer. The supported membranes have self-healing power and minimize defects on the surface on formation[12]. Nissen et al. has studied the spreading kinetics of the self-assembled monolayer over polymer substrates from a large source of lipids using a fluorescent dye. They demonstrated that the spreading continues if the lipid reservoir is available in an air/water interface[13] and tend to self-limiting fingered edges (due to pinning defects) at less supplementation, due to loss of intermolecular interactions within the membrane[14]. The molecules are laterally mobile within the monolayer. This lateral mobility and expansion gives a time-dependent renewability of the surfaces under water. Sackman et al. has immobilized proteins into these monolayers and attempted to evaluate the adhesion induced receptor aggregation and adhesion plaque formation[15].

20.3.2 Optimization of Heterogeneous Phospholipids/ Glycolipid/Cholesterol Ternary Lipid Composition, Lateral Stability Improvement, and Preliminary Blood Compatibility Studies

The authors attempted to immobilize these monolayers over polymeric substrates. The cell membrane components of the endothelial cell membrane, phosphatidylcholine (PTC) for phospholipid, Galactocerebroside (GalC) for glycolipid and cholesterol (Chol) based on the head group structure to represent the major lipid components of the endothelial luminal cell membrane. Further, macromolecules such as protein (albumin), polysaccharide (heparin) and polymer (Polyethylene glycol), and so on, were incorporated into these lipid monolayers. The interfacial behavior of various combinations of lipids as well as the lipid macromolecular combinations have been studied at the air/water interface and deposited on hydrophobic polymer substrates like polycarbonate (PC) and poly methyl methacrylate (PMMA) with the help of the Langmuir-Blodgett (LB) trough. The packing and orientation of the supported monolayers have been varied by means of changing the lipid composition rather than the deposition parameters. This approach seems to be more similar to the *in vivo* conditions. The different supported monolayer surfaces prepared accordingly are: closely-packed ordered hydrophobic surface—polymer (PC) modified with the combination (PTC:Chol:GalC) (1:0.35:0.125); loosely-packed ordered hydrophobic surface—PC modified with the combination (PTC:Chol) (1:0.35); closely packed ordered hydrophilic surface—PC modified with the combination (PTC:Chol) (1:0.7). Such an optimized surface (PTC:Chol:GalC) (1:0.35:0.125) has been identified based on maximum transfer ratio from the air/water interface and characterized by using atomic force microscope (AFM). The concentration of cholesterol has been found to be an important parameter that influences the transfer ratio. The GalC improves the monolayer integrity under reduced Chol concentration. The blood compatibility of these supported monolayers was studied by protein adsorption, blood cell adhesion, and calcification.

The authors have optimized an outer cell mimetic lipid composition (OCMC) containing (OCMC) (PTC:Chol:GalC) (1:0.35:0.125) based on the air/water interfacial studies. Further macromolecular anchors such as albumin (OCMC-A) (PTC:Chol:GalC:Alb) (1:0.35:0.125:0.008), albumin and heparin (OCMC-AH) (PTC:Chol:GalC:Alb:Hep) (1:0.35:0.125:0.008:0.052), as well as albumin, heparin and polyethylene glycol (OCMC-AHP) (PTC:Chol:GalC:Alb:Hep: PEG) (1:0.35:0.125:0.008:0.052:0.15) were incorporated into the lipid layers.

The albumin is treated with organic solvents to do phase inversion and incorporated into the lipid solution to get stabilized itself. The air/water interfacial behavior of the pure as well as the lipid combinations was studied in detail to know the incorporation of the anchors into the monolayer and its stability during compression, with the help of LB trough. A bilayer of the lipid compositions were immobilized into functionalized polymer (PMMA) substrates with the help of LB trough and cross-linked by peptide bonds using carbodiimide chemistry. The surface morphology of the supported lipid systems was studied by using atomic force microscope (AFM). The fundamental interactions that regulate the blood compatibility of these stabilized surfaces have been studied by *in vitro* blood cell adhesion from washed cells, protein adsorption, and calcification studies. The surface pressure area (π-A) isotherm of the pure lipids as well as the different lipid/macromolecular combinations were studied at the air/water interface at ambient temperature.

20.3.3   Air/Water Interfacial Properties of TSF

Figure 20.3A shows the pressure-area isotherm of the lipids using deionized water as the subphase at ambient temperature. The liquid expanded (LE) and liquid condensed (LC) phases of the π-A isotherm of the PTC and GalC as well as the different lipid combinations are coexisting together at the air/water interface. The collapse pressure of the isotherms of the lipid combinations are being regulated by the parent lipid PTC, at 42 mN/m. The π-A isotherm of the cholesterol mono-layer (Figure 20.3A (II)) shows a sharp entry from gaseous (G) to LC phase during compression, and is similar to that of long chain fatty acids. This is due to the strong interaction between the hydrophobic cyclo pentano perhydro phenan-threne ring of the cholesterol, when they are in close proximity. The collapse pres-sure of the GalC is increased (Figure 20.3A (III)) may be due to the stabilization effect of the galactose residues. Furthermore, the incorporation of the GalC into the lipid monolayer under reduced cholesterol concentrations has increased the lateral stability of the monolayer[16].

20.3.4   Macromolecule Incorporation into Lipid Thin Solid Films

Protein incorporation into the lipid monolayer depends on the structure, and the transmembrane proteins with hydrophobic exterior are well incorporated. However, this is not true in the case of hydrophilic soluble globular proteins. The authors have attempted to change the conformation of a model globular protein (albumin) and incorporated into the monolayer. The interaction studies were done at air/water interface with the help of LB apparatus. Incorporation of albumin into the monolayer, OCMC-A (Figure 20.3A (V)), evidenced by the increase in mean molecular area and decrease in collapse pressure of π-A isotherm. This is due to the interaction between the hydrophobic core of the monolayer and hydrophobic core of the conformationally-changed protein[17] molecule. Further incorporation of heparin along with albumin into the mono-layer improved the collapse pressure from 38–42 mN/m along with increase in the mean molecular area. Further incorporation of heparin and PEG along with

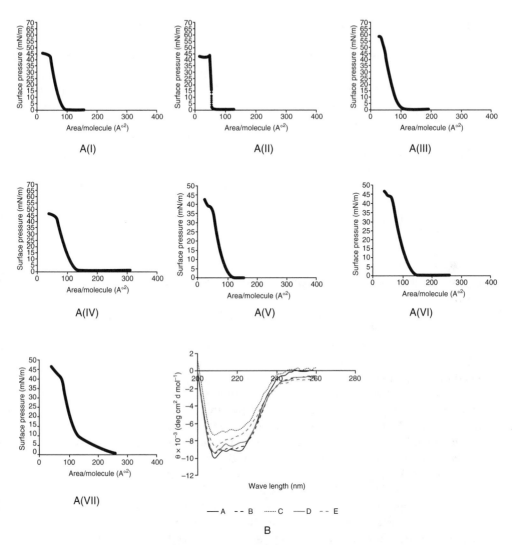

Figure 20.3. **Surface pressure-area (π-A) isotherm (A)**: egg-Phosphatidylcholine (I), Choles-terol (II), Galactocerebroside (III), (PTC:Chol:GalC) (1:0.35:0.125) deposited over PC polymer surface, OCMC-A (C), OCMC-AH (D)., OCMC-AHP (E). **Structure of the Albumin molecule incorporated into lipid bilayer (B)**. CD spectra of albumin in its native (A) and altered state (B), incorporated into PC (C), OCMC-A (D), OCMC-AHP (E).

albumin showed similar phase differences indicating the rearrangement of the macromolecules. The CD spectra indicate that the secondary structure of the native albumin is altered during the phase inversion. This altered structure is retained irrespective of the lipid composition in all the protein lipid mixtures (Figure 20.3B).

20.3.5   Optimization of Deposition Parameters

The deposition parameters of these monolayers depend upon the polarity of the polymeric substrates as well as the composition of the lipids. To optimize the deposition parameters, binary PTC/Chol (1:0.7) compositions at different dipping and withdrawal speeds of the polymer substrate from the air/water interface, were studied with the help of the LB trough. The deposition was done at 30 mN/m in all the studies. In natural membranes, the surface pressure is above 20 mN/m. For an equivalent distribution and packing of the lipids in the model monolayer systems, the surface pressure is expected to be at 30–35 mN/m. Studies at varying dipping speed did not show any difference in the transfer ratio with the speed. It indicates the strong hydrophobic interaction between the monolayer and the polymer films. However, the second monolayer deposition during withdrawal of the polymer substrate has been varying with the speed (Figure 20.4(I)).

At 5 mm and 100 mm/min withdrawal speed, there has been no second monolayer deposition. This ensures a single hydrophilic face exposed monolayer on the polymer substrate. This is schematically represented in Figure 20.4(II) and may be due to the close packing of the deposited monolayer caused by the condensing effect of cholesterol.

The compositions of the monolayer were varied at this juncture to determine the effect of composition on the interaction and packing of the monolayers. Further deposition of various other PTC/Chol/GalC combinations was done at constant deposition parameters (5 mm/min dipping as well as withdrawal speed) at ambient temperature. Figure 20.4(II) shows the composition effect on transfer ratio of the monolayer to the polymer substrates, from the air/water interface. The deposition of the PTC monolayer on this hydrophobic polymer surface showed a tight packed second monolayer deposition during withdrawal (Figure 20.4IIB). This ensures the exposure of the nonpolar face of the monolayer by burying the polar group inside. For the combination of (PTC:Chol) (1:0.7) only a single monolayer deposition is seen on the polymer surface, exposing the hydrophilic phase outside as shown in Figure 20.4IIC. This surface resembles the natural cell membrane where the polar groups are exposed to the aqueous phase. This is due to the condensing effect of cholesterol, which imparts close packing of the deposited monolayer. When the cholesterol concentration is reduced to half (PTC:Chol) (1:0.35) to its original concentration, the interaction between the two monolayers was increased during deposition. This will give a loosely packed second monolayer on the surface that is inversely oriented exposing the hydrophobic face to the aqueous phase (Figure 20.4IID). From this it is evident that the concentration of cholesterol plays an important role in the second monolayer deposition.

The introduction of the Galactocerebroside into the monolayer (PTC:Chol: GalC) (1:0.35:0.125) further improved the transfer ratio during dipping as well as withdrawal to give a more optimized deposition under reduced cholesterol concentrations (Figure 20.4IIE). Therefore the authors chose this monolayer

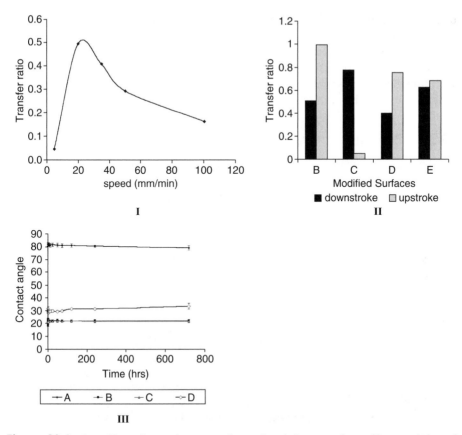

<u>Figure 20.4.</u> **The effect of speed on transfer ratio of the monolayer (I)**; monolayer of (PTC:Chol) (1:0.7) during upstroke, **Transfer ratio of the monolayer with different compositions (II)**; during downstroke and upstroke of the polymer film vertically at the interface; PTC (B), (PTC:Chol) (1:0.7) (C), (PTC:Chol) (1:0.35) (D), (PTC:Chol:GalC) (1:0.35:0.125) (E). The surface pressure was maintained at 30 mN/m for all the monolayers during deposition. **Stability studies under low shear stress conditions (III)**; PMMA Bare (A), OCMC (D). PMMA modified with OCMC-AH (B), OCMC-AHP (C) (B).

for further detailed characterization. This monolayer showed a compact surface, as evident in Figure 20.3D (1).

20.3.6   Surface Properties of Supported Thin Solid Films

The contact angle θ is reduced from 85° to 20° during surface modification. The stability studies were done under low shear conditions. Figure 20.4(III) shows the stability studies of the modified surfaces, represented in terms of the change in contact angle. The polymeric surface modified with the ternary lipid layer shows less stability as compared to the laterally stabilized surfaces. In this surface the contact angle have been stabilized after a certain period, may be due to the improved stability contributed by the Chol and GalC (condensation effect). However, in the case of polymer surface modified with ternary lipids containing anchors (Figures 20.4IIIB and C) the contact angle has not varied significantly with time. This shows that the anchored lipid layers are much more stable on the polymer surface than the unanchored lipid layers.

20.3.7   Biological Interactions onto These Surfaces

Further characterizations of the supported lipid layers are done only for those with improved stability by the lateral stabilization using anchors of albumin, heparin, and PEG. The surface morphology of the optimized PC modified surface was studied using AFM in contact mode in air. Figure 20.5(I) shows the contact mode AFM image of the PC surface modified with optimized lipid composition, in air. The surface shows a smooth texture with domains of the size range of 50–100 nm. No holes or uneven regions were observed on the surface.

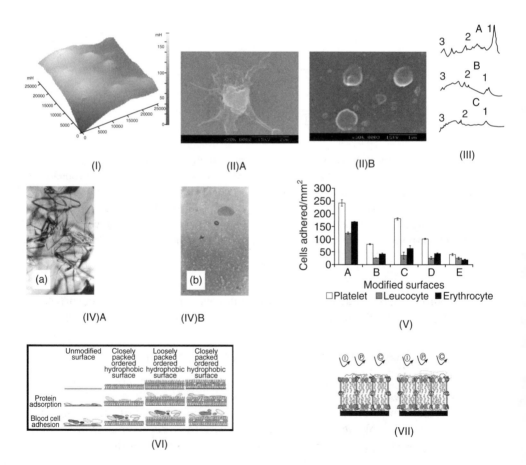

20.4 CALCIFICATION STUDIES

To check the bioactive interaction with ions, calcification studies from metastable salt solution were done on modified surfaces. Calcification to the organized organic–inorganic interface in biological systems has been reported. Apart from the blood compatibility, calcification studies also provide understanding of the orientation and packing density of the supported monolayers. Figure 20.5(IV) shows the calcification to the polymer surfaces. The authors have found that the overall calcification to the modified surfaces reduced significantly with respect to the PC alone.

20.5 PROTEIN INTERACTION STUDIES

The modified surfaces are antifouling, as evident from Figure 20.5(III). The adsorbed proteins onto these ordered monolayers form a gradient at the surface by retaining the natural conformation and hinder further interaction with the blood cells. On surfaces where the protein interaction to the surface is minimal,

---

Figure 20.5. **AFM image of bilayer (I)**: PC polymer surface modified with (PTC:Chol:GalC) (1:0.35:0.125). **Platelet activation on to material surface (II)**; Bare Polymer substrates (A), modified with cell mimetic monolayer (II), Blood cell adhesion studies on lipid modified polymer surfaces, using washed cells. PC bare (A). PC modified with, (PTC) (B), (PTC:Chol) (1:0.7) (C), (PTC:Chol) (1:0.35) (D), (PTC:Chol:GalC) (1:0.35:0.125) (E). **Densitometric diagram of the protein adsorption-desorption studies on lipid modified polymer surfaces (III)**, using mixture of proteins. X axis length in cm (maximum 6cm), and Y axis absorbance (maximum value = 0.5). Polymer bare (A). Polymer modified with lipid bilayer containing albumin and heparin (II), albumin heparin and polyethylene glycol (III). The peaks in figure-III are (1) albumin, (2) γ globulin and (3) fibrinogen. **Calcification studies (IV)**: Bare polymer substrate (A). Polymer modified with lipid bilayer which is anchored with albumin and heparin (B). **Blood cell adhesion studies on lipid modified polymer surfaces (V)**; using washed cells. PC bare (A). PC modified with, (PTC) (B), (PTC:Chol) (1:0.7) (C), (PTC:Chol) (1:0.35) (D), (PTC:Chol:GalC) (1:0.35:0.125) (E). **Schematic representation of the proposed orientation of the deposited mono and bilayers on hydrophobic PC polymer surface and their protein as well as blood cell interaction (VI)**; Horizontally, PC bare (A), PC modified with (PTC:Chol) (1:0.7) (B), PC modified with (PTC:Chol) (1:0.35) (C), PC modified with (PTC:Chol:GalC) (1:0.35:0.125) (D). Vertically, The unmodified and modified substrates (1) Protein adsorption to the substrates (2) Cell adhesion to the substrates (3). PTC (⌇━●), Chol (⌇━●), GalC (⌇⌇‿), protein (◁▬▶), erythrocyte (⬤), leukocyte (◯), Platelets (●) (II). **Schematic representation of Stabilized supported bilayer on polymeric substrate and osmotic exclusion of ions proteins and blood cells from the modified surface (VII)**, Bare polymer (A), OCMC (D), polymer modified with OCMC-AH (B), OCMC-AHP (C), Albumin (◗▬◁), Heparin (⌇⌿), PEG (━━), PC (≋●), Chol (≋◯), GalCC (≋●). Ions., (P) Proteins, (C) Blood cells (II).

the thrombosis may get mediated through the direct interaction between the exposed surface groups and the receptors of the blood cells. Therefore, the authors have studied the blood cell interaction to these surfaces from washed blood cells.

20.6 BLOOD CELL ADHESION STUDIES

Figure 20.5(V) shows the data of blood cell adhesion using washed platelets, erythrocytes and the leukocytes to the bare PC and the modified surfaces. The results show an overall decrease in cell adhesion on to modified surfaces as compared to the bare polymer surface. The orientation as well as packing of the exposed monolayer influences the observed difference in cell adhesion. Furthermore, the optimized surface, PC modified with (PTC:Chol:GalC) (1:0.35:0.125) have been evaluated towards the platelet activation from platelet rich plasma to confirm the anti-thrombogenecity of the surface.

20.7 PLATELET ADHESION AND ACTIVATION STUDIES

Platelet adhesion and activation are two important steps that regulate the formation of the thrombus and medical device rejection. During the initial stage of surface activation, the change in conformation of the adsorbed proteins exposes RGD sequences that are sensitive to the platelet GPIIb/IIIa receptor. When platelets are surface activated, they progress through a sequence of morphological changes. This can be evaluated by using SEM. The surface activation contributes to the change in the organization of the cytoskeleton, in turn increases the surface area of the platelets by the formation of pseudopods. The adhered and activated platelets go through a sequence of cytoskeletal events and rise in endoplasmic Ca++ concentration, polymerization of actin filaments, thrombin activation, release of the cytoskeletal granule contents, and platelet aggregation. The extent of shape change and the spread area have been related to the surface energetic of the polymer materials. Therefore the platelet activation studies are essential to prove the blood compatibility of the surface. The shape change could be correlated with the activation.

The studies were done for two hours with PRP under static conditions. Usually one hour is sufficient to establish the activation of the platelets[18]. The authors' studies show that the platelet activation to the modified surface has been significantly reduced as compared to the bare polycarbonate surfaces (Figure 20.5(II)[16]. The surface mediated shape change of the cells has been related to the physical (interfacial energy) and the chemical (due to specific groups) interactions. More than half of the platelets adsorbed to the bare polymer surface were fully spread and the other platelets were on the verge of spreading. The extended pseudopods of the activated platelets on the bare polymer surface indicate that these platelets can recruit the other platelets still in suspension. (Form surface bound aggregates with time.)

20.8 CONCLUSIONS

Development of thin solid films based on self-assembling of amphiphiles by bio-mimetic approaches has immense potential in controlling the biological interactions. The composition as well as the processing conditions regulates the physical properties of the lipid TSF. This further regulates the integrity of the supported TSF. Calcification, protein adsorption, as well as blood cell adhesion and activation is minimal on these surfaces. Incorporation and lateral stabilization of the proteins as well as other macromolecules into the TSF gives immense opportunity for controlled ligand supplementation.

ACKNOWLEDGMENTS

We express our sincere thanks and gratitude for the financial support by the DST and CSIR as well as Director SCTIMST, and Head BMT Wing for providing the facilities.

REFERENCES

1. Bryce MR, Petty CM. 2002. Electrically conductive Langmuir–Blodgett films of charge-transfer materials. Nature 374:771–776.
2. Ng CY, Chen TP, Sreeduth D, Chen Q, Ding L, Du A. 2006. Silicon nanocrystal-based non-volatile memory devices. Thin Solid Films 504;1–2:25–27.
3. Robert G. 1990. Langmuir-Blodgett Films, Plenum Press, New York.
4. Hayward JA, Chapman D. 1984. Biomembrane surfaces as models for polymer design: the potential for haemocompatibility. Biomaterials 5:135.
5. Svedhem S, Dahlborg D, Ekeroth J, Kelly J, Höök F, Gold J. 2003. In Situ Peptide-Modified Supported Lipid Bilayers for Controlled Cell Attachment. Langmuir 19: 6730.
6. Ishihra K, Aragaki R, Ueda T, Watanabe A, Nakabayashi N. 1990. Reduced thrombo-genicity of polymers having phospholipid polar groups. J Biomed Mater Res 24: 1069.
7. Petty MC. 1992. Possible applications for. Langmuir–Blodgett films Thin solid films 210:211, 417.
8. Langmuir I. 1917. The constitution and fundamental properties of solid and liquids. II. Liquids. J Am Chem Soc 39:1848.
9. Blodgett KB. 1935. Films Built by Depositing Successive Monomolecular Layers on a Solid Surface. J Am Chem Soc 57:1007.
10. Harkins WD. 1952. The physical Chemistry of surface films, Reinhold, NY, 41, 95.
11. Kuhner M, Tampe R, Sackmann E. 1994. Lipid mono- and bilayer supported on poly-mer films: composite polymer-lipid films on solid substrates. Biophys J 67(1):217–226.
12. Boxer SG. 2000. Molecular transport and organization in supported lipid membranes. Current Opinion in Chemical Biology 4:704–709.

13. Nissen J, Gritsch S, Wiegand G, Rädler JO. 1999. Wetting of phospholipid membranes on hydrophilic surfaces—concepts towards self-healing membranes. Eur Phys J B 10:335–344.

14. Cremer PS, Boxer SG. 1999. Formation and spreading of lipid bilayers on planar glass supports. J Phys Chem 103:2554–2559.

15. Kloboucek A, Behrisch A, Faix J, Sackmann E. 1999. Adhesion-induced receptor segregation and adhesion plaque formation: A model membrane study. Biophys J 77(4):2311–2328.

16. Kaladhar K, Sharma CP. 2004. Supported cell mimetic monolayers and their interaction with blood. Langmuir 7;20(25):11115–11122.

17. Kaladhar K, Sharma CP. 2006. ell Mimetic Lateral Stabilization of Outer Cell Mimetic Bilayer on Polymer Surfaces by Peptide Bonding and Their Blood Compatibility. J Biomed Mater Res A 79(1):23–35.

18. Massa TM, Yang ML, Ho JY, Brash JL, Santerre JP. 2005. Fibrinogen surface distribution correlates to platelet adhesion pattern on fluorinated surface-modified polyetherurethane. Biomaterials 26(35):7367–7376.

21

TITANIUM NITRIDE AND DIAMOND LIKE CARBON COATINGS FOR CARDIOVASCULAR APPLICATIONS

C.V. Muraleedharan and G.S. Bhuvaneshwar

Biomedical Technology Wing,
Sree Chitra Tirunal Institute for Medical Sciences & Technology,
Thiruvananthapuram, India

Contents

21.1	Overview	678
21.2	Cardiovascular Devices	678
21.3	Hemocompatibility	680
	21.3.1 Water Adsorption	681
	21.3.2 Protein Adsorption	681
	21.3.3 Blood Cell Interaction	682
	21.3.4 Haemostasis and Coagulation	682
	21.3.5 Complement Activation	683
21.4	Cardiovascular Biomaterials	683
	21.4.1 Heparin and Heparin-Like Coatings	684
	21.4.2 Anti-Adherent Coatings	685
	21.4.3 Inert Coatings	685
21.5	Diamond Like Carbon	686
	21.5.1 Substrates	687
	21.5.2 DLC Coating Process	687
21.6	Titanium Nitride	687

Advanced Biomaterials: Fundamentals, Processing, and Applications, Edited by Bikramjit Basu, Dhirendra S. Katti, and Ashok Kumar

21.6.1 Substrates 688
21.6.2 TiN Coating Process 688
21.7 Coating Characterization 688
21.7.1 Surface Roughness Estimation 688
21.7.2 Adhesive Wear Characteristics 689
21.7.3 Abrasive Wear Characteristics 690
21.7.4 Coating Adhesion Studies 692
21.7.5 Microhardness Measurements 693
21.7.6 Simulated Accelerated Durability Studies 695
21.8 Biological Characterization 697
21.8.1 Cytotoxicity 698
21.8.2 Hemocompatbility 698
21.8.3 Tissue Compatibility 699
21.8.4 Large Animal Experiments 700
21.9 Potential Applications 702
21.10 Future Perspective 703
Acknowledgments 703
References 704

21.1 OVERVIEW

In the current era, the management of cardiovascular diseases is substantially influenced by the research and development in biomaterials. At the same time, the choice of materials intended for this segment has been the most difficult owing to the stringent requirements of blood compatibility. This has led to the researchers look towards surface coatings., The substrate material can be chosen to provide the required strength for structural integrity, while coatings can be employed to enhance the blood compatibility. Titanium Nitride (TiN) and Diamond Like Carbon (DLC) are two such ceramic coatings that seem to offer excellent prospects.

Both DLC and TiN exhibit similar properties such as hardness, low frictional coefficient, high wear and corrosion resistance, chemical inertness, and very good processability. Both coatings can be polished to a high level of surface finish, which is an important parameter in blood contacting applications. Both exhibit very good tissue and blood compatibility and are well tolerated in biological environments. This chapter looks at the processing, characterization, and applications of TiN and DLC coatings, with a focus on cardiovascular applications.

21.2 CARDIOVASCULAR DEVICES

In no area of medical practice have synthetic biomaterials played a more critical role than in the cardiovascular system [Ratner 2004]. Cardiopulmonary bypass with the help of oxygenators and pumps have made possible open heart surgeries. Artificial heart valves are used to replace damaged or diseased natural valves with substantial enhancement of both survival and quality of life. Vascular stents inserted with the help of catheters have provided new dimensions in the treatment of coronary artery disease. Synthetic vascular grafts used to repair weakened blood vessels, while bypass blockages have saved many from massive bleeding or have resulted in enhanced blood flow to severely ischemic organs and limbs. Devices to aid or replace the pumping function of the heart include intra-aortic balloon pump, ventricular assist device, and total implantable artificial heart. Pacemakers and automatic internal defibrillators are widely used to override or correct aberrant, life-threatening cardiac arrhythmias.

Most of these devices either alleviate the conditions for which they were used or provide otherwise enhanced function. Nevertheless, device failure and/or other tissue material interactions frequently cause clinically observable complications. Some important mechanisms of tissue material interactions are similar across device types, and several generic types of device related complications can occur in recipients of nearly all cardiovascular implants [see Table 21.1]. These include thromboembolic complications, infections, dysfunction owning to materials degeneration and improper healing of the luminal surfaces etc. These problems arise from the fact that even after six decades of research, no material has been found to be truly blood compatible and many devices function with low or acceptable risks of complications. The understanding of the complex mechanisms of blood materials interactions is still far from complete.

TABLE 21.1. Major Failure Modes of Cardiovascular Devices

Heart valve	• Thrombus/embolism
	• Anti coagulant related hemorrhage
	• Infection (Endocarditis)
	• Structural dysfunction
	• Non-structural dysfunction
Vascular graft	• Thrombus/embolism
	• Graft infection
	• Perigraft seroma
	• False aneurysms
	• Intimal fibrous hyperplasia
	• Structural failure
Circulatory assist devices	• Thrombus/embolism
	• Infection (endocarditis)
	• Extra luminal infection
	• Hemolysis
	• Structural dysfunction
Coronary stents	• Thrombus/embolism
	• Restenosis
	• Neointimal proliferation
	• Aneurysm formation
	• Structural dysfunction

21.3 HEMOCOMPATIBILITY

The success of any material in the biological environment is defined by its reaction to and from the surrounding environment. But there is no universally accepted definition for biomaterial and biocompatibility. In general, it is understood that a biomaterial is required to perform with *appropriate host response* in a *specific application*. Hence no single test can be used for ascertaining the biocompatibility of a material and a material cannot be categorically stated as a biocompatible. But it can be concluded, through a series of properly selected qualification studies, that a material is suitable for use in a certain specific application. The most popular and accepted standard in this area is ISO 10993: *Biological evaluation of medical devices*, which addresses the issue of biocompatibility by categorizing the materials based on the nature and duration of body contact. In this context, the classification of biomaterials based on the nature of body contact takes practical significance and biomaterials get classified as cardiovascular, orthopedic, dental, wound care materials, etc.

Blood constitutes about 8% of the total body weight of the human and contains mainly water (>90%), proteins such as albumin, globulins, fibrinogen, different types of cells (platelets, white and red cells), ions and different organic nutrients such as lipids and carbohydrates [see Table 21.2] [Moriau et al., 1988]. All these components are implicated in several complex physiological processes related to the multiple functions of blood such as:

- transport of gases, nutrients, waste products, regulatory molecules;
- regulation of pH and osmosis;

TABLE 21.2. Major Constituents of Blood

	Constituent		Primary function(s)
Plasma (55%)	Water 92%		Transport
	Proteins 7%	Albumin (58%)	Capillary colloid; reduces fluid leakage out of capillaries; transport
		Globulin (38%)	Substrate for formation of other molecules; immunity [antibodies]; transport
		Fibrinogen (4%)	Blood clotting
	Other Solutes (1%)		
	$Na^+, K^+, Ca^{2+}, Mg^{2+}, Cl^-, HCO_3^-, HPO_4^{2-}, SO_4^{2-}$		
	Organic nutrients (lipids, carbohydrates, amino acids)		
	Organic wastes (urea, uric acid, creatine, bilirubin)		
Formed Elements	Platelets ($250–400 \times 10^3/mm^3$)		Blood clotting
	WBC ($5–9 \times 10^3/mm^3$)		Immunity
	RBC ($4200–6200 \times 10^3/mm^3$) (>99.9%)		Transport

- maintenance of body temperature;
- protection against foreign substances (complement system);
- clot formation preventing bleeding after injury (haemostasis/coagulation).

The last two processes are the most important in the material tissue interaction, since they dramatically influence the safe and appropriate function of a blood-contacting device. The activation of the complement system is associated with inflammation surrounding the implant, while the activation of the coagulation cascade leads to thrombus formation and all related pathologies.

The interaction of biomaterials with blood constituents leads to many specific reactions. The extent and direction of these reactions determine the blood compatibility of the material. The prominent pathways of blood–material interaction could be classified as:

1. water adsorption
2. protein deposition and adsorption
3. blood cell–material interactions
4. haemostasis and coagulation
5. complement activation

21.3.1   Water Adsorption

The first event on biomaterial in contact with blood is the adsorption of inorganic ions and water molecules. On contact with water, the superficial structure of hydrophobic materials is not changed, but an intermediary layer of water of a few molecules thickness, having a more ordered structure than in pure liquid water, is formed. On the other hand, the surface of hydrophilic materials is greatly modified by water. Water molecules become enmeshed in the macromolecular network and break certain interactions between the polymer chains (Vogler, 1998).

21.3.2   Protein Adsorption

Another early event in blood material interaction is the rapid and selective adsorption of proteins by a multi stage process. The proteins may bind to a surface via three possible mechanisms:

- electrostatic bond formation between charged groups on the protein and oppositely charged surface sites (on ceramics surfaces, for instance),
- hydrogen bonding (on relative polar substrates) and,
- hydrophobic interactions (on low polar polymers), defined as the interaction of non-polar groups in aqueous media.

Adsorption of protein molecules is relatively rapid, but variable, and as much as 75% may get completed in the first five minutes, reaching a maximum in about one hour time period. The surface concentration may depend on the type of protein adsorbed, but could be of the order of $0.1–1.0\,\mu g/cm^2$.

In general it has been found that preferential or selective adsorption occurs so that certain proteins may be enriched in the surface and vice versa. Surface chemistry, time of adsorption, and protein type are major factors in determining the composition of the adsorbed layer. Small proteins, by virtue of their higher diffusion coefficients, will initially adsorb faster than large proteins during competitive adsorption (Ramsden, 1995).

Proteins also undergo conformational changes during the adsorption process. These conformational changes may have a positive consequence (surface passivation with an irreversibly adsorbed protein monolayer) or negative consequence (initiation of blood-enzyme systems, in particular the activation of the coagulation and complement system due to the desorption of the surface activated protein components (Eloy et al., 1990).

21.3.3 Blood Cell Interactions

Cells adhesion occurs at a later stage and is mediated by the proteins initially adsorbed on the surface. Platelets, amongst the other cells present in blood, play the more important role in blood-material interactions. Hemodynamic conditions are of major importance in the adhesion of platelets to material surface and in determining localization, growth, and fragmentation of thrombi. Platelet adhesion to a surface is governed by two independent mechanisms: the transport of platelets to the surface, which depends on the flow conditions, and the reaction of platelets with the surface, which depends on the nature of the surface and the adsorbed proteins (Hanson, 2004).

Red cells can bind weakly to some non-endothelial materials' without spreading. They significantly contribute to blood surface interactions in several ways. Collision of red cells with other blood cells and plasma proteins reduces their adsorption on the materials' surfaces. Leucocytes, particularly neutrophils and monocytes, have a strong tendency to adhere to surfaces. As a result of leukocyte adhesion, several reactions are initiated. These include platelet–platelet and platelet–leukocyte interactions, the detachment of adherent thrombi by the action of leukocyte proteases, the detachment of adherent platelets and adsorbed proteins by leucocytes, and the release of leukocyte products that may rise to both local and systemic reactions.

21.3.4 Haemostasis and Coagulation

Several distinct but interrelated thrombotic and anti-thrombotic systems exist to prevent the formation of intravascular clots that are expected in response to vascular trauma. Haemostasis is the sum of these mechanisms and serves to limit blood loss following injury. Once regulation is initiated, the same mechanisms first combine to localize the clot at the site of injury, then to terminate coagulation, and finally to remove the clot once it has served its purpose. These haemostatic mechanisms include platelet activation, coagulation, and fibrinolysis. The processes of coagulation and fibrinolysis represent a dynamic balance involving the formation and removal of fibrin. If the balance of these processes is upset, either excessive bleeding or thrombosis may occur. The abnormal thrombus formation and related cardiovascular disorders is one of the major challenges in blood–compatible materials design.

21.3.5 Complement Activation

The complement system consists of more than twenty plasma proteins that function either as enzymes or as binding proteins. Complement activation is initiated through different pathways and all of them contain an initial enzyme that catalyses the formation of the assembly of the terminal complement complex. Various complement products (such as C3b, C4b and iC3b) bind to material surfaces, which facilitate their uptake by inflammatory cells. Complement activation also releases anaphylatoxins which are humoral messengers that bind to specific receptors on neutrophils, monocytes, macrophages, mast cells and smooth muscle cells. They produce smooth muscle contraction, mast cell histamine release, affect platelet aggregation, and act as mediators of the local inflammatory process (Hakim, 1992).

21.4 CARDIOVASCULAR BIOMATERIALS

In the study of blood material interactions, a strong contrast exists between natural blood contacting surfaces and artificial material surfaces. The entire blood contacting natural surfaces in human body are lined with the endothelial cells. The most important function of endothelium is to offer a blood-compatible surface to flowing blood. The platelets, erythrocytes, and leucocytes do not adhere to the endothelium. With the help of variety of mechanisms, endothelium prevents adhesion of cells and activation of clotting factors and ensures the removal of thrombus formed on it (Courtney et al., 1998).

The artificial surfaces can neither perform an active role similar to that achieved by the endothelium through the synthesis and release of specific substances, nor provide a surface that blocks the adhesion of proteins and cellular elements from blood. The inability of artificial surfaces to perform an active role means that the application of such surfaces may require simultaneous therapy with anticoagulants, platelet aggregation inhibitors, and/or plasminogen activators. This calls for anti platelet and anticoagulant therapy to be employed with most of the cardiovascular implant devices.

Only very few industrial materials are known to be employed in cardiovascular devices. Certain grades of stainless steels (SS 316L, SS316LVM), cobalt based alloys (Stellite 21, Haynes-25) and titanium alloys (Commercially pure titanium, Ti6Al4V) are widely-used metallic cardiovascular biomaterials. Polyethylene terepththalate (PET), Polytetraflouroethylene (PTFE) and ultra high molecular weight polyethylene (UHMWPE) are well-known polymers. Of these, titanium and its alloys are generally considered to be good blood compatible alloys (Muraleedharan et al., 1995).

Titanium owing to the presence of non-porous titanium oxide layer presents a ceramic surface to blood. Though titanium is one of the most chemically reactive of all metals, it is also one of the most corrosion-resistant because of the lower reactivity of this oxide film. The biocompatibility and specifically blood compatibility of titanium and titanium alloys result from the chemical stability, repassivation ability, and structure of this titanium oxide film that is typically only a few nanometers thick. The film is normally composed of a titanium/titanium-oxide composite close to the bulk material and a titanium-oxide film that could be a few nanometers thick. The surface of the titanium-oxide film may have hydroxide and adsorbed water bond with titanium ions, which forms an extremely blood-compatible interface since it allows adsorption of proteins when exposed to blood. Even when any physical damage occurs to this coating, the interface is rebuild sufficiently fast by minimizing the chance for platelet adhesion. This ability of the coating to repassivate with sufficient speed could be attributed to the blood compatibility of titanium alloys.

Most often, metallic and polymer surfaces are coated with special coatings to enhance their blood compatibility. Much of the efforts in biomaterials research over the past 50 years have been directed toward the development of coatings that do not react with platelets and coagulation factors. Mainly three categories of coatings are employed for enhancing blood compatibility, that is, coating of pharmacological agents (heparin and heparin-like agents), anti-adhering coatings, and inert coatings.

21.4.1 Heparin and Heparin-Like Coatings

Heparin-based coatings have demonstrated substantial improvement in the performance of a variety of blood contacting medical devices. Heparin is a pharmaceutical that has been used clinically for decades as an intravenous anticoagulant to treat inherent clotting disorders and to prevent blood clot formation during surgery and interventional procedures. Heparin molecules are polysaccharides with a unique chemical structure that gives them specific biological activity. When heparin is immobilized on the surface of a medical device material, it improves the performance of the material when it is exposed to blood in several ways:

- It provides local catalytic activity to inhibit several enzymes critical to the formation of fibrin.
- It reduces the adsorption of blood proteins.
- It reduces the adhesion and activation of platelets.

Alternatives to the heparin approach have also been developed for preventing surface-induced thrombus formation. In these approaches, synthetic, non-biological molecules are used to create surfaces with improved blood compatibility. Passivation with hydrophilic molecules to mask the underlying thrombogenic surface from the blood is one method. The passivated surface reduces or prevents the adhesion of thrombogenic cells and proteins onto the underlying substrate or material, thereby preventing surface-induced blood clotting. Another approach involves coatings that actively recruit and bind native albumin from the patient's own blood onto the device surface. This albumin-binding coating acquires a thin, self-regenerating, absorbed albumin layer on the surface. The albumin covered surface minimizes and prevents the adhesion of unwanted thrombogenic cells and proteins.

21.4.2   Anti-Adherent Coatings

For applications requiring short term blood compatibility, it is important only that the device repel platelets, proteins, or cells. It may not be necessary to provide heparin or heparin-like coatings on the surface, since the attachment of blood components must be prevented for a limited time only, and the risk of introducing emboli into the blood stream is minimal. In addition, the patient usually receives systemic anticoagulants during such procedures, further reducing the need for a bioactive coating on the device.

Most of the anti-adherent coatings employed make use of hybrid polymer systems such as hydrogels and hence provide the additional feature of reducing friction on the device surface. Products that can benefit from the use of these anti-adherent coatings are catheters, such as percutaneous transluminal coronary angioplasty (PTCA) catheters, guide catheters, angiography catheters, dilators, introducers, and drug-infusion catheters.

21.4.3   Inert Coatings

Most of the blood-compatible coatings discussed in earlier sections are meant for devices that come in contact with blood for a short span of a few hours to a few weeks. But when it comes to long-term implants, these techniques do not produce very encouraging results. Coatings incorporating pharmacological agents like heparin have limited service life because the activity of the pharmacological agent diminishes with time. Hydrogel coatings can get metabolized by enzymes over time and hence become ineffective in long duration implants.

The best strategy in long-term implant application is to make the substrate itself sufficiently blood compatible or to impart coatings that will stay intact for the life of the implant. The use of ceramic coatings, especially on metallic substrates, becomes more significant in this situation.

Diamond-like carbon (DLC) and Titanium nitride (TiN) are two ceramic materials which offer tremendous potential for use as blood-compatible coatings for long-term applications. Both DLC and TiN exhibit similar properties such as high hardness, low frictional coefficient, high wear and corrosion resistance, chemical inertness, high electrical resistivity, infrared-transparency,

TABLE 21.3. Typical Physical Properties of DLC and TiN Films

Property	Unit	DLC	TiN
Density	g/cc	2.02	5.22
Color	—	Brown to black	Golden yellow
Coefficient of friction (Vs SS 316L)	—	0.06–0.1	0.4–0.65
Modulus of elasticity	GPa	150–250	450–600

and high refractive index. Both coatings can be polished to an extremely high level of surface finish, which is an important parameter in blood contacting applications. Typical physical properties of DLC and TiN coatings are provided in Table 21.3.

21.5 DIAMOND LIKE CARBON

The pioneering work by Aisenberg & Chabot (Aisenberg et al., 1971) on thin films of diamond like carbon (DLC) paved the way to intense research activity in this area. In addition to excellent properties such as low friction, good wear resistance and high hardness, DLC films have been shown to be extremely bio-compatible (Dion et al., 1993; Thomson et al., 1991).

Several methods are used to produce diamond like carbon films, the prominent ones being ion-beam deposition (IBD) of carbon ions, sputter deposition of carbon with or without bombardment by an intense flux of ions (PVD), and deposition from an RF plasma, sustained in hydrocarbon gases, on substrates that are negatively biased (plasma-assisted chemical vapor deposition or PACVD) (Zou et al., 2004).

The Ion beam deposition has the advantage of being able to deposit high-quality coatings at very low temperatures (near room temperature). The disadvantages are that the deposition rate is very low (1 μm/hr maximum) and that being a line of sight deposition technique, even substrates of simple geometry need complex manipulation to ensure uniform coating. PACVD techniques employing radio frequency and direct current glow discharges in hydrocarbon gas mixtures that produce smooth amorphous carbon and hydrocarbon films. The PACVD processes will generally require deposition temperatures of at least 600 °C to give the required combination of properties; however, low temperature deposition is also possible with in certain limits. The CVD technique gives good deposition rates and very uniform coatings and is suited to large-scale production applications.

Another technique, which combines the benefits of both PACVD and IBD, is the closed field sputter ion plating. Low pressure RF plasma CVD is adopted for high rate deposition (>5 μm/hr), in combination with simultaneous ion assistance and physical vapor deposition from unbalanced magnetron sputtering sources, to give very high quality films (Sella et al., 1993).

21.5.1 Substrates

The authors have been working in the area of medical devices, especially cardio-vascular devices, for more than two decades, which included products such as artificial heart valves, oxygenators and other cardio pulmonary support devices (Muraleedharan et al., 2006). As part of these development activities, many ma-terials such as cobalt-based alloys, titanium and its alloys, and ultra-high molecular-weight polyethylene (UHMWPE) were evaluated for their physico-chemical and biological behavior. Based on this experience, commercially-pure titanium (conforming to ISO 5832—Implants for surgery—metallic materials Part 2: Unalloyed titanium) and UHMWPE were selected as substrates.

The titanium samples were machined from annealed rods and polished using a multi-stage process to obtain an average surface finish better than 0.2 micron Ra (Kalyani Nair et al., 2003). UHMWPE samples were machined from extruded rods and then polished using a solid state compaction process to achieve similar levels of surface finish. These samples were cleaned using neutral soap in an ultra-sonic cleaner prior to the coating process.

21.5.2 DLC Coating Process

DLC deposition was done on Ti and UHMWPE substrates using plasma-enhanced chemical vapor deposition (PECVD) technique (M/s. ICC, Le Mée Sur Seine, France). Prior to the coating, the samples underwent an ionic etching process using argon plasma in order to improve the adhesion of the coating on the substrate (Hauert, 2003). This ionic etching process considerably increases the surface energy and liberates the chemical liaison allowing an increase in the adher-ence. A mixture of methane and hydrogen is used as precursor and the process parameters are adjusted to get a coating of thickness between 1 µm to 5 µm.

21.6 TITANIUM NITRIDE

Titanium Nitride (also known as Tinite, TiN) is a hard ceramic material, often used as a coating on metal alloys to improve the substrate's surface properties. It has low coefficient of friction and corrosion rates and hence is used in applica-tions where friction, wear, and erosion are important design considerations. Tita-nium nitride is extensively used in medical applications, especially as orthopedic and dental biomaterials (Wisbey et al., 1987).

Physical Vapor Deposition (PVD), Chemical Vapor Deposition (CVD), and ion implantation are the most widely employed techniques for deposition of TiN coatings. PVD is a vapor deposition process either carried out using vacuum evaporation techniques or using sputtering. In sputtering, a source (cathode) is bombarded in a high vacuum with high energy inert gas ions producing a glow discharge or plasma. Atoms from these are ejected and accelerated using external bias towards the substrate to form the coating.

Chemical Vapor Deposition (CVD) is another very widely-used method for titanium nitride coating. CVD relies on the reaction of metal halide (titanium chloride) gas along with nitrogen. The addition of nitrogen lowers the free energy of the reaction products so that titanium nitride is formed in preference to the titanium metal.

21.6.1 Substrates

Titanium alloy (Ti6Al4V) (conforming to ISO 5832—Implants for surgery—metallic materials: Part 3: Wrought titanium—6 aluminum—4 vanadium alloy) was chosen as substrate for titanium nitride with artificial heart valve cages as one of the prospective applications.

21.6.2 TiN Coating Processes

All samples went through a thorough cleaning process prior to coating. PVD with vacuum evaporation was used for the coating of the samples in this study. Uniform coating thickness in the range of one to two microns was achieved. In evaporation process, the coating material is heated in a vacuum above its boiling point. The molecules in the vapor phase condense on the substrate to form the coating.

21.7 COATING CHARACTERIZATION

Raman spectra of the DLC coatings were recorded by illuminating the samples with a 40 mW power laser whose wavelength was 514.52 nm. The Raman spectra of the DLC coatings indicated a broad maximum around 1525 cm^{-1} and a shoulder like feature at 1223 cm^{-1} but did not show any sharp features normally observed in the case of pure diamond and graphite (Krishnan et al., 2002).

Energy dispersive X-ray microanalysis (EDX) was carried out on the TiN surface (Figure 21.1) and the presence of titanium nitride was confirmed. The elemental composition of the surface was estimated from the EDX as titanium (95.6%), aluminum (0.16%), vanadium (0.81%) and nitrogen (2.64%).

21.7.1 Surface Roughness Estimation

The major factors that affect the blood compatibility of any material are its surface characteristics in terms of surface roughness, free charge, and impurity levels. The surface roughness of the samples was studied using optical profilometer (Talysurf CLI 1000, Taylor Hobson, UK). The average surface roughness was estimated from area profiles of six independent 0.2 mm × 0.2 mm zones, each acquired with 1.0 μm spatial resolution. The waviness of the surfaces was corrected based on the methods described in International standards (ISO 4287 and ISO 4288). Seven equidistant profiles were extracted from the waviness-corrected surface and the average and standard deviation of the Ra values estimated. A

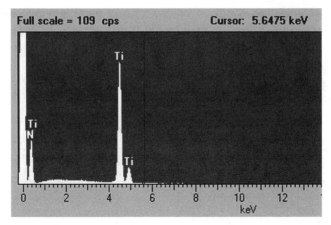

Figure 21.1. Energy Dispersive X-ray spectra (EDX) of TiN surface showing peaks corresponding to titanium and nitrogen elements.

comparison of the profiles of the sample surfaces before and after coating revealed that there is marginal deterioration in surface finish while coating polymer samples. While in the case of metal substrates the surface finish of the substrate was more or less retained after the coating process (see Figure 21.2 and Table 21.4). These measurements correlated well with the surface roughness measurements carried out using mechanical contact profilometry (Surtronic 3+, Rank Taylor Hobson Ltd, UK).

21.7.2 Adhesive Wear Characteristics

A pin-on-wheel test system is used for studying the adhesive wear properties of the material combinations. It consists of platform rotating at a constant speed of 60 rpm and a pin loading arm for provisions for applying a constant load on the pin. The wheel diameter is 25 mm on which the pin with 3 mm diameter contact area is allowed to traverse in circular motion [Muraleedharan et al., 1989]. The test conditions are described in Table 21.5.

Results from the study (see Figure 21.3) show that both DLC and TiN coatings improve the wear characteristics substantially. Moreover, the wear tracks on the UHMWPE surface is found to be more uniform and with less cracks when articulated against coated surfaces than with uncoated metallic surfaces. The weight loss from UHMWPE was lowest when DLC-coated pin is used as the counter face; but TiN surface generated a smoother worn surface with minimal track marks and best surface finish (see Figure 21.4).

UHMWPE wheels used had initial surface finish of the order of 0.15 μm Ra. The wear tracks generated by titanium, DLC coating, and TiN coating were having surface roughness values of 0.47 μm Ra, 0.16 μm Ra, and 0.08 μm Ra, respectively.

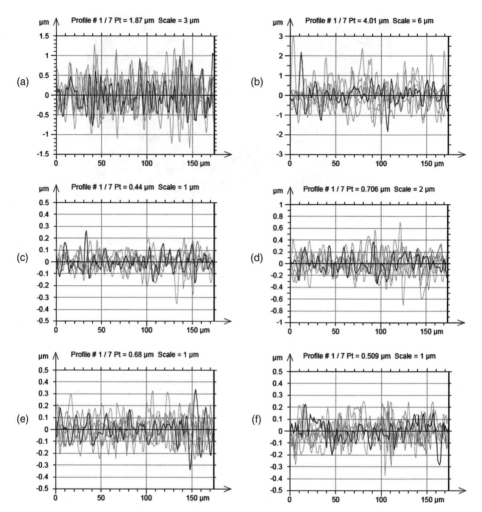

Figure 21.2. Surface profile of coated and uncoated samples (a) UHMWPE (b) DLC coated UHMWPE (c) Ti6Al4V (d) TiN Coated Ti6Al4V (e) CP Titanium (f) DLC-coated CP Titanium. Note that the surface finish of the substrate is reasonably reproduced after the coating.

21.7.3 Abrasive Wear Characteristics

Abrasive wear characteristics of the coatings were studied using a conventional sand slurry test apparatus devised in the Institute. A specially fabricated test specimen is rotated in a slurry or alumina and water (1:1 v/v) at 3000 rpm for six-hour duration and the volume of material lost from the surface is used as a measure of the abrasive wear characteristics of the material (Muraleedharan et al., 1989).

The results indicate that the abrasive wear rates are higher for the coated samples [see Figure 21.5]. This is probably due to the presence of the interface

TABLE 21.4. Surface Roughness Profiles of Coated and Uncoated Samples

	Ra (μm)	
Material surface	Mean	SD
UHMWPE	0.13	0.04
DLC coated UHMWPE	0.25	0.05
Ti6Al4V	0.07	0.01
TiN coated Ti6Al4V	0.08	0.02
Cp Titanium	0.06	0.02
DLC coated Cp Titanium	0.06	0.01

TABLE 21.5. Pin-on-Wheel Test Conditions

Parameter	Unit	Value
Relative motion	—	Circular sliding
Sliding speed	mm/sec	55 ± 2.5
Duration of test	hours	6
Contact stress	Kg/cm^2	14 ± 1
Lubricant	—	None
Temperature	°C	30 ± 3
Initial surface roughness	μm Ra	<0.2

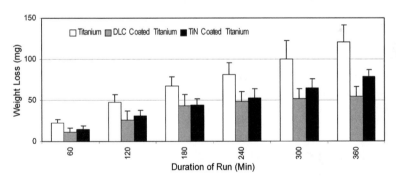

Figure 21.3. Pin-on-Wheel adhesive wear test results: weight loss from UHMWPE wheel when traversed against (a) Titanium (b) DLC-coated titanium and (c) TiN-coated titanium pins. The wear from the UHMWPE is reduced by the introduction of the coating on the counter face.

between the coating and the substrate. The inter-molecular adhesion between the coating material and the substrate will always be lesser than the attractive forces between the substrate molecules. This lower coating adhesion when challenged by an abrasive material tends to give way and causes erosion or peeling of the coating. The adhesion studies were carried out on the coated surfaces to estimate the typical force range in which the coating integrity is maintained.

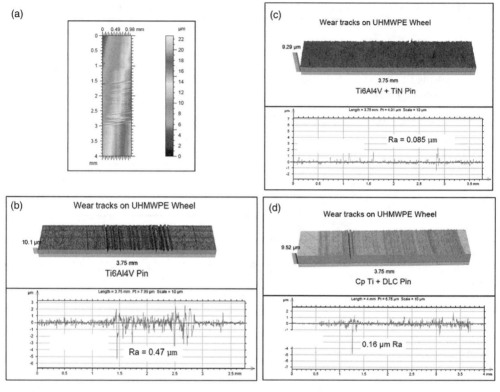

Figure 21.4. Wear surface topography of UHMWPE (initial surface finish 0.15 μm Ra typical) against bare metal and coated counter faces: (a) Wear contour plot (b) Wear tracks generated by Ti6Al4V pin (c) Wear track generated by TiN coated Ti6Al4V pin (d) Wear track generated by DLC-coated Ti pin. The average surface roughness of wear tracks are less when the pin is coated. Titanium nitride counter face generates the smoothest wear tracks and hence could result in minimum wear debris formation. (See color insert.)

21.7.4 Coating Adhesion Studies

The coating adhesion studies were carried out using a micro scratch test system (Micro—Combi Tester, M/s. CSM Instruments, USA). Scratch testing is a comprehensive method of quantifying the adhesion properties of coatings. The technique involves generating a controlled scratch with a diamond tip on the sample under test. The tip, either a Rockwell C diamond or a sharp metal tip, is drawn across the coated surface under either a constant or progressive load. At a certain critical load, the coating will start to fail. The critical loads are used to quantify the adhesive properties of different film–substrate combinations. These parameters constitute a unique signature of the coating system under test.

The test conditions are chosen to ensure that reproducible scratch maps are obtained for the coating under investigation [see Table 21.6]. The critical loads are

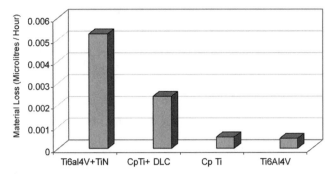

Figure 21.5. Abrasive wear test results: The average quantity of material removed from the test sample during one hour of run in the test system. The results indicate the relatively high wear rates for coated samples. This could limit the applications of these coatings in situations where abrasive or three body wear mechanisms are more prominent such as in orthopedic applications, which may not be a concern in cardiovascular applications where severe abrasive wear conditions are not present.

TABLE 21.6. Micro Scratch Test Conditions

Parameter	Details
Indenter	Rockwell (Diamond) 100 μm radius
Type of test	Linear scratch (progressive)
Loading rate	30 N/min
Start load	0.05 N
End Load	20 N
Scratch length	4 mm
Scratch speed	6 mm/min

detected precisely by means of an acoustic sensor attached to the indenter holder. The same could be cross-checked and verified using the frictional force observed on the indenter, sudden changes in the penetration depth profile as well as with the help of optical microscopy, by examining the scratch profile [see Figure 21.6].

It is observed that TiN coating on Ti6Al4V has better adhesion properties compared to DLC on Cp Titanium [see Table 21.7]. But in both cases, the critical load (LC1) for the initiation of the first crack was better than 4 N, for a 100 μm diamond indenter and is considered as quite good adhesion for most of the adhesive wear conditions. The lower critical loads for DLC could result in high wear during abrasive wear conditions, which corroborates well with the results obtained in the sand slurry abrasive wear studies.

21.7.5 Microhardness Measurements

The microhardness measurements were carried out on the same system used for the evaluation of coating adhesion studies (Micro—Combi Tester, M/s. CSM

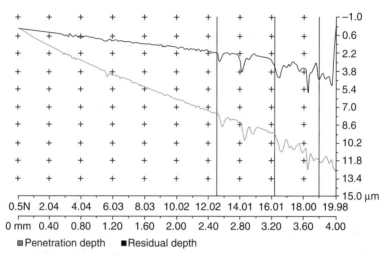

■ Penetration depth   ■ Residual depth

<u>Figure 21.6.</u> Coating adhesion studies using micro scratch test system: The Figure represents the penetration depth and residual depth as a function of applied load. The coating behaves like any ceramic coating on metallic substrates, exhibiting resilience until the first crack (at load $LC_1 = 12.5\,N$) is initiated, leading to complete rupture of the coating (at $LC_2 = 16.2\,N$) and subsequent total delamination as the load is increased (at $LC_3 = 19\,N$).

TABLE 21.7. Critical Loads for TiN and DLC Coatings on CP Titanium and Ti6Al4V Substrates

	Critical loads (N)	
Parameter	TiN coating on Ti6Al4V alloy	DLC coating on Cp titanium
First crack initiation (LC1)	10.8 ± 1.4	4.8 ± 0.7
First de-lamination (LC2)	13.5 ± 1.5	6.9 ± 1.4
Total de-lamination (LC3)	17.6 ± 1.6	9.1 ± 1.0

Instruiments, USA). A Vickers diamond indenter tip is driven into the material by applying a gradually increasing normal load. When the load reaches a preset maximum value, the normal load is reduced until partial or complete relaxation occurs. The position of the indenter relative to the sample surface is continuously monitored with a differential capacitive sensor. For each loading/unloading cycle, the applied load value is plotted with respect to the corresponding position of the indenter. The resulting load/displacement curves provide information specific to the mechanical behavior of the material under examination.

The measurements were taken on a 3×3 matrix with minimum $250\,\mu m$ spatial distance between measurements. The maximum loads were chosen very low to ensure that depth of the indentation is sufficiently low compared to the thickness of the coating [see Table 21.8]. The TiN coating was harder of the two and had higher modulus of elasticity [see Table 21.9].

TABLE 21.8. Micro Hardness Test Conditions

Parameter	Details
Indenter geometry	Triangular pyramid ($\alpha = 136° \pm 0.2°$)
Maximum load	50 mN
Loading cycle	100 mN/min loading, 10 s hold, 100 mN/min unloading
Measurement type	3×3 matrix with 250 μm gap between measurements

TABLE 21.9. Micro Hardness and Elastic Modulus of TiN and DLC Coatings

Parameters	TiN Coating on Ti6Al4V Alloy	DLC coating on Cp Titanium
Micro hardness—Vickers (Hv)	3260 ± 600	2450 ± 480
Elastic modulus of coating (GPa)	346 ± 55	147 ± 18

21.7.6 Simulated Accelerated Durability Studies

Artificial heart valves were identified as one potential application for DLC and TiN-coated materials. One of the primary requirements of artificial heart valves is durability. This calls for extensive studies on candidate materials for their wear properties and fatigue resistance. The adhesive and abrasive wear properties of the DLC/TiN-coated materials have been assessed individually and in combinations using pin-on-wheel and sand slurry tests. The functional durability of the valves is studied using accelerated durability tests.

To test new designs or material combinations at normal heart rates, whether in mechanical systems or in animal models for periods over ten years (as required by the International standards) is unrealistic. Hence, accelerated durability studies are carried out on the valve models. The test system simulates the actual working of a valve in a test chamber (Bhuvaneshwar et al., 1989). The unit at the institute is a hydraulic system capable of testing five valves simultaneously and the cycling rate can be varied between six and twelve times the normal heart rate (see Figure 21.7). The hydraulic pressures and flow rates through the valves can be regulated to simulate the physiological conditions in the heart. The rate of opening and closing of the valve is accelerated to ten times the normal heart rate to obtain meaningful data in a shorter time.

The system incorporates a fluid reservoir containing distilled water which is pumped using a magnetically coupled hydraulic pump through a ten-micron filter to the test chamber. The filter is employed to prevent any wear debris or dust particles reaching the test chamber. A rotating distributor supplies each test valve with the fluid in the required pressure range in a sequential manner so that each valve is opened and closed. The cycling rate is varied by varying the speed of rotation of the distributor, which is driven by a dc motor. The test conditions are listed in Table 21.10.

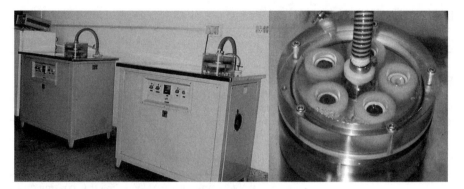

<u>Figure 21.7.</u> Accelerated durability test systems for the evaluation of artificial heart valves. The set up simulates the loading conditions in the heart and is capable of cycling at up to 12 times faster than the heart. Five valves can be tested simultaneously using each system.

TABLE 21.10. Accelerated Durability Test Conditions

Parameter	Unit	Value
Cycling rate	Cycles/min	720 ± 80
Valve closing pressure	mm Hg	120 ± 10
Average flow rate	lpm	3.5 ± 0.5
Test fluid	—	Distilled water + Fungal growth inhibitors
Test temperature	°C	37 ± 5

Four tilting disc type mechanical valves with different material combinations were tested (see Table 21.11). TTK Chitra heart valve, which is already in clinical use, was chosen as the control device in these studies.

The valves were removed from the test system at intervals of 40 million cycles and are examined for evidence of structural deterioration. The valves are weighed accurately in an analytical balance and their weights recorded. The end points in this accelerated durability test were when: there is a failure of any of its components; excessive wear is noticed and there is a likelihood of failure or; when the valve crosses 400 million cycles of operation (Figure 21.8).

At the end of the test, the valves were examined for signs of wear and other structural deterioration. The volume of wear is calculated from the weight loss and the density of the material that is wearing out. The wear rates of all the valves models were comparable with average rates less than 0.5 microlitres/year of run (corresponding to 40 million cycles). The DLC-coated valve showed marginally lower wear rates. Especially in the case of valve with DLC-coated UHMWPE, the disc edge was very uniform and edge surface finish remained extremely good, which indicates smooth rotation of the disc in the valve assembly and is a very important factor. This smooth rotation of the disc ensures uniform distribution of wear in the longer run and can enhance the service life of the valve considerably.

TABLE 21.11. Material Combinations Tested in Accelerated Durability Tester

Valve model	Cage material	Disc material	Sewing ring material
Control (TTK-Chitra)	Haynes-25	UHMWPE	Polyester
Ti + DLC/UHMWPE	Cp Ti + DLC coating	UHMWPE	Polyester
Ti/UHMWPE + DLC	Cp Ti	UHMWPE + DLC coating	Polyester
Ti + DLC/ UHMWPE + DLC	Cp Ti + DLC Coating	UHMWPE + DLC coating	Polyester
Ti + TiN/UHMWPE	Ti 6Al 4V + TiN coating	UHMWPE	Polyester

Accelerated Durability Test Results

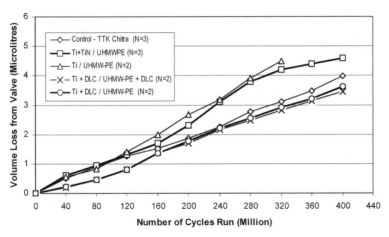

Figure 21.8. Accelerated Durability Results—The volume of material loss during the operation of the valve under accelerated cycling conditions is plotted against the number of cycles. The typical volume loss over 380 million cycles (equivalent to ten years life in the patient) is less than five microlitres. This very small wear rate is essential to ensure that the valves last the life span of the patient. Additionally the complications related to wear debris are minimal in such material combinations. (All valves size #27 mm tissue annulus diameter).

21.8 BIOLOGICAL CHARACTERIZATION

The DLC/TiN-coated materials with their bare metal counterpart as controls were evaluated for their cytocompatibility, hemocompatibility, and tissue compatibility. The biological characterization of the coated surfaces was carried out based on the International standard ISO 10993. Subsequently, two series of large animal experiments were carried out to assess the *in vivo* hemocompatibility of DLC and suitability of use of TiN coating on artificial heart valve cages.

21.8.1 Cytotoxicity

DLC and TiN-coated surfaces were studied for their Cytotoxicity effects using the direct contact, test on extract and agar over lay techniques as per the international standard ISO 10993: Part 5. All these coatings passed the test and hence could be classified as non-cytotoxic material.

Cytocompatibility studies of DLC, TIN on titanium, and UHMWPE were carried out with bare Titanium and UHMWPE, respectively, as controls. L-929 mouse fibroblast cells, osteoblast cells and endothelial cells were used for DLC-coated samples, while L-929 mouse fibroblast cells were used for TiN samples. Both qualitative and quantitative analysis indicates that DLC-coated Ti showed improved cytocompatibility (Kumari et al., 2002).

For better endothelialisation, cells should attach, adhere, spread and proliferate to give a confluent monolayer. The studies indicated that initial number of cells attached and area of spreading of cells are significantly increased on DLC and TiN coated samples compared to the corresponding uncoated surfaces. Adhesion pattern of thickly populated endothelial cells on DLC makes it suitable for vascular application.

21.8.2 Hemocompatbility

The blood compatibility of DLC and TiN coatings was assessed using a number of *in vitro* tests using human blood collected from healthy individual voluntary donors. The tests were chosen from the guidelines given in the standard ISO 10993: Part 4. The hemocompatbility assessment studies included estimation of consumption of blood components during exposure to whole blood, effect of the materials on the activation of coagulation factors and effect of the material on the complement activation characteristics.

The samples are exposed to whole blood for 30 minutes under agitation using an environmental shaker thermo stabilized at $35\,°C \pm 2\,°C$. The count of various formed elements of blood before and after the study were compared to arrive at the blood cell consumption profiles (Krishnan et al., 2002).

The platelet consumption showed a marginal reduction in the coated samples compared to the bare metal surfaces (see Figure 21.9). Quantification of platelet adhesion using radio labeled platelets confirmed this. The WBC consumption was more or less unaffected by the presence of the coating (see Figure 21.10).

The coated surfaces also had lower levels of adsorption of high molecular weight proteins, correlating with the lower platelet adhesion on the coated surfaces. High molecular weight proteins may consist of adhesive proteins that can mediate cell adhesion and thrombus formation. No significant platelet function abnormality was induced due to the material contact; however, the mild activation of platelets seems to have induced a change in plasma coagulation. The observed effect of the materials on plasma proteins on exposure of platelet-poor plasma has shown no significant clotting abnormality (Krishna Prasad et al., 2006).

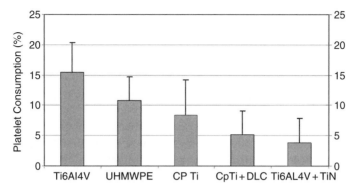

Figure 21.9. Platelet Consumption when exposed to whole blood for 30 minute duration. Lower platelet consumption indicates that less number of platelets are activated by exposure to the material surface and hence less is the chance of thrombus formation.

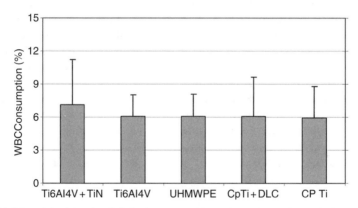

Figure 21.10. White blood cell (WBC) consumption when exposed to whole blood for 30 minute duration. The consumption of the white blood cells is not affected by the presence of the coating.

Hemolysis estimation of the coated and uncoated materials established their non-hemolytic nature. The studies on the effect of material on the complement activation have shown that there is no marked difference between the coated and uncoated samples. In general, the DLC and TiN coatings provide surfaces that are less thrombogenic without compromising the coagulation and complement activation properties.

21.8.3 Tissue Compatibility

The assessment of tissue compatibility included studies related to systemic toxicity, sensitization, intracutaneous reactivity, and chronic toxicity studies involving intramuscular implantation. All these were carried out using ISO 10993 series standards. Both the coated and uncoated materials passed the systemic toxicity, sensitization, and intracutaneous reactivity.

Intramuscular implantation was carried out for studying the effects under various time periods. Skeletal muscle around the coated and uncoated implants was grossly normal at all time periods. There was no evidence of necrosis or inflammation in any specimen. Good healing pattern was observed around both coated and uncoated samples. The light microscopic observations of the various parameters established that the tissue response around both coated and uncoated implants were similar to each other and showed evidence of repair at all time periods. There was no evidence of chronic inflammation in any specimen (Mohanty et al., 2002).

21.8.4 Large Animal Experiments

Two series of large animal experiments were conducted with the DLC and TiN-coated materials. The animal experiments were carried out in sheep with the authorization of the Institute's Animal Ethics Committee and the concerned national agency regulating experiments in animals. The international guiding principles for biomedical research involving animals of the Council for the International Organisation of Medical Sciences (CIOMOS) were adhered to during the animal experiments (Howard, 1985).

The first series was aimed at studying the blood compatibility characteristics of DLC coatings. Circular shaped buttons were implanted in the *inferior vena cava* (IVC) of sheep. The response to DLC-coated commercially-pure titanium (CP Ti + DLC) as the test material was compared against to that of commercially-pure titanium (CP Ti) as control. The buttons are harvested after two hours of implantation and the area of thrombus formed on the surface is assessed. The location of the control and test samples were interposed every experiment to eliminate the effect of implantation site on the results.

Microphotographs (20X) of the explanted samples scanned and digitized to assess the area of the thrombus on the samples using stereo zoom microscope (Nikon Corporation, Japan) and digital microscopy documentation system (DC 120, Kodak Corporation, USA). From these images, the area of the thrombus was estimated using image processing techniques (see Figure 21.11). The area of thrombus averaged over a set of six experiments was found to be marginally more on the bare CP titanium surface over the DLC-coated surface, but the differences were not statistically significant. The thrombus area estimation was validated using radio labeling technique.

The second series of large animal experiments were carried out as part of qualification of TiN coating on Ti6Al4V alloy for use in artificial heart valves. Sheep were chosen as the model based on the previous experience in heart valve evaluation (Bhuvaneshwar et al., 1996). Adult sheep in the weight range 35 to 50 Kg have heart size suitable for implantation of #23 mm size heart valve. Surgery was carried out under general anesthesia through a left thorocotomy in the fourth intercostals space. Cardiopulmonary bypass was established and the animal

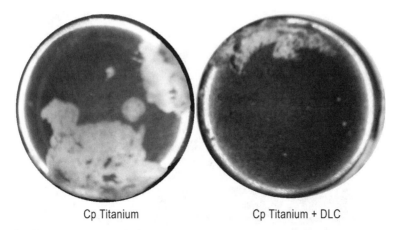

Cp Titanium   Cp Titanium + DLC

<u>Figure 21.11.</u> Thrombus deposits on the material surfaces during the *in vivo* blood compatibility experiments. The coated surface is seen to have marginally lower areas of thrombus deposits. (See color insert.)

cooled to $30\,°C \pm 2\,°C$. The heart was arrested using electrical fibrillation. The native mitral valve was excised and the artificial valve is implanted using 12 to 16 interrupted mattress sutures. Heart was closed and animal warmed back to $38\,°C$ before terminating the CPB. Post-operatively, the animals were administered with anti-platelet drugs during the first two weeks for reducing platelet aggregation and deposition. No anti-coagulants were given during the post-operative period.

A total of 15 animals were implanted with ten test valves and five control valves. Test valves were made of Ti6Al4V cage coated with TiN, UHMWPE disc and polyester sewing ring. The TTK-Chitra heart valve incorporating Haynes-25 alloy cage, UHMW-PE disc and polyester sewing ring was chosen as the control valve. Animals were sacrificed at predefined time periods (Four test valves and two control valves after three months of implantation and similar number of valves at six months of implantation) to assess the healing around the valve and for carrying out detailed histopathological analysis.

The explant analysis of the valves showed that the tissue in growth into the valve orifice area was much less in the case of TiN coated model (see Figure 21.12). Other than this, both test and control valves healed very well and were found to be well integrated to the anatomical site. There were no structural dysfunction or other valve related complications in any of the animals.

The results from these studies correlate well with the literature on tissue, blood, and cytocompatibility of TiN and DLC coatings reported by different investigators. The good blood compatibility of DLC coating is attributed to its hydrophobicity and ability to take an excellent surface finish, resulting in a high albumin deposition compared to fibrinogen deposition (Tsyganov et al., 2004; Sweitzer et al., 2006; Huang et al., 2003). In the case of titanium nitride coatings, it is postulated that the significantly lower interface tension between titanium oxide

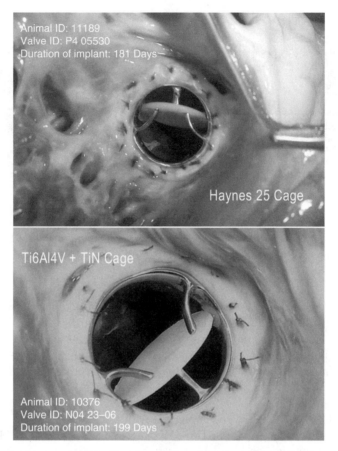

Figure 21.12. Valve explanted after six months of implantation (Mitral position—Inflow view). Very good tissue healing around the valve sewing ring, with minimal tissue overgrowth can be observed in the case of TiN-coated valve cage, compared to uncoated Haynes 25 cage.

and nitride films and plasma proteins and the semi-conducting nature of these films give them their improved hemocompatibility (Jones et al., 2000).

21.9 POTENTIAL APPLICATIONS

Very good blood and biocompatibility coupled with resistance to wear and inherent stability make DLC and TiN ideal materials for a wide range of cardiovascular applications. Artificial heart valves, bearings for blood pumps, left ventricular assist devices, and catheters are potential areas of application (Boguslawski et al., 2001). DLC-coated UHMWPE could be an excellent material for use as a bearing in rotating cardiovascular appliances like centrifugal blood pumps, cell separators, implantable cardiovascular pumps, and so on. Another area that is likely to benefit most from such coatings is the intravascular device segment, where the primary requirement for the coating is to mask the metallic surfaces from coming directly in contact with blood and surrounding tissues, thereby minimizing the release of metallic ions into the surroundings (Muraleedharan and Bhuvaneshwar, 2006).

DLC and TiN coatings with their excellent friction and wear properties make them ideal candidates for articulating orthopedic implantations. The reduction in friction and wear leads to formation of less debris. There can be a substantial improvement over the current metallic biomaterials as one of the most prominent failure modes of articulating orthopedic implants is aseptic loosening due to continuous inflammation caused by wear debris. The debris formed as a consequence of the wear results in tissue inflammation, osteolysis, and finally loosening of the implants. In prosthetic joints, the coating material should be hard and inert enough to prevent the wear out and corrosion. (Allen Mathew et al., 2001).

Diamond-like carbon coatings have been investigated for dental implant applications (Olborska et al., 1994). It was observed that DLC layers showed significant integration with the surrounding bone tissues. DLC coating might offer a solution for infections caused by indwelling urinary tract catheters. Researchers at three institutions are conducting experiments with very thin coatings of carbon applied to urinary catheters that may help alleviate patients' discomfort and infection risk.

21.10   FUTURE PERSPECTIVE

The DLC and TiN coatings are new entrants in the cardiovascular biomaterial segment. Initial indications based on *in vitro* and animal experiments are very encouraging, but use for specific applications will have to be validated, Especially in the case of intravascular device segment, the main challenge is to ensure good coating adhesion even under moderate plastic deformation of the substrate. This will help many balloon mountable devices like vascular stents to be coated with TiN and DLC. Another challenge will be to impart specific functionalities on the surfaces to help loading of drugs for enhancing healing and incorporation.

ACKNOWLEDGMENTS

The authors wish to thank all staff members of the Division of Artificial Organs for their active contribution in this work. We also wish to acknowledge the invaluable contributions the departments/divisions of Thrombosis Research, Histopathology, Tissue culture, Toxicology, Engineering services, *in vivo* models & Testing and Cardiovascular & Thoracic surgery of the Institute during the conduct of various studies.

The authors wish to acknowledge the partial financial support by the Indo-French Center for the Promotion of Advanced Research (IFCPAR) and the Department of Scientific and Industrial Research, Government of India. We wish to place on record the support of our project partners, Dr. R Suryanarayanan, University of Paris-sud and Mr. Yvon Sampeur (formerly ICMC), France, who made these studies possible with the supply of DLC-coated samples.

REFERENCES

Aisenberg S, Chabot R. 1971. Ion beam deposition of thin films of diamond like carbon, J Appl Physics 42:2953

Allen Mathew, Myer Ben, Rushton Neil. 2001. *In Vitro* and *In vivo* investigations into the biocompatibility of Diamond-Like carbon (DLC) coatings for Orthopedic Applications, J Biomed Mater Res 58:319–328

Bhuvaneshwar GS, Muraleedharan CV, Arthur Vijayan Lal G, Sankarkumar R, valiathan MS. 1996. Development of Chitra Tilting Disc Heart valve prosthesis, J Heart Valv Dis 5:448–458

Bhuvaneshwar GS, Muraleedharan CV, Ramani AV. 1989. Accelerated Durability Testing of Prosthetic Heart Valves, Proc. of National Conf. Industrial Tribology, Trivandrum, NCIT-89 VIII:1.1–1.4

Boguslawski G, Couvrat P, Jozwik K, Niedzielski P, Moll J, Nawrat Z, Walkowiak B, Niedzielska A, Szmidt J, Sokolowska A, Mitura S. 2001. Artificial heart valves with NCD coating, Proc. 3rd Inter. Conf. on Novel Applications of DLC, p 174–175

Courtney JM, Irvine I, Gaylor JDS, Forbs CD, Taylor KM. 1998. Blood compatibility in cardiopulmonary bypass, In Hasting GW (Ed), Cardiovascular biomaterials, Springer-Verlag, London p 37–56

Dion I, Baquey C, Monties JR. 1993. Diamond—the biomaterial of the 21st century, Int J Artif Organs 16:623–627

Eloy R, Belleville J. 1990. Biomaterial Blood Interaction, In: Concise Encyclopedia of Medical & Dental Materials; Williams, D. F. Ed.; Newyork, Pergamon Press, p 74–85

Hakim RM. 1992. Complement activation by biomaterials, Cardiovasc Pathol 2:187–197

Hanson SR. 2004. Blood coagulation and blood-materials interactions, In: Biomaterials science: An Introduction to Materials in Medicine, Ratner BD, Hoffman AS, Schoen FJ, Lemons JE, (Eds), Elsevier Academic Press: San Diego, CA, p 332–365

Hauert R. 2003. A review of modified DLC coatings for biological applications, Diamond Related Mater 12:583–589

Howard JN. 1985. A CIOMOS ethical codes for animal experimentation, WHO Chronicle, 39:52–56

Huang N, Yang P, Leng YX, Chen JY, Sun H, Wang J, Wnag GJ, Ding PD, Xi TF, Leng Y. 2003. Hemocompatbility of titanium oxide films, Biomaterials 24:2177–2187

Jones MI, McColl IR, Grant DM, Parker TL. 2000. Protein adsorption and platelet attachment and activation, on TiN, TiC and DLC coatings on titanium for cardiovascular applications, J Biomed Mater Res 52:413–421

Kalyani Nair, Muraleedharan CV, Bhuvaneshwar GS. 2003. Developments in mechanical heart valves, Sadhana, 28:575–58

Krishna Prasad C, Muraleedharan CV, Lissy K Krishnan. 2006. Bio-mimetic composite matrix that promotes endothelial cell growth for modification of biomaterial surface, J Biomedical Materials Research 80A:644–654

Krishnan LK, Varghese N, Muraleedharan CV, Bhuvaneshwar GS, Derange F, Sampeur Y, Suryanarayanan R. 2002. Quantitation of platelet adhesion to Ti and DLC coated Ti *in vitro* using 125I-labelled platelets, Biomolecular Engineering 19:251–253

Kumari TV, Anilkumar PR, Muraleedharan CV, Bhuvaneshwar GS, Sampeur Y, Derange F, Suryanarayanan R. 2002. In vitro Cytotoxicity of diamond-like carbon coatings on titanium, Biomedical Materials and Engineering 12:329–338

Mohanty M, Anilkumar TV, Mohanan PV, Muraleedharan CV, Bhuvaneshwar GS, Derange F, Sampeur Y, Suryanarayanan R. 2002. Long term tissue response to titanium coated with diamond-like carbon, Biomolecular Engineering 19:125–128

Moriau M, Lavenne EP, Scheiff JM, Col Debeys C. 1988. The physiological mechanisms of haemostasis. In Blood Platelets In: Hologramme Ed.: Neuilly-sur-Seine, p 136–141

Muraleedharan CV, Bhuvaneshwar GS. 2006. Titanium Alloys in implant applications, Metals Materials and Processes 18:441–450

Muraleedharan CV, Bhuvaneshwar GS, Ramani AV. 1989. Adhesive and abrasive wear studies on polymers for use in Prosthetic Heart Valves, Proc. of Nat. Conf. on Industrial Tribology, Trivandrum, NCIT-89 VIII:2.1–2.5

Muraleedharan CV, Bhuvaneshwar GS, Valiathan MS. 1995. Materials for Chitra Heart Valve Prosthesis—A Review, Metals Mater and Processes 7:147–158

Olborska A, Swider M, Wolowiec R, Niedzielski P, Rylski A, Mitura S. 1994. Diamond-like carbon coatings for biomedical applications, Diamond Relat Mater 3:899–901

Ramsden JJ. 1995. Puzzles and Paradoxes in Protein Adsorption, Chem Soc Rew 38:73–78

Ratner, BD. 2004. Surface properties and surface characterization of materials, In: Biomaterials Science. An introduction to materials in medicine; Ratner BD, Hoffman AS, Schoen FJ, Lemons JE, (Eds), Elsevier, Academic Press: San Diego, CA p 40–59

Sella C, Lecoeur J, Sampeur Y, Catania P. 1993. Corrosion resistance of amorphous hydrogenated SiC and diamond like coatings by RF plasma enhanced chemical vapor deposition, Surface Coating & Technology, 60:577–583

Sweitzer R, Scholz C, Montezuma S, Rizzo JF. 2006. Evaluation of sub-retinal implants coated with amorphous aluminum oxide and diamond-like carbon, J. Bioactive and Compatible Polymers 21:6–22

Thomson LA, Law FC, Rushton N, Franks J. 1991. Biocompatibility of diamond-like carbon coatings, Biomaterials 12:37–40

Tsyganov I, Maitz MF, Wieser E. 2004. Compatibility of titanium-based coatings prepared by metal plasma immersion ion implantation and deposition, Applied Surface Science 235:156–163

Vogler EA. 1998. Structure and reactivity of water at biomaterial surfaces, Adv Colloid Interface Sci 74:69–117

Wisbey A, Gregson PJ, Tuke M. 1987. Application of PVD TiN to Co-Cr-Mo based surgical implants, Biomaterials 8:477–480

Zou YS, Wang W, Song GH, Du H, Gong J, Huang RF, Wen LS. 2004. Influence of the gas atmosphere on the microstructure and mechanical properties of diamond-like carbon films by arc ion plating, Mater Lett 58:3271–3275

INDEX

A

Abrasion testing
   cardiovascular medical device coatings,
      690–692
   polymer biocomposites, 77–79
Accelerated durability test conditions,
      cardiovascular medical device
      coatings, 695–697
Acetabular cup insert, functionally-graded
      ceramic hip implants
   electrode design, 340
   homogeneous shaping techniques,
      340–344
Acetylcholine receptors (AChR), neurons
      in electric field, 630–633
Acid-base reaction, polyalkenoate
      cements, 412
Acid citrate dextrose (ACD), placental
      umbilical cord blood processing,
      651
Acrylamide monomers, macroporous gels,
      freezing rate and temperature,
      505–508
Action potentials, nervous system
      electrical stimulation, 622–623
Activation studies, thin solid films, 674
Adhesion mechanisms
   blood cell adhesion studies, thin solid
      films, 674

cardiovascular medical device coatings,
      ware characteristics, 689–690,
      692–693
injectable hydrogels, fast chemical
      reaction/physical transitions,
      192–193
nanostructured ceramics, 216–220
titanium dental implants, bone-implant
      interface, 160–163
Agarose, macroporous gels, 523–525
Air/water and air/solid properties, thin
      solid films, 665–667
   interfacial properties, 668
Albumin/fibrinogen adsorption, titanium
      dental implants, bone-implant
      interface, 160–163
Aldehydes, injectable hydrogels, fast
      chemical reaction/physical
      transitions, 192–193
Alginate
   cell-based nanocomposites, 560
   nanofibrous scaffolds, tissue
      engineering, 457–458
Alkali metal ions, ionomer glass structure,
      417–422
Alkaline phosphatase (ALP) activity
   bone regeneration factors, 555–558
   cell-based nanocomposites,
      mesenchymal stem cells, 566–569

Advanced Biomaterials: Fundamentals, Processing, and Applications, Edited by Bikramjit Basu,
Dhirendra S. Katti, and Ashok Kumar
Copyright © 2009 The American Ceramic Society

Alkaline phosphatase (ALP) activity
(*cont'd*)
gene-based nanomaterials, 573
Alumina
hip replacement ceramic implants, 327
zirconia-toughened alumina, 328–329
medical device applications, 359–360
nanostructured ceramics, 213–220
Aluminoborate glasses, 414–415
Alumino-phospho-silicate glasses, 414–415
Alumino-silicate network
ionomer cements, 412–414
Zachariasen Random Network Theory,
415–416
Aluminum-oxygen bioinert ceramics,
70–72
functionally-graded ceramic hip
implants
grain size optimization, 346–348
sintering and microstructure
evaluation, 345–351
hip replacement, basic properties,
326–327
hydroxyapatite-reinforced high-density
polyethylene composites, 75–79
Aluminum/silicon ratio, ionomer glass
structure, 417–422
Ambient conditions
humidity, electrospinning for
nanofibrous scaffold fabrication,
449
temperature, silicon carbide-based
ceramic biomaterials, 375–381
Ammonium persulfate (APS), covalently
cross-linked macroporous gels,
515–516
Amorphous calcium phosphate (ACP)
carbonate apatites, 29–33
in carbonate apatites, 30–33
crystallographic structure, 35
Amorphous phase separation (APS),
ionomer glass crystallization,
423–427
Amphiphilic peptides
air/water and air/solid properties,
665–667
cell-based nanocomposites, 570–572
nanofibrous scaffold self-assembly,
443–444

Anchorage mechanics, titanium dental
implants, 164–167
Anions, apatite incorporation of, 34
Anodic polarization tests, titanium-
niobium-zirconium-tantalum
alloys, LENS-deposited
processing, 296–298
Anodization, nanomaterial processing,
228–231
Anorganic bone mineral (ABM), cell-
based nanocomposites, peptide-
based nanomaterials, 571–572
Anterior cervical fusion, biphasic calcium
phosphate ceramics, 131
Anterior cruciate ligament (ACL), tissue
engineering
design criteria for, 591–593
multi-phased scaffold design, 600–603
nanofibrous scaffolds, 476–479
Anti-adherent coatings, cardiovascular
medical devices, 685
Antibiotics, biphasic calcium phosphate
granules for delivery of, 128–129
Apatites. *See also* Hydroxyapatite (HA)
bioactive coatings, 389–392
biologic apatites and related calcium
phosphates, 39–40
carbonate incorporation, 27–33
cation substitution, 34
ceramic composites, bioactive bonding,
385
fluoride and chloride incorporation,
25–27
lattice parameters, 22–23
overview, 20–23
simultaneous carbonate/fluoride
incorporation, 33–34
structural substitutions in, 25
Area-to-volume ratio, wound healing and,
554
Array technologies, biomedical
applications, 546–547
Articular cartilage, nanofibrous scaffolds,
454–455
Articulating surfaces, orthopedic implants,
wear and fracture complications,
212
Artificial saliva (AS) tests, dental ceramics
dissolution, 68

Ascorbic acid, bone regeneration factors, 555–558

Astrocytes, structure and function, 615

Astroglial cells, nervous system electrical stimulation, 628–629

Auger electron spectroscopy (AES), titanium dental implants, 150–151

Autoimmune disease, placental umbilical cord blood transfusion, 657–658

Autologous bone grafts, current grafts and graft substitutes, 553–554

Axon guidance, neurons in electric field, 629–630

B

Bacteria, nanostructured ceramics and, 216–217

Bacterial polyesters, nanofibrous scaffolds, tissue engineering, 462

Ball-heads, functionally-graded ceramic hip implants, electrophoretic deposition, 339–344

Barium aluminosilicate ionomer glasses, cation substitution, 428

Barium sulfate radiopaque agent, bioactive injectable bone substitutes, 116–118

Bending/fracture behavior, silicon carbide-based ceramic biomaterials, 375–381

β grains, titanium-niobium-zirconium-tantalum alloys, 291–296

Beta-titanium, femoral head implants, LENS™ processing, 285–286

Bioactive bonding, ceramic biomaterials, 385–396

Bioactive materials
biphasic calcium, 107–113
calcium phosphates, *in vivo* testing of, 43–45
host response to, 8
titanium dental implants, anchorage mechanics, 164–167

Bioadhesive materials, medical implants, 541

Bioartificial liver (BAL), 538

Bioceramics. *See* Ceramic biomaterials; Glass ceramic biomaterials

Biochemical binding, titanium dental implants, 157–163

Biocompatibility
cell mimetic monolayer, 548–549
defined, 7
evaluation and testing
in vitro tests, 12–13
in vivo tests, 14–15
heterogeneous phospholipids/glycolipid/cholesterol ternary lipid composition, 667–668
medical device ceramic biomaterials, 396–401
in vitro cell attachment and proliferation testing, 398–400
in vitro cytotoxicity testing, 396–398
in vivo studies, 400–401
tissue engineering scaffolds, 441–442
titanium dental implants, 146–151

Biodegradation
of biomaterials, biocompatibility and, 14–15
injectable hydrogels, photopolymerization and, 186–191
macroporous gels, 522–525
tissue engineering scaffolds, 439–440, 441–442

Bioglass®, bone tissue engineering, 559–560

Bioinert ceramics
cardiovascular medical devices, 685–686
orthopedic applications, overview, 55
processing and properties, 70–72

Biologic apatites
related calcium phosphates, 39–40
simultaneous fluoride/carbonate incorporation, 33–34

Biomaterials
applications
array technologies, 546–547
bioadhesives, 541
cardiovascular devices, 537–538, 678–702
cochlear prosthesis, 542–544
dental implants, 539–541
drug delivery systems, 544–545
extracorporeal artificial organs, 538
ophthalmologic applications, 541–542

Biomaterials (*cont'd*)
  orthopedic implants, 538–539
  overview, 536
  tissue engineering, 545–546
calcium phosphate-based materials,
    40–45
cell-material interactions, 8–11
characterization procedures, 15–16
defined, 5–6
host response to, 7–8
mechanical and biochemical effects,
    4–5
multidisciplinary engineering and
    bioscience research, 4–5
overview, 4–5
processing of
  ceramics, 251–254
  composite materials, 256–260
  future research issues, 269–270
  metals, 248–251
  overview, 247–248
  polymers, 254–255
  scale processing, 260–269
    micro/nano fabrication, 268–269
    micro/nano surface modification,
      260–268
  sterilization, 260–261
Biomechanical binding, titanium dental
    implants, 157–163
Biomedical applications. *See also* Medical
    devices
  array technologies, 546–547
  bioadhesives, 541
  cardiovascular devices, 537–538
  cochlear prosthesis, 542–544
  dental implants, 539–541
  drug delivery systems, 544–545
  extracorporeal artificial organs, 538
  macroporous gels, 522–525
  metallic alloys, 79–86
  ophthalmologic applications, 541–542
  orthopedic implants, 538–539
  overview, 536
  tissue engineering, 545–546
BIOMEMS/BIONEMS technology, micro/
    nano fabrication, biomaterials,
    268–269
Biomimetic surface engineering
  mimetic monolayers

air/water and air/solid properties,
    665–667
air/water interfacial properties, 668
blood cell adhesion studies, 674
calcification studies, 673
dense thin solid films, 664
deposition optimization, 670–671
future research issues, 675
heterogeneous lipid compounds,
    667–668
macromolecule incorporation,
    668–669
overview, 664
platelet adhesion and activation, 674
protein interaction studies, 673–674
surface modification, 664–672
  biological interactions, 672
  supported thin solid films, 671–672
nanofibrous scaffolds, ligaments and
    tendons tissue engineering,
    478–479
nano-HA/collagen-based composites,
    561–565
nanomaterials processing, 230–231
silicon carbide-based ceramic
    biomaterials
  mechanical optimization, 381–384
  medical device applications, 360–365
  tissue engineering scaffolds, 440–442
Biomolecules, nanomaterial interaction,
    232–233
Bionert materials, host response to, 7–8
Biopolymers. *See* Polymers
Bioresorbable materials, host response to, 8
Biotolerant materials, host response to, 7–8
Bioverit® I base glass, processing and
    properties, 69–70
Biphasic calcium phosphate (BCP)
    ceramics
  bioactive injectable bone substitutes,
    radiopacity of, 115–118
  bioactivity and osteogenic properties,
    107–113
  bone tissue engineering, 559–560
  cell proliferation and colonization, 109
  clinical applications
    dentistry, 129–130
    orthopedics, 130–132
  commercial products, 103–104

composition, 109
dissolution properties, 109
drug delivery granules, 128–129
fibrin glue, 127
future research issues, 132
growth plate chondrocyte maturation
    scaffolds, 125
hydroxyapatite:tricalciumphosphate
    ratio and, 61–63
hydroxyapatite-zirconium composites,
    63
injectable bioceramic granules and
    polymers, 125–127
macroporosity and microporosity,
    104–106
macroporous cements, 114–115
mechanical properties, 107
mesenchymal stem cell scaffolds,
    124–125
microstructure improvements, 113–114
overview, 102–104
physical and chemical properties,
    106–107
resorbable osteosynthesis, 118–119
scaffold materials, 120–124
in vivo testing, 109–113
Bismuth oxide radiopaque agents,
    bioactive injectable bone
    substitutes, 116–118
Blended polymers, nanofibrous scaffolds,
    tissue engineering, 462–465
Block co-polymers, injectable hydrogels,
    thermogelling polymers, 193–197
Blood-brain barrier, nanomaterial
    interaction, 232–233
Blood cell interactions
    adhesion studies, thin solid films, 674
    cardiovascular medical device
        hemocompatibility, 683
Blood substitutes, 549. *See also* Placental
    umbilical cord blood
    cord blood, 648–651
    research limitations and trends, 645–648
Bombyx mori silk fibrin, nanofibrous
    scaffolds from, 456
Bone
    biphasic calcium phosphate bonding
        with, 102–103
    tissue engineering scaffolds, 120–124

composition of, 58
resorbable osteosynthesis, biphasic
    calcium phosphates, 118–120
resorption prevention, biphasic
    calcium phosphate ceramics,
    dental applications,
    129–130
structure and properties, 57–59
tissue engineering
    biphasic calcium phosphate scaffolds,
        120–124
    cell-based nanocomposites, 549
        adipose-derived stem cells,
            574–575
        bioceramics, 559–560
        bone marrow-derived stem cells,
            575–576
        cell-material constructs, 566–570
        gene-based materials, 572–573
        grafts and graft substitutes,
            553–554
        mesenchymal stem cells, 576–577
        nanofibrous composites, 565–566
        nano-HA/collagen composites,
            561–565
        peptide-based materials, 570–572
        polymers, 560–561
        regeneration factors, 554–558
    nanofibrous scaffolds, 466–471
        cell sources for, 467–468
        scaffold properties and sources,
            468–471
    nanomaterials, 212–231
        ceramics, 213–220
        chemical processing, 228–231
        composites, 226–228
        future research issues, 231–233
        metals, 220–223
        polymers, 223–226
    titanium dental implants and formation
        of, 147–151
Bone density evaluation, medical device
    biocompatibility, 401
Bone-derived cells, titanium dental
    implants, morphological
    compatibility, 155–157
Bone filler materials
    hydroxyapatite, 61–62
    nanostructured polymers, 223–226

Bone/implant interface
   biological fixation, 549
   tissue engineering, musculoskeletal
         system
      design criteria, 590–593
      future reserach issues, 603
      heterotypic cellular interactions,
            593–596
      multi-phase scaffold design, 599–603
      overview, 589–590
      structure-function relationship,
            596–599
   titanium dental implants, 157–163
Bone marrow cells (BMO)
   cell-based tissue engineering, 575–576
   gene-based nanomaterials, 573
   hydroxyapatie composite with, 61
   micro-macroporous biphasic calcium
         phosphate scaffolds, bone tissue
         engineering, 123–124
Bone morphogenetic proteins (BMPs)
   bone grafts, 553–554
   gene-based materials, 572–573
   mesenchymal stem cell nanocomposites,
         567–569
   nanofibrous scaffolds, 468–469
   nano-HA/collagen-based composites,
         563–565
   peptide-based nanomaterials, 571–572
   regeneration factors, 555–558
Bone sialoprotein-1 (BSP-1), mesenchymal
         stem cell nanocomposites,
         567–569
Boride alloys, titanium boride reinforced
         titanium-niobium-zirconium-
         tantalum metal-matrix
         composites
   LENS™ deposition, 305–309
   tribological behavior, 309–317
   wear resistance, 304–305
Brain, neural progenitor cells in,
         617–618
Brain-derived neurotrophic factor
         (BDNF), neurons in
         electric field, 633
Bridging oxygen (BO)
   ionomer glasses, structural analysis,
         417–422
   ionomer glass formation, 416

Bright-field transmission electron
         microscopy, titanium-niobium-
         zirconium-tantalum alloys,
         292–296
Bromodeoxyuridina, neural progenitor
         cells, 617
"Butterfly" pattern, mica-based glass
         ceramics treatment, 67–68

C
Calcification, thin solid films, 673
Calcite, in biomaterials, 42
Calcium alumino-silicate glass
   ionomer cements, 412–414
   solid state MAS-NMR analysis, 422
   strontium substitution, 427–428
   structural analysis, 417–418
Calcium channels, neurons in electric field,
         633
Calcium chlor-apatite (ClA), structure and
         properties, 23–25
Calcium-deficient apatite (CDA)
   biphasic calcium phosphate
         formation, 108–113
      microstructure improvement, 113–114
   micro/macroporous biphasic calcium
         phosphate composites, 106
   structure and properties, 23–25
Calcium-doped zirconia composites, 70–72
Calcium ions, in apatite structure, cation
         substitution for, 34
Calcium phosphates
   amorphous structures, 35
   bioactive properties of, 8
   biologic apatites and, 39–40
   in biologic systems, 20–21
   in biomaterials, 40–45
   biomaterials processing and properties,
         59–62
   bone tissue engineering, 559–560
   cell-based nanocomposites, 561–565
   classification of, 20–23
   crystallographic properties of, 35–37
   dicalcium phosphate dihydrate, 36–38
   dissolution comparisons, 38
   future research issues, 91
   lattice parameters, 22–23
   medical and dental applications, 44–45
   metallic coating composites, 87–90

molar ratios, 35–36
nanomaterials
  ceramics, 213–220
  composites, 226–228
non-apatitic structures, 35
octacalcium phosphate, 38
overview of, 20–21
synthetic apatites, 21–23
ternary phase diagram, 59
tetracalcium phosphates, 39
titanium dental implants
  bone-implant interface, 159–163
  morphological compatibility,
    156–157
transformation schematic for, 37
tricalciumphosphate, 38–39
Cancellous bone, structure and properties,
    57–59
Capillary radius, silicon carbide-based
    ceramic biomaterials, reaction-
    formation mechanisms, 370–374
Carbohydrates, nanofibrous scaffolds,
    tissue engineering, 456–459
Carbonate hydroxyapatite (CHA),
    biphasic calcium phosphate
    formation, 102–103, 107–113
Carbonates
  apatite incorporation of, 27–33
    bioactivity testing of, 43–45
    simultaneous fluoride/carbonate
      incorporation, 33–34
  in biologic apatites, 39–42
Carbon biomaterials, dental implants,
    539–541
Carbon fiber-carbon polymer composites,
    74
Carbon fiber-poly sialane composites,
    73–74
Carbon nanotubes (CNTs), nanostructured
    composites, 228
Carcinogenicity, *in vivo* biocompatibility
    testing, 14–15
Cardiovascular medical devices, 537–538
  basic properties, 678–679
  biological characterization, 697–702
    cytotoxicity, 698
    hemocompatibility, 698–699
    large animal studies, 700–702
    tissue compatibility, 699–700

biomaterials, 683–684
  anti-adherent coatings, 685
  heparin/heparin-like coatings, 684–685
  inert coatings, 685–686
coating characterization, 688–697
  abrasive wear characteristics, 690–692
  adhesion studies, 692–693
  adhesive wear characteristics, 689–690
  durability studies, 695–697
  microhardness measurements,
    693–695
  surface roughness, 688–689
diamond-like carbon, 686–687
hemocompatibility, 680–683
  blood cell interactions, 682
  complement activation, 683
  hemostasis and coagulation, 682–683
  protein adsorption, 681–682
  water adsorption, 681
overview, 678
potential applications, 702–703
titanium-nitride materials, 687–688
Cartilage regeneration
  biphasic calcium phosphate scaffolds
    for, 125
  injectable hydrogels
    fast chemical reaction/physical
      transitions, 191–193
    photopolymerization and, 186–191
  macroporous gels, 522–525
  nanofibrous scaffolds, 471–474
Cathodal turning, neurons in electric field,
    629–630
Cationic lipid (CL), gene-based materials,
    572–573
Cation substitution, ionomer glasses,
    427–428
Cell-based nanocomposites
  bone tissue engineering, 549
    adipose-derived stem cells, 574–575
    bioceramics, 559–560
    bone marrow-derived stem cells,
      575–576
    cell-material constructs, 566–570
    current grafts and graft substitutes,
      553–554
    gene-based materials, 572–573
    mesenchymal stem cells, 576–577
    nanofibrous composites, 565–566

Cell-based nanocomposites (*cont'd*)
   nano-HA/collagen composites,
      561–565
   peptide-based materials, 570–572
   polymers, 560–561
   regeneration factors, 554–558
  current research issues, 577–578
  historical development of, 552–553
  tissue engineering technology, 554
Cell culture techniques
  bone regeneration factors, 554–558
  macroporous gels, 522–525
Cell fate identification, neural progenitor
   cells, 618–619
Cell-material interactions
  of biomaterials, 8–11
  calcium phosphate biocomposites, 60–62
  cardiovascular medical device
      hemocompatibility, 683
  ceramic biomaterials, medical device
      applications, 359–360
  injectable hydrogels,
      photopolymerization and,
      186–191
  nanomaterials, 232–233
   mesenchymal stem cell-material
      constructs, 566–569
  nervous system electrical stimulation,
      in vitro systems, 628–629
  neurons in electric field, 630–631
  scale processing of biomaterials, 260, 262
  thin solid films, 672
  titanium dental implants, 147–151
   morphological compatibility, 155–157
Cell mimetic monolayer, 548–549
Cell proliferation and colonization
  biphasic calcium, 109
  neural progenitor cells in brain, 617–618
  orthopedic tissue engineering,
      osteoblast-fibroblast interactions,
      594–596
Cell transplantation, tissue engineering
   scaffolds, 439–440
  cartilage regeneration, 472
  ligaments and tendons, 477–479
  skeletal muscle tissue, 475
Cement biomaterials
  biphasic calcium phosphate granules, 129
  macroporous cements, 114–115

polyalkenoate cements
  cation substitution, 427–428
  composition, 414–415
  crystallization, 423–427
  design, 415–416
  future research issues, 429
  overview, 411–414
  structure, 417–422
   solid state MAS-NMR spectroscopy
      characterization, 418–422
Cementless prostheses, metal alloys for,
   85–86
Central nervous system (CNS), damage
   and repair, 620–621
Ceramic biomaterials. *See also* Glass
   ceramic biomaterials
  bone tissue engineering, 553–554,
      559–560
  calcium phosphates in, 40–45
   processing and properties, 59–62
  dental implants, 539–541
  future research issues, 91
  hip implants, functionally-graded
      materials, 285–286
  ceramic hip joint, 324–353
   alumina implants, 327
   ball-heads and cup inserts,
      electrophoretic deposition,
      339–344
   composition gradient, 330–331
   disc formation, electrophoretic
      deposition, 332–339
   electrophoretic deposition, 331–332
   future research issues, 351–353
   historical background, 325–326
   metal implant coatings, 329–330
   overview, 324
   sintering and microstructural
      evaluation, 344–351
   zirconia implants, 327–328
   zirconia-toughened alumina,
      328–329
  hydroxyapatite-ceramic composites,
      processing and properties, 62–63
  hydroxyapatite-titanium composites,
      processing and properties, 63–66
  medical device applications
   bioactive glass coatings, physico-
      chemical properties, 392–396

biocompatibility assessment, 396–401
in vitro cell adhesion and proliferation tests, 398–400
in vitro cytotoxicity testing, 396–398
in vivo studies, 400–401
coating materials, 384–392
bioactive glasses, 386–387
deposition techniques, 387–389
hydroxyapatites and substituted apatites, 385, 389–392
future research issues, 401–403
mechanical properties, 374–384
biomimetic structure optimization, 381–384
microstructure, phase and element distribution, 365–370
overview and background, 358–360
reaction-formation mechanisms, 370–374
silicon carbide, 360–365
nanostructured ceramics, orthopedic and tissue engineering, 213–220
orthopedic applications
mechanical properties, 56
overview, 54–55
osteolysis prevention, 211–212
polymer-ceramic composites, 74–79
processing of, 251–254
electrodeposition, 253–254
formation and sintering of powder, 252
microwave techniques, 253
powder preparation, 251–252
solid freeform fabrication, 253–254
surface treatment, 252–253
vapor phase chemical reactions, 253–254
Ceramic-on-polyethylene implants, osteolysis prevention, 211–212
Cervical spine arthrodesis, biphasic calcium phosphate ceramics, 131
Chemical passivation, titanium dental implants, bone-implant interface, 162–163
Chemical stripping process, titanium dental implants, biocompatibiility and, 149–151

Chemical vapor deposition (CVD), diamond/diamond-like carbon coatings, nanostructured ceramics, 219–220
Chemical-vapor deposition (CVD), diamond-like carbon coatings, cardiovascular medical devices, 686–687
Chitin and chitosan
cell-based nanocomposites, 560
injectable hydrogels, thermogelling polymers, 194–197
macroporous gels, 523–525
nanofibrous scaffolds, tissue engineering, 458–459
cartilage regeneration, 472–474
Chitosan-glycerophosphate mixture, injectable hydrogels, thermogelling polymers, 195–197
Chloride, apatite incorporation of, 25–27
Chondrocyte interactions
cell transplants, cartilage regeneration, 472–474
nanostructured biodegradable polymers, 224–225
orthopedic tissue engineering, osteoblast-fibroblast interactions, 595–596
tissue engineering scaffolds, 441–442
Chondroitin sulfate, injectable hydrogels, photopolymerization, 190–191
Click chemistry, injectable hydrogels, fast chemical reaction/physical transitions, 192–193
Coagulation mechanisms, cardiovascular medical device hemocompatibility, 683–684
Coating biomaterials
cardiovascular medical devices, 683–684, 688–697
abrasive wear characteristics, 690–692
adhesion studies, 692–693
adhesive wear characteristics, 689–690
anti-adherent coatings, 685
diamond-like carbon coatings, 686–687
durability studies, 695–697
heparin/heparin-like coatings, 684–685
inert coatings, 685–686

Coating biomaterials (*cont'd*)
  microhardness measurements,
    693–695
  surface roughness, 688–689
cell-based nanocomposites, 561–565
ceramic biomaterials
  deposition techniques, 387–396
  medical devices, 384–396
    bioactive glasses, 386–387, 392–396
    deposition techniques, 387–389
    hydroxyapatite and substituted
      apatites, 385
    physico-chemical properties,
      389–392
  drug delivery systems, 544–545
  hip implants, ceramic coating on metal
    implants, 329–330
  hydroxyapatite in, 61–62
  metal alloys, 86–90
  metal-on-metal bearings, osteolysis
    prevention, 211–212
  nanostructured ceramics, 219–220
  orthopedic applications, overview, 55–56
  titanium dental implants
    bone-implant interface, 160–163
    integrated implant systems, 163–167
Coaxial electrospinning, nanofibrous
    scaffold fabrication, 451–453
Cobalt-chromium-molybdenum alloys
  metallic coating composites, 90
  nanostructured metals, 221–223
  orthopedic applications, overview, 55
  processing and properties, 85–86
  wear properties, 81
Cochlear implants, biomaterials, 542–544
Co-culture modeling, orthopedic tissue
    engineering
  multi-phased scaffold design, 601–603
  osteoblast-fibroblast interactions,
    593–596
Coefficient of friction, nanostructured
    ceramics, 218–220
Co-efficient of thermal expansion (CTE),
    in coating biomaterials,
    orthopedic applications, 55–56
Collagen fiber
  in bone, 554
  cell-based nanocomposites, 560
    nanofibrous composites, 565–566

nano-HA/collagen-based composites,
    561–565
  peptide-based nanomaterials, 571–572
in hard tissue, 57–59
implant loosening and formation of,
    208–210
macroporous gels, freezing rate and
    temperature, 506–508
nanofibrous scaffolds
  electrospinning fabrication, 450–453
  protein sources, 454–455
Collagenous capsulation
  implant loosening and, 208–210
  nanostructured metals and risk of, 223
Colony-forming uint-fibroblast (CFU-F),
    576–577
Complement activation, cardiovascular
    medical device
    hemocompatibility, 684
Composite materials. *See also* Metal-
    matrix composites; specific
    composites
  alumina-toughened zirconia, 328–329
  nonstructured composites, 226–228
  processing of, 256–260
  zirconia-toughened alumina, 328–329
Compositionally-graded materials
  functionally-graded ceramic hip
    implants, 330–331
  Laser Engineered Net Shaping
    (LENS®) processing technique,
    284–285
Compressive strain
  silicon carbide-based ceramic
    biomaterials, 376–381
  titanium dental implant mechanics,
    152–153
Concanavalin A (ConA), neurons in
    electric field, 630–633
Conductivity, electrospinning for
    nanofibrous scaffold fabrication,
    448
Confocal microscopy (CM), macroporous
    gels, pore structure, 519–521
Coral materials, cell-based
    nanocomposites, 567–569
Cord blood
  clinical applications and safety studies,
    652–656

properties of, 656–658
research limitations, 645–648
stability properties, 648–651
Core-binding alpha factor 1 (Cbfa-1), bone
    regeneration factors, 555–558
Corrosion
    in metallic implants, 81–83
    orthopedic metal implants, 211–212
    titanium dental implants, 146–151
        biocompatibiility and, 147–151
    titanium-niobium-zirconium-tantalum
        alloys, LENS-deposited
        processing, 296–298
Cortical bone
    nano-HA/collagen-based composites,
        563–565
    structure and properties, 57–59
Counter-electrode properties, functionally-
    graded ceramic hip implants,
    electrode design, 340–344
Covalently cross-linked macroporous gels,
    515–516
Cow bone apatite, carbonate apatite
    compared with, 33
Critical concentration of gelation (CCG)
    cryogelation techniques, 502
    macroporous gels, precursor gel
        composition, 509–512
Critical heat treatment experiments,
    mica-based glass ceramics, 67–68
Critical load testing, cardiovascular
    medical device coatings, 694–695
Cross-linked chemistry
    gelatin nanofibrous scaffolds, 455
    injectable hydrogels
        fast chemical reaction/physical
            transitions, 192–193
        photopolymerization and, 186–191
    macroporous gels, 500–502
        covalently cross-linked compounds,
            515–516
        physically cross-linked compounds,
            512–515
        precursor gel composition, 510–512
Cryogelation
    macroporous gels
        biomedical applications, 522–525
        covalently cross-linked MGs, 515–516
        future research, 525

microscopic porous structure
    characterization, 518–521
physically cross-liked MGs, 513–515
pore volume, 516–518
overview, 500–502
polymeric cryostructuration, 502–512
    freezing rate and temperature,
        504–508
    precursor concentration and
        composition, 508–512
    processing techniques, 502–504
Crystalline properties
    carbonate apatites, 29–33
    hydroxyapatite bioceramics, 40–45
    hydroxyapatite-titanium composites, 65
    ionomer glasses, 423–427
    macroporous gels, freezing rate and
        temperature, 504–508
Cup inserts, functionally-graded ceramic
    hip implants, electrophoretic
    deposition, 339–344
Custom-designed implants, Laser
    Engineered Net Shaping
    (LENS®) processing technique,
    284–285
Cyanoacrylate materials, bioadhesives,
    541
Cytoskeleton, cell-material interactions in,
    10–11
Cytotoxicity
    cardiovascular medical device coatings,
        698
    medical device ceramic biomaterials, *in
        vitro* testing, 396–398
    in vitro test of, 12–13

D
DC electric fields, nervous system
    electrical stimulation, *in vivo*
    systems, 623–624
Defect analysis, functionally-graded
    ceramic hip implants, 348–351
Deformation mechanisms, titanium-
    niobium-zirconium-tantalum
    alloys, 290–296
Demineralized bone matrix (DBM), bone
    grafts, 553–554
Density, silicon carbide-based ceramic
    biomaterials, 375–381

Dental applications for biomaterials
　biphasic calcium phosphate ceramics,
　　129–130
　of glass-ceramic biomaterials, 66–70
　implants, 539–541
　mica-based glass ceramics, 66–68
　polyalkenoate cements
　　cation substitution, 427–428
　　composition, 414–415
　　crystallization, 423–427
　　design, 415–416
　　future research issues, 429
　　overview, 411–414
　　structure, 417–422
　　　solid state MAS-NMR spectroscopy
　　　　characterization, 418–422
　structure and properties, 57–59
　titanium implants
　　basic requirements, 146–157
　　biocompatibility, 146–151
　　integrated implant system, 163–167
　　mechanical compatibility, 151–153
　　metal alloys, 84
　　morphological compatibility, 153–157
　　osseointegration and bone/implant
　　　interface, 157–163
　　overview, 144–146
Dentin matrix protein 1 (DMP1),
　　gene-based nanomaterials, 573
Deposition techniques
　bioactive coatings, 387–389
　thin solid films, optimization of, 670–671
Dermabond, 541
Dexamethasone, bone regeneration
　　factors, 555–558
Dextran metacrylate (dextran-MA),
　　macroporous gels
　biomedical applications, 523–525
　precursor gel composition, 510–512
Dextrans, macroporous gels, 523–525
Diameter properties, nanofibrous
　　scaffolds, electrospinning
　　fabrication, 451–453
Diamond/diamond-like carbon coatings,
　　549
　cardiovascular medical devices,
　　685–687
　biological characterization, 695–702
　potential applications, 702–703

metal hip implants, 329–330
nanostructured ceramics, 219–220
Diaspirin-cross-linked hemoglobin
　　(DCLHb), 646–648
Dicalcium phosphate dihydrate (DCPD),
　　36–38
Differential scanning calorimetry (DSC)
　ionomer glasses, crystallization
　　properties, 423–427
　macroporous gels, pore volume
　　calculations, 517–518
　silicon carbide-based ceramic
　　biomaterials, medical device
　　applications, 362–365
　titanium-glass ceramic composites,
　　69–70
Diffusion mechanisms, silicon carbide-
　　based ceramic biomaterials,
　　372–374
1,25-Dihydroxyvitamin D3, bone
　　regeneration factors, 555–558
Direct Laser Forming (DLF) technique,
　　titanium alloy processing, 84
Disc formation, functionally-graded
　　ceramic hip implants
　composition profile, 333–335
　controlled processing, 335–337
　electrophoretic deposition, 332–339
Dissolution properties
　biphasic calcium, 106–107, 109
　calcium phosphates, 38
　dental ceramics, 68
Distance parameters, electrospinning for
　　nanofibrous scaffold fabrication,
　　449
Drug delivery systems
　biomaterials, 544–545
　biphasic calcium phosphate granules,
　　128–129
　nanofibrous scaffolds, 452–453
Durability, cardiovascular medical device
　　coatings, 695–697

E
EDS analysis, dental ceramics, 68
Elastic modulus (E-modulus)
　high-density polyethylene-
　　hydroxyapatite-aluminum oxide
　　hybride composites, 76–79

macroporous gels, 524–525
polymer biomaterials, 73
silicon carbide-based ceramic
   biomaterials, 378–381
titanium dental implant mechanics,
   152–153
integrated implant systems, 163–167
Electrical stimulation, nervous system
   cells, 621–629
cellular response *in vitro,* 628–629
central nervous system, therapeutic
   stimulation, 624–625
DC electric fields *(in vivo),* 623–624
electromagnetic stimulation *(in vivo),*
   624
extracellular stimulation *(in vitro),*
   625–628
physiological endogenous electric fields,
   622–623
Electric field
functionally-graded ceramic hip
   implants, electrode design,
   calculations for, 340–344
nervous system electrical stimulation,
   621–629
   DC electrical fields, 623–624
   electromagnetic stimulation, 625–628
   physiological endogenous fields,
      622–623
   therapeutic applications, 624–625
   in vitro response, 628–629
neurons in, 629–633
   axon guidance, 629–630
   calcium, 633
   cellular-level changes, 630–631
   receptor accumulation and
      autoregulation, 631–633
Electrochemistry, nanomaterial
   processing, 228–231
Electrode materials, nervous system
   electrical stimulation, 627
Electrodeposition techniques, ceramic
   biomaterials processing,
   253–254
Electrolytic deposition (ELD), ceramic
   biomaterials processing,
   253–254
Electromagnetic stimulation, nervous
   system, *in vivo,* 624

Electrophoretic deposition (EPD)
ceramic biomaterials processing,
   253–254
functionally-graded ceramic hip
   implants, 330–331
   ball-heads and cup inserts, 339–344
   disc formation, 332–339
   shaping techniques, 331–332
functionally graded ceramic hip joint,
   overview, 324
Electrospinning
cell-based nanofibrous composites,
   565–566
nanofibrous scaffold fabrication,
   446–453
tissue engineering applications,
   466–480
Electrospraying, nanofibrous scaffold
   fabrication, 447–453
Element distribution, silicon carbide-based
   ceramic biomaterials, medical
   device applications, 365–370
EMEM culture medium, medical device
   biocompatibility, cytotoxicity
   testing, 397–398
Endogenous electric fields, nervous
   system electrical stimulation,
   622–623
Endoplasmic reticulum, cell-material
   interactions in, 8–11
Environmental scanning electron
   microscopy (ESEM),
   macroporous gels, pore structure,
   519–521
Epichlorohydrin (ECH), covalently
   cross-linked macroporous gels,
   515–516
Eukaryotic cell, cell-material interactions
   in, 8–11
External fractionated radiation, tissue
   engineering scaffolds, micro-
   macroporous biphasic calcium
   phosphate, 121–124
Extracellular electrical stimulation, *in vitro*
   systems, 625–628
electrode material, 627
hydrogen concentration, 627–628
methodology, 626
signal selection, 626–627

Extracellular matrix (ECM)
  cell-material constructs
    mesenchymal stem cells, 566–569,
      567–569
    peptide-based materials, 570–572
  cell-material interactions and, 11
  injectable hydrogels
    development of, 182
    nanostructured polymers, 225–226
    photopolymerization and, 188–191
  macroporous gels
    biomedical applications, 524–525
    freezing rate and temperature,
      506–508
  nanomaterials processing, 229–230
  neurons in electric field, 629–630
  tissue engineering scaffolds, 439–440
    bone tissue engineering, 468–469
    cartilage regeneration, 471–474
    ligaments and tendons, 476–479
    natural polymers, 453–459
    overview, 545–546
    self-assembly techniques, 443–444
    three-dimensionality of, 440–442
Extracorporeal artificial organs, 538

F
Fabrication techniques
  biomaterials, micro/nano fabrication,
    268–269
  nanofibrous scaffold synthesis, 442–453
    comparison of techniques, 451–453
    electrospinning, 446–453
    phase separation, 444–446
    self assembly, 443–444
Failure analysis, cardiovascular devices,
    678–679
Fast chemical reactions, injectable
    hydrogels, 191–193
Femoral implants
  composite materials for, 326–327
  femur mechanical properties, 327–328
  Laser Engineered Net Shaping
    (LENS®) processing technique,
    284–285
    functionally-graded materials,
    285–286
Fetal bovine chondrocytes, nanofibrous
    scaffolds, tissue engineering,
    cartilage regeneration, 474

Fiber alignment, nanofibrous scaffolds,
    electrospinning fabrication,
    449–453
Fiber/particle reinforced composites,
    processing of, 256
Fiber reinforced biocomposites, processing
    of, 256
Fibrin composites
  biphasic calcium phosphate, 127
  cell-based nanocomposites, 560
Fibroblast cells, *in vitro* biocompatibility
    testing with, 13
Fibroblast growth factor (FGF), bone
    regeneration, 557–558
Fibrocartilage region
  orthopedic tissue engineering,
    structure-function relationships,
    597–599
  tissue engineering, 591–593
Fibronectin adsorption
  nanofibrous composites, 565–566
  nanostructured biodegradable polymers,
    224–225
Fibrovascular tissue formation, orthopedic
    tissue engineering, 593–596
Finite element analysis, titanium dental
    implant mechanics, 152–153
Fluorapatite (FAP), ionomer glass
    crystallization, 423–427
Fluoride, apatite incorporation of, 25–27
  simultaneous fluoride/carbonate
    incorporation, 33–34
Fluoride-calcium composites, ionomer
    glass crystallization, 426–427
Fluorine containing alumino-phospho-
    silicate glasses
  composition, 414–415
  crystallization properties, 423–427
  design, 415–416
  solid state MAS-NMR analysis,
    419–422
  structure, 417–422
Fluorite, ionomer glass structure,
    417–422
Fluorite-substituted apatite (CFA)
  simultaneous carbonate incorporation,
    33–34
  structure and properties, 23–25
Fluoro-hydroxyapatite (FHA)
  bone tissue engineering, 559–560

nanofibrous tissue scaffolds, bone tissue engineering, 468–469

sintering experiments with, 62–63

Flux growth, of carbonate apatites, 28–33

45S5 bioglass, bioactive properties of, 8

45S5 bioglass ceramics, processing and properties, 69–70

Fourier transform infrared imaging (FTIR-I), orthopedic tissue engineering, structure-function relationships, 597–599

Fourier transform infrared reflection absorption spectroscopy (FTIR-RAS), titanium dental implants, 150–151

Fourier transform infrared (FTIR) spectroscopy

bioactive coatings, physico-chemical properties, 392–396

radiopaque agents, bioactive injectable bone substitutes, 116–118

Four-point bending measurements, silicon carbide-based ceramic biomaterials, 375–381

Fractures

fixation devices, biomaterials, 539

incidence and prevalence, 552

as orthopedic implant complication, 212

silicon carbide-based ceramic biomaterials, 375–381

Fracture toughness, ceramic biomaterials, 74

Freeze-dried materials, macroporous gels, 501–502

Freezing rate and temperature, polymer cryogelation, 504–508

Friction properties

nanostructured ceramics, 218–220

polymer biocomposites, 77–79

titanium boride reinforced titanium-niobium-zirconium-tantalum metal-matrix composites, 309–317

FSZ composites, 71–72

Functionally-graded materials (FGM)

hip implants, 285–286

ceramic hip joint, 324–353

alumina implants, 327

ball-heads and cup inserts, electrophoretic deposition, 339–344

composition gradient, 330–331

disc formation, electrophoretic deposition, 332–339

electrophoretic deposition, 331–332

future research issues, 351–353

historical background, 325–326

metal implant coatings, 329–330

overview, 324

sintering and microstructural evaluation, 344–351

zirconia implants, 327–328

zirconia-toughened alumina, 328–329

hydroxyapatite-titanium composites, 63–66

G

Gadolinium phosphate radiopaque agents, bioactive injectable bone substitutes, 116–118

Galactocerebroside, deposition optimization, 670–671

Gelatin

cell-based nanocomposites, 560

nanofibrous scaffolds, 455

Gelation, nanofibrous scaffold fabrication, 444–446

Gene-based biomaterials, cell-based nanocomposites, 572–573

Genotoxicity, *in vitro* biocompatibility testing, 13

Gentamycin delivery systems, biphasic calcium phosphate granules, 128–129

Giant cell formation, implant loosening and, 208–210

Glass biomaterials. *See also* Ceramic biomaterials

bioactive bonding, 386–387, 392–396

physico-chemical properties, 392–396

ionomer glasses

cation substitution, 427–428

composition, 414–415

crystallization, 423–427

design, 415–416

future research issues, 429

overview, 411–414

Glass biomaterials (*cont'd*)
    structure, 417–422
        solid state MAS-NMR spectroscopy
            characterization, 418–422
    metallic coating composites, 87–90
    orthopedic applications
        mechanical properties, 56
        overview, 55
    processing and properties, 66–70
        mica-based glass ceramics, 66–68
        miscellaneous composites, 69–70
    Zachariasen Random Network Theory,
        415–416
Glass-in-glass phase separation, 423–427
Glutaraldehyde (GTA)
    covalently cross-linked macroporous
        gels, 515–516
    gelatin nanofibrous scaffolds, 455
Glycine-alanine-hydroxyproline units,
    nanofibrous scaffolds, 454
Glycosaminoglycans (GAGs), nanofibrous
    scaffolds, tissue engineering,
    456–457
    cartilage regeneration, 471–474
Gold, bone interfaces with, 83–84
Gradient functional concept (GFC),
    titanium dental implants,
    integrated implant systems,
    165–167
Graft materials. *See* Scaffold materials;
    Tissue engineering
Grain size
    functionally-graded ceramic hip
        implants, optimization, 346–348
    nanostructured ceramics, 217–220
    titanium-niobium-zirconium-tantalum
        alloys, 290–296
Green fluorescent protein (GFP), neural
    progenitor cells, 618–619
"Green ware"
    ceramic biomaterials processing, 252
    functionally-graded ceramic hip
        implants, 351–352
Growth cone changes, neurons in electric
    field, 630–633
Growth factors (GFs)
    bone regeneration, 554–558
    neurons in electric field, 630–631
    tissue engineering scaffolds, 439–440

    nanofibrous scaffold self-assembly,
        443–444
Growth plate chondrocyte maturation,
    biphasic calcium phosphate
    scaffolds for, 125
Guided bone regeneration (GBR),
    nanofibrous scaffolds for,
    469–470
Guided tissue regeneration (GTR)
    membrane, nano-HA/collagen-
    based composites, 561–565

H
Hall-Petch predictions, nanostructured
    ceramics, 218–220
HAPEX™ composite, 74–79
Hardness properties
    nanostructured ceramics, 217–220
    titanium boride reinforced titanium-
        niobium-zirconium-tantalum
        metal-matrix composites,
        305–309
    tribological behavior, 315–317
Hard tissue
    biomaterials replacements for, future
        research issues, 92
    structure and properties, 57–59
    titanium dental implants, integrated
        implant systems, 163–167
Heart valve prostheses, 537–538
Helical rosette nanotubes (HRNs)
    nanostructured injectable hydrogels,
        225–226
    nonstructured composites, 226–228
Hemocompatibility
    cardiovascular medical devices, 680–683,
        698–699
        blood cell interactions, 682
        complement activation, 683
        hemostasis and coagulation, 682–683
        protein adsorption, 681–682
        water adsorption, 681
    in vitro biocompatibility testing, 13
Hemoglobin
    placental umbilical cord blood safety
        and, 654–656
    substitutes for, 645–648
Hemolink, 647–648
Hemopure product, 647–648

Hemostasis, cardiovascular medical device hemocompatibility, 683–684

Heparan sulfate (HS), bone regeneration, 558

Heparin and heparin-like coatings, cardiovascular medical devices, 684–685

Hepatocyte growth factor (HGF), nanofibrous scaffold self-assembly, 443–444

Hertzian contact stresses, titanium boride reinforced titanium-niobium-zirconium-tantalum metal-matrix composites, 305–309
  tribological behavior, 315–317

Heterogeneous phospholipids/glycolipid/cholesterol ternary lipid composition, stability and compatibility studies, 667–668

Heterotypic cellular interactions, orthopedic tissue engineering, 593–596
  multi-phased scaffold design, 600–603

1,1,1,3,3,3-Hexafluoro-2-propanol (HFP), nanofibrous scaffolds, 454–455

High-density polyethylene (HDPE) hydroxyapatite-reinforced composites (HAPEX), 74–79
  orthopedic applications, 56–57
  tricalcium phosphate nanocomposites, 227–228

High-density polyethylene-hydroxyapatite-aluminum oxide hybride composites, 76–79

High-throughput screening, array technologies, 546

High tibial valgisation osteotomy (HTO), biphasic calcium phosphate ceramics, 131–132

Hip implants
  biomaterials, 538–541
  different bearing couples, coefficient of friction, 219–220
  functionally-graded biomaterials
    ceramic hip joint, 324–353
      alumina implants, 327
      ball-heads and cup inserts, electrophoretic deposition, 339–344

composition gradient, 330–331
      disc formation, electrophoretic deposition, 332–339
      electrophoretic deposition, 331–332
      future research issues, 351–353
      historical background, 325–326
      metal implant coatings, 329–330
      overview, 324
      sintering and microstructural evaluation, 344–351
      zirconia implants, 327–328
      zirconia-toughened alumina, 328–329
    laser design, 285–286
  metallic alloys wear properties, 81
  miscellaneous metal alloys for, 85–86
  titanium metal alloys, 84

Homotypic cellular interactions, orthopedic tissue engineering, multi-phased scaffold design, 600–603

Host response
  to biomaterials, 7–8
  cardiovascular medical devices, hemocompatibility, 680–683, 698–699
  implant loosening and, 208–210
  titanium dental implants, 146–151

HP composites, biphasic calcium phosphate, microstructure improvement, 113–114

HPMC-Si composites, self-hardening injectable-mouldable composite, 126–127

Human body parts, synthetic biomaterial compatibility with, 5–6

Human bone morphogenetic protein (hBMP). *See* Bone morphogenetic proteins

Human immunodeficiency virus (HIV), placental umbilical cord blood research, 644–648

Human leukocyte antigen (HLA), placental umbilical cord blood safety and, 648, 654–656

Human ligament fibroblast (HLF), nanofibrous scaffolds, ligaments and tendons tissue engineering, 478–479

Human osteoblast (HOB) cell lines, *in vitro* biocompatibility testing with, 13

Hyaluronan, cell-based nanocomposites, 560

Hyaluronic acid (HA)
  injectable hydrogels
    fast chemical reaction/physical transitions, 192–193
    photopolymerization and, 188–191
  nanofibrous scaffolds, tissue engineering, 457
    bone tissue, 469

Hydrofluoric acid, silicon carbide-based ceramic biomaterials, medical device applications, 363–365

Hydrogels. *See also* Macroporous gels (MGs)
  injectable biomaterials
    fast chemical reaction/physical transitions, 191–193
    nanostructured polymers, 225–226
    overview and basic principles, 180–182
    photo-gelling polymers, 183–191
    research on, 550
    in situ forming gels, 182–197
    thermogelling polymers, 193–197
  peptide-based nanomaterials, 570–572

Hydrogen concentration, nervous system electrical stimulation, 627–628

Hydrophilic polymers
  gelatin nanofibrous scaffolds, 455
  injectable hydrogels, 183
    side group photoactivation, 184–185
  macroporous gels, 500–502
    biomedical applications, 524–525
    microscopic analysis, 518–521
    pore volume, 516–518

Hydrothermal techniques, carbonate apatite preparation, 28–33

Hydroxyapatite (HA)
  bioactive properties of, 8
    coating materials, 389–392
  biomaterials processing and properties, 59–62
  biopolymer composites, orthopedic applications, 56–57
  biphasic calcium phosphate and, 103–104
  in bone, 554
  bone tissue engineering, 553–554, 559–560
  cell-based nanocomposites
    nanofibrous composites, 565–566
    non-mesenchymal stem cell-material constructs, 569–570
  ceramic composites
    bioactive bonding, 385
    in biomaterials, 40–45
    in orthopedic applications, 62–63
  fundamentals of, 23–34
  glass coatings for, 86–90
  in hard tissue, 57–59
  lattice parameters, 22–23
  medical and dental applications, 44–45
  nano-HA/collagen-based composites, 561–565
  nanomaterials
    bone tissue engineering, 468–469
    ceramics, 213–220
    composites, 226–228
  ophthalmologic implants, 542
  orthopedic applications
    mechanical properties, 56, 61–62
    overview, 54–56
  osteoblast composites, 60
  overview, 20
  reinforced HDPE composites and, 74–79
  stoichiometric properties, 24–25
  structure and properties, 23–34
  ternary phase diagram, 59
  titanium-hydroxyapatite composites
    orthopedic applications, 54–56
    processing and properties of, 63–66
  tricalcium-hydroxyapatite ratios, 61–63, 105–106
    BCP scaffolds in mesenchymal stem cells, 124–125
    biphasic calcium phosphate, 109, 112–113

Hydroxy butyl chitosan (HBC), injectable hydrogels, thermogelling polymers, 194–197

Hydroxyethylcellulose (HEC) solution, macroporous gels, precursor gel composition, 509–512

2-Hydroxyethylmethacrylate-L-Lactide (HEMA-LLA), macroporous gels, 523–525

I

Immunocytochemistry, neural progenitor cells, 618–619
Implants. *See also* specific implants
  biomaterials overview, 538–541
  hip implants
    biomaterials, 538–541
    different bearing couples, coefficient of friction, 219–220
    functionally-graded biomaterials
      ceramic hip joint, 324–353
        alumina implants, 327
        ball-heads and cup inserts, electrophoretic deposition, 339–344
        composition gradient, 330–331
        disc formation, electrophoretic deposition, 332–339
        electrophoretic deposition, 331–332
        future research issues, 351–353
        historical background, 325–326
        metal implant coatings, 329–330
        overview, 324
        sintering and microstructural evaluation, 344–351
        zirconia implants, 327–328
        zirconia-toughened alumina, 328–329
      laser design, 285–286
    metallic alloys wear properties, 81
    miscellaneous metal alloys for, 85–86
    titanium metal alloys, 84
  metallic biomaterials
    coatings, 86–90
    corrosion of, 81–83
    wear properties, 81–82
  orthopedic implants
    loosening, 208–210
    osteolysis, 210–212
    problems and failures, 207–212
    wear and fractures, 212
  tissue engineering scaffolds, micro-macroporous biphasic calcium phosphate, 121–124

titanium alloys, 83–84
  dental implants
    basic requirements, 146–157
    biocompatibility, 146–151
    integrated implant system, 163–167
    mechanical compatibility, 151–153
    metal alloys, 84
    morphological compatibility, 153–157
    osseointegration and bone/implant interface, 157–163
    overview, 144–146
  in vivo biocompatibility testing, 14–15
Inflammatory response, titanium dental implants, bone-implant interface, 158–163
Injectable biomaterials
  bone substitute
    biphasic calcium, 104
    radiopacity improvements in, 115–118
  ceramics, BCP granules and polymers, 125–127
  hydrogels
    fast chemical reaction/physical transitions, 191–193
    nanostructured polymers, 225–226
    overview and basic principles, 180–182
    photo-gelling polymers, 183–191
    research on, 550
    in situ forming gels, 182–197
    thermogelling polymers, 193–197
  nanostructured polymers, 223–226
Inorganic phosphate chitosans, injectable hydrogels, thermogelling polymers, 195–197
In situ gel formation, injectable hydrogels, 182–197
  fast chemical reaction/physical transitions, 191–193
  photo-gelling polymers, 183–191
  thermogelling polymers, 193–197
Insulin-like growth factor-1 (IGF-1), bone regeneration, 557–558
Insulinoma cells, macroporous gel attachment, 523–525
Integrated implant systems, titanium dental implants, 163–167

Interface regeneration mechanism
orthopedic tissue engineering, 593–596
current and future research issues,
603
multi-phased scaffold design, 599–603
structure-function relationships,
596–599
thin solid films, air/water and air/solid
properties, 668
International Organization for
Standardization (ISO), ISO
10993 biocompatibility evaluation
guidelines, 12–15
Intraocular implants, 541–543
Inverse Hall-Petch effect, nanostructured
ceramics, 218–220
In vitro testing
of biocompatibility, 12–13
biomaterials characterization, 15–16
biphasic calcium phosphate materials,
109–113
calcium phosphates, 60–61
of calcium phosphates, 43–45
cardiovascular medical device coatings,
hemocompatibility, 698–699
dental ceramics dissolution, 68
gene-based nanomaterials, 572–573
hydroxyapatite-reinforced high-density
polyethylene composites, 75–79
medical device biocompatibility
cell attachment and proliferation
tests, 398–400
cytotoxicity testing, 396–398
metallic coating composites, 86–90,
87–90
nanofibrous materials, cartilage
regeneration, 472–474
nervous system electrical stimulation
cellular response to, 628–629
extracellular stimulation, 625–628
octacalcium phosphate formation, 59–60
orthopedic tissue engineering
multi-phased scaffold design, 601–603
osteoblast-fibroblast interactions,
594–596
osteogenetic markers, 555–558
radiopaque agents, bioactive injectable
bone substitutes, 116–118
titanium dental implants

integrated implant systems, 164–167
morphological properties, 154–157
titanium-niobium-zirconium-tantalum
alloys, LENS-deposited passive
oxide films, 302–304
In vivo testing
aluminum-oxygen bioinert ceramics,
70–72
of biocompatibility, 14–15
biomaterials characterization, 15–16
calcium phosphates, 60–61
of calcium phosphates, 43–45
gene-based nanomaterials, 573
hydroxyapatite implants, 60
medical device biocompatibility,
400–401
nanofibrous scaffold fabrication, bone
tissue engineering, 471
nano-HA/collagen-based composites,
562–565
nanostructured ceramics, 215–220
nervous system electrical stimulation
DC electric fields, 623–624
electromagnetic stimulation, 624
octacalcium phosphate formation, 59–60
orthopedic tissue engineering
multi-phased scaffold design, 601–603
osteoblast-fibroblast interactions,
594–596
osteogenetic markers, 557–558
radiopaque agents, bioactive injectable
bone substitutes, 116–118
of tricalciumphosphates, 61–62
Ion-beam deposition, diamond-like carbon
coatings, cardiovascular medical
devices, 686–687
Ion beam enhanced deposition, titanium
oxide films, dental implants,
159–163
Ionomer glasses
cation substitution, 427–428
composition, 414–415
crystallization, 423–427
design, 415–416
future research issues, 429
overview, 411–414
structure, 417–422
solid state MAS-NMR spectroscopy
characterization, 418–422

J

Joint replacement, biomaterials, 539
Jurin's law, silicon carbide-based ceramic biomaterials, reaction-formation mechanisms, 370–374

K

Keratoprostheses, ophthalmologic implants, 542

L

L929 fibroblast cell cultures
hydroxyapatite-titanium composites, 65–66
polymer biocomposites, 77–80
Langmuir-Blodgett films, air/water and air/solid properties, 665–667
Langmuir-Schaffer technique, air/water and air/solid properties, 666–667
Large animal studies, cardiovascular medical device coatings, 700–702
Laser Engineered Net Shaping (LENS®) processing technique
metal matrix composites, 257–260
micro/nano fabrication, biomaterials, 268–269
orthopedic biomaterials processing, 282–285
future research issues, 318–319
hip implants, 285–286
overview, 270
titanium boride reinforced titanium-niobium-zirconium-tantalum metal-matrix composites, 304–309
titanium-niobium-zirconium-tantalum alloys, 286–304
characterization methods, 286–287
corrosion resistance, 296–298
deformation mechanisms, 290–296
microstructure and mechanical properties, 287–290
in vitro testing, 302–304
x-ray photoelectron spectroscopy of, 298–302
Laser processing
ceramic biomaterials, 252
orthopedic biomaterials, 282–319
functionally-graded hip implant, 285–286

Laser Engineered Net Shaping system, 282–285
metal alloys, 286–304
overview, 278–282
titanium dental implants, integrated implant systems, 163–167
titanium-niobium-zirconium-tantalum alloys, 286–304
characterization methods, 286–287
corrosion resistance, 296–298
deformation mechanisms, 290–296
microstructure and mechanical properties, 287–290
in vitro testing, 302–304
x-ray photoelectron spectroscopy of, 298–302
Ligaments, tissue engineering
interface design, 590–593
nanofibrous scaffolds, 476–479
Lipid thin solid films
air/water and air/solid properties, 665–667
macromolecule incorporation, 668–669
optimization and mechanical properties, 667–668
Liposome-encapsulated hemoglobin (LEH), 648
Liquid Band-Aid, 541
Liquid-liquid immiscibility, ionomer glass crystallization, 424–427
Liver, extracorporeal implants, 538
Load-bearing analysis, orthopedic tissue engineering, structure-function relationships, 597–599
Loewenstein's rules, ionomer glass formation, 415–416
Loosening, of orthopedic implants, 208–210
Low stiffness, polymer biomaterials, 73
Low temperature degradation, yttrium-doped tetragonal zirconia polycrystal ceramics, 328
LP composites, biphasic calcium phosphate, microstructure improvement, 113–114
Lutetium oxide radiopaque agents, bioactive injectable bone substitutes, 116–118

M

Macromeric structures, injectable
　　hydrogels, photopolymerization
　　and, 189–191
Macromolecules, thin solid film
　　incorporation, 668–669
Macrophages, osteolysis in orthopedic
　　implants, 211–212
Macroporosity
　　biphasic calcium phosphates, 104–106
　　　macroporous cements, 114–115
　　　in vivo testing of, 109–113
　　calcium phosphates, 44–45
Macroporous gels (MGs)
　　biomedical applications, 522–525
　　covalently cross-linked MGs, 515–516
　　formation schematic, 503–504
　　future research, 525
　　microscopic porous structure
　　　characterization, 518–521
　　overview, 500–502
　　physically cross-liked MGs, 513–515
　　polymer cryogelation, 504–512
　　　freezing rate and temperature,
　　　504–508
　　pore volume, 516–518
Magic angle spinning, ionomer glass
　　structure, 418–422
Magnesium
　　apatite incorporation of, 34
　　in biologic apatites, 39–40
　　ionomer glass cation substitution, 428
　　in tricalciumphosphates, 39
　　zirconia ceramic composites, 71–72
Malaria, placental umbilical cord blood
　　safety and, 653–656
Mathematical modeling, functionally-
　　graded ceramic hip implants,
　　composition profile, 333–335
MC3T3-E1 cells, radiopaque agents,
　　bioactive injectable bone
　　substitutes, 117–118
Mechanical properties
　　biphasic calcium, 107
　　ceramic biomaterials, 4–5, 56
　　　nanostructured ceramics, 217–220
　　glass ceramics, 56
　　hydroxyapatite, 56, 61–62
　　ionomer glasses, 417–422

macroporous gels, precursor gel
　　composition, 508–512
orthopedic tissue engineering, structure-
　　function relationships, 597–599
polymers, 73
silicon carbide-based ceramic
　　biomaterials, 374–381
　　optimization, 381–384
titanium dental implants, 146–151,
　　151–153
titanium-niobium-zirconium-tantalum
　　alloys, 287–290
Medial collateral ligament (MCL), tissue
　　engineering, structure-function
　　relationships, 597–599
Medical devices. *See also* Biomedical
　　applications
　　cardiovascular medical devices (*See*
　　　Cardiovascular medical devices)
　　ceramic biomaterials
　　　bioactive glass coatings, physico-
　　　　chemical properties, 392–396
　　　biocompatibility assessment, 396–401
　　　　in vitro cell adhesion and
　　　　　proliferation tests, 398–400
　　　　in vitro cytotoxicity testing, 396–398
　　　　in vivo studies, 400–401
　　　coating materials, 384–392
　　　　bioactive glasses, 386–387
　　　　deposition techniques, 387–389
　　　　hydroxyapatites and substituted
　　　　　apatites, 385, 389–392
　　　future research issues, 401–403
　　　mechanical properties, 374–384
　　　　biomimetic structure optimization,
　　　　　381–384
　　　microstructure, phase and element
　　　　distribution, 365–370
　　　overview and background, 358–360
　　　reaction-formation mechanisms,
　　　　370–374
　　　silicon carbide, 360–365
　　nanofibrous scaffolds, 452–453
Melting process, bioactive glasses, 387
Membrane receptors, neurons in electric
　　field, 631–633
Mesenchymal stem cells (MSC)
　　biphasic calcium phosphate scaffolds,
　　124–125

bone marrow-derived stem cells, 576
bone regeneration factors, 555–558
cell-material constructs, 566–569
injectable hydrogels,
    photopolymerization and,
    187–191
micro-macroporous biphasic calcium
    phosphate scaffolds, bone tissue
    engineering, 123–124
nanofibrous scaffolds, 445–446
    bone tissue engineering, 467–468
    cartilage regeneration, 472
    ligaments and tendons tissue
        engineering, 477–479
    orthopedic tissue engineering
        multi-phased scaffold design, 600–603
    osteoblast-fibroblast interactions,
        595–596
    other sources, 576–577
Metal ion treatment, ceramic biomaterials
    processing, 252–253
Metal-matrix composites
    Laser Engineered Net Shaping
        (LENS®) processing technique,
        257–260
    hip implants, 286
    titanium boride reinforced titanium-
        niobium-zirconium-tantalum
        composites, 304–318
        LENS deposition, 305–309
        tribological behavior, 309–317
        wear resistance, 304–305
Metal matrix composites (MMCs),
    processing of, 256–260
Metal-on-metal biomaterials, osteolysis
    prevention, 211–212
Metal-on-polyethylene components,
    nanostructured ceramics vs.,
    219–220
Metals and metallic alloys. See also specific
    alloys, e.g. Titanium and titanium
    alloys
    coating biomaterials, 86–90
    corrosion properties, 81–83
    dental implants, 539–541
    future research issues, 92
    nanostructured metals, 220–223
    non-ferrous metal alloys, 86
    orthopedic biomaterials

Laser Engineered Net Shaping
    (LENS®) processing technique,
    282–285
    overview, 55
    performance limitations, 81–83
    processing and properties, 79–86,
        248–251
    flowchart, 249
    ore-to-raw material processing,
        249–250
    raw material processing, 250
    surface finishing, 250–251
    wear properties, 81
Methyl cellulose, injectable hydrogels,
    thermogelling polymers,
    194–197
MG-63 osteoblast cells, medical device
    biocompatibility, cytotoxicity
    testing, 397–398
Mica-based glass ceramics, processing and
    properties, 66–68
Michael-addition-type reactions, injectable
    hydrogels
    fast chemical reaction/physical
        transitions, 191–193
    photopolymerization, 191
Microcompression testing, orthopedic
    tissue engineering, structure-
    function relationships, 597–599
Microcomputed tomography, macroporous
    gels, pore structure, 519–521
Microfabrication, overview, 546
Microglia, structure and function, 615
Microhardness measurements,
    cardiovascular medical device
    coatings, 693–695
Micro-macroporous biphasic calcium
    phosphate (MBCP)
    future research issues, 132
    injectable bioceramic granules and
        polymers, 125–127
    manufacture of, 106
    orthopedic applications, 130–132
    resorbable osteosynthesis, 118–120
    tissue engineering scaffolds
        bone tissue, 121–124
        growth plate chondrocyte maturation,
            125
    in vivo testing of, 109–113

Micromotion, titanium dental implants, 158–163

Micro/nano fabrication, biomaterials, 268–269

Micro/nano surface modification, scale processing of biomaterials, 260–268

Micron-size silicon carbide-based ceramic biomaterials, phase and element distribution, 367–370

Microporosity
    in bioinert ceramics, 71–72
    biphasic calcium, 104–106
    biphasic calcium phosphates, *in vivo* testing of, 109–113
    of calcium phosphates, 44–45

Microstructure analysis
    functionally-graded ceramic hip implants
        defect analysis, 348–351
        grain size analysis, 346–348
        sintering and evaluation of, 344–351
    improvement in bioceramics, 113–114
    ionomer glass crystallization, 423–427
    silicon carbide-based ceramic biomaterials
        mechanical optimization, 381–385
        medical device applications, 363–365
    titanium-niobium-zirconium-tantalum alloys, 287–290

Microwave processing, ceramic biomaterials, 253

Mimetic monolayers
    air/water and air/solid properties, 665–667
    air/water interfacial properties, 668
    blood cell adhesion studies, 674
    calcification studies, 673
    dense thin solid films, 664
    deposition optimization, 670–671
    future research issues, 675
    heterogeneous lipid compounds, 667–668
    macromolecule incorporation, 668–669
    overview, 664
    platelet adhesion and activation, 674
    protein interaction studies, 673–674
    surface modification, 664–672
        biological interactions, 672
        supported thin solid films, 671–672

Mineral apatites, simultaneous fluoride/carbonate incorporation, 33–34

Minimally invasive surgery (MIS)
    biphasic calcium phosphate and, 102–103
        macroporous cements, 114–115
    injectable bioceramics, BCP granules and polymers, 125–127
    injectable bone substitute, radiopacity improvements in, 115–118
    injectable hydrogels, photopolymerization and, 188–191

Minimum Inhibitory Concentration (MIC), biphasic calcium phosphate granules, 128–129

Monomers, macroporous gels
    biomedical applications, 523–525
    freezing rate and temperature, 505–508
    precursor gel composition, 508–512

Morphological compatibility
    titanium boride reinforced titanium-niobium-zirconium-tantalum metal-matrix composites, tribological behavior, 313–317
    titanium dental implants, 153–157
    titanium-niobium-zirconium-tantalum alloys, 290–296

MTT assay
    medical device biocompatibility, cytotoxicity testing, 397–398
    in vitro biocompatibility testing, 13

Mullite composites
    ionomer glasses, crystallization properties, 423–427
    orthopedic applications, overview, 54–56
    processes and properties of, 63–64

Multi-phased scaffold design, orthopedic tissue engineering, 599–603

Multiphasic calcium phosphate cement (MCPC), macroporous structure, 115

Multi-tissue matrix organization
    ligament-to-bone insertion, tissue engineering, 591–593
    structure-function relationships, 596–599

µCTanalySIS softwarae, macroporous gels, pore structure analysis, 520–521

Muscle-derived stem cells (MDSCs), tissue engineering scaffolds, skeletal muscle tissue, 475

Musculoskeletal system
nanofibrous scaffold tissue engineering in, 466–480
bone, 466–471
cartilage, 471–474
ligaments and tendons, 476–479
skeletal muscle, 474–476
orthopedic tissue engineering
design criteria, 590–593
future reserach issues, 603
heterotypic cellular interactions, 593–596
multi-phase scaffold design, 599–603
overview, 589–590
structure-function relationship, 596–599

Myofibrils, tissue engineering scaffolds, skeletal muscle tissue, 475

N

Nanomaterials
calcium phosphate materials, 91
cell-based nanocomposites
bone tissue engineering, 549
adipose-derived stem cells, 574–575
bioceramics, 559–560
bone marrow-derived stem cells, 575–576
cell-material constructs, 566–570
current grafts and graft substitutes, 553–554
gene-based materials, 572–573
mesenchymal stem cells, 576–577
nanofibrous composites, 565–566
nano-HA/collagen composites, 561–565
peptide-based materials, 570–572
polymers, 560–561
regeneration factors, 554–558
current research issues, 577–578
historical development of, 552–553
tissue engineering technology, 554
of hydroxyapatite, in hard tissue, 58–59
hydroxyapatite-zirconium composites, 63

nanofibrous scaffolds, tissue engineering
cell-based nanocomposites, 565–566
future research issues, 479–480
musculoskeletal system, 466–479
bone, 466–471
cartilage, 471–474
ligaments and tendons, 476–479
skeletal muscle, 474–476
overview, 438–442
polymer structures, 453–465
blended polymers, 462–465
natural polymers, 453–459
synthetic polymers, 459–462
synthesis techniques, 442–453
electrospinning, 446–453
phase separation, 444–446
self assembly, 443–444
orthopedic and tissue engineering
applications, 211–231
ceramics, 213–220
chemical processing, 228–231
composites, 226–228
future research issues, 231–233
metals, 220–223
osteolysis prevention, 211–212
polymers, 223–226
overivew of, 206–207

Nanometer scaling, tissue engineering scaffolds, 442

Natural polymers
cell-based nanocomposites, 560
injectable hydrogels
photo-gelling system, 184–185
photopolymerization, 190–191
thermogelling polymers, 194–197
macroporous gels, 523–525
nanofibrous scaffolds, tissue engineering, 453–459
blended polymers, 463–465
carbohydrates, 456–459
proteins, 454–456

N. clavipes silk fibrin, nanofibrous scaffolds from, 456

Nd:YAG laser, Laser Engineered Net Shaping (LENS®) processing technique, orthopedic biomaterials, 283–285

Near net shape (NNS) forming, titanium dental implants, 163–167

Nernst-Noves-Whitney equation, silicon
     carbide-based ceramic
     biomaterials, diffusion
     mechanisms, 372–374
Nervous system cells
   central nervous system damage and
        repair, 620–621
   electrical stimulation, 621–629
     cellular response *in vitro,* 628–629
     central nervous system, therapeutic
          stimulation, 624–625
     DC electric fields *(in vivo),* 623–624
     electromagnetic stimulation *(in vivo),*
          624
     extracellular stimulation *(in vitro),*
          625–628
     physiological endogenous electric
          fields, 622–623
   future research issues, 634
   neural progenitor cells, 616–620
     applications, 619–620
     in brain, 617–618
     electric fields, 633–634
     fate identification, 618–619
     postnatal neurogenesis, 616–617
   neurons in electric fields, 629–633
     axon guidance, 629–630
     calcium, 633
     cellular-level changes, 630–631
     receptor accumulation and
          autoregulation, 631–633
   overview, 614
   structure and classification, 614–615
Neural progenitor cells (NPCs), 547–548,
     616–620
   applications, 619–620
   in brain, 617–618
   electric fields, 633–634
   fate identification, 618–619
   postnatal neurogenesis, 616–617
Neurons, in electric field, 629–633
   axon guidance, 629–630
   calcium, 633
   cellular-level changes, 630–631
   receptor accumulation and
        autoregulation, 631–633
Neutrophil priming and activation,
     titanium dental implants,
     149–151

Nickel-based alloys
   metallic coating composites, 87–90
   processing and properties, 85–86
Niobium alloys
   LENS-deposited titanium-niobium-
        zirconium-tantalum alloys,
        passive oxide films, 299–302
   metal alloy corrosion, 82–83
   metallic coating composites, 87–90
   titanium-niobium-zirconium-tantalum
        alloys, laser processing of,
        286–304
     characterization methods, 286–287
     corrosion resistance, 296–298
     deformation mechanisms, 290–296
     microstructure and mechanical
          properties, 287–290
     in vitro testing, 302–304
     x-ray photoelectron spectroscopy of,
          298–302
Nitric acid, silicon carbide-based ceramic
     biomaterials, medical device
     applications, 363–365
Non-bridging oxygen (NBO)
   bioactive glasses, 386–387, 392–396
   ionomer glasses
     formation, 416
     solid state MAS-NMR analysis,
          419–422
     structural analysis, 417–422
Non-collagenous proteins, in bone, 554
Non-ferrous metal alloys, properties of, 86
Non-frozen liquid microphase (NFLMP)
   cryogelation process, 502–504
   macroporous gels
     freezing rate and temperature, 504–508
     precursor gel composition, 508–512
Non-mesenchymal stem cell-material
     constructs, 569–570
Non-unions
   bone grafts and, 553–554
   as fracture complication, 212
Notch signaling, bone regeneration, 558
Nucleation-growth kinetics model,
     mica-based glass ceramics
     treatment, 67–68
Nucleation temperatures
   ionomer glass crystallization, 424–427
   polymer cryogelation, 504–508

O

Octacalcium phosphate (OCP), 38
 biphasic calcium phosphate formation
  and, 108–113
 processing and properties, 59–62
Oligodendrocytes, structure and function,
  615
Opthalmologic applications, biomaterials,
  541–542
Optical microscopy (OM), macroporous
  gels, pore structure, 519–521
Organelles, cell-material interactions in,
  8–11
Orientation imaging microscopy (OM),
  titanium-niobium-zirconium-
  tantalum alloys, 290–296
Orthopedic biomaterials
 biphasic calcium phosphate ceramics,
  130–132
  anterior cervical fusion, 131
  cervical spine arthrodesis, 131
  high tibial valgisation osteotomy,
   131–132
 bone/implant interface, 549
 implant problems and failures, 207–212
  loosening, 208–210
  osteolysis, 210–212
  wear and fractures, 212
 Laser Engineered Net Shaping
  (LENS®) processing technique,
  282–285
 nanomaterials, 212–231
  ceramics, 213–220
  chemical processing, 228–231
  composites, 226–228
  future research issues, 231–233
  metals, 220–223
  polymers, 223–226
 overview, 54, 538–539
 tissue engineering, musculoskeletal
  system interface
  design criteria, 590–593
  future reserach issues, 603
  heterotypic cellular interactions,
   593–596
  multi-phase scaffold design, 599–603
  overview, 589–590
  structure-function relationship,
   596–599

Osseointegration
 dental implants, 539–541
 implant loosening and, 208–210
 nanostructured polymers, 223–226
 titanium dental implants, 157–163
  biomechanical bonding, 164–167
Osteoblast-hydroxyapatite composite
 nano-HA/collagen-based composites,
  562–565
 testing of, 60–61
Osteoblast interactions, on bioinert
  ceramics, 70–72
Osteoblasts
 nanofibrous scaffold tissue engineering
  and, 466
 nanostructured metals and morphology
  of, 222–223
 osteolysis prevention, 211–212
 titanium dental implants, bone-implant
  interface, 161–163
Osteocalcin, cell-based nanocomposites,
  mesenchymal stem cells, 567–569
Osteoclast-like cell functions,
  nanostructured ceramics, 215–220
Osteoclasts, nanofibrous scaffold tissue
  engineering and, 466
Osteoconductive properties
 of calcium phosphates, 44–45
 hydroxyapatites, ceramic coatings, 385
 nanofibrous scaffold tissue engineering,
  467
 nanostructured ceramics, 215–220
Osteocytes, nanofibrous scaffold tissue
  engineering and, 466
Osteogenesis
 regeneration factors, 554–558
 stem cell sources for, 574–577
Osteogenesis imperfecta (OI), incidence
  and prevalence, 552
Osteogenic properties
 biphasic calcium, 107–113
 biphasic calcium phosphates, in vivo
  testing of, 111–113
 nanofibrous scaffold tissue engineering,
  467
Osteoinduction, nanofibrous scaffold
  tissue engineering, 467
Osteolysis, orthopedic implants and,
  210–212

Osteopontin gene, bone regeneration, 558

Osteoprogenitor cells, bone grafts, 553–554

Osteosynthesis, biphasic calcium phosphate resorption, 118–120

Outer cell mimetic lipic composition (OCMC), basic properties, 667–668

Oxidation, titanium dental implants, 147–151

Oxide layering, titanium boride reinforced titanium-niobium-zirconium-tantalum metal-matrix composites, tribological behavior, 312–317

Oxide stoichiometry, titanium dental implants, 148–151

Oxygen triangle, carbonate apatite structure, 30–33

P

Paget's disease of bone, incidence and prevalence, 552

Particle-reinforced biocomposites, processing of, 256

Particulate debris, orthopedic implants, 210–212

Passivation parameters, metal alloy corrosion, 82–83

Passive oxide films, titanium-niobium-zirconium-tantalum alloys, LENS-deposited processing, 298–302

PEEK cage, anterior cervical fusion, biphasic calcium phosphate ceramics, 131

PEMF stimulation, central nervous system, 624–625

Peptides
cell-based nanocomposites, 570–572
injectable hydrogels, photo-gelling system, 185
peptide-amphiphiles, nanofibrous scaffold self-assembly, 443–444

Perfluorocarbons, blood substitutes, 647–648

Peripheral nervous system (PNS), damage and repair, 620–621

Phase distribution, silicon carbide-based ceramic biomaterials, medical device applications, 365–370

Phase separation, nanofibrous scaffold fabrication, 444–446

Phosphate buffer saline (PBS), *in vitro* biocompatibility testing with, 13

Phosphates
apatite incorporation of, anion substituions, 34
bone regeneration factors, 555–558
ionomer glass structure, 417–422

Phosphorus-containing ionomer glasses, structural analysis, 417–422

Photo-gelling polymers, injectable hydrogels, 183–191
side group photoactivation, 184–185

Photo initiators, injectable hydrogels, photopolymerization and, 185–191

Photolithography, nanomaterials, electrochemical processing, 229–231

Photopolymerization, injectable hydrogels, 183, 185–191

pH values, cell-material interactions, 8–11

Physically cross-linked macroporous gels, 512–515

Physiological endogenous electric fields, nervous system electrical stimulation, 622–623

Pin-on-wheel testing, cardiovascular medical device coatings, 691–692

Placental umbilical cord blood, 549
clinical experience and safety studies, 651–656
future research issues, 658–659
global research and development, 644–648
medical applications, 649–650
overview, 644
placental wastage and content, 648–649
properties of, 656–658
room temperature and time stability, 650–651

Plasma-assisted chemical vapor deposition (PACVD), diamond-like carbon coatings, cardiovascular medical devices, 686–687

Plasma-enhanced chemical vapor
deposition (PECVD), diamond-
like carbon coatings,
cardiovascular medical devices,
687
Plasmid DNA, injectable hydrogels,
photopolymerization, 189–191
Platelet adhesion studies, thin solid films,
674
PL DLLA polymers, resorbable
osteosynthesis, 118–120
Pluoronics, injectable hydrogels,
thermogelling polymers,
193–197
Poiseuille's law, silicon carbide-based
ceramic biomaterials, reaction-
formation mechanisms,
371–374
Poisson's equation, electric field
calculations, 340
Poly (*N*-isopropylacrylamide), drug
delivery systems, 544–545
Poly-2-hydroxyethyl methacrylate
(pHEMA)
macroporous gels, 522–525
nanostructured injectable hydrogels,
225–226
Polyacrylamide, macroporous gels
freezing rate and temperature, 505–508
precursor gel composition, 508–512
Polyacrylic acid, ionomer cements,
413–414
Poly(α-hydroxy) esters, nanofibrous
scaffolds, tissue engineering,
459–461
Polyalkenoate cements
cation substitution, 427–428
composition, 414–415
crystallization, 423–427
design, 415–416
future research issues, 429
overview, 411–414
structure, 417–422
solid state MAS-NMR spectroscopy
characterization, 418–422
Polycaprolactone (PCL)
cell-based nanocomposites, 560–561
mesenchymal stem cells, 567–569
nanofibrous composites, 565–566

nanofibrous scaffolds, tissue
engineering, 461
bone tissue, 469
cartilage regeneration, 474
Poly DL lactide co-glycolide (PDLG),
resorbable osteosynthesis,
biphasic calcium phosphates,
119–120
Polyesters, nanofibrous scaffolds, tissue
engineering, 462
Poly(ester urethane) urea (PEUU),
nanofibrous scaffolds, ligaments
and tendons tissue engineering,
478–479
Polyethylene (PE) biocomposites,
orthopedic applications,
overview, 55
Polyethylene glycols (PEG)
bone regeneration factors, 555–558
drug delivery systems, 544–545
injectable hydrogels
development of, 181–182
photopolymerization and, 186–191
side group photoactivation, 184–185
thermogelling polymers, 193–197
nanofibrous scaffold fabrication, bone
tissue engineering, 470–471
Polyethylene oxide (PEO), nanofibrous
scaffolds, tissue engineering
alginate incorporation, 458
blended polymers, 463–465
Polyglycolic acid (PGA)
cell-based nanocomposites, 560–561
peptide-based nanomaterials, 570–572
nanofibrous scaffolds, tissue
engineering, 460
nanostructured polymers, 223–226
PolyHeme, 647–648
Polylactic acid (PLA)
cell-based nanocomposites, 560–561
nano-HA/collagen-based composites,
564–565
nanofibrous scaffolds, tissue engineering
bone tissue, 470–471
PLGA-polyethylene glycol blend,
463–465
nanostructured polymers, 223–226
nanofibrous scaffolds, tissue
engineering, 460

Poly(lactic-co-glycolic acid) (PLGA)
cell-based nanocomposites, 560–561
bone marrow-derived stem cells,
575–576
mesenchymal stem cells, 567–569
nano-HA/collagen-based composites,
561–565
drug delivery systems, 544–545
nanofibrous scaffolds, 460–461
cartilage regeneration, 473–474
fabrication
ligaments and tendons tissue
engineering, 478–479
skeletal muscle tissue, 475–476
polyethylene glycol-polylactic acid
blend, 463–465
nanostructured polymers, 223–226
Poly lactide acid (PLLA)
bone tissue engineering, nanostructured
biodegradable polymers, 224–225
cell-based nanocomposites, 560–561
nanofibrous composites, 565–566
non-mesenchymal stem cell-material
constructs, 569–570
nanofibrous scaffold fabrication,
445–446
bone tissue engineering, 470–471
skeletal muscle tissue, 475–476
peptide-based nanomaterials, 572
resorbable osteosynthesis, biphasic
calcium phosphates, 119–120
Poly(lactide-co-glycolide)/nano-
hydroxyapatite (PLGA/NHA)
scaffolds
gene-based nanomaterials, 573
phase separation fabrication, 445–446
Poly-L-lysine (PLL), neurons in electric
field, 629–630
Poly L-ornithine (PLO), neurons in
electric field, 629–630
Polymers
cell-based nanocomposites, 560–561
ceramic composites, 74–79
cryogelation, 504–512
freezing rate and temperature,
504–508
precursor concentration and
composition, 508–512
dental implants, 539–541

drug delivery systems, 544–545
future research issues, 91–92
hydroxyapatite biomaterials and, 43–45
injectable hydrogels
fast chemical reaction/physical
transitions, 191–193
overview and basic principles, 180–182
photo-gelling polymers, 183–191
in situ forming gels, 182–197
thermogelling polymers, 193–197
mechanical properties, 73
nanostructured polymers, 223–226
biodegradable polymers, 223–225
composites, 226–228
injectable hydrogels, 225–226
nanofibrous scaffolds, tissue
engineering, 453–465
blended polymers, 462–465
electrospinning fabrication
technique, 446–453
natural polymers, 453–459
phase separation fabrication,
444–445
synthetic polymers, 459–462
orthopedic applications, overview,
56–57
polymer-polymer composites, 73–74
processing and properties, 72–79,
254–255
surface modification of, 262–268
Polymethylmethacrylate (PMMA)
nanostructured polymers, 223–226
ophthalmologic implants, 541–542
outer cell mimetic lipic composition
(OCMC), 668
Polymorphonuclear leukocytes, titanium
dental implants, 147–151
Poly-N-isopropylacrylamide (pNiPAAm)
injectable hydrogels, thermogelling
polymers, 194–197
macroporous gels, "smart" properties of,
511–512
pore volume, 516–518
Poly(propylene fumarate) (PPF),
nanostructured composites, 228
Poly-SFH, 647–648
Polyurethanes (PU)
carbonate nanostructured composites,
228

nanofibrous scaffolds, tissue engineering, 461–462
Polyvinyl alcohol (PVA), macroporous gels
  physically cross-linked compounds, 512–515
  precursor gel composition, 508–512
Polyvinyl butyral (PVB), bone tissue engineering, 559–560
Polyvinyl pyrrolidone (PVP), bone tissue engineering, 560
Pore volume, macroporous gels, 516–518
  microscopic analysis, 518–521
Porites, in biomaterials, 42
Porosity testing
  cell-based nanocomposites, mesenchymal stem cells, 567–569
  macroporous gels, 518–521
    tissue engineering and, 524–525
  nanofibrous scaffold tissue engineering, bone tissue, 468–469
  silicon carbide-based ceramic biomaterials, 376–381
Porous ceramics
  medical device applications, 359–360
  silicon carbide-based ceramic biomaterials, mechanical optimization, 381–384
Postnatal neurogenesis, neural progenitor cells, 616–617
Potassium channels, nervous system electrical stimulation, 623
Powder-feeder system, Laser Engineered Net Shaping (LENS®) processing technique, 283–285
Powder metallurgy, hydroxyapatite-titanium composites, 65–66
Powder preparation, formation and sintering, ceramic biomaterials processing, 251–252
Precipitation techniques, carbonate apatite nano-crystals, 29–33
Precursor gel composition, macroporous gels, 508–512
Protein interaction studies
  cardiovascular medical device hemocompatibility, adsorption mechanisms, 681–682
  thin solid films, 672–674

Protein kinase C-dependent kinase (PKA), neurons in electric field, 633
Proteins
  adsorption
    cell-material interactions and, 10–11
    titanium dental implants, 157–163
  injectable hydrogels, photopolymerization and delivery kinetics, 189–191
  nanofibrous composites, 565–566
  nanofibrous scaffolds, 454–456
PTC/Chol compositions, deposition optimization, 670–671
Pulsed laser deposition, bioactive coatings, 387–389
  physico-chemical properties, 392–396
Pulse electromagnetic fields (PEMF), hydroxyapatite implant analysis with, 61

Q
Quadrupolar coupling interactions, ionomer glass structure, 418–422
Quaternized chitosan derivatives, nanofibrous scaffolds, tissue engineering, 458–459

R
Radiopaque agents (RAs)
  bioactive injectable bone substitutes, 115–118
  ionomer glass cation substitution, 427–428
Raw materials processing, metal biomaterials, 250
Reaction bonded silicon carbide, mechanical optimization, 382–384
Reaction-formation mechanisms, silicon carbide-based ceramic biomaterials, 370–374
Reaction formed silicon carbide, mechanical optimization, 383–384
Real time neutron diffraction studies, ionomer glass crystallization, 425–427
Receptor accumulation and autoregulation, neurons in electric field, 631–633

Receptor mediated signaling, tissue
    engineering scaffolds, 442
Recombinant hemoglobin, 646–648
Recombinant human bone morphogenetic
    protein (rhBMP). *See* Bone
    morphogenetic proteins
Red blood cells (RBCs), substitutes for,
    645–648
Redox reagents, injectable hydrogels, fast
    chemical reaction/physical
    transitions, 191–193
Regeneration factors, bone tissue,
    554–558
Release testing, silicon carbide-based
    ceramic biomaterials, 370
Repair strategies, central nervous system,
    621
Repetitive freeze-thawing technique,
    macroporous gels, physically
    cross-linked compounds, 514–515
Resorbable osteosynthesis, biphasic
    calcium phosphate, 118–120
Resorption pitting, nanostructured
    ceramics, 215–220
Revision surgery, statistics on, 207
RGD cell binding domain
    nanofibrous scaffolds, 455
    nanomaterials processing, 229–231
    peptide-based nanomaterials, 572
Rho A-Rock signaling pathway,
    mesenchymal stem cell-material
    constructs, 568–569
Rietvelt X-ray structure analysis, of
    carbonate apatite, 32–33
Rotating mandrel device, nanofibrous
    scaffolds, electrospinning
    fabrication, 450–453
RUNX-2 gene expression, bone
    regeneration, 558
Runx-2 protein, nanofibrous composites,
    565–566

S
Safety issues, placental umbilical cord
    blood, 652–656
Saliva composition, titanium dental
    implants, 147–151
Sap channels, micron-size silicon carbide-
    based ceramic biomaterials,

        phase and element distribution,
            367–370
Scaffold materials. *See also* Cell-based
        nanocomposites
    biphasic calcium phosphates
        bone tissue engineering, 120–124
        growth plate chondrocyte maturation,
            125
        mesenchymal stem cells, 124–125
    calcium phosphates for, 43–45
    injectable hydrogels,
        photopolymerization and,
            188–191
    macroporous gels
        biomedical applications, 522–525
        covalently cross-linked MGs, 515–516
        future research, 525
        microscopic porous structure
            characterization, 518–521
        overview, 500–502
        physically cross-liked MGs, 513–515
        pore volume, 516–518
    nanofibrous scaffolds
        future research issues, 479–480
        musculoskeletal system, 466–479
            bone, 466–471
            cartilage, 471–474
            ligaments and tendons, 476–479
            skeletal muscle, 474–476
        overview, 438–442
        polymer structures, 453–465
            blended polymers, 462–465
            natural polymers, 453–459
            synthetic polymers, 459–462
        synthesis techniques, 442–453
            electrospinning, 446–453
            phase separation, 444–446
            self assembly, 443–444
    orthopedic tissue engineering
        design criteria, 592–593
        multi-phased scaffold design,
            599–603
        structure-function relationships,
            596–599
    polymer processing for, 255
Scale processing, biomaterials, 260–269
    micro/nano fabrication, 268–269
    micro/nano surface modification,
        260–268

Scanning electron microscopy (SEM)
  bioactive coatings, physico-chemical
    properties, 395–396
  macroporous gels
    freezing rate and temperature,
      507–508
    pore structure, 519–521
  nanofibrous scaffolds, electrospinning
    fabrication, 449–450
  osteoblast-hydroxyapatite composite,
    60–61
  titanium boride reinforced titanium-
    niobium-zirconium-tantalum
    metal-matrix composites, 306–309
Scratch test conditions, cardiovascular
  medical device coatings, 692–694
Sealants, fibrin glues, biphasic calcium
  phosphate composites, 127
Selected area diffraction (SAD), titanium-
  niobium-zirconium-tantalum
  alloys, 287–290, 292–296
Self-assembly techniques
  nanofibrous scaffold fabrication,
    443–444
  nano-HA/collagen-based composites,
    561–565
Self-hardening injectable-mouldable
  composite, injectable BCP
  bioceramic granules and
  polymers, 126–127
Self-propagating high temperature
  combustion synthesis (SHS),
  cell-based nanocomposites,
  non-mesenchymal stem cell-
  material constructs, 569–570
Sensitization, *in vivo* biocompatibility
  testing, 14–15
Severe combined immunodeficient (SCID)
  mice, gene-based nanomaterials,
  573
Shape-memory alloys, overview, 546
Signal selection, nervous system electrical
  stimulation, 626–627
Silica nanomaterials, nanofibrous scaffolds
  for bone tissue engineering,
  470–471
Silicon, ophthalmologic implants, 542
Silicon carbide (SiC) synthesis
  bioinert ceramics, 72

ceramic biomaterials, medical device
  applications, 360–365
Silicon-nitrogen bioglass composites,
  69–70
Silicon-substituted hydroxyapatite (SiHA)
  coatings, non-mesenchymal stem
  cell-material constructs, 569–570
Silk fibroin
  cell-based nanocomposites, 560
  nanofibrous scaffolds from, 456
    bone tissue engineering, 468–469
Siloxanes, titanium dental implants,
  bone-implant interface, 161–163
Simulated biologic fluid (SBF)
  bioinert ceramic testing in, 71–72
  carbonate apatite bioactivity testing,
    43–45
  high-density polyethylene-
    hydroxyapatite-aluminum oxide
    hybride composites, 77–79
  metallic coating composites, 86–90
  silicon carbide-based ceramic
    biomaterials, 370
  titanium dental implants, integrated
    implant systems, 164–167
  titanium-niobium-zirconium-tantalum
    alloys, LENS-deposited
    processing, 297–298
Single-walled carbon nanotubes (SWNTs),
  nanostructured composites, 228
Sintering techniques, functionally-graded
  ceramic hip implants
  controlled disc processing, 336–337
  microstructural evaluation, 344–351
Sinus lift augmentation, biphasic calcium
  phosphate ceramics, dental
  applications, 130
Skeletal muscle, nanofibrous scaffolds,
  tissue engineering, 474–476
Smad protein, bone regeneration, 557–558
Small angle neutron scattering (SANS),
  ionomer glass crystallization,
  425–427
Smurf protein, bone regeneration, 557–558
Soda lime silica glass microstructure, 424
Sodium channels, nervous system electrical
  stimulation, 623
Sodium-potassium-ATPase pump, nervous
  system electrical stimulation, 623

Soft tissue replacement. *See also*
    Ligaments; Tendons
  orthopedic tissue engineering,
      multi-phased scaffold design,
      600–603
  polymer biomaterials, 72–79
Sol-gel process, bioactive glasses, 387
Solid freeform fabrication (SFF), ceramic
      biomaterials, 253
Solid state magic angle sping nuclear
      magnetic resonance (MAS-NMR)
      studies, ionomer glass structure,
      418–422
  crystallization mechanisms, 424–427
Solubility
  of apatites, 26–27
  carbonate apatites, 30–33
  silicon carbide-based ceramic
      biomaterials, 372–374
Solution parameters, electrospinning for
      nanofibrous scaffold fabrication,
      448
Solution viscosity, electrospinning for
      nanofibrous scaffold fabrication,
      448
Spark Plasma Sintering (SPS),
      hydroxyapatite-titanium
      composites, 64–66
Stability
  cord blood, 648–651
  heterogeneous phospholipids/glycolipid/
      cholesterol ternary lipid
      composition, 667–668
  titanium dental implants, 146–151
Staphylococcus epidermidis,
      nanostructured ceramics and,
      216–217
Steel, corrosion of, 81–83
Stem cells (SCs)
  adipose-derived stem cells, 574–575
  mesenchymal stem cells
    biphasic calcium phosphate scaffolds,
      124–125
    bone regeneration factors,
      555–558
    cell-material constructs, 566–569
    injectable hydrogels,
      photopolymerization and,
      187–191

micro-macroporous biphasic calcium
      phosphate scaffolds, bone tissue
      engineering, 123–124
  nanofibrous scaffolds, 445–446
    bone tissue engineering, 467–468
    cartilage regeneration, 472
    ligaments and tendons tissue
      engineering, 477–479
  muscle-derived stem cells, tissue
      engineering scaffolds, 475
  neural progenitor cells, 619–620
  non-mesenchymal stem cells, 569–570
  osteogenic differentiation, 574–577
  placental umbilical cord blood
      transfusion, 655–658
Stent biomaterials, drug delivery systems,
      544–545
Sterilization, biomaterials processing,
      260–261
Strain hardening, titanium dental implants,
      bone-implant interface,
      162–163
Strength-grain size relationship,
      functionally-graded ceramic hip
      implants, 346–348
Stress distribution, titanium dental implant
      mechanics, 152–153
Stress-strain field
  titanium dental implant mechanics,
      152–153
  titanium-niobium-zirconium-tantalum
      alloys, 287–290
Stroma-free hemoglobin, 646–648
Strontium
  apatite incorporation of, 34
  ionomer glass cation substitution,
      427–428
Structure-function relationships,
      orthopedic tissue engineering,
      596–599
Subgranular zone (SGZ), neural
      progenitor cells, 617–618
Subperiosteal implants, 540–541
Substrate materials
  diamond-like carbon coatings,
      cardiovascular medical devices,
      687
  titanium nitride, cardiovascular medical
      devices, 688

Subventricular zone (SVA), neural
     progenitor cells, 617–618
Supermacroporous biomaterials,
     cryogelation
  macroporous gels
    biomedical applications, 522–525
    covalently cross-linked MGs,
      515–516
    future research, 525
    microscopic porous structure
      characterization, 518–521
    physically cross-liked MGs, 513–515
    pore volume, 516–518
  overview, 500–502
  polymeric cryostructuration, 502–512
    freezing rate and temperature,
      504–508
    precursor concentration and
      composition, 508–512
    processing techniques, 502–504
Supramolecular properties, nanofibrous
     scaffolds, electrospinning
     fabrication, 451–453
Surface adhesion molecules, neurons in
     electric field, 629–630
Surface microstructure
  biphasic calcium, 108–113
  implant loosening and, 209–210
  nanostructured metals, 220–223
  silicon carbide-based ceramic
     biomaterials, reaction-formation
     mechanisms, 371–374
  titanium dental implants
    biocompatibiility and, 149–151
    integrated implant systems, 163–167
    morphological compatibility, 154–157
Surface modification
  biomaterials
    micro/nano surface modification,
      260–268
    surface chemistry, 262–264
    surface topography, 264–268
    tissue interactions, 260, 262
    ceramic biomaterials processing,
      252–253
    composite biomaterials, 260
    implant loosening and, 209–210
    metal biomaterials processing, 250–251
    mimetic monolayers, 664–672

    air/water and air/solid properties,
      665–667
    air/water interfacial properties, 668
    biological interactions, 672
    blood cell adhesion studies, 674
    calcification studies, 673
    dense thin solid films, 664
    deposition optimization, 670–671
    future research issues, 675
    heterogeneous lipid compounds,
      667–668
    macromolecule incorporation,
      668–669
    overview, 664
    platelet adhesion and activation, 674
    protein interaction studies, 673–674
    supported thin solid films, 671–672
  polymer processing, 255
  titanium dental implants, integrated
     implant systems, 163–167
Surface roughness
  cardiovascular medical device coatings,
     688–689
  nanomaterials, ceramics, 213–220
  nanostructured metals, 221–223
  titanium dental implants, 153–157
    bone-implant interface, 159–163
Surface tension, electrospinning for
     nanofibrous scaffold fabrication,
     448
Surface wettability, nanostructured
     ceramics, 213–220
Suspension materials, injectable BCP
     bioceramic granules and
     polymers, 125–126
Swelling ratios, poly-N-
     isopropylacrylamide MGs
     (pNIPAAm-MGs), 511–512
Synthetic biomaterials
  apatites and calcium phosphates, 21–23
  biocompatibility of, 7
  carbonate apatites, 27–33
  polymers
    cell-based nanocomposites, 560–561
    nanofibrous scaffolds, tissue
      engineering, 459–465, 469–471
System parameters, electrospinning for
     nanofibrous scaffold fabrication,
     448–449

T

Tantalum alloys, titanium-niobium-
        zirconium-tantalum alloys
    laser processing of, 286–304
        characterization methods, 286–287
        corrosion resistance, 296–298
        deformation mechanisms, 290–296
        microstructure and mechanical
            properties, 287–290
        in vitro testing, 302–304
        x-ray photoelectron spectroscopy of,
            298–302
        LENS-deposited passive oxide films,
            299–302
Tantalum-based alloys, processing and
        properties, 85–86
Tartrate-resistant acid phosphatase
        (TRAP), nanostructured
        ceramics, 215–220
Taylor cone, electrospinning for
        nanofibrous scaffold fabrication,
        447–453
    needle diameter, 448–449
Teeth
    glass-ceramic biomaterials for, 66–70
    mica-based glass ceramics, 66–68
    structure and properties, 57–59
Temperature stability, cord blood,
        648–651
Tendons, tissue engineering
    interface design, 590–593
    nanofibrous scaffolds, 476–479
TERT subunit, adipose-derived stem cells,
        574–577
Tetracalcium phosphates (TTCP), 39
    processing and properties, 59–62
Tetragonal zirconia polycrystal ceramics
        (TZP)
    hip implants, 327–328
    nanostructured ceramics, 218–220
    processing and properties, 70–72
Tetrahydrofuran (THF), nanofibrous
        scaffold fabrication, 445–446
N,N,N′,N′-Tetra-methyl-ethylenediamine
        (TEMED), covalently cross-
        linked macroporous gels, 515–516
Thermally-induced phase separation
        (TIPS), nanofibrous scaffold
        fabrication, 445–446

Thermal stability, of apatites, 26–27
Thermogelling polymers, injectable
        hydrogels, 193–197
Thermogravimetric analysis, silicon
        carbide-based ceramic
        biomaterials, medical device
        applications, 362–365
Thermoplastics, biomaterials processing
        and properties, 72–79
Thermosets, biomaterials processing and
        properties, 72–79
Thin solid films (TSFs)
    air/water and air/solid properties,
        665–667
    air/water interfacial properties, 668
    blood cell adhesion studies, 674
    calcification studies, 673
    dense thin solid films, 664
    deposition optimization, 670–671
    future research issues, 675
    heterogeneous lipid compounds,
        667–668
    macromolecule incorporation, 668–669
    overview, 664
    platelet adhesion and activation, 674
    protein interaction studies, 673–674
    surface modification, 664–672
        biological interactions, 672
        supported thin solid films, 671–672
Thiol-based systems, injectable hydrogels,
        photopolymerization, 191
Three-dimensionality, tissue engineering
        scaffolds, 440–442
Thrombogenesis, nanostructured metals
        and risk of, 223
Tisseel/TricOs composite, fibrin glues,
        biphasic calcium phosphate
        composites, 127
Tissue compatibility, cardiovascular
        medical device coatings, 699–700
Tissue culture polystyrene (TCPS),
        nanofibrous scaffolds, tissue
        engineering, cartilage
        regeneration, 474
Tissue engineering
    benefits and limitations of, 438–439
    biological fixation, 549
    biomaterials for, 545–546
    bone

biphasic calcium phosphate scaffolds, 120–124

cell-based nanocomposites, 549
adipose-derived stem cells, 574–575
bioceramics, 559–560
bone marrow-derived stem cells, 575–576
cell-material constructs, 566–570
current grafts and graft substitutes, 553–554
gene-based materials, 572–573
mesenchymal stem cells, 576–577
nanofibrous composites, 565–566
nano-HA/collagen composites, 561–565
peptide-based materials, 570–572
polymers, 560–561
regeneration factors, 554–558

ceramic biomaterials, medical device applications, 359–360

injectable hydrogels, photopolymerization and, 188–191

macroporous gels, 522–525

nanofibrous scaffolds
future research issues, 479–480
musculoskeletal system, 466–479
bone, 466–471
cartilage, 471–474
ligaments and tendons, 476–479
skeletal muscle, 474–476
overview, 438–442, 549
polymer structures, 453–465
blended polymers, 462–465
natural polymers, 453–459
synthetic polymers, 459–462
synthesis techniques, 442–453
electrospinning, 446–453
phase separation, 444–446
self assembly, 443–444

nanomaterials, 212–231
ceramics, 213–220
chemical processing, 228–231
composites, 226–228
future research issues, 231–233
metals, 220–223
polymers, 223–226

orthopedic biomaterials, musculoskeletal system interface

design criteria, 590–593
future reserach issues, 603
heterotypic cellular interactions, 593–596
multi-phase scaffold design, 599–603
overview, 589–590
structure-function relationship, 596–599

overview, 545–546

scale processing of biomaterials, 260, 262

Titanium and titanium alloys
cardiovascular medical devices, 684
cell interactions with, 83–84
non-mesenchymal stem cell-material constructs, 569–570
corrosion properties, 82–83
dental implants
basic requirements, 146–157
biocompatibility, 146–151
integrated implant system, 163–167
mechanical compatibility, 151–153
metal alloys, 84
morphological compatibility, 153–157
osseointegration and bone/implant interface, 157–163
overview, 144–146
interdisciplinary research on, 145–146
metallic coating composites, 87–90
nanomaterials
ceramics, 213–220
electrochemical processing, 229–231
metals, 220–223
niobium alloys, corrosion properties, 82–83
orthopedic biomaterials processing, hip implants, 285–286
oxide bioinert ceramics, 70–72
titanium boride reinforced titanium-niobium-zirconium-tantalum matrix metal composites, 304–318
LENS deposition, 305–309
tribological behavior, 309–317
wear resistance, 304–305
titanium-niobium-zirconium-tantalum alloys
femoral head implants, 285–286
future research issues, 318–319
laser processing of, 286–304

Titanium and titanium alloys (*cont'd*)
 characterization methods, 286–287
 corrosion resistance, 296–298
 deformation mechanisms, 290–296
 microstructure and mechanical
  properties, 287–290
 in vitro testing, 302–304
 x-ray photoelectron spectroscopy
  of, 298–302
 titanium-nitride coatings, 329–330, 549
 cardiovascular medical devices,
  685–688
 characterization, 688–697
  abrasive wear characteristics,
   690–692
  adhesion studies, 692–693
  adhesive wear characteristics,
   689–690
  cytotoxicity, 688
  durability studies, 695–697
  hemocompatibility, 698–699
  large animal studies, 700–702
  microhardness measurements,
   693–695
  surface roughness, 688–689
  tissue compatibility, 699–700
 potential applications, 702–703
Titanium-glass ceramic composites,
  processing and properties, 69–70
Titanium-hydroxyapatite composites
 orthopedic applications, overview, 54–56
 processing and properties of, 63–66
Tob protein, bone regeneration, 557–558
Topographic analysis, tissue engineering
  scaffolds, 442
Total hip replacement (THR). *See* Hip
  implants
Toxicity, injectable hydrogels,
  photopolymerization and,
  185–191
Toxic response, cell-material interactions
  and, 10–11
Transforming growth factor beta
 bone morphogenetic proteins, 555–558
 nanofibrous scaffolds, tissue
  engineering, cartilage
  regeneration, 474
Transfusion process, placental umbilical
  cord blood, 650–651

basic properties, 656–658
safety and clinical applicatiosn, 652–656
Transmission electron microscopy (TEM)
 of hydroxyapatite-tricalciumphosphate
  matrix, 63–64
 titanium-niobium-zirconium-tantalum
  alloys, 290–296
Transplantation
 cell transplants, cartilage regeneration,
  472
 hip replacement, 325–327
Tribology
 titanium boride reinforced titanium-
  niobium-zirconium-tantalum
  metal-matrix composites, 309–317
 titanium dental implants, 146–151
Tricalciumphosphate (α-TCP and β-TCP),
  39–39
 bone tissue engineering, 553–554,
  558–559
 cell-material interactions, 60–62
 historical background, 103
 hydroxyapatite composite ratios, 61–63,
  105–106
  BCP scaffolds in mesenchymal stem
   cells, 124–125
  biphasic calcium phosphates, 109,
   112–113
 hydroxyapatite-titanium composites,
  65–66
 nanostructured ceramics, 213–220
 nanostructured composites, 226–228
 processing and properties, 59–62
 resorbable osteosynthesis, 118–120
 resorbable osteosynthesis, biphasic
  calcium phosphates, 119–120
Tri-culture modeling, orthopedic tissue
  engineering, multi-phased
  scaffold design, 601–603
Triethylene glycol diacrylate (TEGDA),
  nanofibrous scaffolds, tissue
  engineering, 459
2,2,2-Trifluoroethanol (TFE), gelatin
  nanofibrous scaffolds fabrication,
  455
TrkB signaling cascade, neuroprogenitor
  cell electric fields, 633–634
Two-dimensional cell culture, tissue
  engineering scaffolds, 440

U

Ultra-high-molecular weight polyethylene (UHMWPE)
femoral head implants, 285–286
titanium boride reinforced titanium-niobium-zirconium-tantalum metal-matrix composites, tribological behavior, 312–327
Ultra-low friction cemented arthroplasty, 207
Umbilical cord blood (UCB), 576–577

V

Vapor phase chemical reactions (VPCR), ceramic biomaterials processing, 253–254
Vascular endothelial growth factor (VEGF), bone regeneration, 557–558
Visible ultraviolet photo-polymerization, injectable hydrogels, 183
Vitronectin adsorption
nanofibrous composites, 565–566
nanostructured biodegradable polymers, 224–225
Voltage, electrospinning for nanofibrous scaffold fabrication, 449
Voltage-gated calcium channels (VGCC), neurons in electric field, 633
Volume fraction, silicon carbide-based ceramic biomaterials, mechanical optimization, 381–384
"Vycor" glass, crystallization properties, 424

W

Water adsorption, cardiovascular medical device hemocompatibility, 681
Wear properties
nanomaterial interaction, 232–233
nanostructured ceramics, 219–220
orthopedic implants and, 210–212
articulating surfaces, 212
polymer biocomposites, 77–79
titanium boride reinforced titanium-niobium-zirconium-tantalum metal-matrix composites, tribological behavior, 309–317

Wear resistance, titanium boride reinforced titanium-niobium-zirconium-tantalum metal-matrix composites, 304–305
Weibull plot, functionally-graded ceramic hip implants, disc properties, 338–339
Wnt signaling, bone regeneration, 558
Wood-derived carbon preforms, silicon carbide-based ceramic biomaterials
medical device applications, 360–365
phase and element distribution, 365–370
World Health Organization (WHO), placental umbilical cord blood research, 644–648
Wound healing, titanium dental implants, 159–163

X

Xenografts, benefits and limitations of, 438–439
X-ray diffraction profiles
biphasic calcium, 109
carbonate apatite, 30–33
of hydroxyapatite-tricalciumphosphate matrix, 63–64
ionomer glasses, crystallization properties, 423–427
radiopaque agents, bioactive injectable bone substitutes, 116–118
titanium-niobium-zirconium-tantalum alloys, 287–290
X-ray photoelectron spectroscopy (XPS)
bioactive coatings, 390–392
physico-chemical properties, 394–396
LENS-deposited titanium-niobium-zirconium-tantalum alloys, passive oxide films, 298–302

Y

Yield strength, titanium dental implants, 152–153
Young's modulus, ionomer glass structure, 418
Y-PSZ particles
bioinert ceramics, 70–72
glass-ceramic composites, 69–70

Yttria doped tetragonal zirconia
polycrystal ceramics (Y-TZP)
nanostructured ceramics, 218–220
processing and properties, 70–72

Z

Zachariasen Random Network Theory,
ionomer glasses and, 415–416
Zero current potential (ZCP), corrosion
properties of metal alloys, 82–83
Zinc, apatite incorporation of, 34
Zinc oxide, nanostructured ceramics,
213–220
Zinc silicate glasses, 414–415
Zirconium alloys
alumina-toughened zirconia, 328–329
hip replacement ceramic implants,
327–328
LENS-deposited TNZT alloys, passive
oxide films, 299–302
medical device applications, 359–360
titanium-niobium-zirconium-tantalum
alloys, laser processing of,
286–304

characterization methods, 286–287
corrosion resistance, 296–298
deformation mechanisms, 290–296
microstructure and mechanical
properties, 287–290
in vitro testing, 302–304
x-ray photoelectron spectroscopy of,
298–302
zirconia oxide-based bioinert ceramics
hip replacements, 326–327
hydroxyapatite-ceramic composites,
62–63
nanostructured ceramics, 213–220
nanostructured composites, 228
orthopedic applications, overview,
55
processing and properties, 70–72
sintering and microstructure
evaluation, 345–351
zirconia-titanium alloys, properties of,
84
zirconium oxide radiopaque agents,
bioactive injectable bone
substitutes, 116–118